Nicole Apelian, Ph.D. & Claude Davis

The Lost Book Of Herbal Remedies

The Healing Power of Plant Medicine

Edited and Written by Nicole Apelian, Ph.D. and copyrighted by Claude Davis

Dedication (Nicole)

In memory of Xanama, Qgum, and Du, whose love, joyful spirits, and ropes of connection live on in so many

Dedication (Claude)

In memory of my grandfather

Disclaimer Page

This book was created to provide information about natural medicines, cures and remedies that people have used in the past. This information is made available with the knowledge that the publisher, editor and authors do not offer any legal or otherwise medical advice. In the case you are ill you should always consult with your caring physician or another medical specialist.

This book does not claim to contain and indeed does not contain all the information available on the subject of natural remedies.

While the authors, editor and publisher have gone to great lengths to provide the most useful and accurate collection of healing plants and remedies in North America, there may still exist typographical and/or content errors.

Therefore, this book should not be used as a medical guide.

The authors, editor and publisher shall incur no liability or be held responsible to any person or entity regarding any loss of life or injury, alleged or otherwise, that happened directly or indirectly as a result of using the information contained in this book. It is your own responsibility and if you want to use a potion, tincture, decoction or anything else from this book you should consult with your physician first.

Some of the remedies and cures found within do not comply with FDA guidelines.

The information in the book has not been reviewed, tested or approved by any official testing body or government agency.

The authors and editor of this book make no guarantees of any kind, expressed or implied regarding the final results obtained by applying the information found in this book. Making, using and consuming any of the products described will be done at your own risk.

The authors, editor and publisher hold no responsibility for the misuse or misidentification of a plant using the contents of this book, or any and all consequences to your health or that of others that may result.

Some names and identifying details have been changed to protect the privacy of the authors and other individuals.

By reading past this point you hereby agree to be bound by this disclaimer, or you may return this book within the guarantee time period for a full refund.

Table of Contents

Introduction – About the Authors

We hope that this book will become a favorite reference for you and serve as a starting place on your health journey. This book is a general guide to herbal treatments as Dr. Nicole Apelian and Claude Davis practice them. We encourage everyone to seek medical help whenever needed and avoid self-diagnosis.

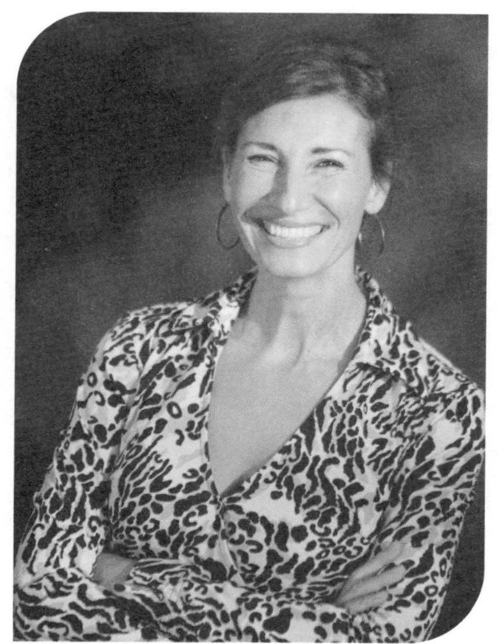

Nicole Apelian, Ph.D.

Dr. Nicole Apelian is an herbalist, a mother, a survival skills instructor, an anthropologist, and a biologist. She graduated with a degree in Biology from McGill University in Canada and has her Master's degree in Ecology from the University of Oregon. She earned her Doctorate through Prescott College while working as an anthropologist and ethnobotanist in Botswana. She is also the author of "A Reference Guide to Surviving Nature: Outdoor Preparation and Remedies". For more about Nicole please visit www.nicoleapelian.com.

Nicole has spent years living in nature with the San Bushmen of the Kalahari Desert, one of the last indigenous peoples who still live as hunter-gatherers. Developing strong relationships within the tribe helped Nicole learn many of the remedies and skills she practices and teaches today.

An unexpected diagnosis of multiple sclerosis in 2000 led Nicole to apply her research skills towards her own personal wellness. She focuses on a healthy living strategy, including deep nature connection and gratitude practices. Through changes in her lifestyle, recognizing profound mind-body linkages, and making and using her own remedies, Nicole went from bedridden to being fully alive and from surviving to thriving.

She believes that there are many more people suffering who need to find their own remedy. This became her life's mission and the main reason for writing this book. In it she poured over 28 years of plant knowledge and her first-hand experiences of making her own poultices, tinctures, decoctions, salves, infused oils, and other herbal remedies.

She has helped thousands of people treat themselves naturally by following her holistic wellness protocols and by using herbal remedies.

In 2015 she was among the first women ever selected for the History Channel's hit TV show "Alone". Despite having MS, she went on to survive solo for 57 days straight in a remote area of Vancouver Island with little more than her hunting knife and the wild foods and medicines she found there.

Dr. Nicole Apelian's knowledge was key to this book. Many of the plants, lichens, and mushrooms you'll find in it are ones that she's used with great results. The remedies you'll find in this book are not, by any means, exhaustive. But she has selected some of the best for people who want to treat themselves naturally with what they can grow and harvest where they live. These remedies are a part of a holistic philosophy of being self-reliant - of connecting your mind with your body and your body with nature. Here's to thriving!

You've taken an amazing first step in learning about herbal remedies by purchasing this book. The next step is using your new knowledge!

I want to help you by inviting you to join my Survive & Thrive community. Go to the link below to join my private email list and become part of the Survive & Thrive Crew. As a bonus, you'll get my free Neighborhood and Backyard Plants E-Course to help you take the first steps in using your new plant knowledge today. Use this link www.nicoleapelian.com to join now!

Claude Davis

Claude Davis is a Wild West history expert and the chief editor at www.askaprepper.com. His main focus is to save the survival skills of our grandparents. He's the author of the bestselling book, "The Lost Ways – Saving Our Forefathers' Skills" – www.thelostways.com.

While most people tend to be obsessed with everything "new"—with technology, smartphones, social media, and cars that drive themselves—he has always been intrigued by what he believes was a happier, wiser, healthier America: a country of more independent people, who took responsibility for themselves, who were proud of being American, and who dreamed of building a better world.

He thinks that progress has brought us so many good things, but in many ways, things used to be much better. We are smarter—but we're not wiser. We own more stuff—but stuff we don't really need. And we live longer lives—but we're not healthier.

Consumerism has reached epic proportions, and people feel aggrieved if they don't own the latest gadget.

The truth is, we have never been more disconnected from life, from the world, from the soil, from the plants, and from our own souls.

Claude's goal with *The Lost Book of Herbal Remedies* was to save the most powerful remedies that we've lost to history, and to separate the true cures from the bogus ones that had no effect.

Acknowledgements

Nicole:

I would first and foremost like to thank my mentors from around the globe. They have taught me well, opened my eyes to the healing powers all around us, and shared their knowledge and wisdom freely. I hope I have done them justice here in these pages as I pass on all that they have taught me, especially for future generations.

Huge thanks to my San community in the Kalahari, and for the way they look at their land as a grocery store and as a pharmacy. They gave me new eyes from which to see our landscape here in North America. Thank you to my sons, Colton and Quinn, especially when I spent long hours writing, for understanding the deep need for this book to come into the world. A huge thanks to my co-author Claude Davis, and to Anne-Marie for her excellent formatting skills, oversight, and hard work.

A big debt of gratitude for the modern researchers around the world who are doing the all-important work of finally bringing forth the scientific evidence that these herbal remedies really do work. Just as important are the storytellers. Without them these oral traditions and remedies would have been lost. My hope is that this book will help keep these remedies alive and that more and more people will realize the power of nature connection, herbal medicine, and traditional wisdom.

Of course, my biggest gratitude is to the plants, lichens, and mushrooms that help us grow and heal. Without them, I wouldn't be here walking amongst you today.

Medicinal Herbal Reference Guide

Bones:

- **Breaks**: Comfrey (64-66), Solomon's Seal (200-202), Wild Teasel (146-148)
- **Osteoarthritis**: Cat's Claw (169-170), Comfrey (64-66), Dandelion (68-70), Diatomaceous Earth (292), Epsom Salts (292-293), Evening Primrose (75-77), Greater Burdock (83-85), Leeks (96-97), Reishi (273-275)
- **Osteoporosis:** Black Cohosh (162), Dandelion (68-70), Diatomaceous Earth (292), Epsom Salts (292-293), Evening Primrose (75-77), Horsetail (181-182), Red Clover (126-127), Sugar Maple (258-259), Wild Teasel (146-148)

Cancer:

- **Cancer Prevention and Treatment**: Ashwagandha (47-48), Balsam Fir (217-219), Bilberry (221-223), Birch (223-224), Bleeding Heart (163-164), Blue and Black Elderberry (227-229), Cabbage (54-55), Calendula (55-56), Cascara Sagrada (229-231), Cat's Claw (169-170), Cattails (279-280), Chaga (268-270), Chokecherry (232-233), Cleavers (171-172), Comfrey (64-66), Cranberry (235-236), Dandelion (68-70), Devil's Club (236-237), Elecampane (74-75), Flax (66-67), Greater Burdock (83-85), Hardy Kiwi (238-239), Holy Basil (86-88), Honey Locust (241-242), Leeks (96-97), Lemon Balm (98-99), Licorice Root (102-103), Lion's Mane (270-271), Mayapple (189), Milk Thistle (110-111), Oregano (116-117), Oregon Grape (247-248), Purslane (125-126), Reishi (273-275), Rosemary (128-129), Self-heal (122-124), Turkey Tail (275-276), Turmeric (295-296), White Mustard (144-145), Wormwood (210-211)
- **Skin Cancer:** Ash (216-217), Bloodroot (164-165), Cabbage (54-55), Chaga (268-270), Lion's Mane (270-271), Mayapple (189), Milk Thistle (110-111), Red Clover (126-127), Sheep Sorrel (131-132), Turkey Tail (275-276)
- **Tumors:** Cabbage (54-55), Chaga (268-270), Cleavers (171-172), Cranberry (235-236), Mullein (114-115), Oregano (116-117), Quaking Aspen (249), Red Root (198-199), Reishi (273-275), Self-heal (122-124), Sheep Sorrel (131-132), Turkey Tail (275-276)

Childhood Diseases and Issues:

- **Bedwetting**: California Poppy (57-58), St. John's Wort (133-135)
- **Colic:** Chamomile (59-60), Dill (70-71), Fennel (77-78), Feverfew (78-79), Lamb's Quarter (93-94), Lemon Balm (98-99), Queen Anne's Lace (129-130), Salal (253-254), Self-heal (122-124), Slippery Elm (257-258), Unicorn Root (204-205), Wild Lettuce (145-146), Wild Yam (208-209), Wintergreen (209-210)
- **Croup**: Bloodroot (164-165), Marshmallow (107-108), Oregano (116-117), Oxeye Daisy (117-118)
- **Teething Pain**: Cattails (279-280), Devil's Club (236-237), Mallow (106-107), Marshmallow (107-108)
- **Well Baby Care**: Cattails (279-280)

Digestive and Intestinal Issues

- **Abdominal Pain**: Agrimony (44-45), Aloe Vera (45-46), American Basswood (215-216), Bayberry and Wax Myrtle (220-221), Bearberry (159-160), Birch (223-224), Black Cohosh (162), Black Walnut (226-227), Bloodroot (164-165),Calendula (55-56), Chamomile (59-60), Chicory (62-63), Chives (63-64), False Solomon's Seal (176-177), Fennel (77-78), Hawthorn (239-241), Kudzu (183-184), Lady's Thumb (92), Leeks (96-97), Lemon

Verbena (101-102), Lungwort Lichen (272-273), Salal (253-254), Slippery Elm (257-258), Thyme (140-141), White Willow (263-264), Wild Yam (208-209)

- **Bloating**: Activated Charcoal (287), Aloe Vera (45-46), Anise Hyssop (46-47), Birch (223-224), Black Cohosh (162), Chamomile (59-60), Chokecherry (232-233), Common Lungwort (105-106), Evening Primrose (75-77), Garlic (80-81), Hawthorn (239-241), Juniper (244), Leeks (96-97), Lemon Verbena (101-102), Lovage (104-105), Lungwort Lichen (272-273), Mugwort (190-191), St. John's Wort (133-135), Sweet Marjoram (137-138), Water Plantain (284), Wild Ginger (206-207), Wild Yam (208-209)
- **Candida**: Anise Hyssop (46-47), Black Walnut (226-227), Cascara Sagrada (229-231), Chicory (62-63), Duckweed (281-282), Fireweed (178-179), Goldenrod (81-83), Lemon Balm (98-99), Moringa (246-247), Oregano (116-117), Turkey Tail (275-276), Usnea (277-278), Wild Teasel (146-148), Wormwood (210-211)
- **Constipation**: Activated Charcoal (287), Aloe Vera (45-46), Black Walnut (226-227), Burning Bush (229), Cabbage (54-55), Cascara Sagrada (229-231), Chickweed (61-62), Club Moss (172-173), Dandelion (68-70), Dill (70-71), Dock (71-72), Fennel (77-78), Feverfew (78-79), Flax (66-67), Garlic (80-81), Hardy Kiwi (238-239), Hawthorn (239-241), Lemon Balm (98-99), Lamb's Quarter (93-94), Leeks (96-97), Lungwort Lichen (272-273), Marshmallow (107-108), Moringa (246-247), Mugwort (190-191), Plantain (119-121), Red Elderberry (251), Sheep Sorrel (131-132), Stone Root (203)
- **Crohn's Disease**: Aloe Vera (45-46), Calendula (55-56), Cat's Claw (169-170), Chamomile (59-60), Kudzu (183-184), Lion's Mane (270-271), Marshmallow (107-108), Peppermint (118-119), Plantain (119-121), Reishi (273-275), Self-heal (122-124), Slippery Elm (257-258), Wild Yam (208-209), Wormwood (210-211)
- **Diabetic Ulcers**: Bleach (288), Honey (294-295)
- **Diarrhea:** Activated Charcoal (287), Agrimony (44-45), Anise Hyssop (46-47), Bayberry and Wax Myrtle (220-221), Bearberry (159-160), Bilberry (221-223), Black Crowberry (225), Black Walnut (226-227), California Buckwheat (167-168), Carolina Geranium (58-59), Cattails (279-280), Chokecherry (232-233), Common Lungwort (105-106), Dandelion (68-70), Dock (71-72), Fireweed (178-179), Goldenseal (179-180), Lungwort Lichen (272-273), Moringa (246-247), Mugwort (190-191), Oregon Grape (247-248), Peppermint (118-119), Plantain (119-121), Quaking Aspen (249), Red Alder (250-251), Red Raspberry (197), Salal (253-254), Self-heal (122-124), Solomon's Seal (200-202), St. John's Wort (133-135), Stone Root (203), Sweet Marjoram (137-138), Thyme (140-141), Unicorn Root (204-205), White Pine (261-262), Wild Rose (264-265), Wild Strawberries (207-208), Wooly Lamb's Ear (149-150)
- **Diverticulitis**: Aloe Vera (45-46), Marshmallow (107-108), Slippery Elm (257-258), Wild Yam (208-209)
- **Duodenal Ulcers**: Bayberry and Wax Myrtle (220-221), Calendula (55-56), Chokecherry (232-233), Garlic (80-81), Wild Rose (264-266)
- **Dysentery**: American Basswood (215-216), Bayberry and Wax Myrtle (220-221), Black Crowberry (225), Cattails (279-280), Oregon Grape (247-248), Saw Palmetto (256), Solomon's Seal (200-202), St. John's Wort (133-135), Wild Strawberries (207-208)
- **Flatulence**: Aloe Vera (45-46), Anise Hyssop (46-47), Angelica (154-156), Bee Balm (161), Club Moss (172-173), Dill (70-71), Fennel (77-78), Garlic (80-81), Juniper (244), Peppermint (118-119), Queen Anne's Lace (129-130), Self-heal (122-124), Stone Root (203), Unicorn Root (204-205), Wormwood (210-211)
- **Food Poisoning**: Activated Charcoal (287), Bee Balm (161), Dill (70-71), Fennel (77-78), Garlic (80-81), Juniper (244), Lovage (104-105), Mugwort (190-191), Queen Anne's Lace (129-130), Unicorn Root (204-205), White Mustard (144-145), Wild Ginger (206-207), Wormwood (210-211)
- **Gastritis & Gastroenteritis**: Black Cohosh (162), Black Crowberry (225), Burning Bush (229), Calendula (55-56), Chamomile (59-60), Chicory (62-63), Chives (63-64), Chokecherry (232-233), Evening Primrose (75-77), Kudzu (183-184), Lion's Mane (281-284), Marshmallow (107-

108), Mullein (114-115), Oregon Grape (247-248), Peppermint (118-119), Saw Palmetto (256), Self-heal (122-124), Sheep Sorrel (131-132), St. John's Wort (133-135), Water Plantain (284), Wild Strawberries (207-208)

- **Heartburn:** Aloe Vera (45-46), American Basswood (215-216), Black Crowberry (225), Chokecherry (232-233), Fennel (77-78), Jerusalem Artichoke (91-92), Juniper (244), Maidenhair Fern (187), Salal (253-254), Saw Palmetto (256), Solomon's Seal (200-202), Slippery Elm (257-258), Stone Root (203), Water Plantain (284), Wormwood (210-211)
- **IBS (Irritable Bowel Syndrome)**: Aloe Vera (45-46), Bilberry (221-223), Borage (51-52), Cat's Claw (169-170), Chamomile (59-60), Dill (70-71), Fireweed (178-179), Hardy Kiwi (238-239), Hops (88-89), Kudzu (183-184), Marshmallow (107-108), Peppermint (118-119), Plantain (119-121), Slippery Elm (257-258), Wild Yam (208-209), Wormwood (210-211)
- **Indigestion**: Agrimony (44-45), Anise Hyssop (46-47), Black Cohosh (162), Burning Bush (229), Cayenne Pepper (289-290), Chamomile (59-60), Chives (63-64), Dandelion (68-70), Evening Primrose (75-77), Fennel (77-78), Greater Burdock (83-85), Honey Locust (241-242), Hops (88-89), Jerusalem Artichoke (91-92), Juniper (244), Lemon Balm (98-99), Lemon Verbena (101-102), Licorice Root (102-103), Marshmallow (107-108), Moringa (246-247), Oregon Grape (247-248), Peppermint (118-119), Quaking Aspen (249), Red Alder (250-251), Rosemary (128-129), Sage (130-131), Saw Palmetto (256), Stone Root (203), Sweet Marjoram (137-138), Turkey Tail (275-276), White Willow (263-264), Wild Ginger (206-207), Wild Violets (142-143)
- **Inflammatory Bowel Disease (IBD):** Aloe Vera (45-46), Calendula (55-56), Lion's Mane (270-271), Lovage (104-105), Plantain (119-121), Reishi (273-275), Slippery Elm (257-258), Sugar Maple (258-259), Wormwood (210-211)
- **Intestinal Colitis**: Bayberry and Wax Myrtle (220-221), Black Walnut (226-227), Calendula (55-56), Fireweed (178-179), Marshmallow (107-108), Peppermint (118-119), Self-heal (122-124)
- **Intestinal Problems**: Cabbage (54-55), Calendula (55-56), Marshmallow (107-108), Peppermint (118-119), Sheep Sorrel (131-132), Thyme (140-141), Wormwood (210-211)
- **Intestinal Worms and Parasites**: Black Walnut (226-227), Black-Eyed Susan (49), Chicory (62-63), Cottonwood (233-234), Diatomaceous Earth (292), Elecampane (74-75), Feverfew (78-79), Garlic (80-81), Lamb's Quarter (93-94), Male Fern (188), Mugwort (190-191), Mullein (114-115), Plantain (119-121), Self-heal (122-124), Sheep Sorrel (131-132), Thyme (140-141), White Pine (261-262), Wormwood (210-211)
- **Leaky Gut**: Fireweed (178-179), Licorice Root (102-103), Lion's Mane (270-271), Marshmallow (107-108), Plantain (119-121), Reishi (273-275), Slippery Elm (257-258), Turkey Tail (275-276)
- **Nausea and Vomiting:** Activated Charcoal (287), Bee Balm (161), Bilberry (221-223), Bloodroot (164-165), Chives (63-64), Mallow (106-107), Peppermint (118-119), Reishi (273-275), Wild Ginger (206-207)
- **Peptic Ulcers**: Calendula (55-56), Chokecherry (232-233), Cranberry (235-236), Licorice Root (102-103), Mallow (106-107), Marshmallow (107-108), Meadowsweet (245-246), St. John's Wort (133-135)
- **Prebiotics**: Chicory (62-63), Dandelion (68-70), Garlic (80-81), Greater Burdock (83-85), Jerusalem Artichoke (91-92), Leeks (96-97), Turkey Tail (275-276)
- **Stomach Flu**: American Basswood (215-216), Bee Balm (161), California Buckwheat (167-168), Chokecherry (232-233), Garlic (80-81), Mallow (106-107), Thyme (140-141), Water Plantain (284)
- **Tapeworm Infection**: Hawthorn (239-241), Male Fern (188), White Pine (261-262)
- **Ulcerative Colitis**: Chaga (268-270), Common Lungwort (105-106), Lion's Mane (270-271), Lungwort Lichen (272-273) Marshmallow (107-108), Plantain (119-121), Reishi (273-275), Rosemary (128-129), Self-heal (122-124), Slippery Elm (257-258), Wild Yam (208-209)

Drug Addiction

- **Alcoholism**: Kudzu (183-184), Skullcap (132-133)
- **Drug Withdrawal**: Parrot's Beak (193-194), Pulsatilla (124-125), Skullcap (132-133), St. John's Wort (133-135)
- **Nicotine Withdrawal**: Lobelia Inflata (184-185), Osha (191-193), Skullcap (132-133), Valerian Root (141-142)
- **Opiate Withdrawal**: California Poppy (57-58), St. John's Wort (133-135)

Ears

- **Earaches**: Black-Eyed Susan (49), Mullein (114-115), Pulsatilla (124-125)
- **Ear Infections**: Boric Acid (288-289), Garlic (80-81), Mullein (114-115), Yarrow (150-151)
- **Hearing Loss**: Pulsatilla (124-125)
- **Inflammation of Ears**: Pulsatilla (124-125)
- **Swimmer's Ear**: Boric Acid (288-289)

Eyes

- **Cataracts**: Bilberry (221-223), Holy Basil (86-88), Pulsatilla (124-125)
- **Conjunctivitis (Pinkeye) and Eye Infections**: Agrimony (44-45), American Basswood (215-216), Blue and Black Elderberry (227-229), Boric Acid (288-289), Chamomile (59-60), Fennel (77-78), Goldenseal (179-180), Oxeye Daisy (117-118), Pulsatilla (124-125), Usnea (277-278), Wooly Lamb's Ear (149-150), Yarrow (150-151)
- **Eye Inflammation**: Blue and Black Elderberry (227-229), Boric Acid (288-289), Calendula (55-56), Cardinal Flower (169), Chamomile (59-60), Chicory (62-63), Fennel (77-78), Holy Basil (86-88), Plantain (119-121), Usnea (277-278), Yarrow (150-151)
- **Glaucoma**: Bilberry (221-223), Holy Basil (86-88), Pulsatilla (124-125)
- **Macular Degeneration**: Bilberry (221-223), Borage (51-52), Cocoplum (254-255), Holy Basil (86-88)
- **Night Blindness**: Bilberry (221-223), Cocoplum (254-255)
- **Sties**: Wooly Lamb's Ear (149-150)
- **Tics**: Pulsatilla (124-125)

Female Issues

- **Amenorrhea (Absence of Menstruation)**: Burning Bush (229), Chicory (62-63), False Unicorn Root (177-178), Motherwort (112-114), Partridgeberry (194-195), Pulsatilla (124-125), Sweet Marjoram (137-138), Unicorn Root (204-205)
- **Breastfeeding**: Cabbage (54-55), Dill (70-71), Fennel (77-78), Spanish Moss (202) , Sweet Marjoram (137-138), Water Plantain (284)
- **Childbirth**: Ash (216-217), Bearberry (159-160), Black Crowberry (225), Blue Cohosh (165-166), Burning Bush (229), Cattails (279-280), Partridgeberry (194-195), Pulsatilla (124-125), Spanish Moss (202) , White Sage (263), Yarrow (150-151)
- **Contraception**: Feverfew (78-79), Juniper (244), Queen Anne's Lace (129-130)
- **Dysmenorrhea**: See "Menstrual Cramps"
- **Endometriosis**: Dandelion (68-70), Evening Primrose (75-77), Flax (66-67), Garlic (80-81), Leeks (96-97), Oregon Grape (247-248), Yarrow (150-151)
- **Fertility, improved**: Evening Primrose (75-77), False Unicorn Root (177-178), Licorice Root (102-103), Rhodiola Rosea (199-200), Saw Palmetto (256), Solomon's Seal (200-202), Sweet Marjoram (137-138), Water Plantain (284)
- **Hemorrhage, Vaginal with Childbirth**: Bearberry (159-160), Cattails (279-280), Male Fern (188)
- **Hormone Regulation**: Blue Cohosh (165-166), Cat's Claw (169-170), Devil's Club (236-237), Evening Primrose (75-77), False Solomon's Seal (176-177), False Unicorn Root (177-178), Fennel (77-78), Flax (66-67), Kudzu (183-184), Milk Thistle (110-111), Mugwort (190-191), Quaking Aspen (249), Reishi (273-275), Rhodiola Rosea (199-200), Sage (130-131), Spanish Moss (202) , St. John's Wort (133-135)
- **Labor: See "Childbirth"**
- **Menopause Symptoms**: Black Cohosh (162), Evening Primrose (75-77), False Unicorn Root (177-178), Flax (66-67), Kudzu (183-184), Lemon Balm (98-99), Licorice Root (102-103), Pulsatilla

(124-125), Quaking Aspen (249), Red Clover (126-127), Sage (130-131), Saw Palmetto (256), Solomon's Seal (200-202), St. John's Wort (133-135), Sweet Marjoram (137-138), Unicorn Root (204-205), Watercress (282-283), White Willow (263-264)

- **Menstrual Cramps**: Amaranthus Caudatus (152), Bloodroot (164-165), Blue Cohosh (165-166), Calendula (55-56), Cattails (279-280), Chicory (62-63), Dill (70-71), Fennel (77-78), Feverfew (78-79), Goldenseal (179-180), Kudzu (183-184), Mugwort (190-191), Partridgeberry (194-195), Peppermint (118-119), Pulsatilla (124-125), Sage (130-131), Sassafras (254-255), Solomon's Seal (200-202), St. John's Wort (133-135), Stinging Nettle (135-136), Sweet Marjoram (137-138), Valerian Root (141-142), Wild Rose (264-265), Yarrow (150-151)
- **Menstrual Cycle**: Amaranthus Caudatus (152), Angelica (154-156), Bee Balm (161), Black Cohosh (162), Black Crowberry (225), Bloodroot (164-165), Blue Cohosh (165-166), Borage (51-52), Burning Bush (229), Cat's Claw (169-170), Cattails (279-280), Chicory (62-63), Comfrey (64-66), False Solomon's Seal (176-177), False Unicorn Root (177-178), Fennel (77-78), Feverfew (78-79), Goldenseal (179-180), Lemon Balm (98-99), Lovage (104-105), Mugwort (190-191), Partridgeberry (194-195), Quaking Aspen (249), Red Raspberry (197), Self-heal (122-124), Stinging Nettle (135-136), Sweet Marjoram (137-138), Unicorn Root (204-205), White Willow (263-264), Wild Ginger (206-207), Yarrow (150-151)
- **Milk Suppression**: Black Walnut (226-227), California Poppy (57-58), Chickweed (61-62), Lemon Balm (98-99), Peppermint (118-119), Sage (130-131), Yarrow (150-151)
- **Miscarriage, habitual**: Unicorn Root (204-205)
- **Miscarriage, threatened**: False Unicorn Root (177-178)
- **Morning Sickness**: False Unicorn Root (177-178), Red Raspberry (197)
- **Pelvic Inflammation**: Echinacea (72-73), False Unicorn Root (177-178), Red Raspberry (197)
- **Polycystic Ovarian Syndrome (PCOS):** Ash (216-217), Black Cohosh (162), Evening Primrose (75-77), Reishi (273-275), Sweet Marjoram (137-138), Unicorn Root (204-205)
- **Post-Partum Aid and Depression**: Bearberry (159-160), Cattails (279-280), Pulsatilla (124-125), St. John's Wort (133-135)
- **Pregnancy & Labor**: False Unicorn Root (177-178), Leeks (96-97), Red Raspberry (197), Western Skunk Cabbage (285-286)
- **Pre-Menstrual Syndrome (PMS):** Black Cohosh (162), Borage (51-52), Calendula (55-56), Evening Primrose (75-77), Fennel (77-78), Hops (88-89), Lemon Balm (98-99), Motherwort (112-114), Licorice Root (102-103), Pulsatilla (124-125), Red Raspberry (197), St. John's Wort (133-135), Sweet Marjoram (137-138), Wild Ginger (206-207), Wild Rose (264-265)
- **Sex Drive, Improved:** Black Cohosh (162), False Unicorn Root (177-178), Spanish Moss (202) , Western Skunk Cabbage (285-286)
- **Urethra inflammation**: Bearberry (159-160), Couch Grass (67-68), Pipsissewa (195-196)
- **Vaginal Infections:** Amaranthus Caudatus (152), Bearberry (159-160), Boric Acid (288-289), Cattails (279-280), False Unicorn Root (177-178), Goldenseal (179-180), Usnea (277-278), Western Red Cedar (259-261)

Glands

- **Adrenal fatigue**: American Ginseng (153-154), Chaga (268-270), Devil's Club (236-237), Reishi (273-275), Rhodiola Rosea (199-200)
- **Endocrine Gland**: Milk Thistle (110-111), Spanish Moss (202)
- **Enlarged Spleen**: Rhodiola Rosea (199-200), Stinging Nettle (135-136)
- **Thyroid Function**: Lemon Balm (98-99), Rhodiola Rosea (199-200)

Hair

- **Hair Loss**: Evening Primrose (75-77), Horsetail (181-182), Rosemary (128-129), Sage (130-131), Saw Palmetto (256)
- **Lice**: Devil's Club (236-237), Lavender (94-96), Listerine (293), Meadow Rue (109), Quaking

Aspen (249), Red Alder (250-251), Sassafras (254-255), Thyme (140-141)

Heart and Circulatory System

- **Anemia**: Dandelion (68-70), Greater Burdock (83-85), Hardy Kiwi (238-239), Lamb's Quarter (93-94), Leeks (96-97), Stinging Nettle (135-136)
- **Angina**: Anise Hyssop (46-47), Hawthorn (239-241)
- **Blood Pressure, High**: American Basswood (215-216), Black Walnut (226-227), Borage (51-52), Cat's Claw (169-170), Chives (63-64), Diatomaceous Earth (292), Evening Primrose (75-77), False Hellebore (174-175), Garlic (80-81), Hardy Kiwi (238-239), Hawthorn (239-241), Honey (294-295), Kudzu (183-184), Lady's Thumb (92), Lavender (94-96), Leeks (96-97), Lemon Balm (98-99), Mugwort (190-191), Red Raspberry (197), Red Root (198-199), St. John's Wort (133-135), Sugar Maple (258-259), Sweet Marjoram (137-138), Turkey Tail (275-276), Turmeric (295-296), Valerian Root (141-142), Water Plantain (284)
- **Blood Pressure, Low**: Blue Cohosh (165-166), Goldenrod (81-83), Goldenseal (179-180), Rosemary (128-129), Turmeric (295-296),
- **Blood Purification**: Chickweed (61-62), Devil's Club (236-237), Feverfew (78-79), Meadow Rue (109), Yarrow (150-151)
- **Blood Thinner**: Red Clover (126-127), Sweet Grass (137), Wild Violets (142-143), Turmeric (295-296),
- **Blood Coagulant**: Agrimony (44-45), Cattails (279-280), Cayenne Pepper (289-290), Common Lungwort (105-106), Yarrow (150-151)
- **Cardiac Insufficiency**: Stinging Nettle (135-136)
- **Cholesterol, Elevated**: Amaranthus Caudatus (152), American Basswood (215-216), Black Walnut (226-227), Cascara Sagrada (229-231), Cinnamon (291), Chives (63-64), Cocoplum (280-281), Cranberry (235-236), Dandelion (68-70), Diatomaceous Earth (292), Evening Primrose (75-77), Flax (66-67), Garlic (80-81), Hardy Kiwi (238-239), Hawthorn (239-241), Honey (294-295), Leeks (96-97), Milk Thistle (110-111), Prickly Pear Cactus (121-122), Purslane (125-126), Red Clover (126-127), Red Mulberry (252), Reishi (273-275), Spanish Moss (202) , Turkey Tail (275-276), Water Plantain (284), Wild Violets (142-143)
- **Circulation, Increased/Vasodilator**: Angelica (154-156), Boneset (50-51), Butterbur (166-167), Cayenne Pepper (289-290), Garlic (80-81), Greater Burdock (83-85), Kudzu (183-184), Prickly Pear Cactus (121-122), Red Clover (126-127), Reishi (273-275), Rosemary (128-129), Stinging Nettle (135-136), Turmeric (295-296)
- **Clotting:** Agrimony (44-45), Amaranthus Caudatus (152), Bilberry (221-223), Cattails (279-280), Cayenne Pepper (289-290), Common Lungwort (105-105), Cranberry (235-236), Hardy Kiwi (238-239), Kudzu (183-184), Leeks (96-97), Lion's Mane (270-271), Mugwort (190-191), Red Clover (126-127), Red Root (198-199), Saw Palmetto (256), Usnea (277-278), Wooly Lamb's Ear (149-150), Yarrow (150-151)
- **Heart Attack**: Bilberry (221-223), Black Walnut (226-227), California Buckwheat (167-168), Chives (63-64), Cocoplum (280-281), Hardy Kiwi (238-239), Hawthorn (239-241), Lion's Mane (281-284), Oregano (116-117), Turmeric (295-296),
- **Heart Disease**: American Basswood (215-216), Black Walnut (226-227), Cat's Claw (169-170), Cinnamon (291), Chives (63-64), Cranberry (235-236), Epsom Salts (292-293), Hawthorn (239-241), Hops (88-89), Juniper (244), Lady's Thumb (92), Leeks (96-97), Lion's Mane (270-271), Milk Thistle (110-111), Prickly Pear Cactus (121-122), Red Clover (126-127), Red Mulberry (252), Sugar Maple (258-259)
- **Irregular Heartbeat**: American Basswood (215-216), Hawthorn (239-241), Reishi (273-275)
- **Myocardial Ischemia**: Kudzu (183-184)
- **Nosebleeds**: Amaranthus Caudatus (152), Stinging Nettle (135-136), Yarrow (150-151)
- **Phlebitis**: Heartleaf Arnica (156-157)
- **Pulse Rate, Lowering**: False Hellebore (174-175), Valerian Root (141-142)
- **Tonic, Heart**: American Basswood (215-216), Bottle Gourd (53), Burning Bush (229), Cayenne Pepper (289-290), Mormon Tea (111-112), Solomon's Seal (200-202), Sugar Maple (258-259),

Wild Ginger (206-207), Wooly Lamb's Ear (149-150)

- **Varicose Veins**: Bilberry (221-223), Chickweed (61-62), Horse Chestnut (242-243), Maidenhair Fern (187), Stone Root (203), Wild Violets (142-143)
- **Vasculitis**: Reishi (273-275)
- **Vasodilator: See Circulation, Increased**
- **Venous Insufficiency, Chronic:** Horse Chestnut (242-243), Salal (253-254)

Immune System

- **Allergies**: Borage (51-52), Butterbur (166-167), Chaga (268-270), Chamomile (59-60), Echinacea (72-73), Evening Primrose (75-77), Garlic (80-81), Goldenrod (81-83), Listerine (293), Lovage (104-105), Mormon Tea (111-112), Reishi (273-275), Self-heal (122-124), Stinging Nettle (135-136), Yerba Santa (213-214)
- **Autoimmune Diseases**: Bilberry (221-223), Cat's Claw (169-170), Chives (63-64), Evening Primrose (75-77), Flax (66-67), Lion's Mane (270-271), Plantain (119-121), Reishi (273-275), Sugar Maple (258-259), Turkey Tail (275-276)
- **Celiac Disease**: Lion's Mane (270-271), Reishi (273-275), Slippery Elm (257-258)
- **Guillain-Barre**: Reishi (273-275)
- **Hashimoto's Thyroiditis**: Reishi (273-275)
- **Lymph Nodes**: Bleeding Heart (163-164), Calendula (55-56), Wild Rose (264-265)
- **Lupus:** Flax (66-67), Reishi (273-275), Turkey Tail (275-276)
- **Multiple Sclerosis (MS):** Evening Primrose (75-77), Flax (66-67), Lion's Mane (270-271), Reishi (273-275), Turkey Tail (275-276)
- **Stimulating the Immune System**: Arrowleaf Balsamroot (158-159), Ashwagandha (47-48), Black-Eyed Susan (49), Blue and Black Elderberry (227-229), Calendula (55-56), Cat's Claw (169-170), Cayenne Pepper (289-290), Chaga (268-270), Chives (63-64), Cocoplum (280-281), Dandelion (68-70), Echinacea (72-73), Goldenseal (179-180), Greater Burdock (83-85), Hardy Kiwi (238-239), Hawthorn (239-241), Lemon Thyme (100), Oregano (116-117), Sheep Sorrel (131-132), Solomon's Seal (200-202), Thyme (140-141), Watercress (282-283)

Infectious Diseases

- **Anti-fungal:** See Fungal Infections
- **Anti-virals**: Anise Hyssop (46-47), Black Walnut (226-227), Blue and Black Elderberry (227-229), Calendula (55-56), Cat's Claw (169-170), Chaga (268-270), Echinacea (72-73), Goldenseal (179-180), Leeks (96-97), Lemon Balm (98-99), Lemon Thyme (100), Licorice Root (102-103), Male Fern (188), Moringa (246-247), Oregano (116-117), Oregon Grape (247-248), Osha (191-193), Peppermint (118-119), Reishi (273-275), Sassafras (254-255), Self-heal (122-124), St. John's Wort (133-135), Thyme (140-141), Turkey Tail (275-276), Usnea (277-278), Western Red Cedar (259-261), Wild Rose (264-265)
- **Bacillus**: Chicory (62-63), Duckweed (281-282), Mugwort (190-191), Reishi (273-275)
- **Chickenpox:** Cleavers (171-172), Club Moss (172-173), Chaparral (231-232), Calendula (55-56)
- **Citrobacter**: Duckweed (281-282)
- **Colds and Flu**: American Ginseng (153-154), Anise Hyssop (46-47), Angelica (154-156), Balsam Poplar (219-220), Bayberry and Wax Myrtle (220-221), Bee Balm (161), Black Crowberry (225), Black-Eyed Susan (49), Bloodroot (164-165), Blue and Black Elderberry (227-229), Boneset (50-51), California Buckwheat (167-168), Cayenne Pepper (289-290), Chaga (268-270), Chokecherry (232-233), Club Moss (172-173), Cranberry (235-236), Devil's Club (236-237), Echinacea (72-73), Feverfew (78-79), Flax (66-67), Garlic (80-81), Goldenrod (81-83), Goldenseal (179-180), Honey Locust (241-242), Horseradish (89-90), Meadowsweet (245-246), Lamb's Quarter (93-94), Lavender (94-96), Licorice Root (102-103), Male Fern (188), Mallow (106-107), Oregon Grape (247-248), Osha (191-193), Quaking Aspen (249), Red Elderberry (251), Reishi (273-275), Sassafras (254-255), Sheep Sorrel (131-132), St. John's Wort (133-135), Sweet Grass (137),Turkey Tail (275-276), Usnea (277-278), Water Plantain (284), White Pine (261-262), White Sage (263), Wild Rose (264-265), Wild Violets (142-143),

Witch Hazel (266-267), Yarrow (150-151), Yerba Santa (213-214)

- **Cholera Prevention**: Potassium Permanganate (293-294)
- **Dengue Fever/ Bone Break Fever**: Boneset (50-51), Cat's Claw (169-170)
- **Diphtheria**: Bloodroot (164-165), Cardinal Flower (169)
- **E. coli**: Cascara Sagrada (229-231), Chicory (62-63), Juniper (244), Mugwort (190-191), Reishi (273-275), Usnea (277-278), Wormwood (210-211)
- **Epstein Barr Virus**: Cat's Claw (169-170), Echinacea (72-73), Garlic (80-81), Lemon Balm (98-99), Oregano (116-117), St. John's Wort (133-135), Turkey Tail (275-276), Usnea (277-278)
- **Fungal Infections (Thrush, Yeast, Athlete's Foot, Jock Itch):** Anise Hyssop (46-47), Angelica (154-156), Arrowleaf Balsamroot (158-159), Black Crowberry (225), Black Walnut (226-227), Boric Acid (288-289), Calendula (55-56), Cat's Claw (169-170), Cattails (279-280), Cinnamon (291), Chives (63-64), Club Moss (172-173), Drumstick Tree (220-221), Duckweed (281-282), Echinacea (72-73), Fireweed (178-179), Garlic (80-81), Goldenrod (81-83), Goldenseal (179-180), Greater Burdock (83-85), Horsetail (181-182), Jewelweed (185-186), Juniper (244), Lady's Thumb (92), Leeks (96-97), Lemon Balm (98-99), Lemon Thyme (100), Listerine (293), Mugwort (190-191), Oregano (116-117), Oregon Grape (247-248), Potassium Permanganate (293-294), Purslane (125-126), Reishi (273-275), Rosemary (128-129), Usnea (277-278), Chicory (62-63), Western Red Cedar (259-261), White Mustard (144-145), Wild Teasel (146-148), Wormwood (210-211), Yarrow (150-151)
- **Gonorrhea**: Balsam Fir (217-219), Bearberry (159-160), Couch Grass (67-68), False Unicorn Root (177-178), Juniper (244) Mormon Tea (111-112), Pipsissewa (195-196), Saw Palmetto (256)
- **H1N1/Swine flu:** Oregon Grape (247-248)
- ***Haemophilus influenzae***: Cranberry (235-236)
- ***Helicobacter pylori**:* Cascara Sagrada (229-231), Cranberry (235-236), Lion's Mane (270-271)
- **Herpes**: Anise Hyssop (46-47), Black Walnut (226-227), Calendula (55-56), Cat's Claw (169-170), Chaga (268-270), Chickweed (61-62), Echinacea (72-73), Greater Burdock (83-85), Honey (294-295), Lemon Balm (98-99), Oregon Grape (247-248), Red Root (198-199), Reishi (273-275), Self-heal (122-124), Slippery Elm (257-258), St. John's Wort (133-135), Turkey Tail (275-276), Usnea (277-278)
- **Human Immunodeficiency Virus (HIV):** Black Walnut (226-227), Cinnamon (291), Licorice Root (102-103), Oregon Grape (247-248), Osha (191-193), Self-heal (122-124), Turkey Tail (275-276)
- **HPV**: Black Walnut (226-227), Cat's Claw (169-170), Osha (191-193), Reishi (273-275), Turkey Tail (275-276), Usnea (277-278)
- **Infections (Viral, Bacterial and Parasitic):** Amaranthus Caudatus (152), Black Walnut (226-227), Boneset (50-51), Boric Acid (288-289), Cattails (279-280), Comfrey (64-66), Cranberry (235-236), Duckweed (281-282), Echinacea (72-73), Garlic (80-81), Goldenseal (179-180), Horseradish (89-90), Leeks (96-97), Lemon Thyme (100), Osha (191-193), Potassium Permanganate (293-294), Self-heal (122-124), Sheep Sorrel (131-132), Turkey Tail (275-276), Usnea (277-278), Western Red Cedar (259-261), White Mustard (144-145), Wild Ginger (206-207), Wild Rose (264-265)
- **Laryngitis**: American Basswood (215-216), California Buckwheat (167-168), Coltsfoot (173-174), Fennel (77-78), Goldenrod (81-83), Lavender (94-96), Lungwort Lichen (272-273), Mormon Tea (111-112), Mullein (114-115)
- **Lymphatic System**: Calendula (55-56), Cleavers (171-172), Greater Burdock (83-85), Red Root (198-199), Watercress (282-283), Wild Violets (142-143)
- **Lyme Disease**: Cat's Claw (169-170), Garlic (80-81), Reishi (273-275), Wild Teasel (146-148), Wormwood (210-211)
- **Malaria**: Boneset (50-51), Burning Bush (229), Chicory (62-63), Club Moss (172-173), Dogwood (238), Hawthorn (239-241), Turkey Tail (275-276), Wormwood (210-211)
- **Measles**: Cleavers (171-172), Honey Locust (241-242), Kudzu (183-184), Yarrow (150-151)

- **Mono/Mononucleosis**: Garlic (80-81), Mugwort (190-191), Red Root (198-199), Reishi (273-275), Usnea (277-278)
- **MRSA**: Oregon Grape (247-248), Usnea (277-278), Wooly Lamb's Ear (149-150)
- **Mumps**: Male Fern (188)
- **Neisseria**: Duckweed (281-282)
- **Parasites and Worms**: Black Walnut (226-227), Black-Eyed Susan (49), Cayenne Pepper (289-290), Chaparral (231-232), Chicory (62-63), Diatomaceous Earth (292), Feverfew (78-79), Garlic (80-81), Hawthorn (239-241), Male Fern (188), Oregano (116-117), Oregon Grape (247-248), Sheep Sorrel (131-132), Thyme (140-141), White Pine (261-262), Wormwood (210-211)
- **Pseudomonas**: Chicory (62-63), Mugwort (190-191), Rosemary (128-129)
- **Roseola**: Chickweed (61-62)
- **Salmonella**: Chicory (62-63), Lungwort Lichen (272-273), Reishi (273-275), Wormwood (210-211)
- **Shingles**: Chickweed (61-62), Echinacea (72-73), Lemon Balm (98-99), Oregano (116-117), St. John's Wort (133-135), Turkey Tail (275-276), Witch Hazel (266–267)
- **Sore Throat**: Amaranthus Caudatus (152), American Basswood (215-216), Angelica (154-156), Arrowleaf Balsamroot (158-159), Balsam Fir (217-219), Bayberry and Wax Myrtle (220-221), Bee Balm (161), Black Walnut (226-227), Borage (51-52), California Buckwheat (167-168), Carolina Geranium (58-59), Cayenne Pepper (289-290), Cleavers (171-172), Comfrey (64-66), Common Lungwort (105-106), Cottonwood (233-234), False Solomon's Seal (176-177), False Unicorn Root (177-178), Fennel (77-78), Fireweed (178-179), Flax (66-67), Garlic (80-81), Greater Burdock (83-85), Heartleaf Arnica (156-157), Honey Locust (241-242), Horsetail (181-182), Lavender (94-96), Licorice Root (102-103), Maidenhair Fern (187), Osha (191-193), Plantain (119-121), Red Root (198-199), Sage (130-131), Self-heal (122-124), Slippery Elm (257-258), Stone Root (203), Sugar Maple (258-259), Sweet Grass (137), Thyme (140-141), White Mustard (144-145), White Pine (261-262), Wild Strawberries (207-208), Wild Violets (142-143), Wintergreen (209-210), Wooly Lamb's Ear (149-150), Lungwort Lichen (272-273)
- **Smallpox**: Honey Locust (241-242)
- **Strep/Streptococcus**: Duckweed (281-282), Mallow (106-107), Mugwort (190-191), Oregon Grape (247-248), Reishi (273-275), Usnea (277-278)
- **Syphilis**: Bearberry (159-160), Mormon Tea (111-112), Red Alder (250-251)
- **Tetanus**: Cardinal Flower (169), Chickweed (61-62)
- **Tonsillitis**: Cardinal Flower (169), Cleavers (171-172), Greater Burdock (83-85), Lavender (94-96), Red Root (198-199)
- **Typhoid**: Boneset (50-51)
- **Venereal Diseases**: Chaparral (231-232), Chickweed (61-62), False Unicorn Root (177-178), Flax (66-67), Mormon Tea (111-112), Sweet Grass (137)
- **Yellow Fever**: Boneset (50-51)
- **Zika**: Oregon Grape (247-248)

Kidneys

- **Kidney Problems, Kidney Disease**: Agrimony (44-45), Bearberry (159-160), Birch (223-224), Chaga (268-270), Chokecherry (232-233), Club Moss (172-173), Common Lungwort (105-106), Goldenrod (81-83), Horsetail (181-182), Mormon Tea (111-112), Queen Anne's Lace (129-130), Sassafras (254-255), Self-heal (122-124), Sheep Sorrel (131-132), Stone Root (203), Usnea (277-278), Water Plantain (284), Wild Ginger (206-207)
- **Kidney Stones**: Bearberry (159-160), Birch (223-224), Black Crowberry (225), Cleavers (171-172), Club Moss (172-173), Couch Grass (67-68), Fennel (77-78), Goldenrod (81-83), Holy Basil (86-88), Horsetail (181-182), Lovage (104-105), Milk Thistle (110-111), Pipsissewa (195-196), Queen Anne's Lace (129-130), Stone Root (203), Water Plantain (284), Watercress (282-283)
- **Nephritis**: Bearberry (159-160)
- **Strengthens Kidneys**: Bilberry (221-223), Cat's Claw (169-170), Club Moss (172-173), Dandelion (68-70), Goldenrod (81-83), Greater Burdock (83-85), Milk Thistle (110-111), Mormon Tea (111-112), Self-heal (122-124)

Liver, Gallbladder, and Spleen

- **Detoxification of Liver**: Calendula (55-56), Chokecherry (232-233), Dandelion (68-70), Dock (71-72), Greater Burdock (83-85), Hops (88-89), Lemon Balm (98-99), Milk Thistle (110-111), Mugwort (190-191), Oregon Grape (247-248), Pipsissewa (195-196), Self-heal (122-124), St. John's Wort (133-135), Stinging Nettle (135-136), Wild Rose (264-265), Wooly Lamb's Ear (149-150)
- **Fatty Liver**: Chicory (62-63), Chokecherry (232-233), Dandelion (68-70), Milk Thistle (110-111), Oregon Grape (247-248), Water Plantain (284)
- **Gallbladder, Liver, Spleen Stimulation**: Cascara Sagrada (229-231), Chicory (62-63), Dandelion (68-70), Dock (71-72), Oregon Grape (247-248), Reishi (273-275), Stinging Nettle (135-136)
- **Gallbladder Diseases**: Agrimony (44-45), Calendula (55-56), Cascara Sagrada (229-231), Chicory (62-63), Couch Grass (67-68), Oregon Grape (247-248), Wild Rose (264-265)
- **Gallstones**: Cascara Sagrada (229-231), Dandelion (68-70), Maidenhair Fern (187), Milk Thistle (110-111), Pipsissewa (195-196), Queen Anne's Lace (129-130)
- **Hepatitis B**: Carolina Geranium (58-59), Cat's Claw (169-170), Self-heal (122-124), Water Plantain (284)
- **Hepatitis C**: Chaga (268-270), Licorice Root (102-103), Self-heal (122-124)
- **Jaundice**: Ash (216-217), Chicory (62-63), Couch Grass (67-68), Dandelion (68-70), Duckweed (281-282), Garlic (80-81), Hops (88-89), Self-heal (122-124), Wild Teasel (146-148)
- **Liver Damage**: Dandelion (68-70), Evening Primrose (75-77), Milk Thistle (110-111)
- **Liver Problems**: Chicory (62-63), Dandelion (68-70), Evening Primrose (75-77), Peppermint (118-119), Pipsissewa (195-196), Self-heal (122-124), Water Plantain (284)
- **Torpid Liver**: Agrimony (44-45), Burning Bush (229)

Male Issues

- **Erectile Dysfunction**: American Ginseng (153-154), Ash (216-217), False Unicorn Root (177-178), Saw Palmetto (256)
- **Hormone Balance**: Ash (216-217), False Unicorn Root (177-178), Flax (66-67), Sage (130-131)
- **Impotence**: Ash (216-217), False Unicorn Root (177-178), Saw Palmetto (256)
- **Nocturnal Emissions**: False Unicorn Root (177-178), Sage (130-131)
- **Premature Ejaculation**: Sage (130-131), Solomon's Seal (200-202)
- **Swollen Prostate and Prostate Cancer**: Cabbage (54-55), Cleavers (171-172), Couch Grass (67-68), Flax (66-67), Leeks (96-97), Milk Thistle (110-111), Reishi (273-275), Saw Palmetto (256)
- **Sexual Potency**: Ash (216-217), Rhodiola Rosea (199-200), Saw Palmetto (256)
- **Sexual Development**: Spanish Moss (202)

Mouth, Oral and Dental Issues

- **Bleeding and Swollen Gums**: Aloe Vera (45-46), Bilberry (221-223), Borage (51-52), California Buckwheat (167-168), Cattails (279-280), Comfrey (64-66), Fennel (77-78), Lamb's Quarter (93-94), Plantain (119-121), Thyme (140-141), Watercress (282-283)
- **Cavities**: Bloodroot (164-165), Calendula (55-56), Dock (71-72), Feverfew (78-79), Holy Basil (86-88), Horsetail (181-182), Thyme (140-141)
- **Cold Sores**: Anise Hyssop (46-47), Balsam Fir (217-219), Black Walnut (226-227), Calendula (55-56), Devil's Club (236-237), Echinacea (72-73), Flax (66-67), Greater Burdock (83-85), Lemon Balm (98-99), Red Root (198-199), Self-heal (122-124), Slippery Elm (257-258), St. John's Wort (133-135), Turkey Tail (275-276), Usnea (277-278)
- **Gingivitis**: Bilberry (221-223), Bloodroot (164-165), Calendula (55-56), Thyme (140-141), Wild Ginger (206-207)
- **Halitosis**: Dill (70-71), Feverfew (78-79), Rosemary (128-129), Watercress (282-283), Yerba Santa (213-214)
- **Mouthwash**: Aloe Vera (45-46), Calendula (55-56), California Buckwheat (167-168), Rosemary (128-129), Thyme (140-141), Watercress (282-283), Wild Ginger (206-207), Yerba Santa (213-214)

- **Sore Mouth**: Amaranthus Caudatus (152), Arrowleaf Balsamroot (158-159), Feverfew (78-79), Watercress (282-283), Wooly Lamb's Ear (149-150), Yarrow (150-151)
- **Thrush**: Garlic (80-81), Goldenrod (81-83), Potassium Permanganate (293-294), Usnea (277-278)
- **Toothache**: Arrowleaf Balsamroot (158-159), Bleeding Heart (163-164), California Poppy (57-58), Cattails (279-280), Chaparral (231-232), Heartleaf Arnica (156-157), Lamb's Quarter (93-94), Plantain (119-121), Red Root (198-199), White Willow (263-264)
- **Toothbrushing**: Diatomaceous Earth (292), Dogwood (238), Horsetail (181-182), Sassafras (254-255), Wild Strawberries (207-208)

Muscles, Joints and Tendons

- **Arthritis**: Balsam Poplar (219-220), Bayberry and Wax Myrtle (220-221), Borage (51-52), Cabbage (54-55), Cayenne Pepper (289-290), Chaparral (231-232), Chickweed (61-62), Cottonwood (233-234), Couch Grass (67-68), Dandelion (68-70), Devil's Club (236-237), Drumstick Tree (220-221), Evening Primrose (75-77), False Solomon's Seal (176-177), Goldenrod (81-83), Heartleaf Arnica (156-157), Henbane (85-86), Horseradish (89-90), Lady's Thumb (92), Lamb's Quarter (93-94), Leeks (96-97), Lemon, Meadowsweet (245-246), Verbena (89-90), Osha (191-193), Partridgeberry (194-195), Peppermint (118-119), Pipsissewa (195-196), Prickly Pear Cactus (121-122), Red Alder (250-251), Reishi (273-275), Rosemary (128-129), Sassafras (254-255), Slippery Elm (257-258), Solomon's Seal (200-202), Spanish Moss (202) , St. John's Wort (133-135), Stinging Nettle (135-136), Turmeric (295-296), Watercress (282-283), Western Skunk Cabbage (285-286), White Mustard (144-145), Wild Teasel (146-148), Wild Strawberries (207-208), Yellow Jessamine (211-212)
- **Bursitis**: Lemon Verbena (101-102)
- **Carpal Tunnel**: Calendula (55-56), Cottonwood (233-234), Osha (191-193), Western Skunk Cabbage (285-286)
- **Joint Pain**: Angelica (154-156), Ashwagandha (47-48), Balsam Poplar (219-220), Bleeding Heart (163-164), Cabbage (54-55), Cayenne Pepper (289-290), Comfrey (64-66), Cottonwood (233-234), Drumstick Tree (220-221), Duckweed (281-282), Goldenrod (81-83), Heartleaf Arnica (156-157), Lemon Verbena (101-102), Lobelia Inflata (184-185), Lovage (104-105), Meadowsweet (245-246), Peppermint (118-119), Prickly Pear Cactus (121-122), Quaking Aspen (249), Sassafras (254-255), Slippery Elm (257-258), Solomon's Seal (200-202), Unicorn Root (204-205), Western Red Cedar (259-261), Western Skunk Cabbage (285-286), White Mustard (144-145), White Pine (261-262), White Willow (263-264), Wild Strawberries (207-208), Wild Violets (142-143)
- **Muscle Aches**: Anise Hyssop (46-47), Ash (216-217), Balsam Fir (217-219), Chamomile (59-60), Dogwood (238), Duckweed (281-282), False Hellebore (174-175), Heartleaf Arnica (156-157), Henbane (85-86), Lavender (94-96), Lobelia Inflata (184-185), Pipsissewa (195-196), Prickly Pear Cactus (121-122), Solomon's Seal (200-202), St. John's Wort (133-135), Stinging Nettle (135-136), Sweet Marjoram (137-138), Unicorn Root (204-205), Western Skunk Cabbage (285-286), Wintergreen (209-210), Witch Hazel (266-267), Yellow Jessamine (211-212)
- **Muscle Spasms**: American Ginseng (153-154), Bayberry and Wax Myrtle (220-221), Bleeding Heart (163-164), Butterbur (166-167), Calendula (55-56), California Poppy (57-58), Chamomile (59-60), Couch Grass (67-68), Dill (70-71), Henbane (85-86), Hops (88-89), Lavender (94-96), Lobelia Inflata (184-185), Mugwort (190-191), Mullein (114-115), Peppermint (118-119), Skullcap (132-133), Stinging Nettle (135-136), Stone Root (203), Sweet Marjoram (137-138), Thorn Apple (138-140), Thyme (140-141), Unicorn Root (204-205), Western Skunk Cabbage (285-286), Wild Ginger (206-207), Wild Yam (208-209), Wooly Lamb's Ear (149-150), Yerba Santa (213-214)
- **Muscle Sprains**: Bleeding Heart (163-164), Blue and Black Elderberry (227-229), Butterbur (166-167), Cardinal Flower (169), Cayenne Pepper (289-290), Comfrey (64-66), Heartleaf Arnica

(156-157), Henbane (85-86), Stinging Nettle (135-136), Yarrow (150-151)

- **Rheumatoid Arthritis and Rheumatism**: Ashwagandha (47-48), Balsam Poplar (219-220), Birch (223-224), Cat's Claw (169-170), Cayenne Pepper (289-290), Chaparral (231-232), Chickweed (61-62), Chives (63-64), Club Moss (172-173), Couch Grass (67-68), Epsom Salts (292-293), Evening Primrose (75-77), False Hellebore (174-175), Feverfew (78-79), Greater Burdock (83-85), Heartleaf Arnica (156-157), Henbane (85-86), Horseradish (89-90), Lady's Thumb (92), Leeks (96-97), Lemon Verbena (101-102), Osha (191-193), Peppermint (118-119), Prickly Pear Cactus (121-122), Quaking Aspen (249), Reishi (273-275), Rosemary (128-129), Slippery Elm (257-258), Spanish Moss (202) , St. John's Wort (133-135), Stinging Nettle (135-136), Unicorn Root (204-205), White Mustard (144-145), White Pine (261-262), White Willow (263-264), Wild Strawberries (207-208), Wild Violets (142-143), Wild Yam (208-209), Yellow Jessamine (211-212), Yerba Santa (213-214)
- **Tendonitis**: Solomon's Seal (200-202), Stinging Nettle (135-136)

Nervous System, Brain, and Head Issues

- **Alzheimer's Disease**: Ashwagandha (47-48), Bilberry (221-223), Borage (51-52), Bottle Gourd (53), Cinnamon (291), Drumstick Tree (220-221), Horsetail (181-182), Lemon Balm (98-99), Lion's Mane (270-271), Red Mulberry (252), Reishi (273-275), Turmeric (295-296), Skullcap (132-133)
- **Anxiety**: Anise Hyssop (46-47), Angelica (154-156), Ashwagandha (47-48), Black Cohosh (162), Bleeding Heart (163-164), California Poppy (57-58), Hops (88-89), Watercress (282-283), Lavender (94-96), Lemon Balm (98-99), Lemon Verbena (101-102), Lion's Mane (270-271), Lobelia Inflata (184-185), Motherwort (112-114), Parrot's Beak (193-194), Partridgeberry (194-195), Pulsatilla (124-125), Reishi (273-275), Rhodiola Rosea (199-200), Skullcap (132-133), St. John's Wort (133-135), Stone Root (203), Valerian Root (141-142), Yarrow (150-151)
- **Appetite Stimulation**: Bleeding Heart (163-164), Burning Bush (229), Chives (63-64), Peppermint (118-119), Unicorn Root (204-205), Wormwood (210-211)
- **Concentration**: American Ginseng (153-154), Ashwagandha (47-48), Lion's Mane (270-271), Rhodiola Rosea (199-200), Rosemary (128-129)
- **Concussions**: Lion's Mane (270-271)
- **Confusion**: Spanish Moss (202)
- **Coordination**: Cranberry (235-236)
- **Creutzfeldt-Jakob Disease (CJD)/Prions**: Lungwort Lichen (272-273)
- **Dementia**: Bilberry (221-223), Bottle Gourd (53), Horsetail (181-182), Lemon Balm (98-99), Lion's Mane (281-284), Pulsatilla (124-125), Rosemary (128-129), Spanish Moss (202)
- **Depression**: American Ginseng (153-154), Ashwagandha (47-48), Bottle Gourd (53), Drumstick Tree (220-221), Evening Primrose (75-77), Holy Basil (86-88), Lemon Balm (98-99), Lion's Mane (270-271), Lobelia Inflata (184-185), Motherwort (112-114), Moringa (246-247), Pulsatilla (124-125), Reishi (273-275), Rhodiola Rosea (199-200), Skullcap (132-133), Spanish Moss (202) , St. John's Wort (133-135), Sugar Maple (258-259), Turmeric (295-296), Valerian Root (141-142), Wild Rose (264-265)
- **Epilepsy, Seizures**: American Basswood (215-216), Black Crowberry (225), Cardinal Flower (169), Hops (88-89), Lavender (94-96), Mugwort (190-191), Reishi (273-275), Skullcap (132-133), Thyme (140-141), Valerian Root (141-142), Western Skunk Cabbage (285-286)
- **Headaches and Migraines**: Agrimony (44-45), Bottle Gourd (53), Butterbur (166-167), California Buckwheat (167-168), Cottonwood (233-234), Duckweed (281-282), Feverfew (78-79), Fireweed (178-179), Oregon Grape (247-248), Osha (191-193), Parrot's Beak (193-194), Peppermint (118-119), Pulsatilla (124-125), Quaking Aspen (249), Red Alder (250-251), Rosemary (128-129), Sassafras (254-255), Skullcap (132-133), Sweet Marjoram (137-138), Watercress (282-283), White Willow (263-264), Wintergreen (209-210), Yarrow (150-151), Yellow Jessamine (211-212)
- **Hyperactivity**: Evening Primrose (75-77), Lemon Balm (98-99), Pulsatilla (124-125)

- **Hypnotic**: Henbane (85-86), Pulsatilla (124-125)
- **Insomnia**: Agrimony (44-45), American Basswood (215-216), Black Cohosh (162), Chamomile (59-60), Drumstick Tree (220-221), Hardy Kiwi (238-239), Hops (88-89), Lemon Balm (98-99), Lion's Mane (270-271), Motherwort (112-114), Moringa (246-247), Mugwort (190-191), Parrot's Beak (193-194), Partridgeberry (194-195), Pulsatilla (124-125), Reishi (273-275), Skullcap (132-133), St. John's Wort (133-135), Valerian Root (141-142), Wild Lettuce (145-146)
- **Memory Loss**: American Ginseng (153-154), Ashwagandha (47-48), Bottle Gourd (53), Cranberry (235-236), Lemon Balm (98-99), Lion's Mane (281-284), Rhodiola Rosea (199-200), Rosemary (128-129), Sage (130-131), Spanish Moss (202) , Turmeric (295-296)
- **Myasthenia Gravis**: Reishi (273-275)
- **Multiple Sclerosis**, see Immune System
- **Nerve Pain**: American Basswood (215-216), Angelica (154-156), Bleeding Heart (163-164), Cayenne Pepper (289-290), Chickweed (61-62), Evening Primrose (75-77), Henbane (85-86), Lavender (94-96), Peppermint (118-119), St. John's Wort (133-135), Stinging Nettle (135-136)
- **Neuralgia**: Henbane (85-86), Peppermint (118-119), St. John's Wort (133-135)
- **Obsessive Compulsive Behaviour**: St. John's Wort (133-135), Valerian Root (141-142)
- **Pain Relievers**: Aloe Vera (45-46), Black Crowberry (225), Bleeding Heart (163-164), California Buckwheat (167-168), Cattails (279-280), Chicory (62-63), Comfrey (64-66), Cottonwood (233-234), Devil's Club (236-237), Feverfew (78-79), Heartleaf Arnica (156-157), Henbane (85-86), Holy Basil (86-88), Unicorn Root (204-205), Wild Lettuce (145-146), Wild Yam (208-209), Wintergreen (209-210), Yarrow (150-151)
- **Panic Attacks**: Pulsatilla (124-125), Reishi (273-275), Valerian Root (141-142)
- **Parkinson's Disease**: Ashwagandha (47-48), Cinnamon (291), Flax (66-67), Lion's Mane (270-271), Red Mulberry (252), Skullcap (132-133), Thorn Apple (138-140)
- **Post-Traumatic Stress Disorder (PTSD):** California Poppy (57-58), Rhodiola Rosea (199-200)
- **Restlessness**: Lemon Balm (98-99), Parrot's Beak (193-194), Reishi (273-275), St. John's Wort (133-135), Wild Lettuce (145-146)
- **Schizophrenia**: California Poppy (57-58), Pulsatilla (124-125)
- **Sciatica**: Cayenne Pepper (289-290), Peppermint (118-119), St. John's Wort (133-135), Stinging Nettle (135-136), Wintergreen (209-210)
- **Sedatives**: American Basswood (215-216), Black Cohosh (162), Bleeding Heart (163-164), California Poppy (57-58), Chicory (62-63), Hops (88-89), Lavender (94-96), Parrot's Beak (193-194), Partridgeberry (194-195), Saw Palmetto (256), Solomon's Seal (200-202), Unicorn Root (204-205), Wild Lettuce (145-146), Yellow Jessamine (211-212)
- **Seizures**: See Epilepsy
- **Stress**: American Ginseng (153-154), Ashwagandha (47-48), Borage (51-52), Chaga (268-270), Epsom Salts (292-293), Holy Basil (86-88), Lavender (94-96), Lemon Balm (98-99), Lemon Verbena (101-102), Lion's Mane (270-271), Parrot's Beak (193-194), Reishi (273-275), Rhodiola Rosea (199-200), Skullcap (132-133), Stone Root (203), Sugar Maple (258-259), Sweet Marjoram (137-138)
- **Stroke**: Bilberry (221-223), Cocoplum (280-281), Lion's Mane (270-271), Oregano (116-117), Motherwort (112-114)

Pancreas

- **Diabetes**: Aloe Vera (45-46), Amaranthus Caudatus (152), American Ginseng (153-154), Bilberry (221-223), Bottle Gourd (53), Cabbage (54-55), Cascara Sagrada (229-231), Cayenne Pepper (289-290), Cinnamon (291), Chicory (62-63), Drumstick Tree (220-221), Elecampane (74-75), Evening Primrose (75-77), Garlic (80-81), Goldenseal (179-180), Greater Burdock (83-85), Horse Chestnut (242-243), Horsetail (181-182), Kudzu (183-184), Leeks (96-97), Lemon Balm (98-99), Lion's Mane (281-284), Milk Thistle (110-111), Pipsissewa (195-196), Plantain (119-121), Prickly Pear Cactus (121-122), Purslane (125-126), Red Mulberry (252), Reishi (273-275), Self-heal (122-124), Sheep Sorrel (131-132), Spanish Moss (202) ,

Sugar Maple (258-259), Sweet Marjoram (137-138), Turkey Tail (275-276), Water Plantain (284), Wild Ginger (206-207)

Respiratory Issues and Lungs

- **Asthma**: Angelica (154-156), Bloodroot (164-165), Butterbur (166-167), Chamomile (59-60), Coltsfoot (173-174), Comfrey (64-66), Common Lungwort (105-106), Cranberry (235-236), Echinacea (72-73), Elecampane (74-75), Evening Primrose (75-77), Holy Basil (86-88), Hops (88-89), Lavender (94-96), Lemon Thyme (100), Lobelia Inflata (184-185), Lungwort Lichen (272-273), Marshmallow (107-108), Mormon Tea (111-112), Mugwort (190-191), Mullein (114-115), Oregano (116-117), Osha (191-193), Oxeye Daisy (117-118), Purslane (125-126), Reishi (273-275), Salal (253-254), Self-heal (122-124), Stinging Nettle (135-136), Thorn Apple (138-140), Western Skunk Cabbage (285-286), Wild Rose (264-265), Yerba Santa (213-214)
- **Bronchitis**: Anise Hyssop (46-47), Angelica (154-156), Balsam Fir (217-219), Balsam Poplar (219-220), Bloodroot (164-165), Boneset (50-51), Cardinal Flower (169), Chamomile (59-60), Chokecherry (232-233), Coltsfoot (173-174), Common Lungwort (105-106), Devil's Club (236-237), Echinacea (72-73), Elecampane (74-75), Garlic (80-81), Holy Basil (86-88), Horsetail (181-182), Lavender (94-96), Lemon Verbena (101-102), Lobelia Inflata (184-185), Lungwort Lichen (272-273), Maidenhair Fern (187), Mallow (106-107), Marshmallow (107-108), Mormon Tea (111-112), Mullein (114-115), Osha (191-193), Pipsissewa (195-196), Red Root (198-199), Slippery Elm (257-258), Sugar Maple (258-259), Sweet Grass (137), Thyme (140-141), Usnea (277-278), Western Skunk Cabbage (285-286), White Mustard (144-145), Wild Rose (264-265)
- **Congestion**: Anise Hyssop (46-47), Arrowleaf Balsamroot (158-159), Bee Balm (161), Bilberry (221-223), Boneset (50-51), Chamomile (59-60), Club Moss (172-173), Coltsfoot (173-174), Comfrey (64-66), False Solomon's Seal (176-177), Fireweed (178-179), Flax (66-67), Garlic (80-81), Goldenrod (81-83), Horsetail (181-182), Lavender (94-96), Lemon Thyme (100), Lemon Verbena (101-102), Lungwort Lichen (272-273), Maidenhair Fern (187), Marshmallow (107-108), Oxeye Daisy (117-118), Quaking Aspen (249), Reishi (273-275), St. John's Wort (133-135), Sweet Grass (137), Sweet Grass (137), Usnea (277-278), White Mustard (144-145), White Pine (261-262), Yarrow (150-151)
- **Cough**: American Basswood (215-216), Angelica (154-156), Arrowleaf Balsamroot (158-159), Balsam Fir (217-219), Balsam Poplar (219-220), Butterbur (166-167), California Buckwheat (167-168), Coltsfoot (173-174), Comfrey (64-66), Devil's Club (236-237), False Solomon's Seal (176-177), Flax (66-67), Greater Burdock (83-85), Honey Locust (241-242), Lavender (94-96), Licorice Root (102-103), Mallow (106-107), Oxeye Daisy (117-118), Quaking Aspen (249), Red Root (198-199), Salal (253-254), Saw Palmetto (256), Slippery Elm (257-258), Sugar Maple (258-259), Sweet Grass (137), Thorn Apple (138-140), Thyme (140-141), White Pine (261-262), White Sage (263), Wild Violets (142-143), Witch Hazel (266-267)
- **Emphysema**: Butterbur (166-167), Chaparral (231-232), Coltsfoot (173-174), Ginger (211-212), Mallow (106-107), Mormon Tea (111-112), Mullein (114-115), St. John's Wort (133-135)
- **Expectorant/Mucus** – Arrowleaf Balsamroot (158-159), Balsam Poplar (219-220), Bloodroot (164-165), Blue and Black Elderberry (227-229), Boneset (50-51), Cardinal Flower (169), Chaparral (231-232), Coltsfoot (173-174), Cottonwood (233-234), Evening Primrose (75-77), Elecampane (74-75), Fennel (77-78), Horseradish (89-90), Lobelia Inflata (184-185), Lovage (104-105), Lungwort Lichen (272-273), Maidenhair Fern (187), Marshmallow (107-108), Mullein (114-115), Osha (191-193), Plantain (119-121), Red Root (198-199), Saw Palmetto (256), Solomon's Seal (200-202), St. John's Wort (133-135), Sugar Maple (258-259), Thyme (140-141), Watercress (282-283), Western Skunk Cabbage (285-286), White Pine (261-262), Wild Violets (142-143), Witch Hazel (266-267), Yerba Santa (213-214)
- **Inflammation of Respiratory Tract**: Balsam Poplar (219-220), Chaparral (231-232), Club Moss (172-173), Goldenseal (179-180), Juniper (244),

Lamb's Quarter (93-94), Plantain (119-121), St. John's Wort (133-135), Sweet Marjoram (137-138)

- **Pleurisy**: Horseradish (89-90), Lobelia Inflata (184-185), Marshmallow (107-108), Slippery Elm (257-258)
- **Pneumonia**: Bloodroot (164-165), Borage (51-52), Cottonwood (233-234), False Hellebore (174-175), Juniper (244) Lobelia Inflata (184-185), Lungwort Lichen (272-273), White Mustard (144-145), Usnea (277-278)
- **Tracheitis**: Mormon Tea (111-112), Mullein (114-115)
- **Tuberculosis**: Arrowleaf Balsamroot (158-159), Balsam Fir (217-219), Black-Eyed Susan (49), Bloodroot (164-165), Devil's Club (236-237), Elecampane (74-75), Lungwort Lichen (272-273), Mormon Tea (111-112), Mullein (114-115), Quaking Aspen (249), Red Alder (250-251), Rhodiola Rosea (199-200), Salal (253-254), Slippery Elm (257-258), Solomon's Seal (200-202), St. John's Wort (133-135), Usnea (277-278), Watercress (282-283), Western Skunk Cabbage (285-286)
- **Whooping Cough**: Arrowleaf Balsamroot (158-159), Bloodroot (164-165), Butterbur (166-167), Chamomile (59-60), Coltsfoot (173-174), Common Lungwort (105-106), Cottonwood (233-234), Elecampane (74-75), Evening Primrose (75-77), Flax (66-67), Garlic (80-81), Honey Locust (241-242), Lavender (94-96), Lungwort Lichen (272-273), Oxeye Daisy (117-118), Pipsissewa (195-196), Red Root (198-199), Thorn Apple (138-140), Wild Violets (142-143)

Skin

- **Abrasions and Irritations**: Aloe Vera (45-46), Balsam Fir (217-219), Black-Eyed Susan (49), Bottle Gourd (53), Calendula (55-56), Cardinal Flower (169), Cattails (279-280), Chickweed (61-62), Dock (71-72), Feverfew (78-79), Goldenrod (81-83), Goldenseal (179-180), Juniper (244), Lamb's Quarter (93-94), Lobelia Inflata (184-185), Lovage (104-105), Marshmallow (107-108), Peppermint (118-119), Quaking Aspen (249),Red Elderberry (251), Salal (253-254), Sassafras (254-255), Slippery Elm (257-258), Wild Rose (264-266)Witch Hazel (266-267), Wild Violets (142-143)
- **Abscesses**: Cattails (279-280), Cleavers (171-172), Flax (66-67), Male Fern (188), Moringa (246-247), Potassium Permanganate (293-294), Red Elderberry (251), Yarrow (150-151)
- **Acne**: Activated Charcoal (287), Angelica (154-156), Black Crowberry (225), Black Walnut (226-227), Calendula (55-56), Chaparral (231-232), Chickweed (61-62), Chicory (62-63), Cleavers (171-172), Evening Primrose (75-77), Fireweed (178-179), Flax (66-67), Garlic (80-81), Greater Burdock (83-85), Juniper (244), Listerine (293), Lovage (104-105), Milk Thistle (110-111), Moringa (246-247), Oregon Grape (247-248), Plantain (119-121), Reishi (273-275) Solomon's Seal (200-202), Sugar Maple (258-259), Thyme (140-141), Wild Rose (264-265)
- **Bedsores**: Bleach (288), Hops (88-89)
- **Boils**: American Basswood (215-216), Bottle Gourd (53), Cattails (279-280), Chickweed (61-62), Chicory (62-63), Cleavers (171-172), Common Lungwort (105-106), Devil's Club (236-237), False Hellebore (174-175), Flax (66-67), Goldenrod (81-83), Goldenseal (179-180), Greater Burdock (83-85), Hops (88-89), Lobelia Inflata (184-185), Male Fern (188), Oregon Grape (247-248), Osha (191-193), Red Elderberry (251), Slippery Elm (257-258), Thorn Apple (138-140), White Pine (261-262), Western Red Cedar (259-261)
- **Bruises**: Arrowleaf Balsamroot (158-159), Balsam Poplar (219-220), Bleeding Heart (163-164), Cardinal Flower (169), Cattails (279-280), Chaparral (231-232), Comfrey (64-66), Evening Primrose (75-77), Greater Burdock (83-85), Heartleaf Arnica (156-157), Hops (88-89), Jewelweed (185-186), Mallow (106-107), Oxeye Daisy (117-118), Slippery Elm (257-258), Solomon's Seal (200-202), St. John's Wort (133-135), Water Plantain (284), Western Skunk Cabbage (285-286), Wild Comfrey (205-206), Wild Violets (142-143), Yarrow (150-151)
- **Burns**: American Basswood (215-216), Anise Hyssop (46-47), Arrowleaf Balsamroot (158-159), Balsam Poplar (219-220), Birch (223-224), Calendula (55-56), Cattails (279-280), Chaparral (231-232), Chokecherry (232-233), Cleavers (171-172),

Comfrey (64-66), Common Lungwort (105-106), Cottonwood (233-234), Devil's Club (236-237), Echinacea (72-73), Feverfew (78-79), Fireweed (178-179), Flax (66-67), Goldenrod (81-83), Greater Burdock (83-85), Honey (294-295), Jewelweed (185-186), Lamb's Quarter (93-94), Mallow (106-107), Mugwort (190-191), Salal (253-254), St. John's Wort (133-135), Stinging Nettle (135-136), Thorn Apple (138-140), Western Skunk Cabbage (285-286), Wild Comfrey (205-206), Wild Strawberries (207-208)

- **Carbuncles**: Flax (66-67), Male Fern (188), Western Red Cedar (259-261)
- **Chilblains**: Heartleaf Arnica (156-157), Horseradish (89-90), Quaking Aspen (249), White Mustard (144-145),
- **Corns**: Dandelion (68-70), Garlic (80-81), White Willow (263-264)
- **Cuts**: Balsam Fir (217-219), Balsam Poplar (219-220), Black-Eyed Susan (49), Calendula (55-56), Cattails (279-280), Cayenne Pepper (289-290), Cleavers (171-172), Common Lungwort (105-106), Cottonwood (233-234), Dogwood (238), Goldenrod (81-83), False Solomon's Seal (176-177), Marshmallow (107-108), Mullein (114-115), Plantain (119-121), Slippery Elm (257-258), St. John's Wort (133-135), Yarrow (150-151), Wild Strawberries (207-208)
- **Dandruff**: Chaparral (231-232), Devil's Club (236-237), Moringa (246-247), Usnea (277-278), Western Red Cedar (259-261)
- **Dermatitis**: Chickweed (61-62), Club Moss (172-173), Watercress (282-283), Lovage (104-105), Wild Violets (142-143), Red Root (198-199)
- **Diaper Rash**: Calendula (55-56), Cattails (279-280)
- **Eczema**: Aloe Vera (45-46), Arrowleaf Balsamroot (158-159), Birch (223-224), Black Walnut (226-227), Bleach (288), Bloodroot (164-165), Calendula (55-56), Chamomile (59-60), Chaparral (231-232), Chickweed (61-62), Cleavers (171-172), Club Moss (172-173), Coltsfoot (173-174), Comfrey (64-66), Common Lungwort (105-106), Dandelion (68-70), Evening Primrose (75-77), Fireweed (178-179), Flax (66-67), Greater Burdock (83-85), Hawthorn (239-241), Heartleaf Arnica (156-157), Horsetail (181-182), Jewelweed (185-186), Lamb's Quarter (93-94), Lavender (94-96), Licorice Root (102-103), Milk Thistle (110-111), Oregon Grape (247-248), Prickly Pear Cactus (121-122), Quaking Aspen (249), Red Alder (250-251), Red Clover (126-127), St. John's Wort (133-135), Stinging Nettle (135-136), Watercress (282-283), Wild Violets (142-143)
- **Foreign Objects**: Marshmallow (107-108), Plantain (119-121)
- **Frostbite**: Birch (223-224), Heartleaf Arnica (156-157)
- **Hemorrhoids and Piles**: Bilberry (221-223), Blue and Black Elderberry (227-229), Calendula (55-56), Cascara Sagrada (229-231), Common Lungwort (105-106), Evening Primrose (75-77), Henbane (85-86), Horse Chestnut (242-243), Maidenhair Fern (187), Meadow Rue (109), Mullein (114-115), Quaking Aspen (249), Red Root (198-199), Self-heal (122-124), Self-heal (122-124),Solomon's Seal (200-202), Spanish Moss (202) , St. John's Wort (133-135), Stinging Nettle (135-136), Stone Root (203), Wild Violets (142-143), Witch Hazel (266-267), Wooly Lamb's Ear (149-150), Yarrow (150-151)
- **Hidradenitis Suppurativa**: Fennel (77-78)
- **Hives**: Chickweed (61-62), Club Moss (172-173), Prickly Pear Cactus (121-122)
- **Impetigo**: Greater Burdock (83-85)
- **Infections**: Aloe Vera (45-46), American Basswood (215-216), Anise Hyssop (46-47), Balsam Fir (217-219), Black-Eyed Susan (49), Borage (51-52), Bottle Gourd (53), Cabbage (54-55), Calendula (55-56), Cattails (279-280), Chamomile (59-60), Chaparral (231-232), Comfrey (64-66), Couch Grass (67-68), Echinacea (72-73), Fireweed (178-179), Holy Basil (86-88), Hops (88-89), Horseradish (89-90), Juniper (244), Marshmallow (107-108), Mormon Tea (111-112), Meadowsweet (245-246), Mullein (114-115), Osha (191-193), Red Raspberry (197), St. John's Wort (133-135), White Pine (261-262), Yarrow (150-151)
- **Insect bites**: Activated Charcoal (287), Black Crowberry (225), Cattails (279-280), Club Moss (172-173), Echinacea (72-73), Greater Burdock (83-85), Jewelweed (185-186), Listerine (293), Oxeye Daisy (117-118), Plantain (119-121), Quaking Aspen (249), Red Alder (250-251), Salal (253-

254), Self-heal (122-124), Stinging Nettle (135-136), Western Skunk Cabbage (285-286), Wild Violets (142-143), Wooly Lamb's Ear (149-150)

- **Lip Chapping**: Balsam Fir (217-219), Calendula (55-56), Cottonwood (233-234)
- **Mouth Ulcers**: Amaranthus Caudatus (152), Borage (51-52), Common Lungwort (105-106), Goldenseal (179-180), Watercress (282-283)
- **Pain Relief**: Aloe Vera (45-46), American Basswood (215-216), Balsam Fir (217-219), Black Crowberry (225), Cattails (279-280), Chicory (62-63), Cottonwood (233-234), Heartleaf Arnica (156-157), Wild Lettuce (145-146), Wintergreen (209-210), Yerba Santa (213-214)
- **Poison Ivy itchiness**: Anise Hyssop (46-47), Black Walnut (226-227), Lady's Thumb (92), Mugwort (190-191), Red Alder (250-251), Self-heal (122-124)
- **Psoriasis**: Aloe Vera (45-46), Black Walnut (226-227), Calendula (55-56), Chaparral (231-232), Cleavers (171-172), Club Moss (172-173), Comfrey (64-66), Dandelion (68-70), Evening Primrose (75-77), Fireweed (178-179), Flax (66-67), Greater Burdock (83-85), Hawthorn (239-241), Honey (294-295), Lavender (94-96), Listerine (293), Lovage (104-105), Milk Thistle (110-111), Oregon Grape (247-248), Prickly Pear Cactus (121-122), Red Clover (126-127), Reishi (273-275), Turkey Tail (275-276), Valerian Root (141-142)
- **Rashes**: Balsam Poplar (219-220), Bee Balm (161), Black Crowberry (225), Calendula (55-56), Chaparral (231-232), Chickweed (61-62), Cleavers (171-172), Comfrey (64-66), Common Lungwort (105-106), Cottonwood (233-234), Fireweed (178-179), Goldenseal (179-180), Greater Burdock (83-85), Hawthorn (239-241), Holy Basil (86-88), Lady's Thumb (92), Lamb's Quarter (93-94), Licorice Root (102-103), Listerine (293), Lovage (104-105), Mugwort (190-191), Oxeye Daisy (117-118), Plantain (119-121), Quaking Aspen (249), Queen Anne's Lace (129-130), Red Alder (250-251), Sassafras (254-255), Self-heal (122-124), Western Skunk Cabbage (285-286)
- **Ringworm**: Arrowleaf Balsamroot (158-159), Black Walnut (226-227), Calendula (55-56), Chicory (62-63), Common Lungwort (105-106), Dandelion (68-70), Greater Burdock (83-85), Holy Basil (86-88), Oregano (116-117), Purslane (125-126), Red Mulberry (252), Western Red Cedar (259-261), Usnea (277-278)
- **Shingles**: Chickweed (61-62), Echinacea (72-73), Garlic (80-81), Lemon Balm (98-99), St. John's Wort (133-135), Turkey Tail (275-276)
- **Staph Infections**: Cascara Sagrada (229-231), Chaparral (231-232), Chicory (62-63), Duckweed (281-282), Juniper (244), Lemon Verbena (101-102), Lungwort Lichen (272-273), Mallow (106-107), Mugwort (190-191), Oregano (116-117), Oregon Grape (247-248), Reishi (273-275), Rosemary (128-129), Usnea (277-278)
- **Sunburn**: Aloe Vera (45-46), American Basswood (215-216), Calendula (55-56), Cleavers (171-172), Club Moss (172-173), Cottonwood (233-234), Mullein (114-115), St. John's Wort (133-135), Stinging Nettle (135-136), Wild Strawberries (207-208)
- **Ulcers, Skin**: Bilberry (221-223), Bloodroot (164-165), Cabbage (54-55), Calendula (55-56), Coltsfoot (173-174), Goldenseal (179-180), Honey (294-295), Marshmallow (107-108), Mullein (114-115), Red Raspberry (197), Self-heal (122-124), Sugar Maple (258-259), Wintergreen (209-210)
- **Warts**: Black Walnut (226-227), Bloodroot (164-165), Dandelion (68-70), Garlic (80-81), Mayapple (189), Moringa (246-247), Mullein (114-115), Thyme (140-141), Western Red Cedar (259-261), White Willow (263-264), Wild Lettuce (145-146)
- **Wounds**: Agrimony (44-45), Aloe Vera (45-46), Anise Hyssop (46-47), Arrowleaf Balsamroot (158-159), Balsam Fir (217-219), Balsam Poplar (219-220), Black-Eyed Susan (49), Borage (51-52), Cabbage (54-55), Calendula (55-56), California Buckwheat (167-168), Cattails (279-280), Chaparral (231-232), Club Moss (172-173), Comfrey (64-66), Common Lungwort (105-106), Dandelion (68-70), Dock (71-72), Dogwood (238), Echinacea (72-73), Evening Primrose (75-77), False Hellebore (174-175), False Solomon's Seal (176-177), Fireweed (178-179), Goldenrod (81-83), Hawthorn (239-241), Heartleaf Arnica (156-157), Honey (294-295), Hops (88-89), Horseradish (89-90), Horsetail (181-182), Juniper (244), Listerine (293), Meadow Rue (109), Mullein (114-

115), Oregon Grape (247-248), Osha (191-193), Oxeye Daisy (117-118), Plantain (119-121), Potassium Permanganate (293-294), Quaking Aspen (249), Red Elderberry (251), Red Raspberry (197), Red Root (198-199), Sage (130-131), Salal (253-254), Sassafras (254-255), Self-heal (122-124), Slippery Elm (257-258), St. John's Wort (133-135), Stinging Nettle (135-136), Stone Root (203), Thorn Apple (138-140), Turmeric (295-296), Usnea (277-278), Western Skunk Cabbage (285-286), White Mustard (144-145), White Pine (261-262), Wild Strawberries (207-208), Wild Teasel (146-148), Witch Hazel (266-267), Wooly Lamb's Ear (149-150)

Poisons

- **Inducing Vomiting**: Activated Charcoal (287), Lobelia Inflata (184-185), Unicorn Root (204-205)
- **Mushrooms**: Activated Charcoal (287), Milk Thistle (110-111)
- **Poison Ingestion**: Activated Charcoal (287), Lobelia Inflata (184-185), Unicorn Root (204-205), White Mustard (144-145)

Urinary Tract

- **Cystitis**: Bearberry (159-160), Birch (223-224), Chaparral (231-232), Common Lungwort (105-106), Couch Grass (67-68), Feverfew (78-79), Henbane (85-86), Juniper (244), Lavender (94-96), Marshmallow (107-108), Plantain (119-121), Red Mulberry (252), Slippery Elm (257-258), Water Plantain (284), Wild Rose (264-266)
- **Irritable Bladder**: Henbane (85-86), Hops (88-89), Juniper (244), Salal (253-254)
- **Obstructions**: Cleavers (171-172), Meadow Rue (109)
- **Urinary Tract Infections**: Bearberry (159-160), Bilberry (221-223), Cattails (279-280), Chaparral (231-232), Cleavers (171-172), Club Moss (172-173), Common Lungwort (105-106), Couch Grass (67-68), Cranberry (235-236), Dandelion (68-70), Duckweed (281-282), Echinacea (72-73), Fennel (77-78), Goldenrod (81-83), Goldenseal (179-180), Horseradish (89-90), Horsetail (181-182) Juniper (244), Lavender (94-96), Leeks (96-97), Lovage (104-105), Maidenhair Fern (187), Mallow (106-107), Marshmallow (107-108), Oregon Grape (247-248),Plantain (119-121), Pulsatilla (124-125), Red Mulberry (252), Reishi (273-275), Saw Palmetto (256), Sheep Sorrel (131-132), Slippery Elm (257-258), Usnea (277-278)

Whole Body

- **Adaptogens**: American Ginseng (153-154), Cat's Claw (169-170) Chaga (268-270), Devil's Club (236-237), Reishi (273-275), Rhodiola Rosea (199-200)
- **Altitude Sickness**: Osha (191-193), Reishi (273-275), Wild Ginger (206-207)
- **Anti-Oxidant**: American Ginseng (153-154), Bilberry (221-223), Black Crowberry (225), Borage (51-52), Bottle Gourd (53), Cat's Claw (169-170), Cattails (279-280), Cinnamon (291), Chaga (268-270), Chaparral (231-232), Cocoplum (280-281), Common Lungwort (105-106), Cottonwood (233-234), Cranberry (235-236), Dandelion (68-70), Flax (66-67), Goldenrod (81-83), Hardy Kiwi (238-239), Hawthorn (239-241), Horsetail (181-182), Juniper (244), Leeks (96-97), Lemon Balm (98-99), Lion's Mane (281-284), Lungwort Lichen (272-273), Maidenhair Fern (187), Milk Thistle (110-111), Moringa (246-247), Oregano (116-117), Plantain (119-121), Purslane (125-126), Reishi (273-275), Rosemary (128-129), Salal (253-254), Skullcap (132-133), Sugar Maple (258-259), Thyme (140-141), Turkey Tail (275-276), Turmeric (295-296), Western Red Cedar (259-261), Wild Ginger (206-207), Wild Rose (264-265), Wild Violets (142-143)
- **Detoxification**: Activated Charcoal (287), American Ginseng (153-154), Bilberry (221-223), Calendula (55-56), Cat's Claw (169-170), Chickweed (61-62), Chives (63-64), Chokecherry (232-233), Cleavers (171-172), Common Lungwort (105-106), Dandelion (68-70), Diatomaceous Earth (292), Dock (71-72), Duckweed (281-282), Epsom Salts (292-293), Fennel (77-78), Goldenseal (179-180), Greater Burdock (83-85), Holy Basil (86-88), Leeks (96-97), Meadow Rue (109), Mugwort (190-191), Osha (191-193), Oxeye Daisy (117-118), Sheep

Sorrel (131-132), Solomon's Seal (200-202), St. John's Wort (133-135), Stinging Nettle (135-136), Wild Violets (142-143)

- **Diuretics**: Amaranthus Caudatus (152), Ash (216-217), Bayberry and Wax Myrtle (220-221), Bearberry (159-160), Birch (223-224), Black Walnut (226-227), Bleeding Heart (163-164), California Poppy (57-58), Cascara Sagrada (229-231), Chicory (62-63), Chives (63-64), Cleavers (171-172), Common Lungwort (105-106), Couch Grass (67-68), Dandelion (68-70), Fennel (77-78), Greater Burdock (83-85), Hardy Kiwi (238-239), Henbane (85-86), Horseradish (89-90), Horsetail (181-182), Jerusalem Artichoke (91-92), Juniper (244), Lady's Thumb (92), Lavender (94-96), Mormon Tea (111-112), Mullein (114-115), Oxeye Daisy (117-118), Pipsissewa (195-196), Plantain (119-121), Red Elderberry (251), Reishi (273-275), Salal (253-254), Sassafras (254-255), Saw Palmetto (256), Sheep Sorrel (131-132), Solomon's Seal (200-202), St. John's Wort (133-135), Sugar Maple (258-259), Unicorn Root (204-205), Water Plantain (284), Watercress (282-283), White Mustard (144-145), Wild Ginger (206-207), Wild Rose (264-265), Wild Teasel (146-148), Wild Strawberries (207-208), Wooly Lamb's Ear (149-150)
- **Edema**, Dropsy: Birch (223-224), Burning Bush (229), Horsetail (181-182), Juniper (244), Moringa (246-247), Pipsissewa (195-196), Sassafras (254-255), Stone Root (203), Watercress (282-283), Water Plantain (284)
- **Fatigue**: American Ginseng (153-154), Cat's Claw (169-170), Chaga (268-270), Devil's Club (236-237), Lion's Mane (281-284), Moringa (246-247), Mugwort (190-191), Prickly Pear Cactus (121-122), Reishi (273-275), Rhodiola Rosea (199-200), Spanish Moss (202) , St. John's Wort (133-135), Stinging Nettle (135-136), Turkey Tail (275-276)
- **Gout**: Bearberry (159-160), Couch Grass (67-68), Duckweed (281-282), Goldenrod (81-83), Henbane (85-86), Juniper (244), Lamb's Quarter (93-94), Leeks (96-97), Peppermint (118-119), Pipsissewa (195-196), Queen Anne's Lace (129-130), Slippery Elm (257-258), St. John's Wort (133-135), Stinging Nettle (135-136), Watercress (282-283), Wild Strawberries (207-208)
- **Inflammation/Anti-inflammatory**: Agrimony (44-45), Bilberry (221-223), Birch (223-224), Black Crowberry (225), Bleach (288), Bottle Gourd (53), Butterbur (166-167), Cabbage (54-55), Cascara Sagrada (229-231), Cat's Claw (169-170), Cinnamon (291), Chaga (268-270), Chicory (62-63), Chives (63-64), Cleavers (171-172), Coltsfoot (173-174), Comfrey (64-66), Common Lungwort (105-106), Dandelion (68-70), Drumstick Tree (220-221), Epsom Salts (292-293), Fireweed (178-179), Goldenrod (81-83), Hawthorn (239-241), Heartleaf Arnica (156-157), Holy Basil (86-88), Honey (294-295), Hops (88-89), Horsetail (181-182), Lemon Balm (98-99), Lion's Mane (270-271), Lovage (104-105), Lungwort Lichen (272-273), Mallow (106-107), Marshmallow (107-108), Mullein (114-115), Osha (191-193), Oxeye Daisy (117-118), Pipsissewa (195-196), Plantain (119-121), Prickly Pear Cactus (121-122), Queen Anne's Lace (129-130), Reishi (273-275), Rosemary (128-129), Sassafras (254-255), Self-heal (122-124), Sheep Sorrel (131-132), Stinging Nettle (135-136), Stone Root (203), Thorn Apple (138-140), Thyme (140-141), Turkey Tail (275-276), Turmeric (295-296), Usnea (277-278), Wild Ginger (206-207), Wild Rose (264-265), Wild Violets (142-143), Wild Yam (208-209), Wintergreen (209-210), Witch Hazel (266-267)
- **Smoking, Quitting**: Lobelia Inflata (184-185), Osha (191-193), Parrot's Beak (193-194), Pipsissewa (195-196), Skullcap (132-133), St. John's Wort (133-135), Valerian Root (141-142)
- **Physical Endurance, Increase**: Ashwagandha (47-48), Chaga (268-270), Juniper (244), Rhodiola Rosea (199-200)
- **Stimulates Metabolism**: Bleeding Heart (163-164), Oregano (116-117)
- **Weight Gain**: Cocoplum (280-281), Saw Palmetto (256)

Emergency Care

- **Bleeding, external**: Agrimony (44-45), Amaranthus Caudatus (152), Cattails (279-280), Cayenne Pepper (289-290), Cleavers (171-172), Duckweed (281-282), Goldenseal (179-180), Red Elderberry (251), Water Plantain (284), Western Red

Cedar (259-261), Witch Hazel (266-267), Yarrow (150-151)

- ❖ **Fevers**: Ash (216-217), Bee Balm (161), Bayberry and Wax Myrtle (220-221), Boneset (50-51), Cayenne Pepper (289-290), Chaparral (231-232), Cleavers (171-172), Cottonwood (233-234), Devil's Club (236-237), Dogwood (238), Feverfew (78-79), Garlic (80-81), Hawthorn (239-241), Horseradish (89-90), False Hellebore (174-175), Lamb's Quarter (93-94), Male Fern (188), Meadow Rue (109), Mormon Tea (111-112), Oregon Grape (247-248), Osha (191-193), Pipsissewa (195-196), Quaking Aspen (249), Red Alder (250-251), Red Elderberry (251), Red Root (198-199), Sweet Grass (137), Water Plantain (284), White Willow (263-264), Wild Rose (264-265), Wooly Lamb's Ear (149-150), Yarrow (150-151), Yellow Jessamine (211-212), Yerba Santa (213-214)
- ❖ **Internal Bleeding**: Cattails (279-280), Goldenseal (179-180), Lungwort Lichen (272-273), Male Fern (188), Self-heal (122-124), Wooly Lamb's Ear (149-150), Yarrow (150-151)
- ❖ **Snake Bites**: Activated Charcoal (287), Black-Eyed Susan (49), Black Walnut (226-227), Echinacea (72-73), Mullein (114-115), Plantain (119-121), Prickly Pear Cactus (121-122)
- ❖ **Spider Bites**: Activated Charcoal (287), Black Walnut (226-227), Echinacea (72-73), Plantain (119-121)

Other

- ❖ **Antibiotic/ Antibacterial properties:** Agrimony (44-45), Comfrey (64-66), Balsam Fir (217-219), Bilberry (221-223), Black Crowberry (225), Bloodroot (164-165), Bottle Gourd (53), Calendula (55-56), Cascara Sagrada (229-231), Cat's Claw (169-170), Cinnamon (291), Chaparral (231-232), Chicory (62-63), Chives (63-64), Cleavers (171-172), Common Lungwort (105-106), Cottonwood (233-234), Cranberry (235-236), Duckweed (281-282), Echinacea (72-73), Garlic (80-81), Goldenrod (81-83), Goldenseal (179-180), Greater Burdock (83-85), Heartleaf Arnica (156-157), Honey (294-295), Horseradish (89-90), Horsetail (181-182), Juniper (244), Lavender (94-96), Leeks (96-97), Lemon Balm (98-99), Lemon Thyme (100), Lungwort Lichen (272-273), Maidenhair Fern (187), Male Fern (188), Mallow (106-107), Meadowsweet (245-246), Mugwort (190-191), Oregano (116-117), Osha (191-193), Plantain (119-121), Peppermint (118-119), Pipsissewa (195-196), Reishi (273-275), Rosemary (128-129), Sage (130-131), Slippery Elm (257-258), Sugar Maple (258-259), Stone Root (203), Turkey Tail (275-276), Usnea (277-278), Wild Ginger (206-207), Wild Rose (264-265), Wild Strawberries (207-208), White Mustard (144-145), White Sage (263), White Pine (261-262), Wooly Lamb's Ear (149-150), Wormwood (210-211), Yarrow (150-151)
- ❖ **Lowering Blood Sugar:** Aloe Vera (45-46), Amaranthus Caudatus (152), American Ginseng (153-154), Bottle Gourd (53), Cabbage (54-55), Cayenne Pepper (289-290), Cinnamon (291), Chaga (268-270), Dandelion (68-70), Devil's Club (236-237), Garlic (80-81), Greater Burdock (83-85), Goldenseal (179-180), Horsetail (181-182), Horse Chestnut (242-243), Jerusalem Artichoke (91-92), Leeks (96-97), Lemon Balm (98-99), Lion's Mane (270-271), Moringa (246-247), Oregon Grape (247-248), Red Mulberry (252), Reishi (273-275), Sugar Maple (258-259), Turkey Tail (275-276)
- ❖ **Restless Legs Syndrome:** Reishi (273-275), Valerian Root (141-142), Skullcap (132-133)
- ❖ **Scabies, Crabs, Mites:** Meadow Rue (109), Quaking Aspen (249), Red Alder (250-251), Thyme (140-141)
- ❖ **Ticks:** Epsom Salts (292-293), Listerine (293)
- ❖ **Water Purification:** Bleach (288), Moringa (246-247), Potassium Permanganate (293-294)

How to Harvest the Healing Power from Plants

Introduction

When compared to the timeline of human history, modern medicine hasn't been around that long. Medicine has a much longer history than the modern pharmaceutical industry. Humankind has used medicines for thousands of years. But the medicines used before our modern knowledge of science were natural medicines, making use of the medicinal qualities of what nature provides for us.

The herbal medicines that have always existed still work today, just as they have throughout history. What was once our sole medicine still exists, even though the number of people who have knowledge of these natural remedies has dwindled. It is our hope that this book will help you relearn and pass on this lost knowledge.

Herbal medicine is often scoffed at by the pharmaceutical industry and yet it is the grandparent of much of that same modern medicine. Many of today's pharmaceuticals try to replicate what nature provides. Most of what we call "medicines" are artificial creations that have been slightly chemically altered from nature. This is necessary, as patent laws don't permit filing a patent on something that exists naturally. Thus, the large pharmaceutical labs have to come up with a suitable alternative and many of their products have serious side effects. This isn't to say that modern-day medicine and herbal medicine can't coexist. They can. But many new medicines can be easily replaced by herbs at a fraction of the cost and risk – to both our wallets and our bodies.

In a post-apocalyptic world, these herbal medicines may be the only thing available to us. If modern manufacturing and distribution methods become unavailable, we will have to rely on what can be grown locally. Many of those who have knowledge of herbal medicine are already growing and tending the necessary plants and have learned how to turn those plants into usable medicines.

One of the advantages of growing and using your own herbs, as opposed to buying herbal supplements at the local health food store, is that you know how fresh they are and how they've been grown. The sooner you can prepare and store your herbs for use, often the more potent they are. At the same time, you will know exactly what is in any herbal mixture that you create, giving you the peace of mind that there are no additives or fillers, and only the herbs you want and need.

How to Harvest Herbs

All herbal medicines start as living beings. They are not always what most people traditionally think of as herbs. Medicines come from trees, flowers, roots, mushrooms, lichens, and more. While those who are interested in herbal medicines tend to grow an herb garden, some are harvested from plants that grow in the wild. It is a useful skill to learn how to identify medicine in the wild.

When looking at pictures for plant identification, be sure to look at pictures that depict plants in the various stages of their life cycle. A good plant identification guide for your area is essential.

Many people know flower identification; but when the plants are not in flower, they can't identify them. Considering how short the flowering season is for most plants, that severely limits the amount of time for harvest.

Before even thinking about harvesting herbs, it is necessary to understand how the herb will be used; specifically, what part of the plant will be used for medicinal purposes. Never assume that the whole plant carries the same chemical compounds. Often, only the leaves or the flower will provide what you need; but in some cases, it will be the bark of a tree or a piece of root that you will need to harvest.

It is best to harvest herbs early in the day, after the dew has gone, but before the hot sun can dry out the essential oils. Whenever possible, avoid harvesting the whole plant, unless it is a plant that needs to be collected whole.

If you are harvesting leaves you will usually cut off small branches, making it easier to dry them. For flowers, wait until they develop fully and harvest them as soon as possible after they have fully opened. If you are harvesting only the seeds, you'll need to wait until the seeds mature and the seed pod dries on the stem before harvesting. We give harvesting instructions for almost every herb in this book.

If you are cutting part of a stem, such as harvesting stinging nettle, be sure to leave at least a few inches of leafy stem, with at least two sets of leaves on it, so that the plant doesn't die. Always cut right above the point where the leaves are. With many plants, like basil, you can cut the plant down to a third its original size without killing it. Always reseed, replant, and tend the wild when possible. Harvest ethically and with great care.

How to Dry Herbs

Traditionally, herbs are air-dried without the use of any additional heat source. Bundle them together by tying the stems with string or a rubber band and hang in a warm, dry place. It is usually easiest to hang them upside-down by the bundled stems to dry.

Drying racks may be used for individuals who are drying a lot of herbs or doing so regularly. But you can accomplish the same thing by hanging them from a coat hanger, a nail in the wall or on a curtain rod over the window. I often spread flowers or leaves on a cookie sheet or pizza pan and let them dry.

If you are collecting the seeds, tie a paper bag over the bundled stems and hang them. The bag will catch the seeds as the seed pods dry and they fall out.

Drying in this manner can take as long as three weeks (though is often accomplished much faster) depending on the plant and its moisture content.

If you are drying something that dries extremely slowly, like rosemary, it is easier to strip the leaves off of the stems and spread them on a drying rack, as the coating of the leaves will hold in the moisture. They need to be fully dry before storing.

It is possible to dry herbs with a dehydrator if you have one of the better ones that has temperature control. Ideally, it should have a fan to circulate the warm air,

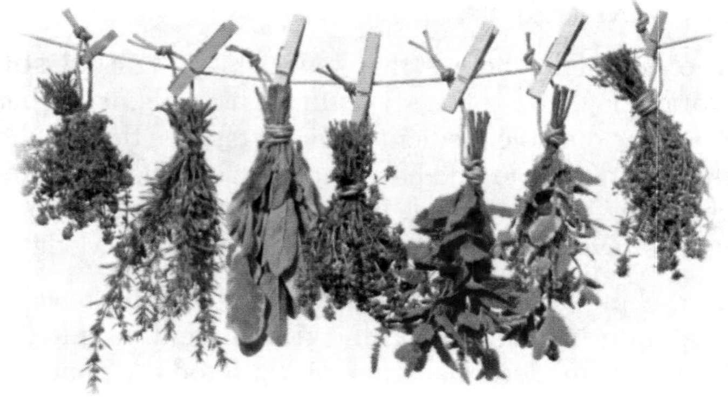

allowing the entire batch to dry evenly. To avoid singing or burning the herbs you are drying, you'll need to use the lowest possible temperature. I have used this method successfully many times. If using a dehydrator, it is very important to keep a close eye on your herbs so that you don't leave them to dry too long.

Once dried, remove the leaves from the stems. In the case of smaller leaves, you can strip them from the stem by lightly pinching the stem between your thumb and forefinger and running it down the stem, from top to bottom.

However, in the case of larger leaves with thicker stems, you will need to cut or pinch them off individually, cutting the stems as near the leaf as possible.

Store your dried herbs in sealed glass jars until you are ready to use them.

Encapsulating Powdered Herbs

If you go to the health food store to buy herbs, you'll often find them offered in powdered form, encapsulated. This is a convenient way to store and use herbs, especially if you are using them with people who are unaccustomed to taking herbal remedies.

There are two ways of encapsulating your herbs, but to start you need to turn the herbs into powder. This is most easily done by grinding them in a food processor or electric coffee mill. If you want to go for a more traditional method or are trying to encapsulate them during a time when there is no electrical power, use a mortar and pestle.

If you are going to make any sort of herbal mix, you'll need a scale to measure out your various herbs. Be sure to mix the powdered herbs well, so that your capsules all have the same herbal concentration.

Capsules come in three sizes; "0," "00" and "000." They can be filled by hand or with the aid of a simple filling machine.

The least expensive method is to fill them by hand. To start, put the powder in an oversized bowl. Open the capsules individually by hand, and scoop up the powder in both sides of the capsule, trying to get them reasonably full. Then push the sides of the capsule together. The powder will compress as the capsule slides closed.

This is a very boring and time-consuming operation, although effective. You might want some company or some assistance while doing this task.

Capsule Filling Machines

For a slightly more efficient operation, you can buy a simple capsule-filling machine. These are available in 50 or 100 capsule sizes and must be bought to match the size capsules you are using. The machine consists of several plates, which have holes to hold the capsule halves and a base.

Separate the capsules, putting the two parts into separate bowls. The thinner, longer part goes into the base plate on the machine. There is a funnel-like device used to fill this plate. Simply place the funnel over the base plate and pour a quantity of the capsule halves onto it. Shake the machine, until the capsule halves fall into the holes in the plate, ready to be filled. The same basic operation is done with the top plate.

The part of the capsules that is in the bottom plate is the part being filled. Pour a quantity of the powdered herbs onto this plate and move it around with the supplied scraper, allowing it to fill the capsules. Once filled, remove any extra powder by scraping it off.

To close the now-filled capsules, place the top plate over the bottom one. The machine will have aligning pins to ensure that the two halves of the capsules are aligned. Then push down on the plates, several times, seating the capsules. Remove your finished capsules and put them in a jar for storage.

Herbal Water Infusions: Cold and Hot Methods

Tea and coffee are both infusions; usually hot infusions. Cold versions of these drinks are often still infused hot, and then chilled in the refrigerator or with ice; however it is possible to make cold infused coffee and tea; the process is just slower. This cold-infusion process takes time.

The properties of the herbs are simply extracted from the leaves or beans into the water. This same process can be used with just about any herb.

The typical means of hot infusing herbs is to make a tea out of it. Herbal teas can be made from individual herbs, but it is more common to use a mixture of herbs that work well to treat the condition you are seeking to heal.

The advantage of hot infusion over cold is that it often extracts more of the essential ingredients from the plant tissue. The heat breaks down cell walls, creating a stronger infusion. On the other hand, a hot infusion may also extract ingredients that are not desirable, such as those that give the infusion a bitter flavor. In that case, a cold infusion may be better. Mucilaginous herbs tend to extract better cold, leaving the mucilage intact. Some common herbs we do cold infusions with are lemon balm, marshmallow, slippery elm, and comfrey.

Sun tea is probably the most common "cold" infusion made. Leave the herbs loose (and strain later) or put the crushed leaves in a cheesecloth or muslin bag (you can find these sold as reusable tea bags) and tie it to the top of your jar or cup. For tea, most people simply use 1 to 2 teaspoons of dried herb to 8 ounces (250ml) of water. Moisten dried herbs before putting them in the cold infusion – this is not necessary for fresh herbs. Leave the cold infusion for at least 48 hours to fully extract the beneficial compounds from the herbs.

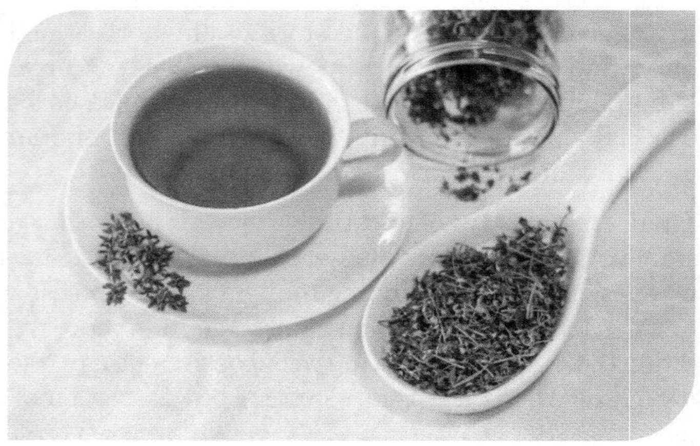

Teas

Herbal tea is a very common way that herbs are used for medicinal purposes. As mentioned above, an herbal tea is a "hot infusion," which works extremely well to extract the beneficial components from many herbs. Hot infusions can be made in a matter of minutes, unlike cold infusions, which take longer.

Teas can be made from either fresh or dried herbs, producing different results. Each particular herb will react differently whether it is dry or fresh, so you will want to know what is recommended for that herb or for that herbal mixture.

Decoctions

A decoction is a concentrated form of a hot infusion or tea. This can be an extremely useful method for herbs that don't give up their beneficial chemicals easily or for woody parts or roots. It is also a great way of creating a more concentrated form of an herbal supplement, and for use with children, animals, or anyone else who it is unlikely to drink enough of a hot infusion to do them any good.

To make a decoction, start with cold distilled or purified water. Cold water is important, to help ensure you extract the maximum amount of beneficial nutrients from the herbs. It is best to make your decoction in an earthenware, glass, or glazed ceramic cooking pot, so that you don't end up with the metal pots reacting to the astringent herbs, affecting the final flavor.

Use a ratio of 1 oz.(28g) of dried herbs per 16 ounces (500ml) of water. Decoctions are normally made in a quantity that can be used within a couple of days, as they don't keep well in the refrigerator for more than three days. If you do need to keep one for more than three days, keep it in a tightly sealed container or freeze them (ice cube trays work well). You may also add two tablespoons of alcohol (like vodka, rum, or brandy) per cup (8oz) for better preservation.

1. Crush, chop or grind the herbs, as appropriate, into small pieces and place them in the cold water in your cooking pot.
2. Allow the herbs to cold soak for a few hours.
3. Cover the pot and bring to a slow boil. Once the water is boiling, reduce the heat to a simmer.
4. Keep simmering until the volume of liquid has been reduced to ½ of what you started with (about 15-20 minutes).
5. Strain (cheesecloth works well). Once cooled, squeeze the herbs left behind, to ensure that you have removed all the liquid from them.
6. Pour the decoction into a jar with a lid for storage. Use within 48 hours or freeze.

Decoctions contain four times more medicine than a tea. Adults in good health can take up to 1 cup of a decoction, three times per day, depending on the herb. Children's dosages should be cut, based upon their weight.

Double Decoctions: Double Decoctions are the same as decoctions, with the exception that they are simmered until the final volume equals ¼ of the original volume of liquid, increasing your final medicinal concentration. Adults should only take 1 TB of a double decoction and children up to ½ tsp for most herbs.

Double decoctions are especially useful when decocting shredded bark and dried roots, where the useful compounds come out of the herbs slowly. When working with these herbs, allow them to soak for 12 hours in cold water before bringing it to a boil and simmering.

Oil Infusions

The hot and cold infusion methods outlined below are used to infuse herbs into oil. For cold extractions in oil, cold actually means at room temperature. This method takes time. It takes 6 to 8 weeks to infuse herbs into a carrier oil using only time. The "hot" method is actually a "warm" method of extracting herbs into a carrier oil. Some herbs need the heat to extract and this method also shortens the amount of time needed if you need the remedy sooner. Be careful not to boil or overheat the oil, as this alters the chemical compounds of the herbal properties you are extracting.

Carrier Oils and "Cold" & "Hot" Infusions:

To cold-infuse oil use only dried herbs to start (with a few exceptions), as moisture can make your oil turn rancid or mold. Many carrier oils will work. I prefer organic olive oil as it is temperature stable, well-priced, and works well for salve-making. It is important to purchase organic oils from somewhere with strict labeling laws (like California). Other good carrier oils are sweet almond oil, coconut oil (although it changes consistency with temperature), jojoba oil, baobab oil, tamanu oil, castor oil, grapeseed oil, argan oil, avocado oil, apricot kernel oil, emu oil, and many more. Rendered fat or tallow, like bear fat, can also be used.

"Cold" Oil Infusion:

1. Tear or crush the dried herbs then lightly pack into a clean, sterilized glass jar. Fill a glass jar 1/3rd full with dried herb (for some herbs, like cottonwood buds, I fill it well over half-full).
2. Pour your high-quality organic olive oil (or other natural plant oil) over the herbs. Fill to within ½ inch (1.25 cm) of the top with your carrier oil. Mix well, removing all air bubbles. Cap and label with herb and date.
3. Store your jar for 6 to 8 weeks. Make sure you don't go longer than 8 to 10 weeks or your oil may go rancid (cottonwood buds are an exception to this). I often kickstart certain herbs with a little heat by placing my glass jars in a water bath on low (see warm infusions below) for a day or two and then storing for 6 to 8 weeks.
4. After 6 to 8 weeks strain out the herbs using cheesecloth or a tincture press. Squeeze the cheesecloth to get all of the herbal oil out. Pour into a clean, sterile bottle or jar. This oil can be used directly for medicine or for making salves. Lasts about 1 to 2 years.

"Hot" Oil Infusion: To infuse oils using heat use a crock pot that has a "warm" or very low setting or use a water bath on low on the stovetop. This works well for infusing several oils at once.

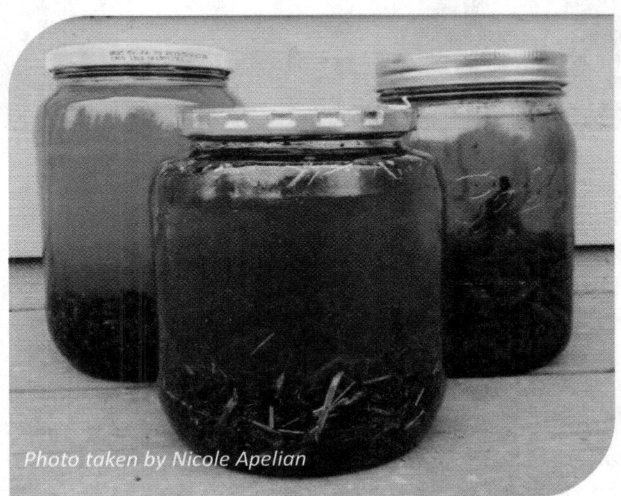

Photo taken by Nicole Apelian

1. Tear or crush the dried herbs then lightly pack into a clean, sterilized glass jar. Fill a glass jar 1/3rd full

with dried herb (for some herbs, like cottonwood buds or *Usnea*, I fill it over half-full).

2. Pour your high-quality organic olive oil (or other natural plant oil) over the herbs. Fill to within ½ inch (1.25 cm) of the top with your carrier oil. Mix well, removing all air bubbles. Cap and label with herb and date.
3. Place your glass jars in the crock pot and cook on low for 4 to 7 days, depending on the herb, making sure the water in your water bath/crock pot stays full. If you are using fresh herbs leave the caps off the jars letting the moisture evaporate out and make sure no water gets in from your water bath.
5. Once cooled, strain herbs using cheesecloth or a tincture press. Pour into a clean, sterile bottle or jar. This oil can be used directly for medicine or for making salves. Lasts about 1 to 2 years.

Salve-making

Salves are a useful way of applying herbs to the skin. They are useful for treating burns, rashes, skin irritations, bites, wounds, eczema, sore muscles, arthritis, nerve pain, and more. Turning herbal oil infusions into salves provides a good way to apply herbs and to take them with you when not at home.

In order to make a salve, you have to already have turned the herbs into an infused oil (see above). You may also use the "fast method" below:

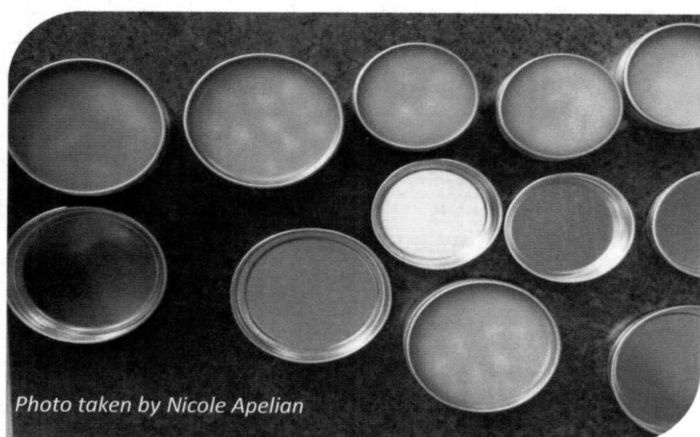

Photo taken by Nicole Apelian

The quickest method for making herbal salves combines the infusion and salve-mixing steps into one. It uses a lot of dried herb. Combine your herbs and enough oil to cover the herbs in the top of a double-boiler being sure there is water in the bottom half of your double boiler. Simmer for a few hours (don't overheat – about 100 degrees). Stir, cool slightly, and strain through cheesecloth. Pour back into your double-boiler and add melted beeswax (about 1/4 cup to 1/5 cup per cup of oil) to the oil. Then add 15 to 20 drops or more of each of your essential oils for every 8 oz of oil. Vitamin E can be added to help rancidity. Mix well, pour into containers, and let set.

To make a simple salve out of your infused oil and beeswax:

1. Measure and pour your infused oil(s) into the top part of a double boiler.
2. Add beeswax and melt. I usually use a 1 part beeswax to 4 parts infused oil mixture and common usage is 1/4 cup to 1/5 cup per cup of oil. For 8 oz (250ml) of oil I use 2 oz (48g) of beeswax.
3. Mix together thoroughly until the beeswax has melted.
4. Add 15 to 20 drops or more of each of your essential oils for every 8 oz (250ml) of infused oil. Vitamin E can be added to help rancidity (1/2 tsp for 16 oz (250ml) oil). Add essential oils just before pouring.
5. Before you pour into your containers (jars/tins) to set you may add just a few drops to your container to test the consistency. If it's too hard add more oil and if it's too soft add more beeswax. Then complete pouring, label, and date.

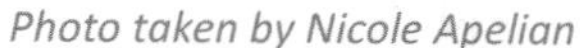

Photo taken by Nicole Apelian

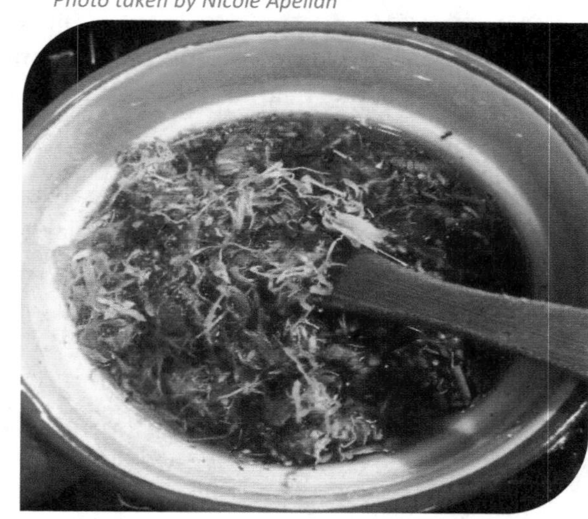

Tinctures/Extracts

Tinctures are medicinal extracts of any herb or herbal concoction in an alcohol, vinegar, or glycerin base. Because alcohol is a universal solvent, it is usually able to extract the essential oils from herbs, as well as extract most of the other chemical compounds that water is able to extract (note that some herbs need a double-extraction in water and alcohol to access all of the medicinal compounds).

But alcoholic tinctures have another, much more important attribute. They absorb into the body faster than any other means of using herbal medicines. This is due to the alcohol base, which starts absorbing through the stomach wall and even through the mouth upon taking the tincture. Rather than being digested, like other things that are eaten and drunk, the herbs are absorbed right into the bloodstream.

Another benefit of tinctures is that they last virtually forever, as long as they are stored in a well-sealed container. The alcohol is uniformly fatal to any microorganisms might that come into contact with it, so there is no possibility of the tincture decomposing. The biggest risk is evaporation.

To make a tincture you will need some sort of consumable alcohol that is at least 80 proof (40% alcohol). Vodka is the preferred alcohol to use, because it has no flavor, but rum, gin, brandy, and whiskey will work as well. You can also use apple cider vinegar or food grade vegetable glycerin, although these often don't work as well for many herbs and they don't last as long.

1. Fill a glass jar 1/3 to 1/2 full of the dried herbs you are using for your tincture, but don't pack it down (amount of the herb used depends on the surface area and extractability of the herb). You can also use fresh herbs – use 2x the amount of dried herbs.
2. Fill the jar with the alcohol, leaving ½ inch (1.25 cm) of headspace. Stir well.
3. Close the lid on the jar, label and date, and store in a cool, dry place. Tinctures can take anywhere from 4 weeks up to 6 months to fully extract, depending on the herbs you are using. 2 months works well for most herbs. Shake the jar once a day if possible.
4. Once your tincture is complete, usually around 8 weeks, strain out the herbs and rebottle the finished product. The alcohol renders it very shelf-stable and tinctures can last up to 7 years. Many people put tinctures in dropper bottles for ease of use, but any small glass bottle will work. ½ to 1 teaspoon is a normal dose for adults. For children dosage is about 1/4 to 1/3 of the adult dose, depending on weight.

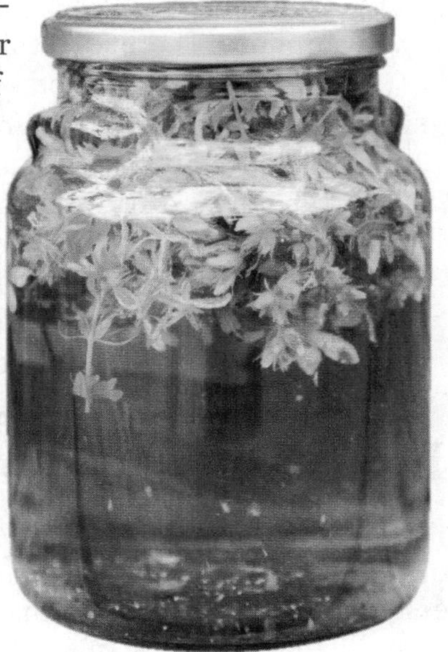

Double Extractions

A double extraction is a combination of a tincture and a decoction, often used for mushrooms and lichens. In recent years, the medicinal value of various types of mushrooms has been researched heavily. If only a water-based decoction is used with Reishi Mushroom, for example, it extracts the beneficial polysaccharides (including the beta-glucans) and the glycoproteins but not the triterpenes (like ganoderic acid in Reishi), as they are not soluble in water. Both water and alcohol are needed to extract all of the medicinal compounds.

For this tincture, alcohol and water are required. There are two methods. Both are below and different herbalists prefer different methods. Final alcohol percentage should be 25% to 30% or higher. The recipes below give you that percentage but you may also start with a higher proof alcohol. If you see cloudiness in your final product that is OK - it is just the polysaccharides coming out of solution. Simply shake before use.

Method #1: Starting with the alcohol extraction

Feel free to scale down this recipe. You'll need: 8 ounces (224g) or more of dried mushroom or lichen, 24 ounces (750ml) of 80 to 100 proof alcohol (40 to 50 % alcohol), 16 ounces (500ml) distilled water.

1. Fill a quart-sized (1 liter) canning jar half-full with diced dried mushrooms, then fill it to about ½ inch (1.25 cm) of the top with alcohol. Stir and cap it, shaking it every day for 2 months. Then strain out the alcohol and set it aside.
2. Make the decoction. Put 16 ounces (500ml) of water into a ceramic or glass pot with a lid and put the mushrooms into it. Cover and simmer the mixture until half of the water has boiled off. This will take a few hours. If the water level drops too quickly, add more so that you can continue simmering your mushrooms. The end result should be 8 ounces (250ml) of your decoction.
3. Allow the water to cool, and then strain out the mushrooms. Mix the water and alcohol (you should have about 24 oz (710ml) of alcohol tincture) together to create the finished double-extraction. It has a high enough alcohol content (30%) that it should be shelf-stable for many years, as long as it is stored in a sealed container.

Method #2 Starting with the water extraction

I like to use a small crockpot for this recipe. You may also place the herbs and water into a jar, which is then covered and placed into a crockpot of water on low or a pot of water on low on the stove. Feel free to scale down this recipe. You'll need: 8 ounces (230g) or more of dried mushroom or lichen, 24 ounces(710ml) of 80 to 100 proof alcohol, 16 ounces (500ml) distilled water.

1. Cut up the herbs into very small pieces. Place the distilled water and the dried herbs into the crockpot and stir well. Cover and cook on the lowest possible setting for 3 days. It will cook down to about 8 oz (250ml) of medicinal decoction (water).
2. Allow the herb and water mixture to cool and pour it into a large glass jar. Add the alcohol while the mixture is still quite warm, but not hot. Make sure the jar is large enough that you are adding 24 ounces (710ml) of alcohol or split everything evenly between 2 jars.
3. Cap the jar tightly, label and date the jar and allow it to macerate for 6 to 8 weeks, shaking the jar daily.
4. Strain out the herb (cheesecloth works well for this) or carefully decant the tincture off. Store it in tightly capped glass jar. Label and date.

Distillation

Distillation is a process used for extracting essential oils from herbs or other plants. Not all plants provide essential oils; but for those that do, this is one of the surer methods of extracting the essential oil.

Distillation is something that should only be undertaken by someone who wants to make a lot of essential oils, due to the equipment investment and the amount of plant matter you need. The amount of essential oil that is distilled out of plants is very small and it takes a pretty good size still to get enough oil to make the effort worthwhile. You may want to simply purchase organic essential oils from a reputable source to have on hand.

There are three basic types of distillation, requiring minor differences in the still:

- **Water distillation** – The herbs are immersed in water and the water is boiled. This works best for herbs that don't break down easily.
- **Water and steam distillation** – The only difference in the equipment for this and water distillation is the insertion of a rack inside the still, which holds the herbs up out of the water and only allows the steam to have contact with it. This method produces essential oils much more quickly than water distillation.
- **Direct Steam Distillation** – A different sort of still is needed for this method, so that the steam can be created in a separate chamber. The steam is then injected into the retort/still that is holding the herbs, below a rack holding the herbs. This allows a lower temperature to be used, reducing the potential for heat damage to the essential oil. This is the most common method used commercially, especially for essential oils like rosemary and lavender.

Much expertise is needed for distillation as the amount of plant material, distillation times, and temperatures are specific to the still and the herb from which you are trying to extract the essential oil.

Medicinal Syrups

Herbal syrups are a great way of getting children to take herbal medicines and supplements. Made with raw honey, they store extremely well, taste good, and can also soothe a sore throat. Making a medicinal honey syrup for treating colds, sore throats, or the flu will have the added benefit that the raw honey brings.

Before starting, decide how sweet you want your syrup. Some people like a sweeter syrup, using a 1:1 ratio of honey to decoction, while others use a 1:2 ratio, using less honey. The 1:1 ratio will store longer, as honey doesn't spoil easily. You can add glycerin in place of some of the honey to extend shelf-life.

To make any medicinal syrup, start out by making a decoction. You want to end up with a known amount of decoction, so that you'll know how much honey to add. This is easy, as you will need to strain out the herbs before adding the honey. When you do this, measure using a Pyrex glass measuring cup.

Typically, these syrups will last about six months in the refrigerator if you use a 1:2 ratio. You can also extend the life by adding a tincture to the mixture, as the alcohol in the tincture will act as a preservative, or by adding glycerin.

Poultices

Poultices may be one of the oldest ways in which herbal medicines are used. They provide an excellent way of applying healing herbs directly to the afflicted area. Usually used for first-aid field situations, such as dealing with burns, bee stings, cuts, and infections, they are also useful for deeper problems, like joint problems and bruises. They can even be applied to the chest to aid with congestion.

Normally, poultices are made of fresh herbs, picked on the spot. This means that they are at their most potent, able to provide the maximum possible benefit. They are also able to help draw out splinters, bee stingers, and other infection-causing foreign matter that has embedded itself into the skin.

One of the great things about poultices is that they are made on the spot to deal with a specific need. There is little preparation and they are not stored. Rather, they are often made of whatever herbs are readily available at the time. Of course, that requires the ability to recognize those herbs growing in the wild so that they can be harvested and put to use immediately.

How to Make a Poultice: To make a poultice, select the necessary fresh herbs and tear or cut them finely. If you don't have the ability to cut them, crushing them between the fingers will work too. Doctors carried a mortar and pestle in ancient times for this purpose. The idea is to have the leaves broken, so that the sap of the plant can come out, contacting the skin. Chewing also works but make sure the herbs are safe to chew.

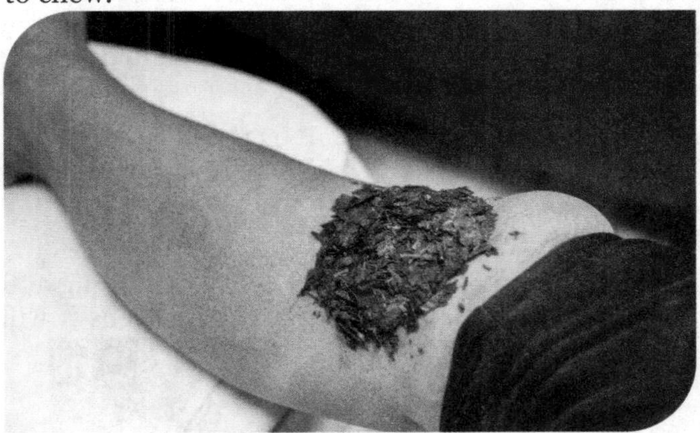

A generous quantity of the poultice is applied to the afflicted area of the skin and bound in place with a bandage. Gauze is normally used for this, but an elastic bandage or a large leaf are other options. The poultice must be kept damp to work, so it is usually changed out a couple of times per day.

Poultices can be made from dried herbs as well. In that case, the crushed or chopped herbs are soaked in warm water, softening them so that they won't irritate the skin and to draw out their medicine.

A little fine-tuning can be applied by using either hot or cold water with it. A hot poultice (not hot enough to burn) helps to increase the circulation in the area where it is applied. This can help get the medicinal properties of the herbs to the cells needing it more quickly. Using cold water, on the other hand, reduces circulation, while also reducing swelling.

How to Make a Field Poultice

Poultices have been used as field bandages and dressings for countless generations. In wartime, poultices helped manage many serious traumatic wounds and prevented as well as treated infection.

I have used poultices on both others and myself many times in the field. My most common go-to poultice herbs are Plantain, Yarrow, Mullein, and *Usnea*. I always carry dried Yarrow and Plantain with me in the winter when these plants are not readily available. These herbs are all in this book, so rest assured you'll have no problem identifying them. You can use these as single-herb poultices or mix them together.

One of my favorites is a plant growing in many back yards and probably yours as well: Plantain (*Plantago* spp.).

Plantain has a powerful antibacterial effect. It also contains allantoin, which is a phytochemical (a chemical found in plants) that speeds up wound healing and stimulates the growth of new skin cells. Plantain stops bleeding and helps relieve pain and itching. We use it for immediate relief for bites and stings.

Another common poultice herb is the plant known as "The Cowboy's Toilet Paper": Mullein. Mullein works in two different ways to enhance the effects of the plantain already in the poultice.

Mullein is an analgesic and thus lessens the pain, and it works as an astringent as well. That means it will contract your skin and, in doing so, will help close the wound. This plant has the added benefit of being used as, well, toilet paper if you ever run out. It's very soft.

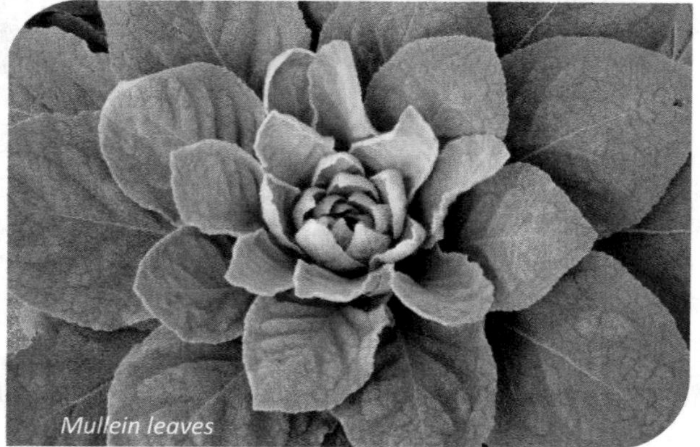

Mullein leaves

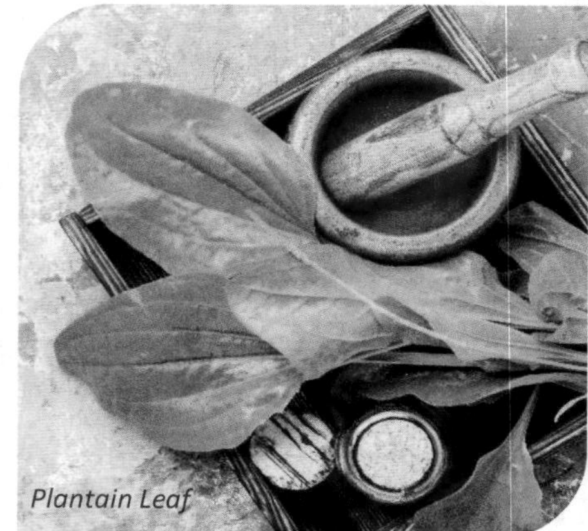

Plantain Leaf

Another plant you can use alone or mix into your field poultice is Yarrow. Yarrow is a very strong anti-bacterial and is also a blood coagulant and thus helps stop bleeding.

Usnea Lichen is my other fantastic go-to for applying to a wound. It is very absorbent and has anti-microbial, anti-bacterial, anti-viral and anti-fungal properties. It is ready to go as is!

A strong herbal field poultice:

1. Gather plantain, mullein, and yarrow in equal quantities.
2. Grind the leaves together until you get a paste-like mixture. Add clean water if needed.
3. Apply it to your wound or cut.
4. Leave it on for one to two hours; then reapply as needed.
5. Keep the paste in place by using a non-toxic plant that has big leaves and high flexibility or normal bandages if you have some around. Burdock leaves are perfect for this if you don't have normal bandages.

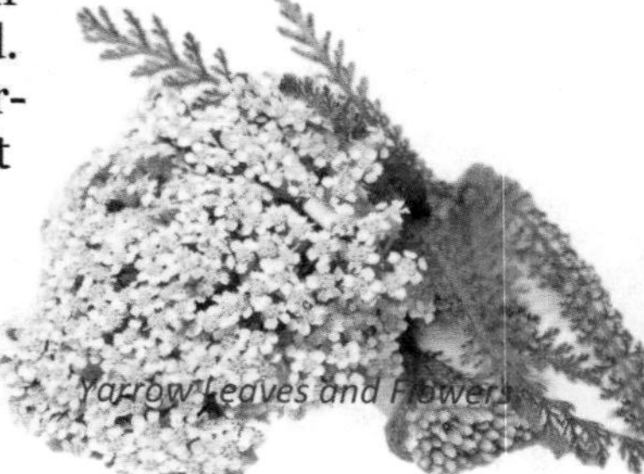

Yarrow Leaves and Flowers

How I Manage Multiple Sclerosis (Nicole Apelian)

I do a lot to manage Multiple Sclerosis. This page is also available (with products links for your convenience) at www.nicoleapelian.com. I believe that a lot of this information can be extrapolated for other autoimmune conditions as well.

The first thing I did was get an IGG food sensitivity test to see how I needed to alter my diet for optimum health. I don't eat gluten. I also stick to a low sugar diet with few processed foods. I alternate an anti-inflammatory diet with a ketogenic diet and practice intermittent fasting. This works well for me. For some, a modified paleo diet is ideal. I find that adding freshly ground flax seeds into my diet is helpful. I have progressive Multiple Sclerosis (though it is not currently progressing!). Diet is really important in managing MS and health in general.

Here are some of the things I incorporate into my MS management in addition to diet:

I give gratitude daily and I try to stay in the present moment the best I can. (This is very important! The mind-body connection is huge.)

I spend time in nature daily. Nature connection is a big piece of total health for me.

I spend time away from media and carry a personal anti-EMF device and have another one for my home.

I take these specific vitamins and herbal remedies:

- High-dose Biotin & Alpha-Lipoic Acid. Personally, I take 100mg Biotin three times every day (300mg a day total) for progressive MS.
- 4000 units Vitamin D drops
- Omega 3s (and incorporate these into my diet)
- Multi--Vitamin + Ca/Mg blend
- Tru Niagen (nicotinamide riboside)
- Probiotics
- Vitamin B12 if my levels get low

For preventing general illness (which causes the dreaded immune response that then causes MS to flare up) I rely on my healing trinity of Elderberry Tincture, Usnea Spray, and First Aid Salve. You can make all of them using the information in this book.

The 3 tinctures that I take daily for MS are:

- Lion's Mane Mushroom Tincture. Lion's Mane is known to boost mental functioning and stimulate Nerve Growth Factor (NGF). Studies show great potential for myelination and regeneration of nerves.

- Reishi Mushroom Tincture. I make this tincture as a double-extraction. I take this daily as Reishi mushrooms are adaptogens, which help us deal with the negative effects of stress, address issues such as increased inflammation, depleted energy levels, damaged blood vessels, and various types of hormonal imbalances. Reishi has been shown to have neuroprotective effects and, because many autoimmune illnesses are inflammatory in nature, I also take it for its anti-inflammatory properties.

- Turkey Tail Mushroom Dual-extracted Tincture. I always make all of my products with locally sourced and/or organic ingredients. It works well for leaky gut, as turkey tail has prebiotics that helps balance the digestive system and helps with *Candida* overgrowth. It is also been shown to be a great cancer preventative, an anti-inflammatory, and more.

I keep leaky gut at bay. Plantain tincture works well for me for this as does Turkey Tail and probiotics. I do make a Leaky Gut Tincture, which can be found in my apothecary, and drink organic bone broth for my gut.

I keep internal inflammation down with my Reishi Mushroom Tincture and Turmeric.

Wishing you the best on your journey to health.

For more information and links to everything I discuss above please see www.nicoleapelian.com

Backyard Plants

Agrimony, *Agrimonia eupatoria*

Agrimony, also called sticklewort, cocklebur, or church steeples, is native to Europe and is now found across North America. It is a pretty plant with spikes of tiny yellow flowers. It is in the Rosaceae (Rose) Family.

Identification: This dark green perennial has a rough stem. It is covered with soft hairs that help it spread its seeds. It grows to a height of 2 feet (0.6meters).

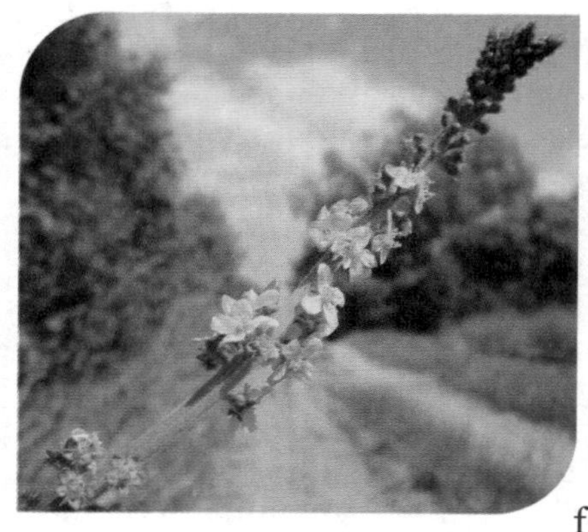

The leaves are serrated and pinnate. They are large (7 inches) (17.5 cm) at the base and get smaller at the top of the stem. Its roots are deep woody rhizomes.

The short-stemmed flowers have a sweet, apricot-like scent. They bloom from June to September on long terminal spikes. Each flower is a cup with rows of hook-shaped bristles on the upper edge. Flowers have five sepals and five yellow, rounded petals, each with 5 to 20 stamens.

The fruit has hooked bristles called cockleburs that attach to animals, thus spreading the seeds.

Edible Use: The leaves are used for tea, and the fresh flowers are often added to home-brewed beer or wine to enhance flavor.

Medicinal Use: Both the leaves and seeds are used in medicinal preparations. It is astringent, anti-inflammatory, and antibacterial.

To Induce Sleep: While lying in bed, place a few of this plant's leaves under your head to induce sleep.

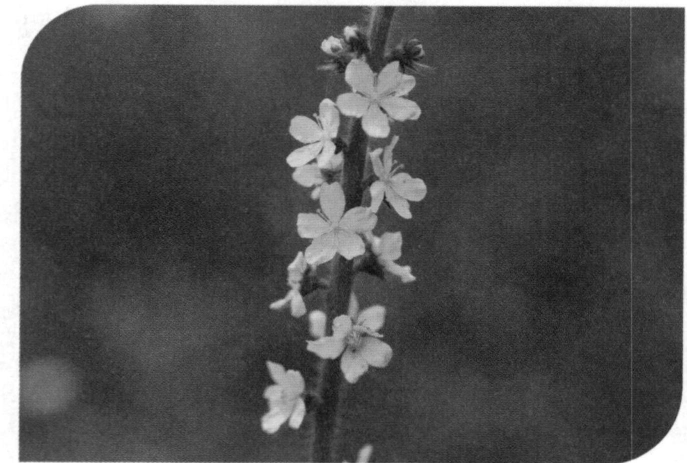

Anti-inflammatory, Wound and Skin Care: Agrimony is effective for wound care. It stops excessive bleeding by promoting the formation of clots. It contains tannins and is an astringent. It also has antibacterial and anti-inflammatory properties. Agrimony tea can be used as a wash for wounds and all types of skin diseases or the fresh leaves can be pounded and applied directly to a wound as a poultice.

Digestive Problems and Diarrhea: Agrimony Tea is used for digestive problems. The tea acts as a tonic to the digestive system and heals underlying problems.

Migraines: An herbal poultice made from fresh agrimony leaves and applied to the head is a good topical treatment for migraines. Use it at night as it may also induce deep sleep.

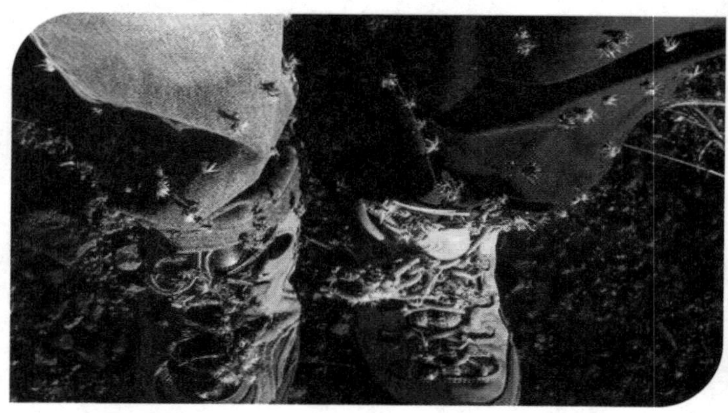

Conjunctivitis and Eye Infections: For application as an eye wash, mix equal parts of Agrimony Tea with boiled and cooled water.

Harvesting: Harvest agrimony in the late spring to early summer when the herb is in full bloom. Pick the leaves, flowers, and stems. Use the herbs fresh or dry them for later use.

Warning: Some people develop an allergic rash with sun exposure while using agrimony. Do not use if taking anti-coagulant therapy or taking blood-pressure medications. Avoid using agrimony if pregnant or nursing.

Recipes: Agrimony Tea. 1 to 2 teaspoons of powdered agrimony leaves or 3 teaspoons of crushed fresh leaves, 1 cup boiling water, raw honey, to taste, if desired. Steep the agrimony leaves in boiling water for 5 to 10 minutes. Cool and strain. Take one cup, three times daily.

Aloe Vera

Aloe Vera is edible and is incredibly effective for many afflictions. It's not native to North America, but it's been naturalized in many places. I find it readily in the southwest where the weather is warm and it is easy to grow in pots around the house. It is in the *Asphodelaceae* (Aloe) Family.

Identification: Aloe Vera plants have succulent leaves that grow to 2 to 3 feet (0.6 meters to 0.9 meters) tall. The plant is stemless or has very short stems. Aloe Vera leaves are thick, fleshy, and filled with gelatinous sap. The leaves grow in clumps, and are green to grey-green and may have white flecks on the leaf surfaces. The leaf margins are serrated with small white teeth. Flowers appear in the summer on a tall spike growing from the center of the plant. Flowers range in color from white and yellow to orange and red.

Edible Use: Eat aloe vera leaves raw or cooked. The outer green skin can also be eaten, but is bitter and tough. Removing the skin with a sharp knife leaves the meat and gel inside the plant; both are edible.

Aloe is good poached or otherwise gently cooked. Fully cooked, it loses its slimy texture. Some people enjoy raw aloe as juice or by putting a chunk in their water.

Medicinal Use: Aloe Vera gel, the gelatinous substance inside the leaf, is used as a relief for sunburn, wounds, and other minor skin irritations. It also has internal uses.

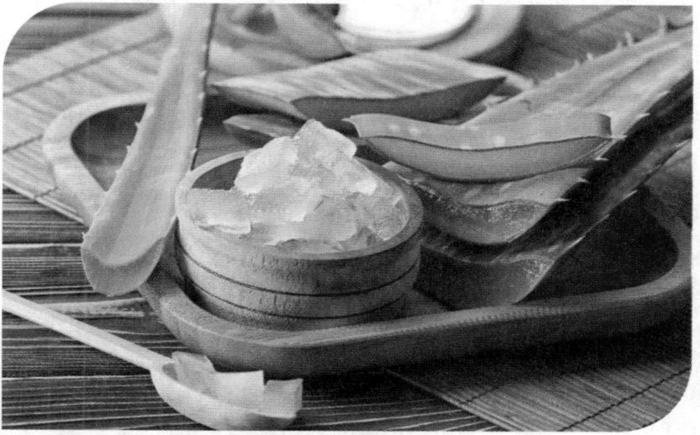

How to Use Aloe Vera: For external use, split the leaf long ways with a knife and scrape the gel from the leaf's interior. I most often use it as a soothing salve directly on the skin. For internal use, try 1 to 3 ounces (28-85g) of the gel added to juice, since the gel can be unpleasant and bitter when taken alone.

Heartburn Relief and Irritable Bowel Syndrome: Consuming 1 to 3 ounces (28g to 85g) of aloe vera gel with each meal reduces the severity of acid reflux and the associated heartburn. It also helps the cramping, abdominal pain, flatulence, and bloating caused by irritable bowel syndrome. However, there are some safety concerns and it may cause irritation, so use internally with care for these conditions.

Bleeding or Swollen Gums: Aloe Vera extract makes a safe and effective mouthwash that reduces swelling, soothes, and provides relief from bleeding or swollen gums. Try adding the gel to the final rinse water and swishing it around, holding it in the mouth for a minute, then spitting it out.

Lowering Blood Sugar in Diabetics: If you suffer from type 2 diabetes, you can regulate your blood sugar levels by simply ingesting two tablespoons of Aloe Vera juice or pulp extract daily.

Laxative: Aloe Vera gel relieves constipation but should be used sparingly.

Skin Care, Sunburn, Eczema: Aloe gel is soothing on the skin and an excellent remedy for sunburn, skin abrasions, eczema, and other mild skin irritations. It also keeps skin clear and hydrated. Excellent as a moisturizer and pain reliever.

Warning: Long term internal use of Aloe Vera is not recommended due to the latex found in Aloe Vera. Do not use internally while pregnant. Do not use if you have hemorrhoids or kidney issues.

Anise Hyssop, *Agastache foeniculum*

Anise Hyssop is also known as blue giant hyssop, lavender giant hyssop, elk mint, and licorice mint. It belongs to the Lamiaceae (Mint) Family. It is native to northern and central North America.

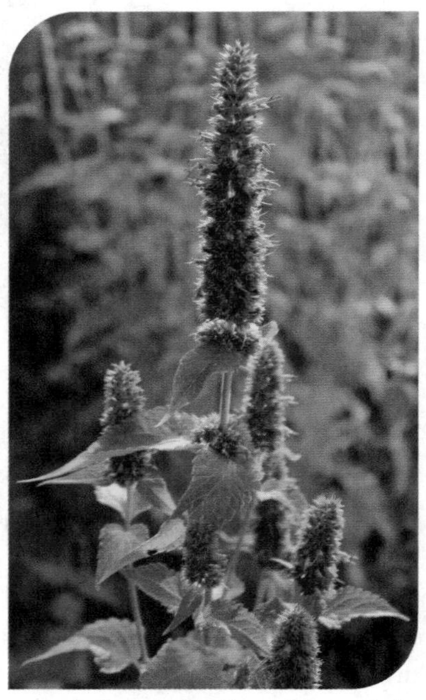

Identification: Anise hyssop grows from 2 to 5 feet (0.6 to 1.5m) tall, with bright green leaves that are notched at the edge and covered with fine white hairs on the underside. New growth has a purple tint. The plant has an aroma suggestive of mint and anise. The herb is partially woody with branched and usually hairless stems. The fibrous roots are also branching. Clusters of small lilac-blue flowers appear on elongated flower spikes from July through September.

Edible Use: Anise hyssop can be used as a sweetener and to make tea. It can be used as a flavoring or seasoning. The leaves and flowers can be eaten fresh, cooked, or dried.

Medicinal Use. Heart Healthy, Angina Pain: An infusion of anise hyssop is a tonic for the heart and a quick remedy for angina pain.

Sores, Wounds, and Burns: For skin infections, wounds, and burned skin, use a poultice of anise hyssop leaves. Soak dried leaves or bruise fresh leaves and flowers and apply them directly on the affected area. Cover with a clean cloth. Anise hyssop leaves have anti-bacterial and anti-viral properties.

Facilitates Digestion: Drinking Anise Hyssop Tea with meals eases digestion and prevents excessive gas and bloating.

Diarrhea: Anise hyssop tea is helpful in relieving diarrhea. The tea works best if continued throughout the day even after the diarrhea has been successfully eliminated. Continuing to sip occasionally prevents the return of diarrhea.

Sore Muscles and Anxiety: Try gathering 3 to 4 tablespoons of anise hyssop leaves in a square of cheesecloth and hang it from the faucet while drawing a bath. The scent released as the water flows calms the spirit. When the bath is ready, drop the herbs into the bathwater and soak your sore muscles in the bath.

Colds, Flu, Bronchial Congestion: Anise hyssop tea helps expel mucus from the lungs, making it a good choice for treating colds, flu, and congestion.

Herpes: Try Anise Hyssop Essential Oil externally as an antiviral treatment for Herpes Simplex I and II and drink the tea to treat the virus internally.

Poison Ivy: Wash the skin in Anise Hyssop Infusion to help relieve the itchiness of poison ivy.

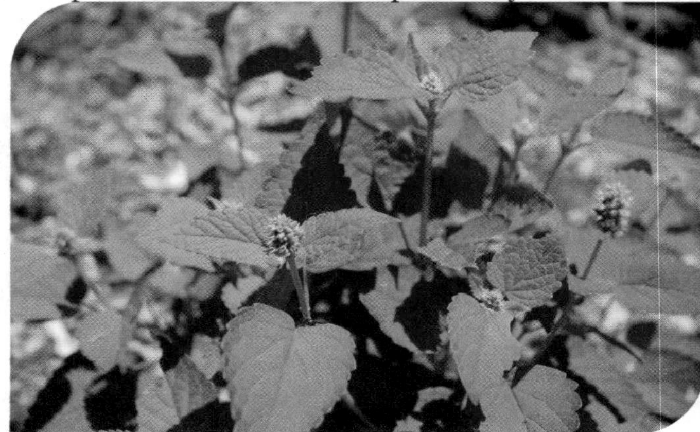

Saiberiac, Attribution 2.0 Generic (CC BY 2.0)

Athlete's Foot, Fungal Skin Infections, Yeast Overgrowth: Soak the foot or infected area in a bath with a strong infusion of Anise Hyssop. Soak daily until the infection is cured.

Recipes: Anise Hyssop Tea or Infusion. You'll need one cup of boiling water and raw honey to your liking. Add one teaspoon of dried leaves and flowers or one tablespoon of fresh leaves and flowers.

Add them to the boiling water and cover tightly. Allow the leaves to steep for 15 minutes.

Strain the tea through a fine sieve. Add raw honey to sweeten, if desired.

Ashwagandha, *Withania somnifera*

Ashwagandha, *Withania somnifera*, is a member of the nightshade family. It is sometimes called Winter Cherry or Indian Ginseng, due to its importance in Ayurvedic medicine. Ashwagandha is considered a rejuvenating adaptogenic herb, useful for treating many debilitating conditions.

Identification: Ashwagandha is native to India but can be grown in herb gardens across the United States. It is a perennial in warm climates with no frost. Ashwagandha likes sandy or rocky soil, full or partial sunlight, and moderately dry conditions.

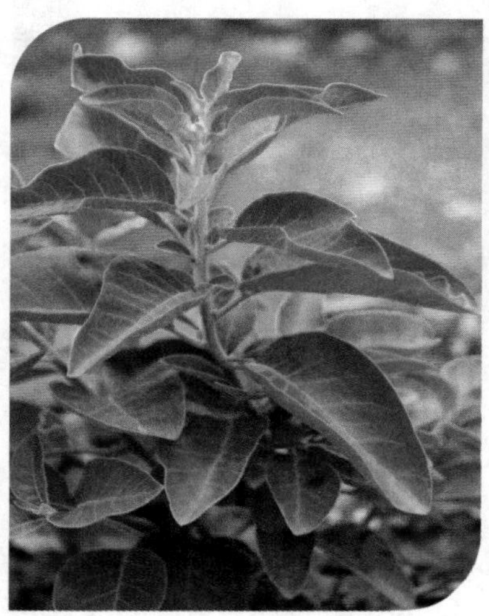
Photo By Hari Prasad Nadig, CC BY 2.0

The bush grows to a height of 2 to 3 or more feet (0.6m-0.9m), with dull green leaves. Light green, bell-shaped flowers appear in midsummer and orange to red berries in the fall. Branches grow radially from a center stem.

Edible Use: The plant is not generally eaten, but its seeds are used in the production of vegetarian cheeses. The leaves are used to make Ashwagandha Tea.

Other Uses: The fruits are rich in saponins are can be used as a substitute for soap. The leaves repel insects.

Medicinal Uses: Ashwagandha is an adaptogenic herb that has been in use for thousands of years. It is highly valued for its ability to strengthen the immune system, balance hormone levels, and for its anti-anxiety, anti-depressant, and anti-inflammatory properties. Roots and leaves of the ashwagandha plant are used for their medicinal properties.

Root extracts in powdered or capsule forms are effective as are leaf extracts and tinctures. Powders can be added to food or drinks thought they have a strong taste. Ashwagandha tea made from the leaves is also used. Adding a little honey improves the flavor.

Expect it to take two weeks or more to begin to notice the benefits of ashwagandha. Long-term use has not been studied and may not be safe, but many patients do well taking the herb long-term.

"Adrenal Fatigue" (= HPA Axis Dysregulation – HPA-D): Ashwagandha supports adrenal function and overcoming "adrenal fatigue", though this term is really a summary of stress response symptoms that are often caused by a hypothalamic–pituitary–adrenal (HPA) axis dysfunction. Essentially, HPA-D is our stress response system and a more accurate term for adrenal fatigue. Ashwagandha helps balance this.

Combats Stress, Fight or Flight, Anxiety, and Depression: Ashwagandha has long been used to relieve anxiety, improve mental health, concentration, vitality, and overall improve the quality of life. It also acts as a mood stabilizer and relieves symptoms of depression. It provides benefits similar to anti-anxiety and anti-depressant drugs without drowsiness, insomnia, or other side effects.

Reduces Cortisol Levels: Cortisol is a stress hormone implicated in controlling blood sugar levels and fat storage in the abdomen. Studies show that ashwagandha helps significantly reduce cortisol levels in chronically stressed adults.

Balances Blood Glucose Levels: Ashwagandha is particularly beneficial to diabetic patients in reducing blood glucose levels. It may help improve insulin sensitivity and reduce inflammation.

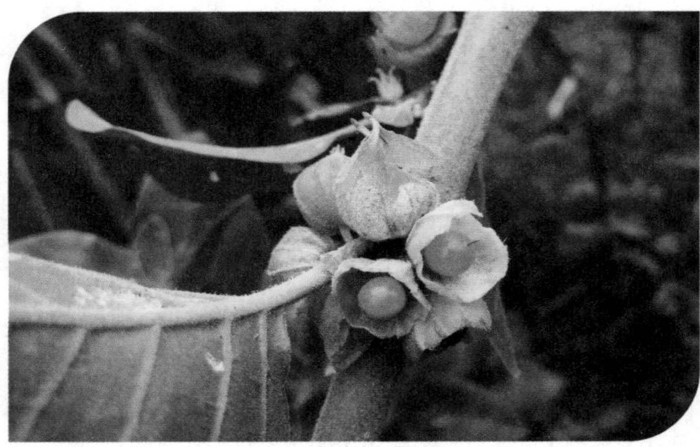

Cancer: Research shows that ashwagandha has anti-tumor effects. It reduces cancerous tumors by preventing cell growth and killing cancerous cells. Ashwagandha is useful in treating breast, lung, stomach, ovarian, and colon cancer cells. These benefits are due to its antioxidant abilities and their effects in helping the immune system.

In addition to reducing the growth of cancer cells, it can also help the body deal with the side effects of conventional anti-cancer drugs in boosting immunity and improving the quality of life. Ashwagandha stimulates the production of white blood cells and helps cancer patients fight infections.

Memory and Brain Cell Degeneration: Research suggests that ashwagandha protects the brain from the damaging effects of emotional, physical, and chemical stress. It protects the brain from cell degeneration, which may help in treating neurodegenerative diseases like Alzheimer's and Parkinson's Disease.

Ashwagandha contains naturally occurring steroids and antioxidants that protect the brain and improve cognitive function. Patients notice an improvement in attention, processing speed, and mental acuity.

Stamina, Endurance, and Muscle Performance: Studies suggest that ashwagandha boosts endurance and reduces muscle pain. It calms stress, energizes the brain, and enhances cardiorespiratory endurance in athletes. It increases muscle mass and strength in athletes engaging in resistance training and strenuous exercise when taken for 8-weeks or longer.

Anti-inflammatory: Joint Pain and Arthritis: Patients taking ashwagandha for eight weeks or longer experience improvement in joint function and a reduction in joint pain related to rheumatoid arthritis.

Sexual Function and Fertility: Ashwagandha helps improve sexual function. It boosts testosterone levels and improves male fertility. When used for a period of 3 months, ashwagandha increases sperm count, sperm volume, and sperm motility. In women, it improves arousal, lubrication, and orgasm.

Immune Function: Ashwagandha helps regulate immune function by reducing the body's stress hormones, reducing inflammation, increasing the white blood cell count, and increasing immunoglobulin production.

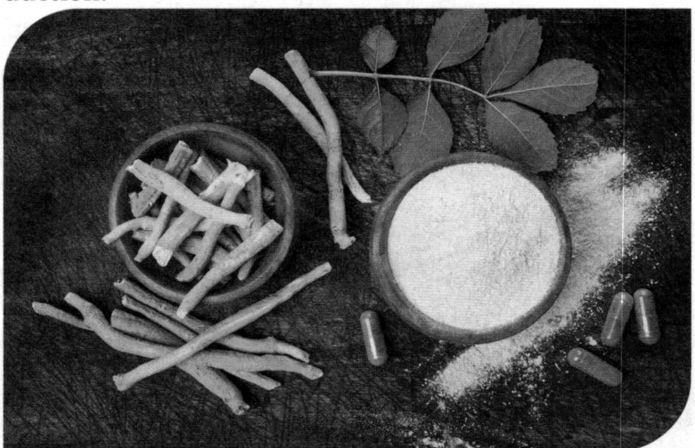

Harvesting: Pick berries in the fall when red and fully ripe, then dry them for planting in the spring. For medicinal use, dig up the roots in the fall and clean thoroughly. Slice, dry, and powder for future use. Leaves are used fresh or can be dried to use in tea.

Warning: The herb is generally believed to be safe and has an extensive history of use. However, there are no long-term studies on the safety and long-term use may make it more likely that side effects will be experienced. Consult your doctor and watch for side-effects when using ashwagandha over the long term.

Black-Eyed Susan, *Rudbeckia hirta*

Black-eyed Susan is a member of the Aster/Sunflower Family, and is found throughout eastern and central North America. It is also called brown-eyed Susan, hairy coneflower, gloriosa daisy brown betty, yellow daisy, yellow ox-eye daisy coneflower, poor-land daisy, and golden Jerusalem. It prefers full sun and moist to moderately-dry soil.

Identification: Black-eyed Susan is usually an annual; but sometimes a perennial, growing up to 3 feet (0.9m) tall and up to 1 ½ feet (0.5m) wide.

The leaves are alternate, 4 to 7 inches (10 cm to 20 cm) long, and covered by coarse hair. The branched stems grow from a single taproot.

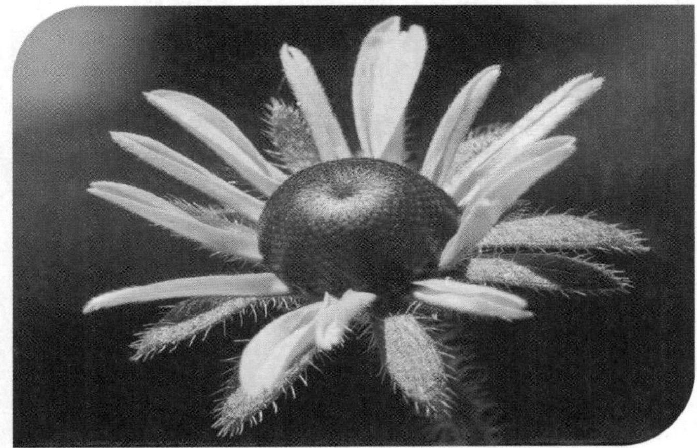

There is no rhizome and reproduction is by seed only. Be on the lookout for these flowers during late summer and early autumn. They are about 4 inches (10 cm) in diameter, with a brownish black dome in the middle, circled by yellow petals.

Medicinal Use: Black-eyed Susan is a traditional herb used for colds, flu, infection, swelling, and snake bite. The roots and sometimes the leaves are used to boost immunity and fight colds, flu, and infections.

Colds and Flu: A root infusion treats colds and the flu. Common usage is to drink the root infusion daily until all symptoms are gone.

Parasites: The Chippewa people have traditionally used Black-eyed Susan Root Tea to treat worms in children.

Poultice for Snake Bites: A poultice of black-eyed Susan is said to treat snakebites. Moisten the hopped leaves or ground root and place over the affected area as a poultice. Wrap with a cloth and keep it on the wound until the swelling is reduced.

Skin Irritations: Black-eyed Susan root infusions are soothing on irritated skin including sores, cuts, scrapes, and swelling. Use a warm root infusion to wash the irritated skin.

Earaches: If you have fresh roots, use the sap or juice as drops to treat earaches. One or two drops in the affected ear treat the infection and relieves pain. Place the drops in the ear morning and night until the infection is completely cleared up.

Stimulates the Immune System: Like Echinacea, Black-eyed Susan roots have immune-stimulant activity and boost the immune system to treat colds, flu, and other minor illness. Those with autoimmune issues should be careful using this herb internally due to its immune-stimulating properties.

Tuberculosis: Black-eyed Susan contains compounds that act against the bacterium that causes tuberculosis.

Harvesting: To harvest the taproot, wait until the plant has produced seeds, then dig the plant up by the root. Black-eyed Susan has one central taproot with hairs, but no other rhizomes. Dig deeply to get the entire root. Use it fresh in season and also dry some root for future use.

Warning: Black-eyed Susan plants are toxic to cats and are reported to be poisonous to cattle, sheep, and pigs. The seeds are poisonous. Those with autoimmune conditions should be careful with internal use of this herb due to its immune-stimulating properties.

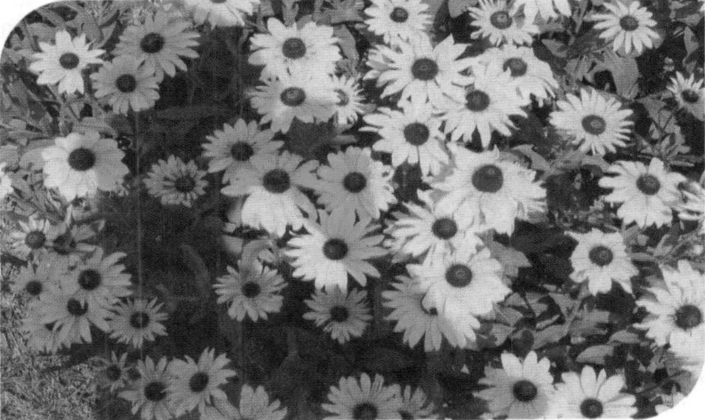

Boneset, *Eupatorium perfoliatum*

This herb supposedly got the name boneset due to its use treating dengue fever, also known as break-bone fever. It is excellent for treating fevers and is a great choice for chest colds and flu. The herb is a perennial native to North America. It is a member of the Aster/Sunflower family. It is also known as feverwort.

Identification: Boneset has erect, hairy stems that grow 2 to 4 feet (0.6m to 1.2m) high and branch at the top. The leaves are large, opposite, and united at the base. They are lance-shaped, finely toothed and have prominent veins. Leaves are 4 to 8 inches (10 cm to 20 cm) long with the lower ones larger than the upper ones. The blades are rough on the top and downy, resinous, and dotted on the underside.

The leaves of boneset are easily distinguished. They are either perforated by the stem or connate; two opposite leaves joined at the base.

The numerous large flower heads of boneset are terminal and slightly convex, with 10 to 20 white florets, and have bristly hairs arranged in a single row.

The fragrance is slightly aromatic, while the taste is astringent and strongly bitter. Flowering from July to September, this plant's size, hairiness and other aspects can vary greatly.

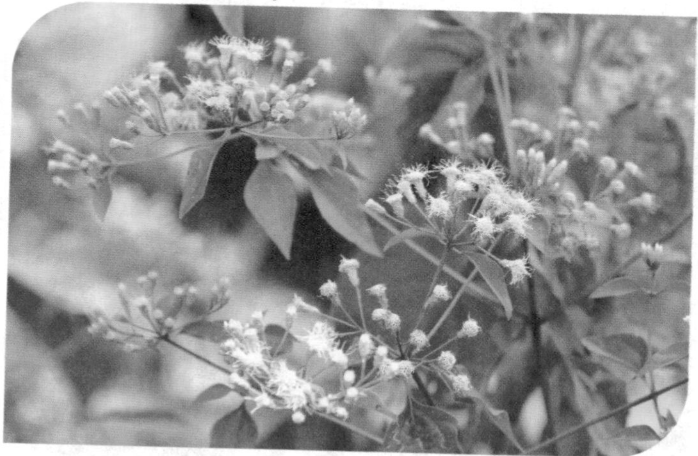

Medicinal Use: The flowers and leaves are used. Best to let dry rather than use fresh due to some degree of toxicity. The major medicinal properties of boneset include use as an antispasmodic, sweat inducer, bile-producer, emetic, fever-reducer, laxative, purgative, stimulant, and as a vasodilator.

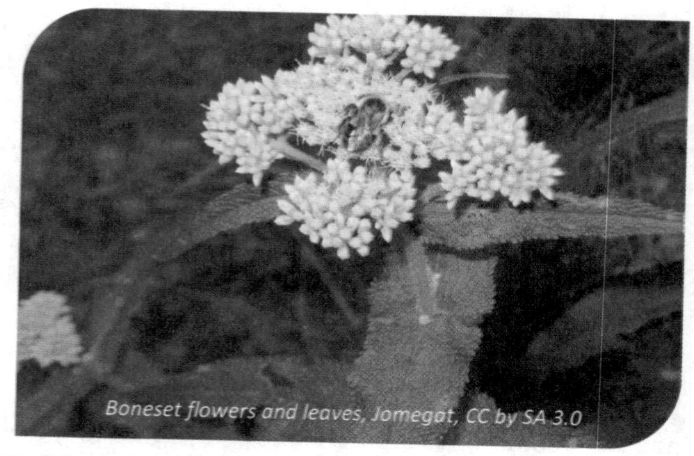

Boneset flowers and leaves, Jomegat, CC by SA 3.0

Colds, Flu, Bronchitis, Congestion and Excess Mucus: Boneset is an excellent choice for the treatment of the common cold, flu, and respiratory infections. It discourages the production of mucus, loosens phlegm and helps eliminate it from the body, fights off both viral and bacterial infections, and encourages sweating, which helps reduce the associated fever.

People given boneset early in the disease process have milder symptoms and get well faster. A tincture is the easiest form to use.

Dengue Fever, AKA Break Bone Fever: Dengue fever thrives in tropical environments, and while it is not yet a problem here in the United States, it is probably only a matter of time before it arrives.

Boneset is the herb of choice for fighting dengue, a painful mosquito-borne disease that results in high fevers and terrible muscle and bone pain. It reduces the fevers and fights the underlying causes of the disease. It also gives the patient some relief from the "bone-breaking" pain.

Malaria: Native Americans have commonly used boneset to treat malaria. It promotes sweating, which helps relieve the fever associated with malaria and lessens the severity of the disease.

Yellow Fever and Typhoid: Boneset is helpful in the treatment of yellow fever and typhoid, although it is not as effective as it is for treating dengue fever and malaria. Its main use here is its ability to reduce the accompanying fevers.

Harvesting: Harvest the leaves and flowering stems of boneset during the summer, just before the buds have opened. Dry them for later use. Seeds of boneset ripen about a month after flowering and are collected when the heads are dry, split, and the fluffy seed begins to float away. If seeds are collected earlier, dry the seed heads for 1 to 2 weeks in open paper bags.

Warning: Do not use boneset for pregnant or nursing mothers or for young children. Not for long-term use.

Recipes: Boneset Infusion. Take Boneset Infusion hot to relieve fevers and treat colds, flu, and similar diseases. Use it cold as a tonic or tincture.

Ingredients: 1-ounce dried boneset leaf, 1-quart (1 Liter) boiling water, 1-quart (1 Liter) jar with a tight-fitting lid.

Instructions: Put the dried boneset leaves into the jar and pour the boiling water over it to fill the jar. Tightly cap the jar and shake it gently to distribute the herb.

Let the infusion steep for 4 hours. Strain through a coffee filter or a fine sieve. Warm it before drinking. It is very bitter, but warming it helps.

Borage, *Borago officinalis*

Common Borage is an annual frequently found in gardens. Bees are attracted to the flowers and make an excellent honey from the nectar.

Identification: The entire borage plant is covered with stiff white hairs. The stems are round, branched, hollow, and succulent. The plant grows to about 1 1/2 feet tall. Its deep green leaves are alternate, wrinkled, oval and pointed. Each is about 3 inches long and about 1 1/2 inches across. The lower leaves have tiny hairs on the upper surface and on the veins on the lower side. Leaf margins are wavy, but entire.

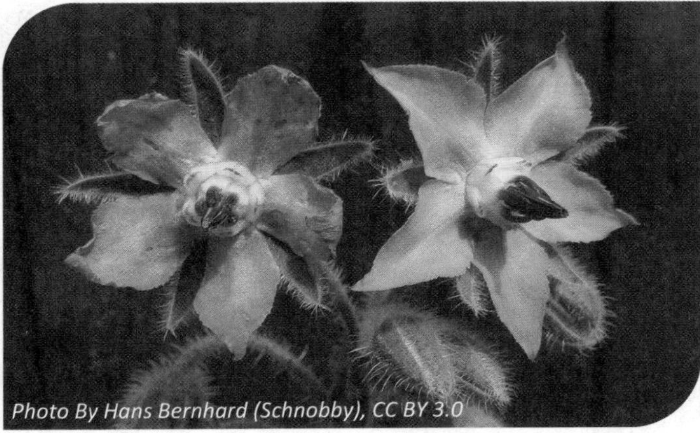
Photo By Hans Bernhard (Schnobby), CC BY 3.0

The flowers are a vivid blue and star-shaped, with prominent black anthers. The anthers form a cone in the center that is referred to as a beauty spot. The flowers start pink and turn blue, hanging in clusters.

The flowers produce four brown-black nutlets.

Edible Use: The leaves, flowers, dried stems, and seeds are all edible and nutritious. You can eat the leaves raw or cooked. I use them in salads or cooked as a pot-herb. The leaves have a salty flavor similar to a cucumber. It is best to use the leaves while young. The more mature raw leaves are very hairy, which some people find unpleasant.

The flowers are nice used raw as a decorative garnish for salads and drinks. They make a refreshing drink when the leaves are brewed as a tea.

Dried stems are often used as a flavoring. The seeds are a healthy source of gamma-linolenic acid (GLA), a beneficial Omega-6 fatty acid, but it is difficult to collect enough for regular use.

Medicinal Use. Regulates Hormones, PMS and Menstrual Issues: Borage treats hormonal imbalances and regulates metabolism. Eating borage with meals regularly helps keep your metabolism running smoothly.

Borage reduces symptoms of premenstrual syndrome (PMS), menopause, and regulates the menstrual cycle.

Stress and HPA-Dysfunction ("Adrenal Fatigue"): Borage is a calming herb and is taken to relieve stress. It also helps balance cortisol levels in the body, this aiding the stress response and HPA-Dysfunction (often called Adrenal Fatigue).

Anti-Oxidant Properties: Anti-oxidants in borage helps destroy free radicals in the body, protecting it against aging and cancers caused by free radicals.

Digestive Problems and Irritable Bowel Syndrome: Borage has a soothing effect on the stomach muscles and is a good treatment for irritable bowel syndrome.

It reduces inflammation in the intestinal tract and treats gastritis and other digestive problems. It promotes digestion and stabilizes the stomach. Borage also has a mild laxative effect.

Pneumonia: Borage Leaf and Flower Tea or Tincture reduces the symptoms of pneumonia, relieves congestion, and helps the body get rid of excess mucus. However, there are better herbs for these symptoms.

Mouth Ulcers and Sore Throats: Use borage as a mouthwash or gargle to kill bacteria in the mouth and throat. It prevents and treats sore throats and mouth sores.

Urinary Tract and Kidney Infections, Diuretic Properties: Borage acts as a diuretic, removing excess water and toxins from the body. It also works to improve bladder function. Borage flushes the bladder, removing bacteria and relieving bladder infections. Borage also relieves kidney inflammations and restores health of the kidneys. However, I prefer other herbs to treat these, such as Usnea, Oregon Grape and Uva Ursi.

Protects the Brain: The GLA in borage seed oil improves the brains protection against neuro-degeneration. It protects the brain against synaptic failure in Alzheimer's disease and improves resistance to the disease.

Lowers Blood Pressure: Eat borage or drink the juice daily to treat high blood pressure. The GLA content helps to significantly lower blood pressure. Recent studies have confirmed the benefits of Borage for treating hypertension.

Allergies: The anti-oxidants in borage help subdue allergies, reduce inflammation, and suppress the allergic response.

Reduces Fevers: Borage stimulates the sweat glands to produce sweat and cool the body. This property is beneficial for treating fevers in colds, and respiratory illnesses.

Arthritis and Gout: Borage is useful for treating inflammation, reducing swelling, and thereby reducing pain. It is effective for reducing inflammation caused by arthritis and gout.

Skin Infections, Wounds, and Rashes: The anti-inflammatory and anti-bacterial properties of borage help keep your skin clear. It is useful in treating wounds and fighting infections or rashes. Use borage tea as a skin wash or use borage as a poultice to treat wounds. A poultice of borage leaves also reduces itching and inflammation from rashes or stings and insect bites. It clears up skin inflammations and the unpleasant symptoms of skin rashes.

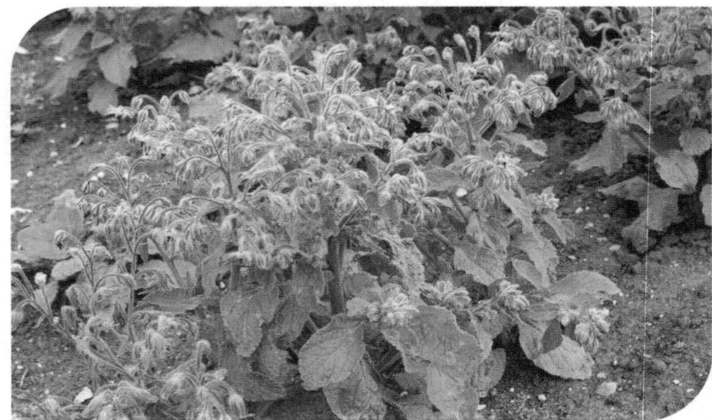

Photo By David Wright, Geograph project, CC BY 2.0

Treating Bleeding Gums: Borage fights the infections that cause bleeding gums. Borage helps kill the mouth pathogens and restores health to the gums and mouth.

Macular Degeneration: One cause of macular degeneration is a lack of fatty acids. Borage seeds contain up to 30% GLA, a beneficial fatty acid for treating and preventing macular degeneration.

Improves Milk Production for Nursing Mothers: Borage tea is used to improve milk production in nursing mothers.

Treat Hangovers: Borage Tea made from a combination of dried leaves and flowers is an effective treatment for hangover.

Harvesting: Harvest borage leaves in the late spring and early summer before the plant flowers. Use the leaves fresh or dry them for use throughout the year. Dried leaves lose their medicinal properties over time, so dry a new batch each year. Harvest flowers in the morning in the summer.

Warning: Borage leaves contain a small amount of pyrrolizidine alkaloids and other compounds that are toxic to the liver.

The levels are low and are not a problem for healthy people, but people with liver disease should not use borage in any form. Pregnant women should avoid using borage. In some people, borage causes skin dermatitis. Persons with schizophrenia or epilepsy should avoid using borage.

Bottle Gourd, *Lagenaria siceraria*

Also known as calabash, white-flowered gourd, and long melon, the bottle gourd is often cultivated for its fruit. When harvested young, the fruit is used as a vegetable. When mature, it is dried, and it can be scraped and used as a bottle, container, or pipe. Bottle gourd is in the cucumber family. It is hard to find in the wild, but easy to cultivate.

Identification: This annual vine grows to be 15 feet (4.5m) long or more. The fruit has a smooth light-green skin and white flesh. It grows in a variety of shapes and sizes. It has long densely packed hairs on the stems.

These hairs are tipped with glands that produce a sticky sap. The leaves grow on long stalks and are oval to heart-shaped. Leaves can be unlobed or have 3 to 5 irregular shallow lobes. The flowers are white, growing alone or in pairs. They open at night during the summer and close again in the morning.

Edible Use: Although it is safe to eat in moderate amounts, be aware that young gourds can be bitter. If you think the plant has grown too old or tastes too bitter, throw it away because it might have a buildup of toxins or it may have spoiled. Otherwise, the fruit can be steamed, boiled, fried, used in soups and stir-fries. Young shoots and leaves are cooked as a pot herb.

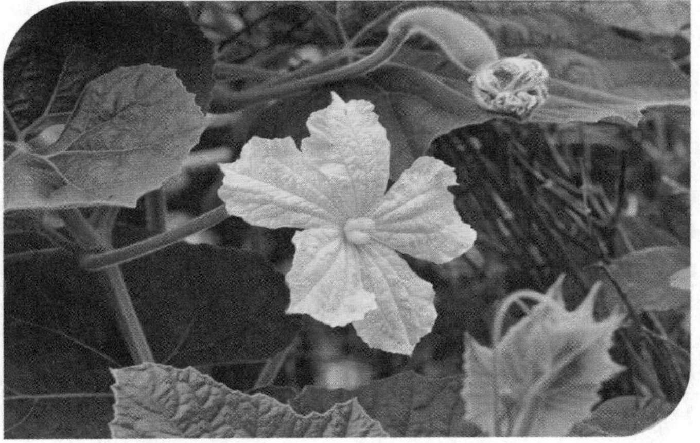

Medicinal Use: This plant is mainly used for blood sugar control in diabetics, but I know of healers who use it as a heart tonic and as a sedative. It is anti-inflammatory, antioxidant, anti-bacterial, pain relieving, and a tonic for the internal organs.

Diabetes: Bottle gourd helps to lower blood sugar readings in diabetics when taken regularly. Eat a piece of bottle gourd at each meal for blood sugar control. One or two large bites of the gourd are enough to provide the desired benefit.

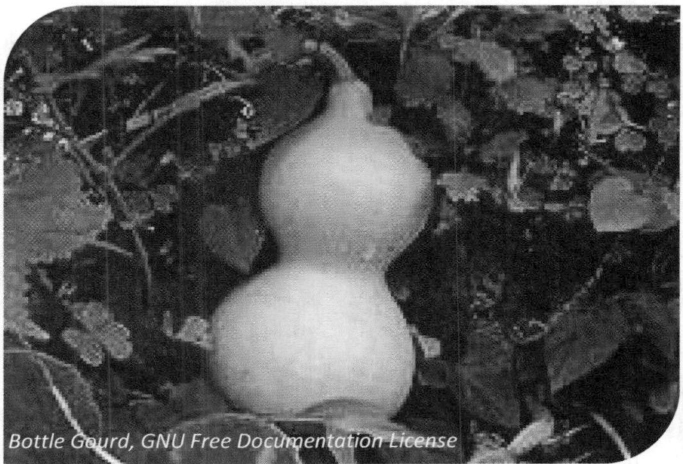

Bottle Gourd, GNU Free Documentation License

Headaches: A poultice made by crushing the leaves and applying it to the head over the painful area is useful for relieving the pain of headaches.

Boils, Skin Infections, and Irritations: Bottle gourd has anti-bacterial and anti-inflammatory effects. For these external uses, make poultice from the boiled seeds of the gourd for skin irritations and infections.

Cover the poultice with a clean cloth and leave in place as long as possible to reduce swelling and prevent the spread of the infection.

Memory Loss, Depression and Senility: Studies have been done demonstrating bottle gourd for mild depression and memory improvement, including patients with Alzheimer's Disease and age-related senility.

Cabbage, *Brassica oleracea*

The common cabbage is familiar to gardeners across the country, but many don't realize how valuable it is as a medicinal plant. The plant is a biennial or perennial, forming a round head that can reach up to 8 feet (2.4m) when fully mature. Most cabbages are harvested long before they reach such a size. It is in the Brassicaceae (Mustard) Family.

Identification: The leaves are gray with a thick stem. Yellow flowers with four petals appear in the spring. The leaves form a head during the late summer of the first year. Cabbage can also be reddish-purple, green, or white. All varieties have the health-giving benefits detailed below.

Edible Use: The cabbage is a common vegetable, especially in the winter because it keeps well in the root cellar. It is eaten raw and cooked.

Medicinal Use. Mastitis and Painful Breasts in Nursing Mothers: This is my number one use for cabbage leaves. For painfully engorged breasts and mastitis, use a poultice made from cabbage leaves. Cut out the vein from the cabbage leaf and crush or pound the leaf with a hammer. You'll want your leaf intact but badly bruised to access the healing sulfur compounds and the juice. Apply the bruised leaf to the breast or line the bra cup with the leaf. Repeat as needed until the infection clears.

Treatment for Wounds, Leg Ulcers, Joint Pain, Arthritis, Skin Cancers: Cabbage leaves work well to clean wounds and prevent infection. They are also useful in reducing swelling in painful joints and treating skin tumors.

Chop the leaves and crush them to release the health-giving juices and heat them in a very small amount of water. Apply the leaves as a poultice over the affected area. The cabbage detoxifies the skin and underlying tissue, prevents bacterial growth, and reduces inflammation.

Intestinal Problems: Cabbage is useful for treating intestinal problems due to its sulfurous compounds. Fermented cabbage in the form of sauerkraut is even more effective for treating intestinal problems of all kinds.

Diabetes: Sauerkraut juice, mixed with a little lemon juice, helps people control their diabetes and stabilize their blood sugars. The sauerkraut juice stimulates the digestion and pancreas.

Constipation: Cabbage, cabbage juice, and sauerkraut juice all have laxative properties.

Treating Cancer: For treating cancer, especially cancers of the stomach, intestines, pancreas, and prostate, drink cabbage juice or sauerkraut juice twice daily. Finely chopped cabbage should also be eaten as tolerated. Both cabbage juice and sauerkraut juice have many different beneficial compounds that fight cancer and help heal the body.

Recipes: Sauerkraut. Equipment: Large glass jar or crock. I prefer using a fermentation crock, but a glass jar will work, a fermentation weight or a plate that fits in the container, a large bowl or tub for mixing, a plate or tray. Ingredients for 1 gallon (4 liters) of Sauerkraut: 1 large head of cabbage, shredded fine, a few large leaves from the outside of the cabbage, 3 tablespoons pickling salt and 1 tablespoon caraway seeds, optional.

Shred the cabbage finely and add 2 TBS of salt. Let the cabbage stand for about 10 minutes to draw out juices. Knead the cabbage for 10 minutes or more to bruise it and release more juices.

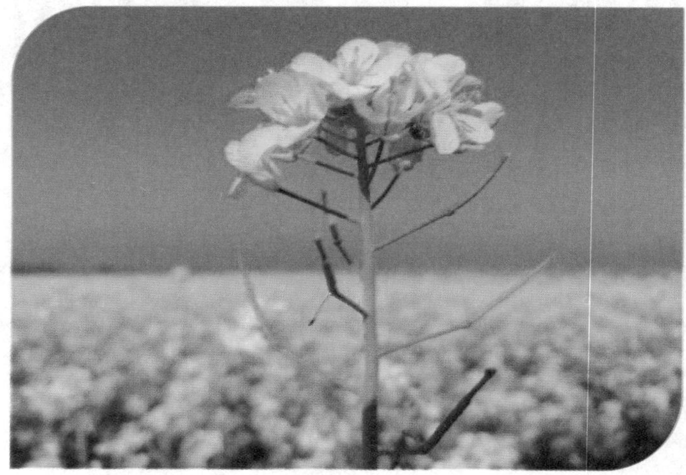

Cabbage, By Taken byfir0002, GFDL 1.2

Add the remaining salt and the caraway seeds. Pack the cabbage into a large glass jar or crock and add the juices. Cover the top of the shredded cabbage with the whole cabbage leaves. Add a weight to the top of the cabbage to keep it beneath the liquid.

Fermenting crocks use fermenting weights, but a clean plate or another dish can be used. Cover the container with its lid. Place the container in a cool spot on a tray or plate to catch any spills. Leave the cabbage overnight and check it the next day to make sure that all the cabbage is submerged in liquid and skim off any scum that forms.

Continue checking the sauerkraut every other day for 4 weeks. Transfer the sauerkraut to the refrigerator and use within 6 months. Sauerkraut can be canned for longer storage. However, I believe this destroys some of the beneficial enzymes as well as the live culture. I recommend using the sauerkraut with live culture.

Calendula, *Calendula officinalis*

Calendula or Pot Marigold is a perennial plant in the Aster/Daisy family that is often grown as an annual. It is not originally native to North America but is widely cultivated in flower gardens, self-seeds, and is easy to grow.

Identification: Calendula usually grows 12 to 24 inches (30 cm to 60 cm) tall with branched sprawling or erect stems. The leaves are oblong and lance-like, approximately 2 to 7 inches (5 cm to 18 cm) long, and hairy on both sides. The margins can be smooth, wavy, or even weakly toothed.

The flowers are yellow or orange with a 2 to 3-inch (5 cm to 7.5 cm) flower head with two rows of hairy bracts. Flowers appear year-round in warmer climates. Some flowers have multiple rows of ray florets while others have only one. High resin varieties and multi-row flowers are said to be better for medicine. The fruit is a small curved achene.

Edible Use: Calendula flowers are edible raw in salads or dried and used as a seasoning. They can be used as a saffron substitute for color but not taste. Tea is made from the petals. The leaves are edible, but are bitter and unpalatable.

Medicinal Use: Calendula can be used as a tea, infused oil, salve, compress, or poultice.

Skin Diseases, Cuts, Rashes, Wounds, Burns, Cold Sores, Herpes, Chicken Pox, and Irritations: Calendula leaves and flowers are soothing to the skin, and I use them to treat all kinds of skin problems like acne, sunburn, and rashes, including diaper rash. The leaves make a healing poultice for minor cuts, scratches, bites, and skin irritations.

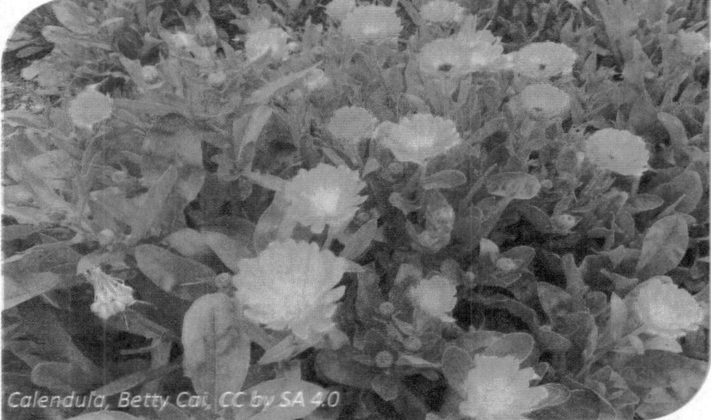
Calendula, Betty Cai, CC by SA 4.0

Place the bruised leaves directly on the skin. The leaves soothe inflamed skin and help it heal. I use the flowers to make a healing salve for skin irritations. The leaves and flowers have anti-bacterial, anti-fungal, anti-microbial, and anti-viral effects as well being an immunostimulant. To treat skin infections, including ringworm, athlete's foot, thrush, diaper rash, and cradle cap, I use Calendula Oil or Salve applied to the affected area several times a day. Note that Calendula is a tonic anti-fungal, weaker than many. I prefer to use a stronger anti-fungal such as black walnut hull powder, Oregano Oil, or Usnea to treat the primary infection and save calendula as a preventative or for chronic situations.

Anti-aging and Collagen Production: Calendula stimulates the immune system, induces collagen production and inhibits collagen degradation. I make an anti-aging blend with Calendula and Cottonwood Buds infused in organic almond oil and use it on my face and neck every day in place of a commercial face cream.

Soothes Muscle Spasms: Calendula relaxes muscles and can prevent spasms. Calendula tea treats abdominal cramping caused by constipation and menstrual cramping.

It is also effective in relieving body aches and pains due to muscle spasms.

Helps Heal Ulcers, Wounds, and Hemorrhoids: Slow healing wounds such as ulcers and hemorrhoids are soothed by the application of calendula as an ointment, gel, or salve. It speeds up healing and wound closure while improving skin firmness and hydration. Calendula increases the blood and oxygen availability in the infected area, which encourages rapid healing. It is antimicrobial and antibacterial.

Stomach and Intestinal Diseases: Calendula works to heal a variety of gastro-intestinal problems including intestinal colitis, GERD, esophageal irritation, peptic ulcers, and inflammatory bowel disease. It soothes the inflammation from infections and irritations while helping heal the underlying problems.

Immune System and Lymphatic System: Calendula stimulates the functioning of the immune system and the lymphatic system, including swollen lymph nodes and tonsillitis, and helps to prevent infections.

Additionally, the astringent and antiseptic properties help the body fight off infections and viruses. Calendula also reduces congestion and swelling in the lymph glands.

Menstruation and PMS: Calendula Tea is an effective aid in easing the painful side effects of menstruation. It helps induce the menses, relieves painful cramping, relaxes the muscles, and improves blood flow. Some people claim that it also helps with hot flashes.

Improves Oral Health: Calendula has powerful antibacterial and antimicrobial properties and treats gingivitis, plaque, oral cavities and many other oral health issues.

Inhibits Cancer: Calendula has anti-inflammatory properties which aid the body in fighting cancer, as well as irritations caused by cancer treatments. It activates the lymphatic system against the cancer and helps kill off the cancer cells. It also effectively soothes the skin after radiation treatments.

Liver, Gallbladder, and Whole-Body Detoxification: Calendula helps remove toxins from the body and helps cleanse the liver and gallbladder. The detoxification properties also have a positive effect on the skin and help clear up chronic skin problems such as eczema and acne caused by the body's efforts to rid itself of toxins. For detoxification, try an internal Calendula Extract.

Harvesting: To promote flowering, pick the flowers every two days. Dry them on screens or hang them in a well-ventilated warm area.

Warning: Some people are allergic to calendula. Do not use it if you are allergic to marigold, ragweed, daisies, chrysanthemums, chamomile, echinacea and other plants in the Aster/Daisy family. If you are not sure, start with a small test patch on the skin and increase use gradually if you have no reactions. Do not use calendula internally if you are pregnant or breastfeeding, since safety is unknown. Do not take calendula internally if you are taking prescription medications without the advice of your doctor.

Recipes: Soothing Calendula Salve (Fast Method). Ingredients: half a cup of organic olive oil, 1/3 cup solid organic coconut oil, 3 tablespoons dried calendula flowers, 1 1/2 tablespoons dried chamomile flowers, 1 to 2 ounces (28g to 56g) beeswax. In a double boiler, melt the olive oil and the coconut oil together.

Add the flower petals and allow the mixture to steep for 2 to 3 hours making sure it does not get too hot. Strain out the flower petals. Return the pan to the heat and add the beeswax, stirring. Once the wax melts pour into your containers (adjust amount of beeswax to get the consistency you want). Allow the salve to cool completely before use.

Calendula Extract: Take 1-pint (500ml) loosely packed calendula flowers and 1-pint (500ml) 80 proof vodka or other drinking alcohol of 80 proof or higher. Place the flowers in a pint (500ml) jar with a tight fitting lid.

Fill the jar with alcohol so that the flowers are completely covered.

Allow the extract to steep in a cool, dark place for 4 to 6 weeks. Shake daily. Strain out the flowers and store the extract tightly covered in a cool, dark place. Use within 3 years.

California Poppy, *Eschscholzia californica*

The California poppy has sedative and healing effects but is not psychoactive or narcotic like some poppy species.

The California poppy is a species of flowering plant in the Papaveraceae (Poppy) Family, It is native to Western North America. It occurs across a variety of habitats including coastal, foothill, valley, and desert regions, at elevations below 7000 feet (2133m). It is also known as Golden Poppy and Cup of Gold due to its golden color.

Identification: The California poppy is a flowering annual or deep-rooted perennial. It is 1/2 to 2 feet (0.6m) tall, and its foliage is blue-green in color. Its leaves are compound, with three finely divided lobes, and are nearly smooth with no hair.

California poppy produces upright flowers on branching stems with four bright orange to yellow petals. The flowers often have distinct, darker orange centers.

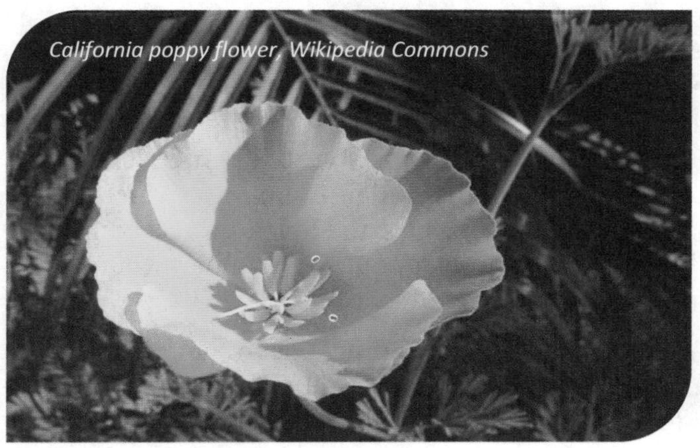
California poppy flower, Wikipedia Commons

The seed capsules of California poppy are cylindrically shaped and burst open from the base when ripe. These capsules open explosively to aid in seed dispersal, ejecting the small seeds up to 6 feet (1.83m) from the parent plant. Its tiny round seeds are usually gray to gray-brown in color when mature.

Edible Use: Its leaves are edible if cooked. Caution is advised because other plants in the family are poisonous.

Medicinal Use: The California poppy is a diuretic, relaxes spasms, relieves pain, promotes perspiration,

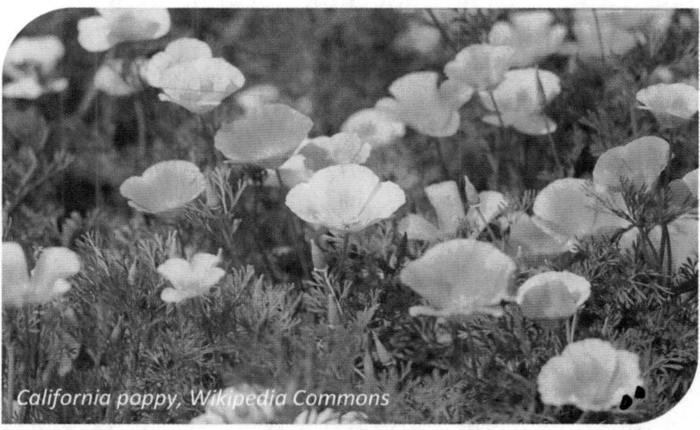
California poppy, Wikipedia Commons

and is sedative. It is non-addictive and can help with opiate withdrawal. It most likely works with GABA receptors. The entire plant is used medicinally, with the root being the most potent part.

Sedative Properties and Antispasmodic: California poppy is a mild sedative that also works well for incontinence, especially for children. It aids in treating sleep deprivation, anxiety, and nervous tension. The sap is somewhat narcotic and works well for alleviating toothaches. Unlike opium poppy, it does not depress the nervous system and it's much milder in action. Take it at bedtime since it induces sleep. It is also an antispasmodic.

Normalizes Psychological Function, PTSD, and Anxiety: California poppy seems to normalize the thinking patterns of people with psychological issues, and is mild enough to use for children. It does not have a narcotic effect, but helps calm the spirit and helps people regain normal function. It works well for anxiety disorders and PTSD.

Suppresses the Milk in Nursing Mothers: When lactation is not desired, apply California Poppy Tea made from the roots as a wash on the breasts to suppress the flow of milk. It helps the milk dry up quickly.

Harvesting: Harvest the entire plant when it is flowering from June to September and dry for use in tinctures and infusions.

Warning: Do not drive or operate heavy machinery, as it is a sedative.

Recipes. California Poppy Infusion: 1 to 2 teaspoons of dried California poppy plant or root, 1 cup boiling water. Make a strong tea by infusing the dried herb in boiling water for 10 minutes and allowing it to cool. Drink one cup of the infusion at night before going to bed. It induces sleepiness.

California Poppy Tincture: 1-pint (500 ml) of 80 proof vodka or other alcohol, or substitute apple-cider vinegar, dried or fresh California poppy plant. Place the chopped fresh herbs or dried plant into a pint (500ml) jar with a tight-fitting lid, filling the jar 3/4 full. Cover the herbs with alcohol, filling the jar. Store the jar in a cool, dark place such as a cupboard. Shake the jar daily for 4 to 6 weeks. Strain the herbs out of the liquid, cover it tightly and use within seven years.

Carolina Geranium, *Geranium carolinianum*

Geranium carolinianum, known as Carolina Geranium, Carolina Cranesbill, Crane's Bill Geranium, and Wild Geranium, is native across the US, Canada, and Mexico.

This plant is often found in areas with poor soil, clay, and limestone. I often see it near roadsides, abandoned fields, and farmland.

Identification: The Carolina geranium is a winter annual or biennial herb. It is low-growing, usually under 12 inches tall. It has earned the name cranesbill because of the beak-like appearance of the fruit. Its palmate leaves have 5 to 7 toothed lobes, with each lobe divided again.

Leaves are 1 to 2.5 inches (2.5 cm to 6 cm) wide, grayish-green and covered in fine hair. Each leaf usually has five segments, edged with deep teeth. Its pinkish-red stems grow erect and are covered in hairs.

White, pink, or lavender flowers appear in small clusters on stalks growing off the main stems in April through July. Each flower has five sepals and five notched petals.

One-half inch long fruits, with a longer style, ripen in the fall. Ripe seeds are covered in pits/depressions.

The plant has a taproot system that grows close to the surface.

Edible Use: Carolina Geranium is edible raw, cooked, or as a tea. The roots are best boiled for 10 minutes to soften. The cooking water can be used as a tea to relieve stomach upsets.

The leaves are astringent and have a strong bitter flavor caused by their high tannin level. Using them young helps relieve some of the bitterness, or change the water out once when you cook them.

The tea is often consumed with milk and cinnamon to improve the flavor.

Medicinal Use: The astringent tannic root is the part most often used medicinally, though leaves are also used.

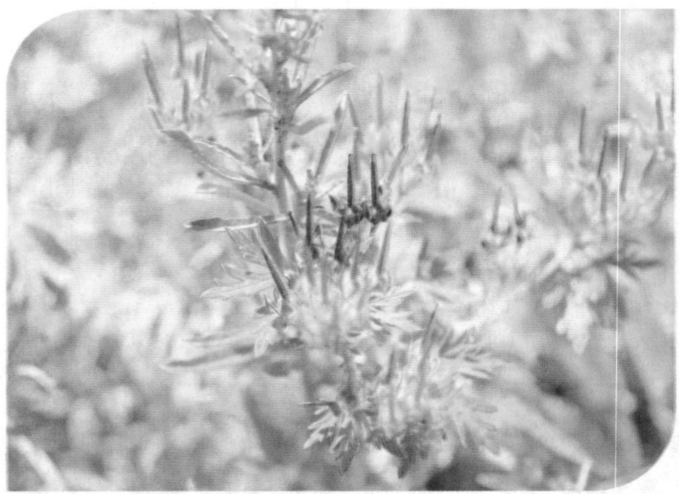

Stops Bleeding, Dries out Tissue: The entire plant is astringent and high in tannins, which causes the contraction of tissues and helps stop bleeding. Use the root or leaves as a poultice on moist wounds and for drying out tissues.

As a styptic (to stop bleeding), clean the root or leaves and apply to the wound. Hold the compress tightly for a few minutes until bleeding stops, and then bind the poultice with gauze or a clean cloth.

The plant is excellent for use in skin salves to promote skin healing.

Diarrhea and Stomach Upset: Tea made from the root is ideal for treating stomach upsets and diarrhea.

Canker Sores: Wash the canker sore with Carolina Geranium Tea or cover it with a root poultice. The astringent root is drying and reduces canker sores quickly.

Treats Sore Throats: The root is soothing for sore throats. It may have anti-viral properties as well.

Hepatitis B: Tinctured Carolina Geranium root has been shown to have the anti-Hepatitis B (HBV) compounds geraniin and hyperin.

Harvesting: Harvest young leaves and use them fresh or dry them for future use. Dig up roots in the late fall when they are plump with stored starch, or if necessary, in the early spring. Clean the roots, slice them thinly and dry for future use or use them fresh.

Recipes: Carolina Geranium Leaf Tea.
2 Tablespoons dried leaves and stems, 2 cups boiling water. Pour the boiling water over the dried leaves and allow the tea to steep, off the heat, for 10 minutes or more. Strain and enjoy.

Carolina Geranium Root Tea: The roots make the most effective medicinal tea. Bring 2 cups of water to a boil and add 2 tablespoons of chopped, dried root. Reduce the heat and simmer the tea for 10 to 15 minutes. Remove from the heat and steep for another 10 minutes. Take up to 3 cups daily.

Carolina Geranium Tincture: Sterilized glass jar with tight fitting lid, ¾ jar cleaned, chopped fresh root or ½ jar dried root, 80 proof vodka or other alcohol to fill jar.

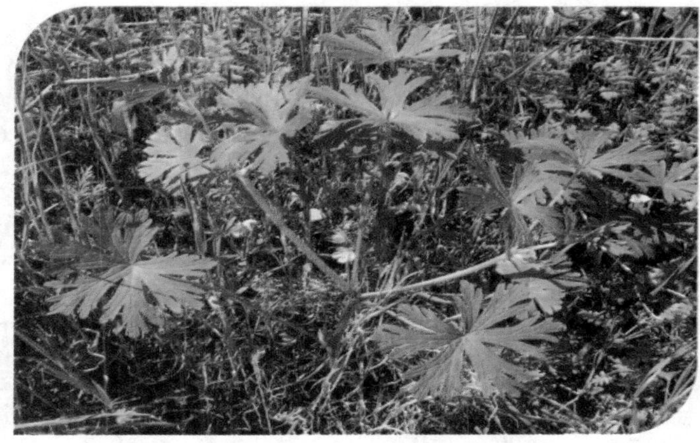

Cheese cloth or fine mesh strainer, glass bowl for straining.

Sterilize all jars, utensils, and bowls with boiling water.

Pack the jar with herbs: ¾ full for fresh root or ½ full for dried herbs, fill the jar with alcohol, making sure all herbs are covered. Cover tightly with lid.

Store the jar in a cool, dark place. Shake the jar daily for 6-8 weeks. Strain out the root and all sediment. When clean, pour into amber bottles and seal tightly. Label and date the containers

Store the bottles in a cool, dark location for up to 10 years.

Chamomile, *Matricaria chamomilla*

Chamomile is a commonly used useful herb. It is a calming plant, and has sedative properties. It is in Aster/Daisy family.

Identification: Chamomile has daisy-like flowers with a hollow, cone-shaped receptacle. Its yellow cone surrounded by 10 to 20 downward-curving white petals. You can distinguish the plant from similar flowers by the pattern in which the flowers grow, each flower on an independent stem.

The most common way of identifying chamomile is by plucking a small amount of the blossom and crushing it in between your fingers. Chamomile has a faintly fruity scent. Chamomile grows wild and it is also easy to cultivate in the garden. It thrives in open, sunny locations with well-drained soil. It does not tolerate excessive heat or dry conditions.

Matricaria chamomilla is German chamomile. English chamomile has similar medicinal uses. The two plants can be distinguished by their leaves. German chamomile leaves are very thin and hairy while those of the English Chamomile are larger and thicker. The leaves of the German chamomile are also bipinnate; each blade can be divided again into smaller leaf sections. German chamomile stems are somewhat feathery while English Chamomile is hairless. Depending on the growing conditions chamomile can grow to between 2 feet (0.6m) and 3 feet (0.9m) tall.

Edible Use: I collect both flowers and leaves for medicinal use, but the flowers make the best tea. The flowers have an apple-like flavor, and the leaves have a grassy flavor. You can make a nice liqueur with dried chamomile flowers and vodka.

Medicinal Use: Chamomile is most often taken as a tea but it may also be taken as a tincture or as a dried encapsulated herb.

Digestive Issues: Chamomile relaxes the muscles, including the digestive muscles. This makes it a good treatment for abdominal pain, indigestion, gastritis and bloating. It is also used it for Crohn's disease and irritable bowel syndrome.

Colic: Chamomile is known to be safe for use with babies. Adding a cup of tea to the baby's bath at night soothes colic and helps with sleep.

Muscle Aches: The antispasmodic action of chamomile relieves muscle tension. It soothes aching muscles and body aches.

Insomnia: Chamomile is soothing and sedative. One cup of chamomile tea, taken at bedtime or during the night, helps with sleep. If more help is needed, use a tincture.

Eyewash, Conjunctivitis, and Pinkeye: For eye problems, try an eyewash made by dissolving 5 to 10 drops of Chamomile tincture in some boiled and cooled water or by making a strong chamomile tea.

This mixture relieves eyestrain and treats infections. I often pair it with other herbs like Yarrow and Usnea.

Asthma, Bronchitis, Whooping Cough, and Congestion: Use a steam treatment for congestion. Add two teaspoons of chamomile flower petals to a pot of boiling water. Inhale the steam until the phlegm is released. Or add 2 to 3 drops of Chamomile Essential Oil to a vaporizer and use overnight.

Allergies and Eczema: For allergic conditions, including itchy skin and eczema, try Chamomile Essential Oil. The steam distillation process alters the chemical properties of the remedy, giving it anti-allergenic properties. Dilute the essential oil in a carrier oil to use directly on the skin or inhale it.

Harvesting: It is best to harvest chamomile during its peak blooming period. I prefer to pick chamomile in the late morning, after the dew has evaporated and before the real heat of the day. Select flowers that are fully open and pinch or clip the flower head off at the top of the stalk. Dry for future use.

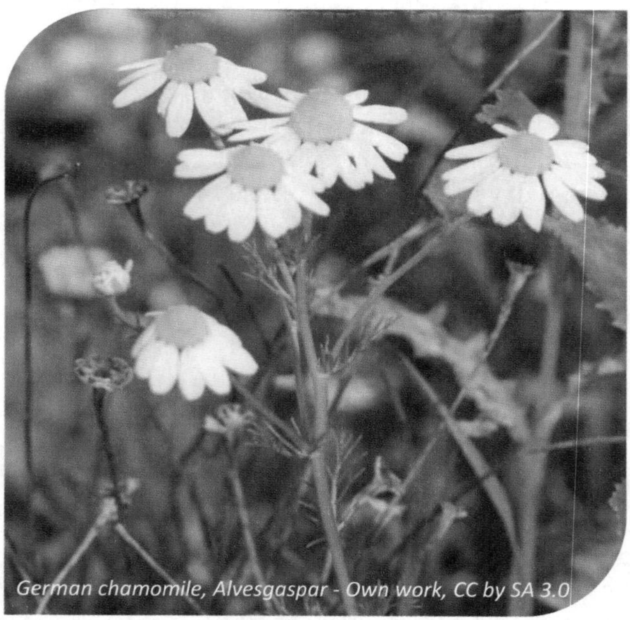
German chamomile, Alvesgaspar - Own work, CC by SA 3.0

Warning: While it is uncommon, some people have an allergic reaction to chamomile. People with allergies to the Asteraceae family, including ragweed and chrysanthemums, should not take chamomile.

Recipes: Chamomile Tea. Ingredients: 1 to 2 teaspoons of dried chamomile flowers or leaves and 1 cup boiling water. Pour 1 cup of boiling water over the chamomile flowers or leaves. Let the herb steep for 5 to 10 minutes. Strain.

Chamomile Liqueur: Ingredients: 1 pint (500 ml) of 80 proof vodka, 1 cup chamomile flowers, 2 tablespoons raw honey or to taste and zest of one lemon. Combine all ingredients in a tightly covered jar and allow the mixture to steep for two to four weeks. Strain.

Chickweed, *Stellaria media*

Chickweed is an annual plant in the Caryophyllaceae (Pink) Family. This herb is naturalized to many parts of North America. It is sometimes referred to as common chickweed to distinguish it from other plants with the same name. It is also referred to as winterweed, maruns, starweed, and chickenwort among others. It is commonly grown as feed for chickens.

Identification: Common chickweed grows from 2 to 20 inches (5 cm to 50 cm) in height. Its intertwined manner of growing usually covers large areas. Its flowers are white and shaped similarly to a star. The oval leaves have cup-like tips with smooth and slightly feathered edges. Its flowers are small, white, and star-shaped. They are produced at the tip of the stem. The sepals are green in color.

Edible Use: The leaves, stem, and flowers are edible raw or cooked.

Medicinal Use. Arthritis: A tea or tincture from this herb is used as a remedy for arthritis. It relieves the inflammation and pain of rheumatoid arthritis. Also try adding a strong tea to a warm bath and soaking to relieve pain, especially on the knees and feet.

Roseola and Other Rashes: Children and adults suffering from roseola are plagued by an itchy rash. Use a poultice of moistened crushed chickweed leaves applied to the rash for relief of pain and itching. Adding a strong tea to the bathwater also helps.

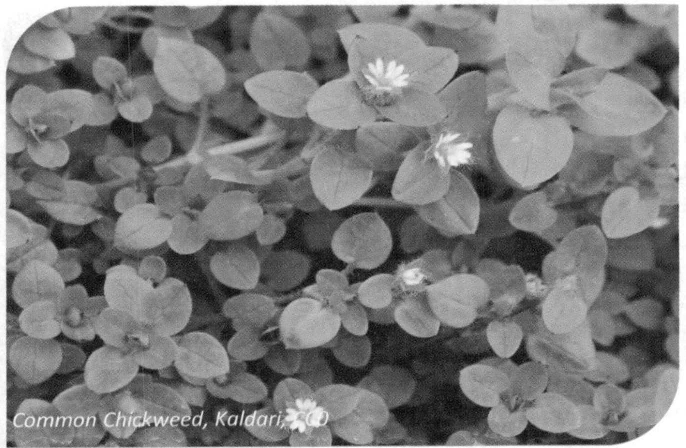

Common Chickweed, Kaldari, CC0

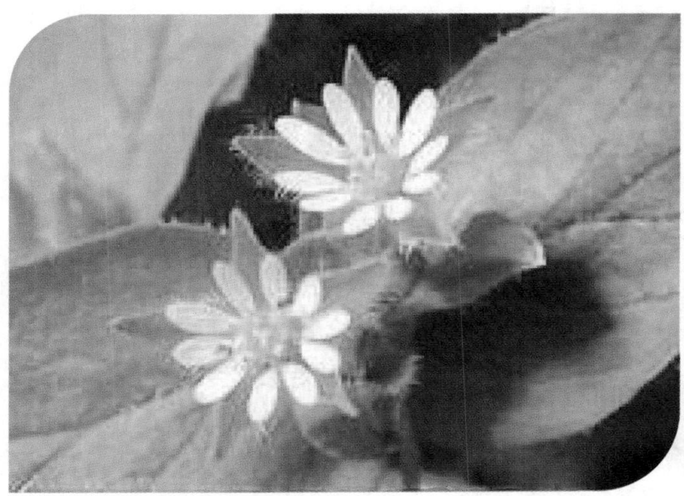

Nerve Pain: Chickweed applied as a poultice or salve helps relieve the pain and tingling caused by surface nerves misfiring.

Constipation and Digestive Problems: Chickweed tea treats constipation. Be careful not to overdo it with the decoction; it has a strong purgative action.

Chickweed also has analgesic properties that act on the digestive system to relieve pain, but it does not treat the underlying causes.

Skin Irritations, Dermatitis, Eczema, Hives, Shingles, and Varicose Veins: A salve or poultice made from chickweed works well for skin irritations, especially on itches and rashes. It is also useful for varicose veins, hives, dermatitis, and eczema. You can add the decoction to your bath if the affected area is larger.

Detoxification, Blood Purification, Tetanus, Boils, Herpes, and Venereal Diseases: Chickweed is an excellent detoxification agent and blood purifier. It draws poisons out of the body in cases of blood poisoning, tetanus, or from poisons entering the bloodstream through a wound.

For these purposes make a poultice from equal parts chickweed, ginger root, and raw honey. Blend the mixture to a smooth paste and apply it directly to the wound and the surrounding area.

Cover the poultice and replace it every six hours. Also take chickweed powder or tea to treat the problem from the inside out. This same protocol works for the treatment of boils, herpes sores, and other venereal diseases. Take both internal and external remedies for best results.

Harvesting: Harvest this herb early in the morning or late in the evening. Snip off the upper branches. Use them fresh or dry them for future use.

Warning: Some people are allergic to chickweed. The herb is considered safe, but should not be used by nursing women or pregnant women without the approval from a healthcare professional.

Recipes. Chickweed Decoction: Use fresh chickweed whenever possible to make this herbal decoction. It is an excellent internal cleanser and makes a good wash and external agent. You need 1 cup freshly picked chickweed leaves and 1 pint (500 ml) of water. Bring the water to a boil and add the chickweed leaves. Reduce the heat to low and simmer the leaves for 15 minutes. Cool the decoction and use it internally or externally. The internal dose is 1 to 2 ounces (30 to 60ml).

Chicory, *Cichorium intybus*

Common chicory is an annual or biannual plant in the Aster/Daisy Family. It originated from Eurasia and is found throughout North America, where it is known as an invasive species in several places. Common chicory is also called blue daisy, blue dandelion, blue sailors, blue weed, coffeeweed, cornflower, succory, wild bachelor's buttons, wild endive, and horseweed.

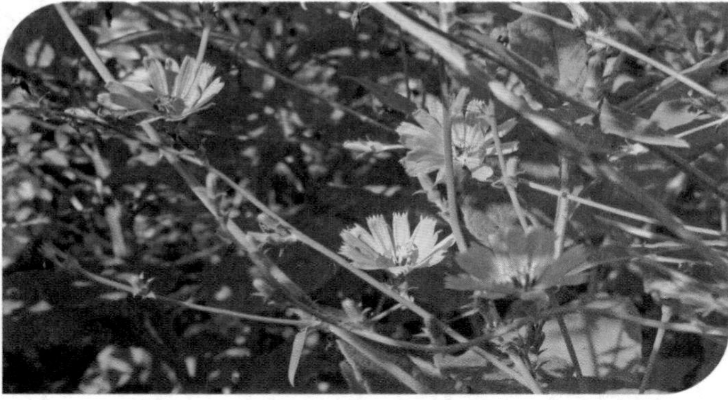

It is sometimes confused with Curly Endive (*Cichorium endivia*), a closely related plant often called chicory.

Identification: Chicory is easy to identify by its purple flowers when in bloom. Its stems are rigid with hairy lower stems. Its alternate lobed leaves are coarsely toothed and similar to dandelion leaves in appearance. The lower leaves are covered with hairs and grow up to 8 inches (20 cm) in length. The stems and leaves both exude a milky latex when cut.

The plant grows 1 to 3 feet (0.3m to 0.9m) tall and has numerous flower heads, each around 1 to 1 1/2 inches (2.5 cm to 3.75 cm) wide, appearing in clusters of two or three. Light blue-purple (and rarely pink or white) flowers bloom from July thru October. Petals grow in two rows with toothed ends. The blooms are open in the morning but close during the heat of the day. Its root is a thick, fleshy bitter taproot.

Edible Use: The leaves have a bitter taste, which can be reduced by boiling and draining. I prefer young leaves boiled, then sautéed with garlic and butter. The most famous use of chicory is as a coffee additive or substitute. Roast the roots and grind them. Roots may be eaten raw or cooked.

Medicinal Use: Chicory roots and seeds help eliminate intestinal worms and parasites, are antibacterial, antifungal, and hepatoprotective. Roots are being studied for use in cancer. The flowers and leaves are also used medicinally. It is a mild diuretic.

Sedative and Analgesic: The milky juice from the fresh root of chicory is similar to the milky sap of Wild Lettuce (*Lactuca* spp.), also in this book. They contain lactucin and lactucopicrin, which are sedative and analgesic (pain-killing). They are sesquiterpene lactones, so it is recommended to use the latex as is or, if you want a liquid form, to dry them and then extract the medicine in high proof alcohol or oil versus in water. Pain-relief is similar to ibuprofen.

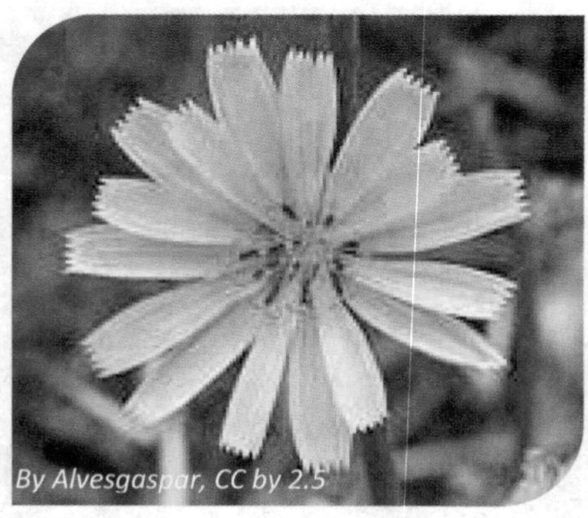
By Alvesgaspar, CC by 2.5

Antibacterial and Anti-Fungal (*Candida*): Chicory seed and root extracts are antibacterial and anti-fungal. Seeds work against *Staphylococcus*,

Pseudomonas, E. coli, and *Candida*. Roots work to kill *Staphylococcus, Bacillus, Salmonella, E. coli,* and *Micrococcus* as well as athlete's foot, ringworm, and jock itch. It can be taken internally and externally.

Anti-Parasitic and Malaria: Chicory root alcoholic extractions eliminate intestinal worms and the protozoan responsible for cerebral malaria (Plasmodium falciparum). The roots contain lactucin and lactucopicrin, both anti-malarials.

Liver and Gallbladder Disorders: The leaves, seeds, and roots of chicory are used to treat liver disorders. They are hepatoprotective. They promote the secretion of bile, treat jaundice, and treat enlargement of the spleen. They help fatty liver and to detox the liver.

Diabetes: Chicory leaf tincture, leaf powder, or a whole-plant alcoholic extraction helps regulate insulin levels, stimulate insulin secretion, and lower blood glucose levels.

Digestive Problems and Ulcers: Chicory coffee or tea made from the roots helps treat digestive problems and ulcers.

Skin Eruptions, Swellings, and Inflammations: For external use, wash blemishes with a chicory leaf infusion or apply crushed leaves as a poultice to areas of inflammation. Many people report that chicory infusion used as a wash nourishes the skin and gives it a more radiant and youthful appearance. It can be used as a face and body wash daily.

Harvesting: Only harvest plants that have not been exposed to car fumes and chemical spray along roadsides.

Leaves and flowers are easily picked throughout the season. Harvest the roots in the late autumn. Loosen the soil around the base of each plant, grab the plant at the base, and pull up as much of the tap root as possible. Clean and use them fresh or cut and dry them for future use.

Warning: Chicory can cause contact dermatitis in some people. It also causes skin irritations and rashes in some people if taken internally. Avoid chicory during pregnancy; it can stimulate menstruation. Chicory can interfere with beta-blocker drugs for the heart.

Recipes. Chicory Coffee: Clean the roots and chop them into small pieces. Lay them out on a cookie sheet to roast. Roast them in a very slow oven or over a fire. When the roots are completely roasted and dried throughout, grind them into a powder. Store the powder sealed in a cool, dry place. Brew like you would coffee.

Chives, *Allium schoenoprasum*

Allium schoenoprasum belongs to the Amaryllidaceae (Amaryllis) Family. It is a close relative of garlics, shallots, and leeks. These herbs are often cultivated in home gardens, but also occur wild in many areas. They are widespread across North America, Europe, and Asia. They are mostly used as a culinary herb.

Identification: Chives are bulb-forming plants that grow from 12 to 20 inches (30 cm to 50 cm) tall. Their slender bulbs are about an inch (2.5 cm) long and nearly 1/2 inch (1.25 cm) across. They grow from roots in dense clusters. The stems are tubular and hollow and grow up to 20 inches (50 cm) long and about an inch across. The stems have a softer texture before the emergence of the flower. Chives have grass-like leaves, which are shorter than the stems. The leaves are also tubular or round in cross-section and are hollow, which distinguishes it from garlic chives, *Allium tuberosum*.

Chives usually flower in April to May in southern regions and in June in northern regions. Its flowers are usually pale purple and grow in a dense inflorescence of 10 to 30 flowers that is ½ to 1 inch (1.25 cm to 2.5 cm) wide. Before opening, the inflorescence is typically surrounded by a papery bract. Fruits are small, 3-sectioned capsules. The seeds mature in the summer.

Edible Use: The leaves, roots, and flowers are all edible. Leaves have a mild onion flavor.

Medicinal Use: Chives have similar medical properties to those of garlic but are weaker overall. For this reason, it is used to a limited extent as a medicinal herb. Chives are also a mild stimulant, and have antiseptic and diuretic properties.

Digestion: Chives contain sulfide compounds, antibacterial compounds, and antifungal compounds that are effective in easing digestion and an upset stomach. They also stimulate the appetite.

Lowers Blood Pressure, Cholesterol, and Promotes Heart Health: Like other plants in the onion family, chives contain allicin, which helps reduce the levels of bad cholesterol in the body and improves the circulatory system and heart health. Regular consumption of chives reduces arterial plaques, relaxes the blood vessels, lowers high blood pressure, and decreases the risk of heart attacks and strokes.

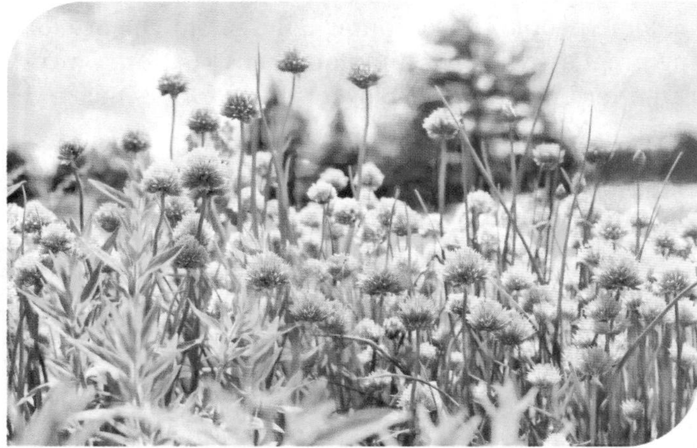

Detoxing the Body and Diuretic: The mild diuretic properties of chives help flush toxins from the body and encourage urination.

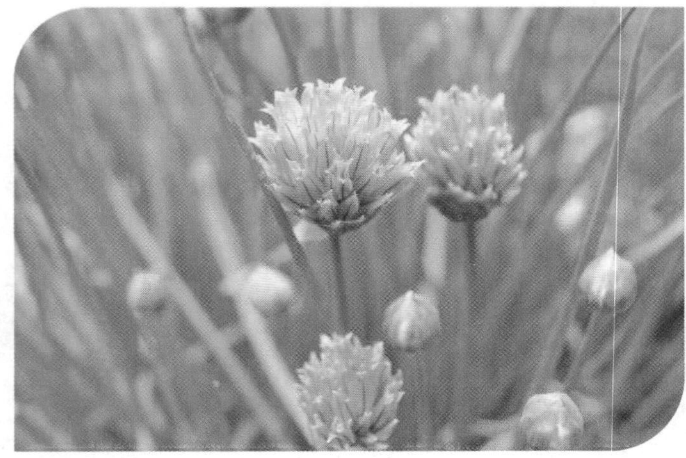

Anti-inflammatory: Chives have mild anti-inflammatory properties and are a good addition to the diet for people with diseases that involve inflammation, such as arthritis, autoimmune conditions, and inflammatory skin conditions.

Boosts the Immune System: Chives contain a wide range of vitamins and minerals, including vitamin C, which helps boost the immune system and stimulates the production of white blood cells.

Harvesting: Chives can be harvested as soon as they are big enough to clip and use. Snip off the leaves at the base. The plant will continue to grow and can be harvested 3 to 4 times a year when young (the first year) and even monthly as they mature. Store them fresh in the refrigerator or dry them for future use.

Comfrey, *Symphytum officinale*

Comfrey, is a member of the borage family. The herb is easily grown in your home garden and grows like a weed in many areas. It is also known as knit bone, boneset and slippery root.

Identification: Comfrey is a vigorous perennial herb with long lance-like leaves, each 12 to 18 inches (30 cm to 45 cm) long. The hairy leaves grow from a central crown on the ends of short stems. The plant reaches 2 to 5 feet (0.6m to 1.5m) in height and spreads to over 3 feet (0.9m) in diameter. It can be propagated from cuttings but is not invasive once planted. Comfrey flowers begin as a blue to purple bell, fading to pink as

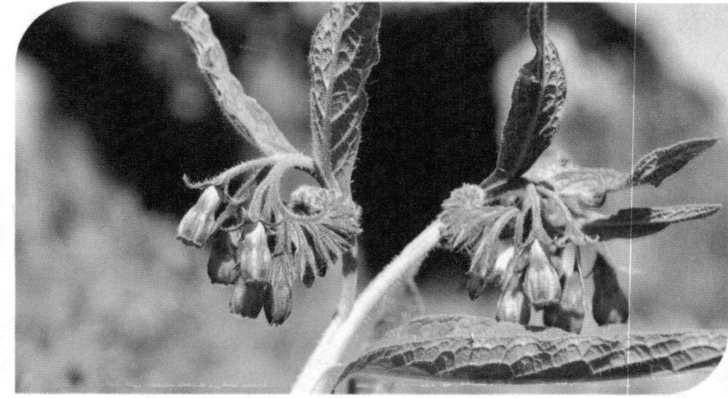

they age. The thick, tuberous roots have a thin black skin.

Edible Use: Comfrey leaves and roots are not edible because they contain small amounts of toxins that should not be consumed. The leaves can be used to make a medicinal tea or gargle.

Medicinal Use: This herb is a valuable remedy that accelerates healing of the skin and wounds. A compress of the roots or leaves can be applied directly to the skin or made into a salve. It inhibits the growth of bacteria, helping to prevent infections, and minimizes scarring. It is mucilaginous and contains the compound allantoin, which boosts cell growth and repair. It also is an excellent anti-inflammatory and relieves pain, inflammation, and swelling in joints and muscles. Comfrey tea is best used to alleviate stomach problems, heavy menstrual bleeding, bloody urine, breathing problems, cancer, and chest pain. Be careful with internal use (see Warning section). It can also be gargled to treat gum disease or sore throat.

Sprains, Bruises and Breaks: Comfrey Salve or comfrey compresses are one of the best remedies for sprains, strains, bruised muscles and joints, and fractured bones. The herb speeds up healing while increasing mobility and relieving the pain and swelling. Apply the salvet or a poultice made from crushed comfrey root up to four times a day. Make sure that a broken bone is set before applying comfrey.

Back Pain: Use comfrey root salve to treat back pain. Applied three times a day, it relieves bone and joint pains.

Osteoarthritis: Likewise, external Comfrey Salve is beneficial for knee and joint pain due to osteoarthritis.

Coughs, Congestion, and Asthma: Comfrey Tea treats coughs, congestion, and asthma. The herb reduces the inflammation and soothes the irritation.

Minor Skin Injuries, Burns, Rashes, Eczema, Psoriasis and Wounds: One of the best uses for comfrey is in healing minor injuries to the skin. Rashes, eczema, burns, and skin wounds heal quickly when the herb is used. I prefer to use the root for this purpose, but leaves can also be used. Apply Comfrey Salve three times a day or use bruised leaves or crushed root to make a poultice for the damaged skin. I also use Comfrey Tea or Comfrey Root Decoction as a wash for the area, especially for rashes, acne, eczema, and psoriasis. Do not use for deep wounds or puncture wounds as it heals them too quickly, blocking in infection.

Stomach Upsets, Ulcers of the Stomach and Lungs: Comfrey is used to treat internal ulcers and the bleeding they cause. The comfrey stops the bleeding and helps the wounded tissue heal. You can drink the tea or use the decoction.

Harvesting: Comfrey leaves are best harvested in the spring or early summer, before the plant blooms. They can be harvested in several cuttings and dried for later use. The roots can be dug at any time as needed. Leave behind part of the roots to encourage continued growth and an additional crop the next year.

Warning: Harmful toxins in comfrey are believed to cause liver damage, lung damage, or cancer when used in highly concentrated doses. For this reason, many healers do not recommend internal use of comfrey. However, small doses have been used safely in herbal medicines for hundreds of years with no reported ill effects. Use internally with caution or under care.

Comfrey should not be used by pregnant or breastfeeding women.

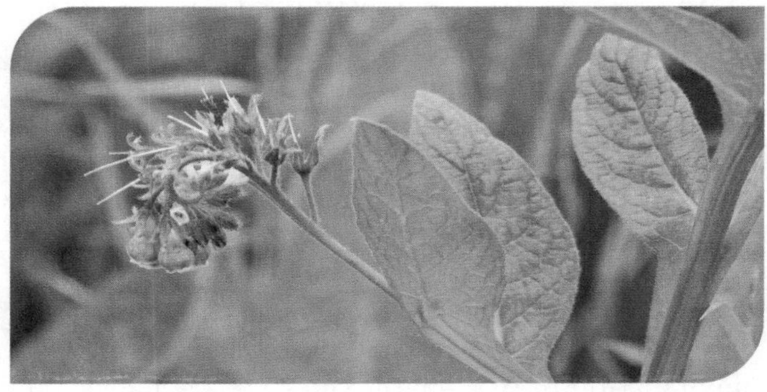

Both oral use and skin application could be hazardous and could cause birth defects. Do not use comfrey if you have liver disease or any liver problems. Comfrey heals wounds very quickly. As such, it is recommended that bone fractures and bone breaks are properly set before using it. This also applies for puncture wounds, as its rapid healing can seal in the bacterial infection.

Recipes. Comfrey Salve.: You'll need: Comfrey root and/or leaves to fill a pint (500ml) jar, 1 cup Organic Olive Oil and 1/4 cup of beeswax, or more.

Allow the comfrey leaves and root to dry, removing excess moisture. This can be done in a low oven, dehydrator, or by leaving them out in a warm place for a few days. Turn the oven on to its lowest setting.

Place the dried leaves and chopped root pieces into a pint (500ml) jar. Add 1 cup of olive oil and place the open jar in the oven. Allow the oil to warm and infuse for 90 minutes. Remove the jar from the oven and cover with a cloth to cool. When cool, place the lid on the jar and allow it to steep for 2 to 3 weeks in a cool, dark place. Strain the oil, removing the leaves and roots.

Combine the oil and the beeswax in a pot and warm gently until the beeswax is melted (4:1 ratio of oil to beeswax). Test the consistency of the oil by dipping a small amount onto waxed paper or aluminum foil and place in the freezer for five minutes. If the oil is thick enough, pour the mixture into a jar or wide mouth container. If not add a little more beeswax and test again.

Continue until desired consistency is reached. If the mixture is too thick you can warm it again and stir in a little more oil. Note: use an old non-aluminum pot to heat the oil and wax. It is difficult to clean. I have a small pot that I use only for this purpose.

Common Flax, *Linum usitatissimum*

Also known as Linseed, this is a useful plant for making medicine, oil, and fabric. Many people take it as a nutritional supplement. It is in the *Linaceae* (Flax) Family.

Identification: Common Flax is an annual. While rarely found growing wild, it is usually easy to find a cultivated crop or to grow yourself. The mature plant is 3 to 4 feet (0.9m to 1.2m) tall. A loose cluster of blue-purple stalked flowers grows at the tips of the branching stems. Each ¾ to 1 inch (2 cm to 2.5 cm) wide flower has 5 ovate petals surrounded by 5 erect, blue-tipped stamens with a green ovary. The 5 sepals have a lance-shape. Flax has simple, alternate, erect green leaves that are 1/2 to 1 1/2 inches (1.25 cm to 3.75 cm) long and very narrow. They are stalkless and have smooth margins. Its stems are mostly unbranched and erect, and has multiple round, smooth stems growing from its base. Flax fruit is a round, dry, 5-lobed capsule that is 1/4 -1/2 (0.75 cm to 1.25 cm) inch in diameter.

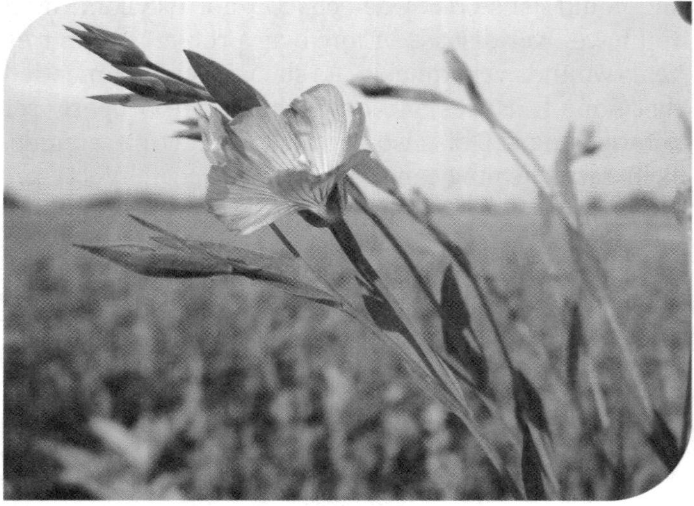

Edible Use: The sprouts and seeds can be eaten raw or cooked. Careful eating the sprouts raw as they can stop up the bowel. Chew seeds well to access their nutrition, as they don't digest well whole.

Medicinal Use. As a Nutritional Supplement: Flax seed is rich in dietary fiber, protein, omega-3 fatty acids, and other nutrients. I grind flax and chia seeds fresh and eat them daily for health. I find that the fresh seeds are better as oil goes rancid quite quickly.

Cholesterol Control: Ingesting crushed flaxseeds on a daily basis is a good way to lower your cholesterol and LDL.

Autoimmune Issues: Flax seeds are high in omega 3 fatty acids, alpha-linolenic acid (ALA), and lignans. These compounds help regulate immune response, suppress inflammation, have neuroprotective effects, act as antioxidants, and modulate hormonal influences in autoimmune conditions.

Respiratory Problems: Flax seed oil helps with respiratory problems, including ARDS (acute respiratory distress syndrome). Its anti-inflammatory effects help coughs, sore throat, and congestion.

Constipation: For constipation, try two teaspoons of ground flax seed every morning, taken with a full glass of water.

Skin, Boils, Abscesses, Herpes, Acne, Burns: A warm poultice of flax seed oil on a cotton ball or applied directly helps heal these common skin problems. Flax is an excellent anti-inflammatory both internally and externally. For boils, add *Lobelia inflata* root to flax seed oil and apply it directly to the boil or use as a poultice.

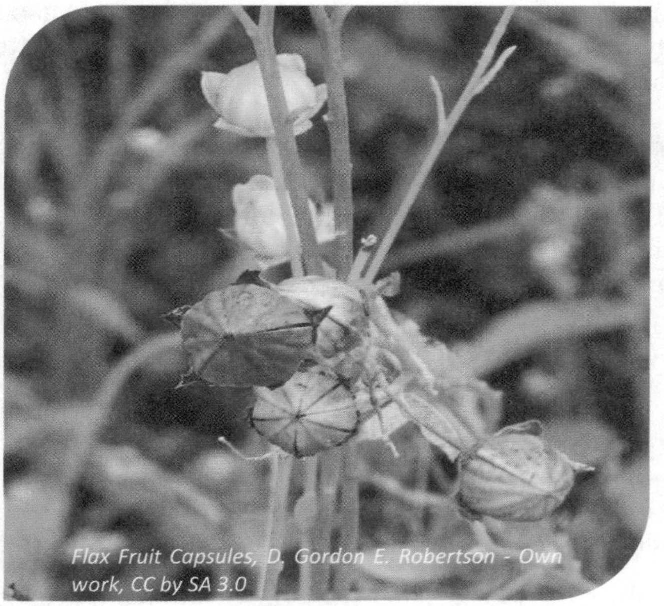
Flax Fruit Capsules, D. Gordon E. Robertson - Own work, CC by SA 3.0

Balancing Hormones: Flax seed contains lignans, a type of phytoestrogen. This helps balance female hormones, especially in post-menopausal women, and helps with symptoms of menopause.

Cancer: Flax seed and flax seed oil work as a complementary treatment as well as for the prevention of breast cancer and prostate cancer, where they seem to reduce PSA (prostate specific antigen) levels. Flax seeds help decrease breast cancer risk, lower the risk of metastasizing, and help to kill cancer cells in post-menopausal women. Consult with your oncologist.

Harvesting: Flax seed is harvested in the same manner as wheat. Harvest when the plant and fruits are dry and the seedpods begin to split. Shake over a sheet and sift. You may have to crush the seedpods to access the seeds.

Warning and Recommendations: Ground and powdered flax seed go rancid very quickly. I keep my flax seed whole until I need them, then grind or crush only the needed amount. Drink plenty of water with flax seeds.

Couch Grass, *Agropyron (Elymus) repens*

Couch Grass is often considered a simple weed and a nuisance; however, it has a list of medicinal properties that can't be ignored. It is also called dog grass, witchgrass, quack grass, and twitch grass. It can grow up to 3 feet (0.9m) tall and is part of the Poaceae (Grass) Family.

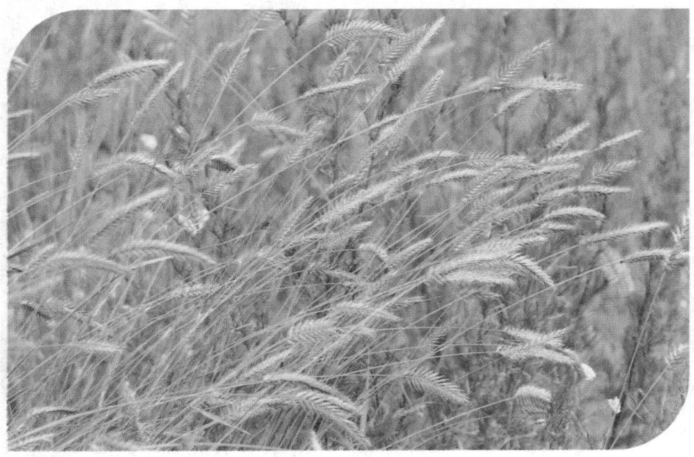

Identification: The crawling tubular root is elongated while the leaves are slender. Each short stem produces five to seven leaves and possibly a flower spike at the terminal. Each flower spike is composed of oval-shaped spikelets less than an inch (2.5 cm) long. The flowers appear in late June through August. The seed heads look like a stalk of grain. The roots are elongated, thin, tubular and whitish in color with yellow ends. Couch grass grows aggressively and is capable of crowding out agricultural crops and is often found on cultivated land. It likes loose and sandy soils and will die out as the soil becomes compacted.

Edible Use: The grain has food value as fodder for animals, and I am told that the root is sometimes eaten when food is scarce. I've never tried it. The roots can also be ground and roasted to make a coffee substitute.

Medicinal Use: Use the rhizomes of this plant to make a tincture, infusion, or decoction.

Urinary Tract Problems, Kidney Stones, Cystitis, Gallbladder Diseases: Couch grass is effective at treating urinary tract problems including inflammations, infections, and slow and painful urination caused by muscle spasms of the bladder and urethra. It soothes the mucous membranes and relieves the pain. It is a diuretic that increases the production of urine. It also works to dissolve kidney stones and gravel and treat cystitis and diseases of the gallbladder. Try using couch grass in combination with Usnea and bearberry to treat urinary tract infections.

Swollen Prostate: The herb is effective for treatment of swollen prostate glands, especially from gonorrhea. It is often combined with saw palmetto for this use.

Gout: Try couch grass decoction for treating gout.

Rheumatoid Arthritis: The diuretic properties, anti-inflammatory properties, and analgesic properties of couch grass make it effective in treating rheumatoid arthritis.

Jaundice: The anti-inflammatory properties and diuretic properties, combined with the benefits to the urinary tract and gallbladder, make couch grass a good choice for treating jaundice. It helps the body eliminate toxins and allows it to heal.

Recipes. Couch Grass Decoction: Ingredients: 4 ounces (113g) couch grass roots, chopped and 1-quart (1 Liter) water. Bring the water and the roots to a boil and reduce the heat to a simmer. Simmer the roots, uncovered, until the liquid is reduced by half, leaving approximately 2 cups of liquid. Store in the refrigerator for 3 days or freeze for longer periods.

Dandelion, *Taraxacum officinale*

Most children relish the opportunity to blow a puff of dandelion seeds into the wind. This wonderful plant is commonly regarded as a weed and can be found growing in sidewalk cracks and across untended roadsides and lawns. There are some look-alike flowers, so be sure of your identification before harvesting the plant. It is in the Aster/Daisy Family.

Identification: Dandelion is a perennial herbaceous plant native to North America. It grows from a tap-root that reaches deep into the soil. The plant grows up to a foot in height and flowers from April to June. It produces a yellow flower head consisting of florets. Leaves grow from the base of the plant in an elongated shape with highly jagged edges. The edges are said to resemble a lion's tooth, giving the plant its name.

Edible Use: The entire plant is edible and nutritious. The young leaves are best for greens, since the leaves grow more bitter with age. Young leaves can be cooked or eaten raw. Dandelion root is sometimes dried and roasted for use as a coffee substitute. The roots can also be cooked and eaten. They are bitter, with a taste similar to a turnip. Dandelion flowers make a nice salad garnish or can be battered and fried. Unopened flower buds are prepared into pickles similar to capers. Flowers can also be boiled and served with butter. Dandelion leaves and roots make a pleasant, but bitter tea. Flowers are fermented to make dandelion wine. Leaves and roots are used to flavor herbal beers and soft drinks.

Medicinal Use: The entire dandelion plant is used medicinally. The bitter roots are good for gastrointestinal and liver problems, while the leaves have a powerful diuretic effect. The plant makes a great general tonic and benefits the entire body. It is high in vitamins, minerals, and antioxidants. I use dandelion tea and tincture for internal use.

Digestion Problems, Liver and Gallbladder Function: Dandelion root is used to aid digestion and benefits the kidneys, gallbladder, and liver. It stimulates bile production, helping with the digestion of fats and toxin removal. Use it to treat jaundice and raise energy levels after infections. It removes toxins from the body and restores the electrolyte balance, which improves liver health and function.

I do a 2-week liver cleanse with my homemade Liver Tonic – a Dandelion Root and Milk Thistle seed tincture blend – every 6 months for general health. It also helps prevent gallstones. Dandelion contains inulin, a carbohydrate that helps maintain healthy gut flora and helps to regulate blood sugar levels. The plant is rich in fiber, which adds bulk to the stool, reducing the

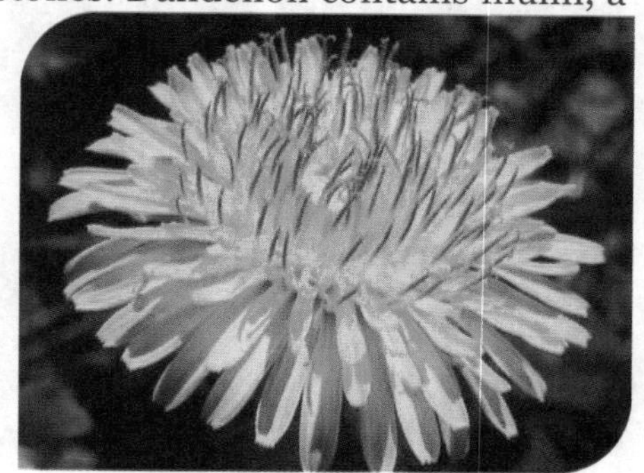

Dandelion FlowerGreg Hume, CC BY-SA 3.0

chances of constipation, diarrhea, and digestive issues.

Liver Protection and Healing: Vitamins and antioxidants in dandelion protect the liver and keep it healthy. It helps protect the liver from toxins and treats liver hemorrhages. Dandelion tea is used to treat non-alcoholic fatty liver disease. My Liver Tonic Blend (Dandelion Root and Milk Thistle Seed extract) reversed a patient's liver disease to the point that she no longer needs a liver transplant. This blend is also good for cirrhosis and hepatitis.

Diuretic and Detoxifying the Body: Dandelion leaves are a powerful diuretic and blood purifier. They stimulate the liver and gallbladder while eliminating toxins through the production and excretion of urine. They also help flush the kidneys. Even though dandelion is a diuretic it helps replace lost potassium and other minerals that are lost when water and salts are expelled.

Skin Wounds, Corns, and Warts: Fresh dandelion juice applied to the skin helps wounds heal and fights the bacteria and fungi that would otherwise cause infections. Dandelion sap, sometimes called dandelion milk, is useful to treat itches, ringworm, eczema, warts, and corns. Apply dandelion sap directly to the affected skin. Dandelion tea can be used as a wash on the skin to help healing. Dandelion sap is also useful in treating acne. It inhibits the formation of acne blemishes and reduces scarring. Some people are allergic to dandelion sap, so watch for signs of dermatitis on first use.

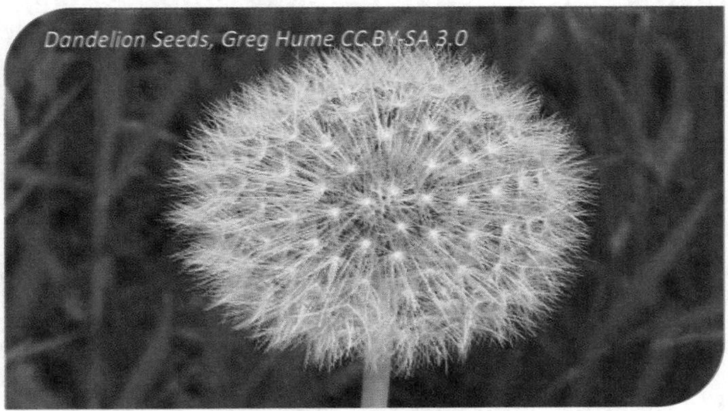
Dandelion Seeds, Greg Hume CC BY-SA 3.0

Osteoporosis and Bone Health: The calcium and vitamin K found in dandelion can protect bones from osteoporosis and arthritis. It helps stabilize bone density and strengthen the bone.

Controls Blood Sugar: Dandelion has several effects that are beneficial to diabetics. Dandelion juice stimulates the production of insulin in the pancreas, which helps regulate blood sugar levels and prevent dangers blood sugar swings. The plant is a natural diuretic which helps remove excess sugars from the body. It also helps control lipid levels.

Urinary Tract Disorders: The diuretic nature of dandelion helps eliminate toxins from the kidneys and urinary tract. The herb also acts as a disinfectant, inhibiting bacterial growth in the urinary system.

Prevents and Treats Cancer: Dandelion extracts are high in antioxidants, which reduce free radicals in the body and the risk of cancer. Its role in removing toxins from the body is also helpful. Researchers have shown that Dandelion Root coupled with Burdock Root have potential in treating cancer.

Prevents Iron Deficiency Anemia: Dandelions have high levels of iron, vitamins, and other minerals. Iron is an important part of the hemoglobin in blood and essential for healthy red blood cell formation. Using dandelion and eating the greens helps keep iron levels high.

Treating Hypertension: As a diuretic, dandelion juice helps eliminate excess sodium from the body and bring down blood pressure. It also helps reduce cholesterol ratios and raises the "good" HDL levels.

Boosts the Immune System: Dandelion boosts the immune system and helps fight off microbial and fungal agents.

Mastitis and Lactation: Dandelion has traditionally been used to enhance milk production and for treatment of mastitis. Check in with your doctor for this use.

Fights Inflammation and Arthritis: Dandelion contains antioxidants, phytonutrients and essential fatty acids that reduce inflammation in the body. This relieves swelling and related pain in the body. Inflammation is the root cause of many diseases, such as arthritis. Taraxasterol, found in dandelion roots, has shown great promise for Osteoarthritis.

Harvesting: I prefer to gather dandelion leaves in the spring when they are young and less bitter. I dry them for later medicinal use. Often, they grow in lawns or parks that have been sprayed so be careful where you harvest them.

For roots, I prefer the roots of plants that are 2-years old or older. The roots are larger and more medicinally potent. Grab the plant at the base and pull the entire plant up. The root is a deep taproot and will require some force.

You can also dig around the plant at a modest distance to help remove the entire root. As many gardeners know, leaving just a bit of the root will allow the plant to regrow.

So, if you want more dandelions simply leave part of the root intact. Plants dug in the autumn have more medicinal properties and higher levels of inulin.

Warning: Dandelion is generally considered safe, although some people may be allergic to it. Do not take dandelion if you are allergic to plants from the same family, or similar plants such as ragweed, chrysanthemum, marigold, yarrow, or daisy. Do not take dandelion if you are pregnant and consult your doctor if nursing.

Consult your doctor before taking if you are taking prescription medicines. Some people have reported dermatitis as a result of touching the plant or using the sap. Do not use dandelion if you are allergic.

Recipes: Dandelion Tea. Ingredients: 1/2 to 2 teaspoons of roasted dandelion root, in small pieces and 1 cup of boiling water. Pour boiling water over roasted or dried dandelion root and allow it to steep for 20 minutes. Strain the tea and drink.

Do not add sweeteners, as they reduce the herb's effectiveness. Milk may be used to taste, if desired.

Drink 3 cups per day for general medicinal use.

Dill, *Anethum graveolens*

Dill is a familiar aromatic herb cultivated in herb gardens across the country. It is in the Apiaceae /Umbelliferae (Celery/Carrot) Family.

Identification: Dill grows to 30 inches (75 cm) tall with a slender, hollow, and erect stem and feathery leaves. Leaves are finely divided and delicate in appearance, and are 4 to 8 inches (10 cm to 20 cm) long. They are similar to fennel in appearance.

Numerous tiny yellow or white flowers appear on umbrellas that are 3/4 to 3 1/2 inches (1.875 cm to 8.75 cm) in diameter as soon as the weather turns hot.

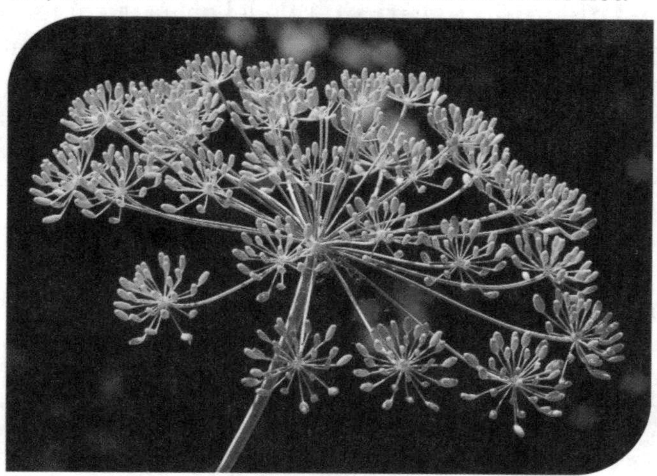

The seeds are small, up to 1/5 of an inch (0.625 cm) long with a ridged surface.

Edible Use: Dill is widely enjoyed as an herb, especially with fish and in pickles. The leaves, seeds, and stems are edible.

Medicinal Use. Colic: Colicky babies respond well to a dill infusion. The dill soothes the stomach and calms the baby. This is a popular colic remedy because it is easily attained, effective, and known to be safe for children.

Digestive Issues, Irritable Bowel Syndrome, Menstrual Cramps, and Muscle Spasms: Dill Leaf Infusion relieves cramping and muscle spasms including those in the digestive tract. It relieves the symptoms of painful spasms without treating the underlying cause. Use it to give immediate relief while looking for the cause of the problem. A Dill Seed Infusion or Dill Tincture may also be used.

Stimulates Milk Flow: Dill Infusion helps nursing mothers increase their milk flow. It has a beneficial calming effect on both mother and child.

Halitosis: Temporary bad breath is easily solved by chewing on dill leaves or seeds, but the problem can be completely alleviated by chewing the seeds daily. Over the long term the seeds attack the causes of the problem causing a permanent solution.

Flatulence: For abdominal flatulence, take Dill Seed Infusion before each meal.

Harvesting: Harvest leaves throughout the summer until the flowers appear in late summer. Gather leaves in the late morning after the dew has dried and use them fresh, freeze them, or dry them for later use. I collect the seed heads once the flowers are fully open, if needed, or I allow them to completely ripen for seed collection. The brown seeds are collected and dried for storage.

Warning: Consumption of dill can cause sensitivity to the sun in some people. People sometimes have a rash appear after exposure to sunlight.

Recipes. Dill Leaf Infusion: Ingredients: 1 Tablespoon chopped dill leaves and 1 cup boiling water. Pour the boiling water over the dill leaves and cover the cup. Let it steep until cool enough to drink, then strain out the leaves.

Dill Seed Infusion: You need 1 to 2 tablespoons dill seeds and 1 cup water. Bring the seeds and water to a boil, turn off the heat and cover the pot. Allow the infusion to steep for 15 minutes. Cool and strain out the seeds. Take one cup before each meal for digestive issues.

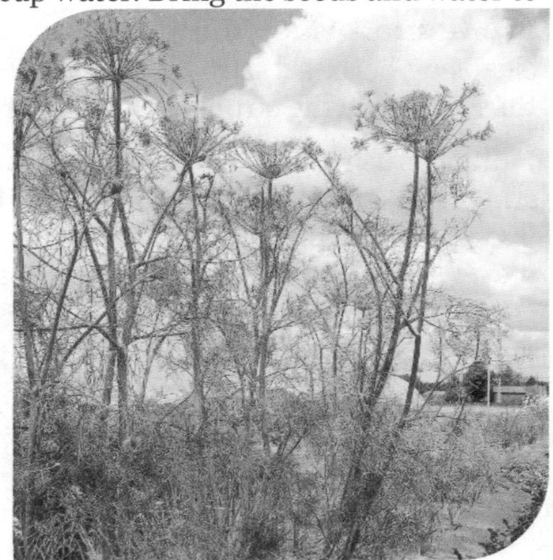

Dock (Curly/Yellow), *Rumex crispus*

Docks and Sorrels, genus *Rumex*, is a group of over 200 different varieties in the Polygonaceae (Buckwheat) Family. Here I am referring specifically to *Rumex crispus* and its medicinal use, but broad-leaved dock, *Rumex obstusifolius*, is used in a similar manner. Curly Dock is a biennial herb that grows across the globe. The plant is also called yellow dock, sour dock, narrow-leaved dock, and curled dock.

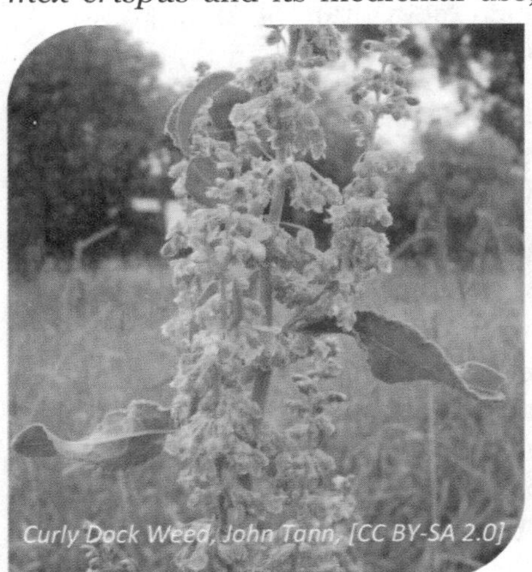

Curly Dock Weed, John Tann, [CC BY-SA 2.0]

Identification: Flower stalks grow from the base (similar to a rosette) with smooth, leathery, fleshy leaves growing in a large cluster at the apex. Leaves are wavy or curly on the edges and have a coarse texture. These leaves can grow up to 2 feet (0.6m) long and are only 3 inches (7.5 cm) wide, making them long, narrow and wavy. Small veins curve out toward the edge of the leaf and then turn back towards the central vein. Leaves farther up the plant may vary in size and appearance. On older leaves the central vein is sometimes tinged with red.

The flower stalk is approximately 3 feet (0.9m) in height with clustered flowers and seeds. Tiny green flowers grow in dense heads on the flower stalk during the second year.

The 3-sided seeds are brown, shiny, and covered by a papery sheath that looks like heart-shaped wings. The root is a long yellow, forking taproot that regenerates the plant each year.

Edible Use: Curly dock has a lemony flavor and its leaves are used as a cooked vegetable. Young leaves can

1Curly Dock Weed, By Olivier Pichard [CC BY-SA 3.0]

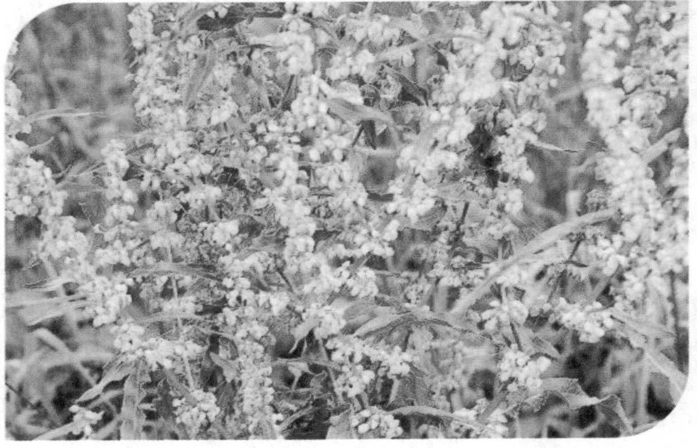

be eaten raw (old ones can too but they don't taste as good). Leaves contain varying amounts of oxalic acid and tannin. The seeds can be pounded into a flour. The root is generally not eaten but it is used for medicine.

Medicinal Use: Curly dock is a purifying and cleansing herb. All parts of the plant can be used, but the roots have the strongest healing properties.

I often crush dock leaves to put on stinging nettle stings. My grandmother showed me this trick when I was a child visiting her in England and I've been using it ever since. They tend to grow near each other, which is very useful.

Constipation and Diarrhea: Curly dock is a gentle and safe laxative for the treatment of mild constipation. It can also cause or relieve diarrhea, depending on the dosage and other factors such as harvest time and soil conditions.

Skin Problems: Curly dock weed is useful externally to treat a wide variety of skin problems due to its cleansing properties.

Taken internally, it is a tonic. Its dried or pounded root can be used as a poultice, salve, or powder applied to sores, wounds, or other skin problems.

Liver, Gall Bladder and Detox: Curly dock root is a bitter tonic for the gall bladder and liver. It increases bile production, which helps the body with detoxification. It is helpful for any condition that can benefit from purifying and cleansing the body from toxins. It is often combined with Greater Burdock to create a stronger detoxifying effect.

Harvesting: Harvest the root early in autumn and dry it for later use. Dig up the entire plant and root if possible and wash the root lightly. Cut before drying. Harvest leaves from spring through summer as needed. Look for leaves that are fresh and curled. Avoid leaves that are brown or full of bug holes. Also avoid areas that are near highways or that have been sprayed with pesticides.

Recipes. Curly Dock Tincture: You need fresh curly dock root, grated, 80-proof vodka or other drinking alcohol and a glass jar with tight-fitting lid. Place the grated root in a clean glass jar. Fill the jar, covering the root completely, with 80-proof alcohol.

Allow the tincture to steep for 6 to 8 weeks, shaking gently every day. Strain out the root pieces and place the tincture in a clean glass jar. Store in a cool, dark place for up to 7 years.

Echinacea angustifolia and *E. purpurea*, Purple Coneflower

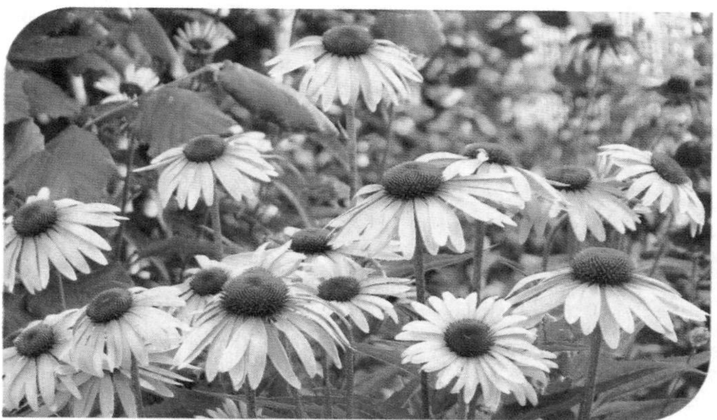

Close up of flower disc, Photo by Bernie, CC by SA 3.0

Echinacea is commonly called Purple Coneflower. It is a pretty, purple sunflower-like flowering plant that has strong medicine. It is native to North America and belongs to the Asteraceae (Daisy) Family. It is widespread and easy to cultivate in the garden. Echinacea grows wild in open rocky prairies and plains.

Identification: Purple coneflower is a perennial herb that is 6 to 24 inches (15 cm to 60 cm) tall with a woody, often branching taproot. This plant has one to several rough-hairy stems that are mostly unbranched.

The leaves are alternate, simple, and narrowly lance-shaped. The stem leaves are widely spaced and attached alternately to the lower half of the stem. Edges of leaves are toothless and have three distinct veins along its length. Stem and leaves are rough and hairy to touch. Its stems may be purple or green tinged. Echinacea Flowers look like lavender sunflowers. Its flowerheads are 1 ½ to 3 inches (3.75 cm to 7.5 cm) wide and are at the ends of long stalks. They bloom in summer. The disk flowers are 5-lobed, brownish-purple in color, and are situated among stiff bracts with yellow pollen. Its fruits are small, dark, 4- angled achenes.

Medicinal Use: This herb has a modulating effect on the body's natural immune system, encouraging it

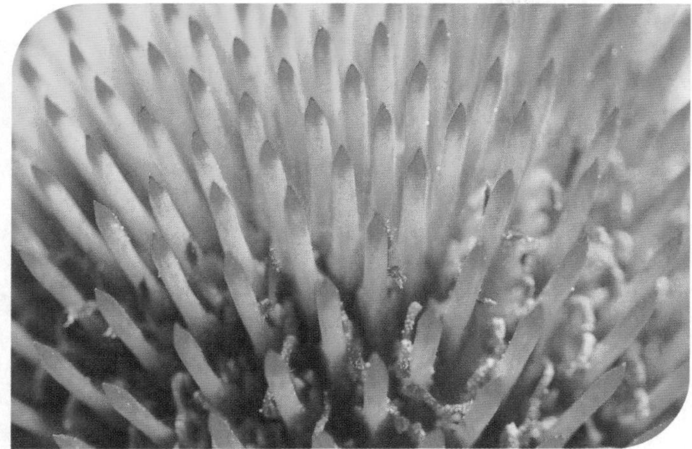

to operate more efficiently. It raises the body's resistance to bacterial and viral infections by stimulating the immune system. It also has anti-inflammatory and pain-relieving functions.

Do not use internally if you have an autoimmune condition. Most people seem aware that Echinacea is an herb for preventing and healing colds and the flu, but these plants can do a lot more. The root and leaves are used medicinally.

Urinary Tract Infections: The anti-microbial and anti-inflammatory effects of Echinacea make it an ideal choice for the treatment of urinary tract infections. It is a standard UTI treatment and is often combined with goldenseal root. Do not take either of these herbs if you have an autoimmune condition.

Colds and the Flu: Echinacea is known to reduce the impact of the common cold and the flu. People who begin taking Echinacea extract or tea immediately upon feeling sick heal much more quickly than those who do not.

In general, people who take Echinacea get well up to 4 days faster than those who don't (note that the same holds true for blue elderberry). For best results, they should begin taking Echinacea as soon as they notice symptoms, taking a double dose three times on the first day and then take three regular doses each day during the illness.

Allergies and Respiratory Diseases: Echinacea helps to relieve allergies by stimulating and balancing the immune system. It is especially helpful in relieving asthma attacks. While it doesn't cure asthma, it reduces the severity of the attack and helps the patient get over attacks. It is also useful for treating bronchitis.

For Infections, Burns, Wounds and as an Anti-Fungal: Echinacea is an antibiotic, antifungal antiviral, and it stimulates the immune system. It is helpful to relieve infections of all kinds. It is used both externally and internally.

Snakebite, Insect and Spider Bites, and Stings: Echinacea is used to treat spider bites and insect stings. It does a good job of neutralizing the poison and reducing the pain. It is said to be useful for snakebites, as it is a strong anti-inflammatory.

Harvesting: Harvest the roots in autumn when the plant has died back. Dig up the entire plant, watching for branched roots. Scrub the dirt from the root and dry it for later use.

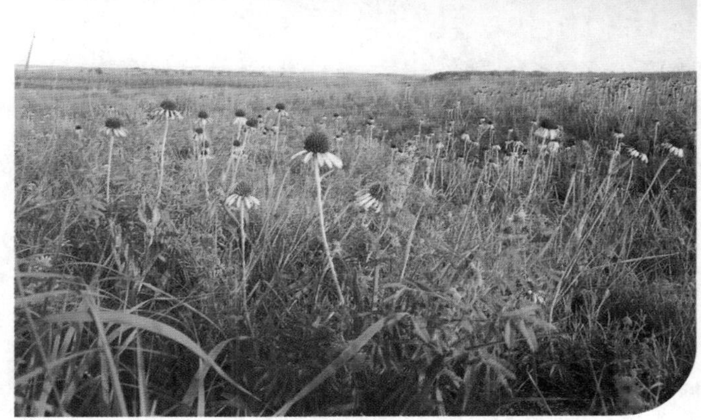

Warning: Do not use internally long-tem as it may cause digestive upset. People with autoimmune conditions should not use Echinacea internally as it is an immune-system booster and may lead to a flare-up.

Recipes. Echinacea Tincture: 1-pint (500ml) of vodka or rum, at least 80 proof, 1 cup of loosely packed Echinacea leaf and root, chopped fine, 1-pint(500ml) glass jar with a tight-fitting lid.

Put the loosely packed Echinacea leaf and finely chopped root into the jar. Fill with 80 proof vodka or rum and tightly fasten the lid. Keep the herb covered and shake the jar daily for 2 months. Add more alcohol when needed to keep the jar full. Strain the herbs. Keep the extract covered in a cool, dark place.

Elecampane, *Inula helenium*

Elecampane, a member of the sunflower family Asteraceae, is also commonly known as horse-heal, horse-elder, wild sunflower, starwort and elfdock. According to legend, the plant sprung up where the tears fell from Helen of Troy. The plant was considered sacred to the Celts and was thought to be associated with the fairy folk.

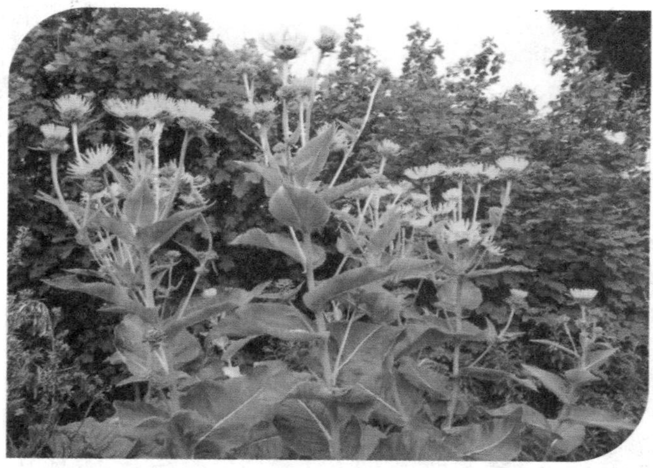

Elecampane is found in moist soil and shady places. It is cultivated in North America and is naturalized in the eastern United States growing in pastures, along roadsides, and at the base of eastern and southern facing slopes.

Identification: Elecampane is an upright herb that grows up to 6 feet (2m) in height. The large rough leaves are toothed and can be egg-shaped, elliptical, or lance-shaped. Lower leaves have a stalk, while the upper ones grow directly on the stem. Each leaf is up to 12 to 20 inches long (15cm-30cm) and 5 inches (12cm) wide. The upper side of the leaf is hairy and green, while the underside is whitish and velvety.

Flower heads are up to 3 inches (7 cm) in diameter and contain 50 to 100 yellow ray flowers and 100 to 250 yellow disc flowers. Elecampane blooms from June to August. The flowers are large, bright yellow, and resemble a double sunflower. The brown aromatic root branches below ground. It is large, thick, mucilaginous, and bitter with a camphoraceous odor and a floral background scent.

Edible Use: The root has been used in the making of absinthe and as a condiment. It stimulates pungent and bitter tastes, but it also has a sweet flavor due to its high polysaccharide content (inulin). Inulin, not to be confused with insulin, is a prebiotic that is used to feed and support healthy gut bacteria.

Medicinal Use: The elecampane root is the part most often used medicinally. Asian traditions also use the flowers, but I have had best results with the roots.

Elecampane root is useful fresh and dried. It can be infused into honey, extracted in alcohol, made into cough syrup, or made into a tea.

In most cases, it is best to start with a small dose and slowly increase it until the best results are obtained without nausea or overly drying effects.

Elecampane contains alantolactone and isoalantolactone, which is antibacterial, antifungal, and acts as a vermifuge (against parasites). These compounds also demonstrate anti-cancer activity, helping with apoptosis (programmed cell death).

Asthma, Bronchitis, Mucus, Whooping Cough, Influenza, and Tuberculosis: Elecampane root is useful as an expectorant and cough preventative in asthma, bronchitis, whooping cough, and tuberculosis. It lessens the need to cough by loosening phlegm and making the cough productive. It is beneficial for any respiratory illness with excess mucus discharge. Not recommended for dry coughs. It soothes bronchial tube linings, reduces swelling and irritation of the respiratory tract, cleanses the lungs, and fights harmful organisms in the respiratory tract. For acute coughs, use small, frequent doses. It is also useful to support lung health in asthma patients (as is mullein).

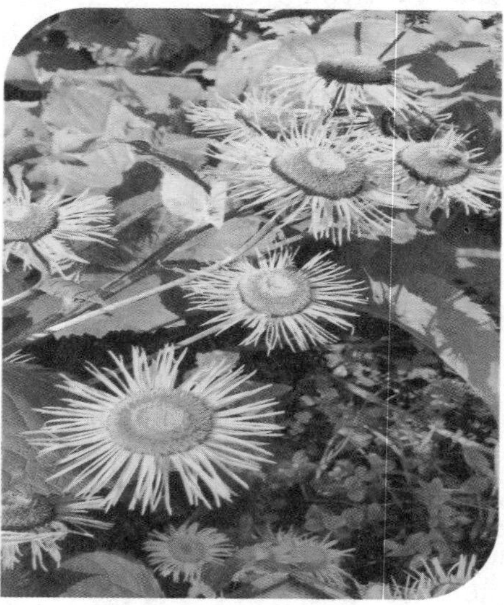

Stimulates Digestion and Appetite: While elecampane is mostly valued for its effects on the respiratory system, it is also valuable for treating digestive system problems. It is warming, draining, and bitter.

Use elecampane for poor digestion, poor absorption, poor appetite, mucus in the digestive system, excess gas, and lethargy or sluggishness of the digestive system.

Elecampane strengthens digestion and improves absorption which is beneficial in malnourished or undernourished patients. It also treats nausea and diarrhea.

Type 2 Diabetes: The high inulin content in elecampane is helpful for patients with high blood sugar and for type 2 diabetes patients. Inulin slows down sugar metabolism, reduces blood glucose spikes and decreases insulin resistance. It may also reduce inflammation associated with diabetes.

Intestinal Parasites: Elecampane is a vermifuge that eliminates intestinal parasites from the body, including hookworm, roundworm, threadworm, and whipworm.

Cancer: Elecampane contains alantolactone and isoalantolactone, which have been shown to help with programmed cell death (apoptosis) for certain cancers.

Harvesting: Harvest fresh elecampane root in the fall after the plant has produced seed, or in the early spring before leaves appear. I prefer roots that are two to three years old. Older roots are too woody, and younger roots lack their full medicinal potential. It is best to dig up some of the larger horizontal roots and leave the remaining roots so the plant can continue growing.

Warning: Large doses of elecampane can cause nausea, vomiting, and diarrhea.

Avoid use of elecampane during pregnancy since it can cause contractions and is a uterine stimulant.

Skin rashes have been reported in sensitive people. Persons with known allergies to plants in the Aster family should avoid using elecampane.

Elecampane can lower blood sugar and could interfere with blood sugar control in diabetics.

There are indications that elecampane may interfere with blood pressure control in some patients. Monitor blood pressure carefully while using elecampane.

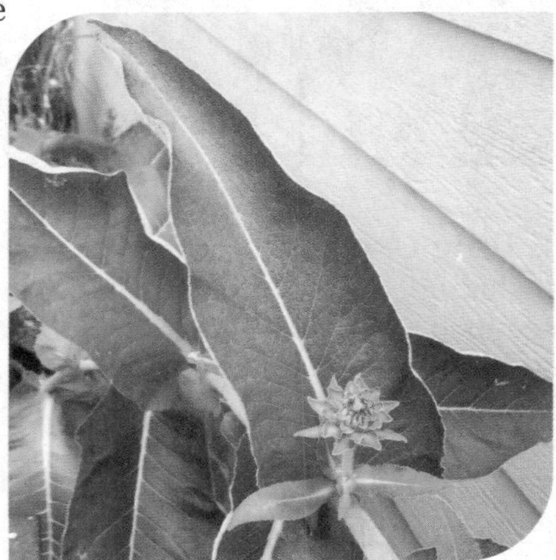

Do not use elecampane within 2 weeks before or after a scheduled surgery.

It may cause drowsiness – no not use with sedatives.

Evening Primrose, *Oenothera biennis*

Evening primrose is also known as evening star and sun drop. Evening primrose gets its name because its flowers usually open at dusk, after the sun is no longer on them. It grows in eastern and central North America and has naturalized to Europe. It is in the Onagraceae (Evening Primrose) Family.

Identification: *Oenothera biennis* is a biennial plant. In its first year, the leaves can grow up to 10 inches (25 cm) long. Leaves are lance-shaped, toothed, and form a rosette. In its second year, the flower stem has alternate, spirally-arranged leaves on a hairy, rough flower stem that is often tinged with purple.

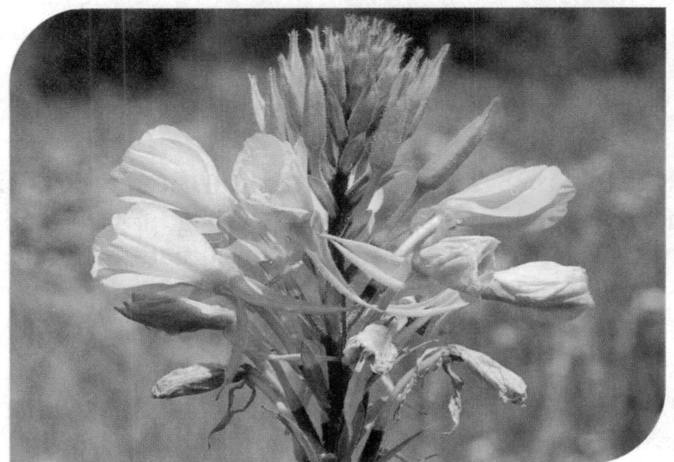

The leaves are reminiscent of willow leaves. This erect flower stem sometimes branches near the top of the plant and grows from 3 to 6 feet (0.9m to 1.8m) tall. It flowers from June to October.

The bright yellow flowers are partially to fully closed during the heat of the day. Flowers have four petals and are 1 to 2 inches (2.5 cm to 5 cm) across. They grow in a many-flowered terminal panicle. The fragrant flowers last only 1 to 2 days. Seedpods are long and narrow.

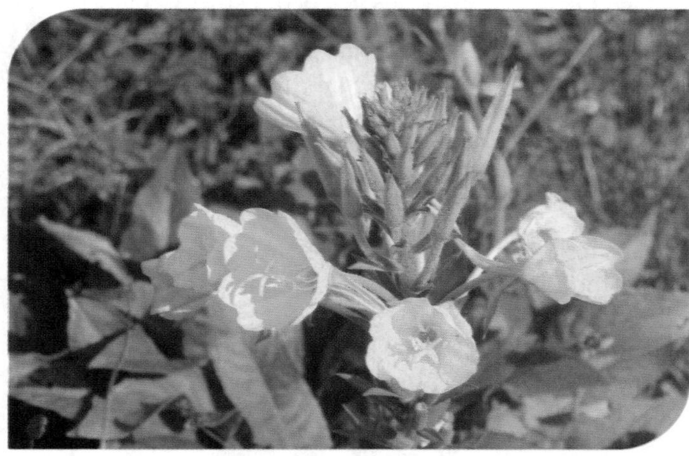

Edible Use: All parts of evening primrose are edible, including the flowers, leaves, stalks, oil, root, and seedpods. Roots can be eaten either cooked or boiled. Its flowers and flower buds are good raw in salads. Young seedpods can be cooked or steamed. Second year stems can be peeled and eaten fresh. Its seeds are edible and oily. Leaves aren't usually eaten due to their texture but they can be if boiled a few times.

Medicinal Use: Evening primrose oil comes from the seeds of the evening primrose, which contain gamma linolenic acid (GLA) - an omega 6 fatty acid also found in borage. Flowers, roots, bark, and leaves are also used medicinally.

Balancing Women's Hormones, PCOS, PMS, and Menopause: Evening primrose oil helps balance hormones in women. It naturally treats symptoms of PMS, including breast tenderness, water retention and bloating, acne, irritability, depression, moodiness, and headaches.

It is also useful in the treatment of polycystic ovarian syndrome (PCOS), helping with fertility and in normalizing the menstrual cycle. It helps ease the symptoms of menopause as well, like hot flashes, moodiness, and sleep disturbance.

Hair Loss in Men and Women: Evening primrose attacks the hormonal causes of male pattern baldness and androgenetic alopecia in women. By balancing the hormones, it prevents further hair loss and, in some people, helps hair grow back. It is best used both internally and externally (rub on the scalp daily along with diluted rosemary essential oil).

Skin Diseases, Eczema, Psoriasis, Acne: Evening primrose oil works well for people with skin problems such as acne, eczema, dermatitis, and psoriasis. It balances the hormonal causes of these diseases, reduces inflammation, and promotes healing while reducing symptoms such as itching, redness, and swelling.

Arthritis and Osteoporosis: Evening primrose oil is a good supplement for people with rheumatoid arthritis and osteoporosis. It is anti-inflammatory and reduces pain and stiffness. It also balances the hormones that cause bone loss in osteoporosis. It also seems to help with calcium absorption and is best combined with fish oil.

Gastro-Intestinal Disorders: The bark and leaves are astringent and healing. They are effective in treating gastro-intestinal disorders caused by muscle spasms of the stomach or intestines. They calm the spasms and allow better digestion.

Whooping Cough: Evening primrose is an expectorant. A syrup made from the flowers helps treat whooping cough symptoms and is easier than a tincture or tea to get young children to swallow. Boil the flowers in a small amount of water, strain, and sweeten with raw honey.

Asthma and Allergies: Use leaf and bark tea to treat asthma. The tea relieves bronchial spasms and opens the airways. It does not cure the asthma, only treats the symptoms. It seems to work best for asthma with allergic causes.

Blood Pressure and Cholesterol: Regular consumption of evening primrose oil helps reduce blood cholesterol levels and lowers blood pressure.

Best results are achieved by long-term use; it is not intended for acute situations.

Diabetic Neuropathy: Evening primrose oil helps treat nerve pain specifically due to diabetes.

Harvesting, Preparation, and Storage: The seeds of evening primrose ripen from August to October. Collect them when ripe and press for oil before they dry out. Flowers must be picked in full bloom.

Gather the leaves and stem "bark" when the flowering stems have grown up. Strip the "bark" of evening primrose and dry for later use; the leaves are also harvested and dried at that time. Dig the roots in the second year when they are larger and more potent.

Recipes. How to Make Cold-Pressed Evening Primrose Seed Oil: Grind fresh seeds. You can use a flourmill, sausage grinder, auger type juicer, coffee grinder, or blender to grind the seeds into a paste. It may take several passes through the grinder to get a fine grind. Add a tiny amount of water only if necessary, to facilitate grinding. Roll the ground seeds into a ball and knead them by hand to release the oil, catching it in a small bowl. Knead and squeeze the seeds until the oil is released, this may take some time. Place the seed paste into a seed bag or use a coffee filter and tighten it to release even more oil into the bowl. When you have gathered as much oil as possible, filter it through a fresh filter to remove any remaining seed remnants. The standard dosage for internal use is 1 gram of oil daily, broken into 2 to 3 doses.

Strong Evening Primrose Tea. (1-ounce bark and leaves, crushed or chopped into small pieces, 1-pint (500 ml) of water). Bring the water and herbs to a boil and reduce the heat to a low simmer. Simmer the herbs for 10 minutes. Allow the tea to cool and strain out the herbs. Keep the tea refrigerated until needed and use within three days.

Fennel, *Foeniculum vulgare*

Fennel is a commonly used vegetable in the Apiaceae /Umbelliferae (Celery/Carrot/Parsley) Family. It has a licorice flavor and is very fragrant. It is found across the United States and Canada. I grow it in my garden, but am also able to find it along roadsides, riverbanks, and pasture lands.

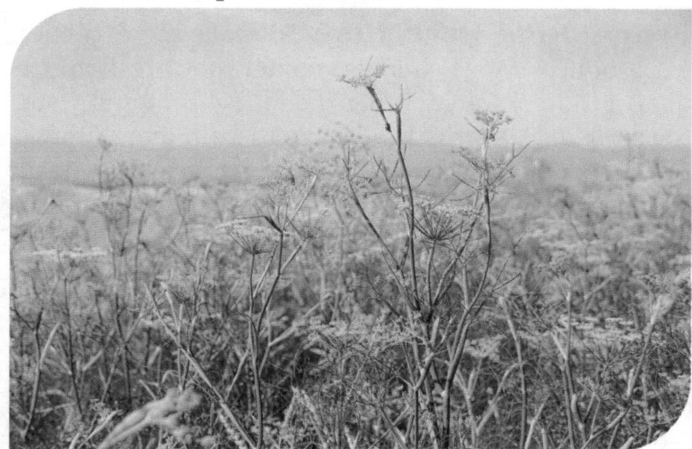

Identification: Fennel is a flowering perennial herb with yellow flowers. It looks a lot like dill, except for the bulb. The leaves are feathery, and finer than dill leaves. The stems are erect, smooth and green and grow to a height of eight feet (2.4m).

The leaves are finely dissected with threadlike segments. Most, but not all varieties form a stem-bulb that sits on the ground or is lifted by a segment of stem. Leaf branches fan out from the stem, forming the bulb. Flowers appear on umbels, 2 to 6 inches (5 cm to 15

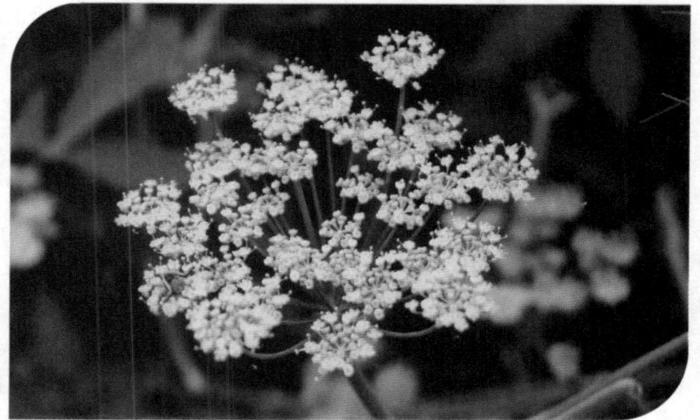

cm) in diameter. The umbels are terminal and compound, with each section containing 20 to 50 tiny yellow flowers. The fruit is a small seed, approximately 1/5 to 1/3 inch-long (0.6 cm to 0.9 cm) with grooves along its length.

Edible Use: The stems, leaves, and seeds are edible. I prefer to roast the bulbs and use the seeds for seasoning.

Medicinal Use: The seeds and root are used to prepare remedies, but eating the plant is also healthy.

Digestive Problems: An infusion made from the seeds is effective in the treatment of digestive problems. Take it after meals for the treatment of indigestion, heartburn, and flatulence.

It is also effective for constipation and stomach pains. In addition to using the infusion, if you have digestive problems add fennel seeds to your cooking.

Nursing Mothers and Colic: For the treatment of colic, have the mother drink Fennel Infusion. It not only relieves the baby's colic, but it also increases the milk flow. Non-nursing babies can take a spoonful of the infusion to relieve the symptoms.

Sore Throats, Laryngitis, Gum Problems: I also use Fennel Infusion as a treatment for sore throats. Gargle with the infusion to treat the infection and pain. This treatment is also effective for sore gums.

Urinary Tract Problems, Kidney Stones: For urinary tract infections, kidney stones, and other urinary tract problems, use a decoction of the fennel root.

Menstrual Problems and Premenstrual Tension: Fennel has the ability to regulate the menstrual cycle and the hormones affecting it. I prescribe Fennel Seed Tea for a variety of menstrual problems including cramping, PMS, pain fluid retention and other menstrual symptoms. Fennel contains estrogen-like chemicals that work to restore the hormonal balance

Detoxifying, Diuretic: Fennel is a strong diuretic and detoxifier. It cleans toxins from the body and flushes them out through the urinary tract. Drink Fennel Seed Tea up to three times daily to detoxify the body and remove excess fluids.

Eyesight, Eyewash, Conjunctivitis, Eye Inflammations: To strengthen eyesight, eat fennel with your meals.

For inflammations and eye infections, use Fennel Seed Tea as an eyewash. It treats conjunctivitis, infections and reduces inflammations of the eye.

Harvesting: Harvest fennel seeds in autumn when they are fully mature. Dry them and store in an air-tight container in a cool, dark place.

Warning: Rarely people have had problems with photo-dermatitis while taking fennel seed. Fennel has hormonal effects and should not be consumed by pregnant women.

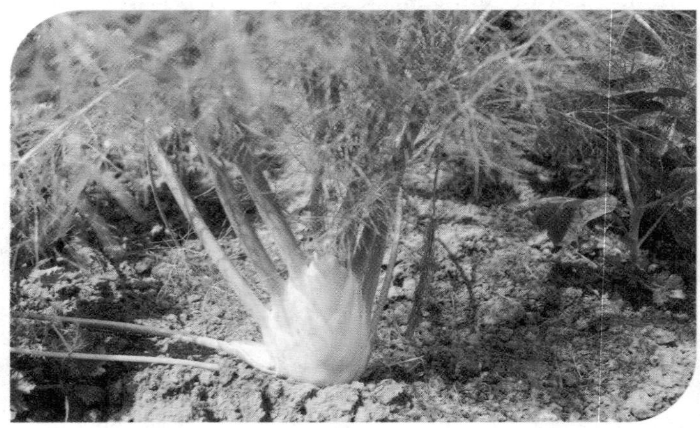

Recipes. Fennel Infusion: You need 1 teaspoon crushed fennel seeds and 1 cup boiling water. Pour the boiling water over the fennel seeds and allow the infusion to steep, covered, for 10 to 15 minutes. Drink 3 cups daily. Take after meals for digestive issues.

Fennel Root Decoction: To make the decoction get 2 ounces (56g) chopped fennel root, fresh and 1-quart (1 Liter) water. Bring the fennel root and water to a boil and turn the heat down to a simmer. Simmer the decoction for 1 hour. Turn off the heat and strain out the root. Store the decoction in the refrigerator for up to 1 week.

Feverfew, *Tanacetum parthenium*

Feverfew is an herb that is widely used for migraines. It grows along roadsides, in rocky and disturbed soil, and is cultivated in some home herb and ornamental gardens. Also known as Chrysanthemum parthenium, wild chamomile, and bachelor's buttons. It is a member of the Aster/Daisy Family.

Identification: Feverfew grows into a bushy shape approximately 1 to 3 feet (0.3m to 0.9m) tall. It has round, leafy stems that grow from a taproot. The leaves

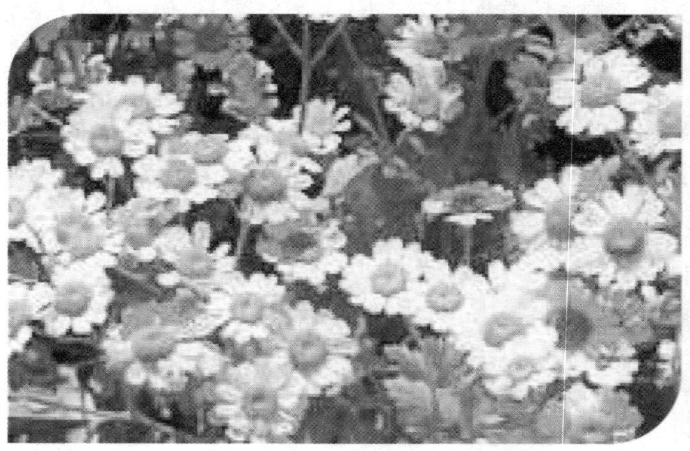

Flower of Feverfew 1Feverfew by Vision, CC 2.5

are yellow-green and pinnately divided into slightly rounded divisions. The upper leaves are more lobed and toothed than lower leaves. Leaves have a distinctive bitter aroma and taste. Flowers bloom in summer.

The flowers look like small daisies with a large yellow disk and short white rays. The center disk is flat, unlike chamomiles, which have conical central disks.

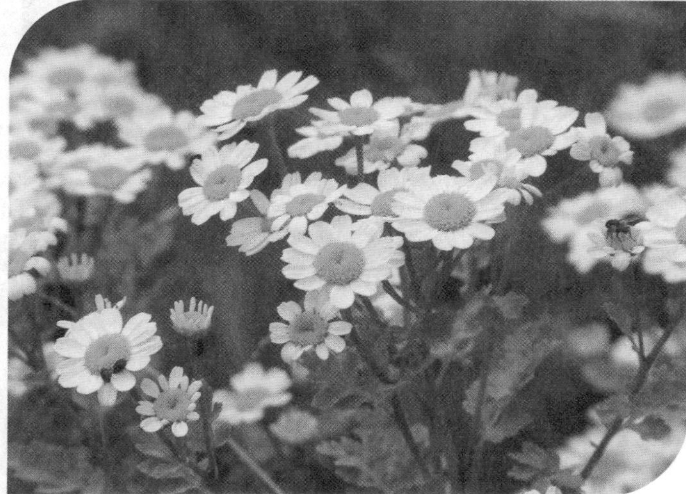

Edible Use: Feverfew leaves are edible but are very bitter.

Medicinal Use: The leaves and flowers are used medicinally. Typical doses are 2 to 3 leaves per day, with a proportionally reduced dose for children over the age of three.

Migraines and Tension Headaches: Taking feverfew regularly works well as a preventative for migraine headaches, as does butterbur. It must be taken regularly to work.

Feverfew may work in a few ways: as an anti-inflammatory, by inhibiting smooth muscle contraction, as an analgesic, and by inhibiting blood platelet aggregation. It may also help via other mechanisms still being studied.

Use the flowers and leaves fresh or dried. To prevent migraines, chew 1 to 4 leaves per day, or drink 1 cup of Feverfew Leaf Tea daily, or use a daily tincture.

For people with migraines simply keep dried leaves or a feverfew tincture on hand with you.

If mouth sores develop from chewing leaves regularly, switch to a powdered or tinctured form. The tea, leaf, or tincture may also be used as a treatment for tension headaches.

Fevers, Cold and Flu Pain (and Colic): Feverfew gets its name from its traditional use treating fevers. Hot Feverfew Tea helps break a fever and treats the aches and pains associated with cold and flu. It is anti-inflammatory and analgesic. For colic in babies and young children, try just a few drops of a cold infusion.

Menstrual Cramps and to Regulate the Menses: Feverfew is both a uterine stimulant and a pain reliever and is particularly good at relieving painful menstrual cramping and in bringing on menses.

Feverfew shouldn't be used if you are pregnant, as it can stimulate uterine contraction and directly affect the baby.

Harvesting: Harvest feverfew leaves and flowers shortly after the flowers appear in early summer. Dry a supply for future use. You can also powder the dried leaves and encapsulate them.

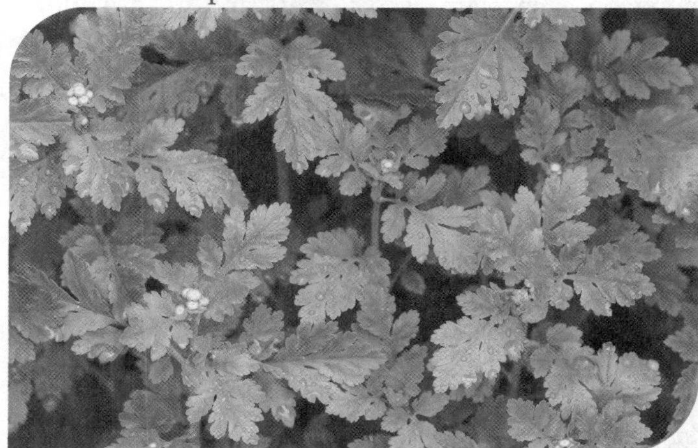

Warning: Some people have an allergic reaction to feverfew and dermatitis can also occur with skin contact. Chewing the leaves can cause mouth sores in some people. If you are allergic to ragweed, marigold, or chrysanthemum, you may also react to feverfew.

Do not use during pregnancy as it causes contractions. Do not use on people who have blood coagulation problems.

Recipes. Feverfew Tea: Steep 1 heaping teaspoon of feverfew leaves and flowerheads in 1 cup of hot water. Allow the infusion to cool to lukewarm, then drink it or apply as directed.

Garlic, *Allium sativum*

Garlic has strong medicinal value, and it tastes great. Most people would benefit greatly by eating more garlic, no matter how good or bad their health. I use garlic for nearly everything.

Most of the garlic that I use now is cultivated. It is found in nearly every herb garden and kitchen garden across the country and is easily found at supermarkets. Don't fall for prepared garlic, however. Chop it fresh and make your own garlic products for maximum health.

Identification: The garlic plant grows to about 2 feet (0.6 meters) tall. It is a bulbous herb with four to twelve long, flat, sword-shaped leaves growing from an underground stem. The bulbs are rounded and contain approximately 15 smaller cloves. Each clove and the bulb is covered by a thin white or pinkish papery coat. Flowers appear in a cluster at the top of a 10-inch (25 cm) flower stalk. Flower stalks grow from a common point on each plant. The flowers are green-white or pinkish with six sepals and petals. Propagation is primarily by bulbs. Seeds are rarely produced.

Edible Use: The bulbs are the only part of the garlic eaten and are usually used for seasoning or as a condiment.

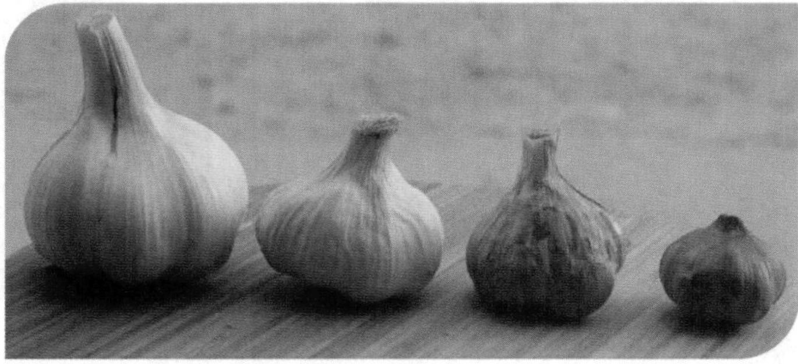

Medicinal Use: For internal use, I usually recommend that people simply eat more garlic in their foods. For best results, garlic should be chopped fine and allowed to rest for 10 minutes or so before cooking. Eating it raw is even better.

Chopping, and allowing time for the sulfurous compounds to develop in the garlic, will make it more potent. Some people complain of a strong garlic smell in the sweat when consuming garlic. This is a natural response and indicates that the body is using the beneficial components. To alleviate this complaint, eat fresh parsley with the garlic.

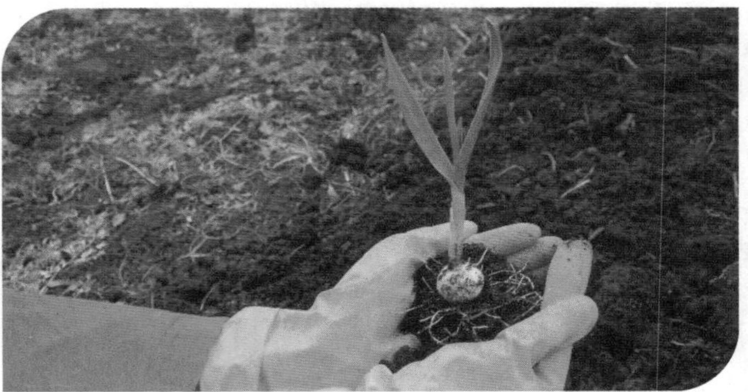

Taking Garlic as Medicine: In general, use garlic in any way that best suits you. People who don't like the strong flavor can put it into capsules, but I like using it fresh and chopped fine or crushed to release the beneficial sulfurous compounds.

You can also take it as a tincture. For people who like garlic, try chewing one whole raw clove at each meal or drinking garlic juice daily.

Treating Viral, Bacterial, and Parasitic Infections: Garlic is a potent antibiotic, antifungal, and anti-parasitic plant. Use garlic to treat infections of all kinds, including colds, flu, sore throats, bronchitis, stomach flu, and intestinal worms.

Thrush, Yeast, and Fungal Infections: Use garlic preparations topically to treat thrush infections and other types of yeast or fungal infections. Spread a paste of garlic on the affected area several times a day and eat garlic regularly to clear the infection internally.

Digestive Problems: Garlic improves digestion and is useful to relieve excessive gas, bloating, and other digestive upsets.

Lowers Blood Sugars in Diabetics: Garlic helps lower blood sugar in diabetics by improving the function of the pancreas and increasing the secretion of insulin.

This helps the body regulate blood sugar levels and alleviates the problems associated with high blood sugar. To be effective, garlic needs to be eaten at every meal in significant quantities. Adding a couple of cloves of pickled garlic to the meal is usually enough to get the full benefits.

Bronchitis, Whooping Cough, Congestion of All Causes: Garlic has a strong decongestant effect and expectorant action. It is useful for maladies where phlegm or mucous is a problem. Garlic also reduces fevers and kills off the underlying infection. It is also useful for bronchial asthma where the breathing passages have swollen making breathing difficult.

Elevated Blood Cholesterol Levels and Blood Pressure: Garlic effectively lowers blood cholesterol levels and blood pressure when consumed regularly.

Corns, Warts, and Acne: For corns, warts, and acne, rub a paste made from fresh mashed garlic on the affected spot. Garlic actually softens and soothes the skin and kills the viral or bacterial infection causing the problem.

Recipes: Garlic Infusion. Chop or grind garlic cloves and allow them to rest for 10 to 15 minutes before continuing. Place the garlic into a pot and cover with water. Heat the water gently to a simmer, then turn off the heat. Allow the garlic and water to steep overnight. Use 2 to 4 ml of this infusion, 3 times a day with meals. Keep the Infusion in the refrigerator for up to three days or in the freezer for up to a month.

Garlic Tincture: Chop 1 cup of garlic cloves fine and allow to rest for 10 to 15 minutes. Place the garlic cloves in a pint (500ml) jar with a tight-fitting lid. Cover the chopped garlic with apple cider vinegar, preferably with the mother (live vinegar). Allow the jar to steep for 4 to 6 weeks, shaking it several times a week. Take 1 tablespoon of garlic tincture with each meal.

Goldenrod, *Solidago* spp.

Goldenrods comprise about 100 species or more that grow throughout North America in open areas like meadows, prairies, and savannas. I primarily use *Solidago canadensis*, which is the most common goldenrod in North America. It is in the Aster/Daisy Family and is also known as goldruthe, woundwort, and solidago. Goldenrods take the blame for a lot of allergies, but most of it is undeserved. There are people allergic to goldenrod and they should not use the plant. However, most of the allergies are caused by ragweed and other similar flowering plants. Goldenrod are pollinated by bees and do not release pollen into the air like the ragweeds. Furthermore, Goldenrod can be used against allergies caused by ragweed.

Identification: I often find goldenrod in open areas and along trailsides. I identify it by its unique aroma, taste, and its visual properties – like its height and its large sprays of yellow flower clusters. Crushing a goldenrod leaf releases a salty, balsam-like fragrance. Any goldenrod species can be used medicinally; however, it is necessary to differentiate the plant from similar toxic plants, including ragwort and groundsel. If you are unsure of your identification, use a local field guide. Goldenrod plants have alternate, simple leaves that are usually toothed. They can also be smooth or hairy.

The leaves at the base of the plant are longer, shortening as they climb the plant, with no leaf stem and 3 distinct parallel veins. The shape can vary from species to species. The stems are unbranched, until the plant flowers. Flower heads are composed of yellow ray florets arranged around disc florets. Each flower head may contain a few florets per head or up to 30, depending on the species. The flower head is usually 1/2 inch (1.25 cm) or less in diameter, although some varieties are larger. The inflorescence is usually a raceme or a panicle. Plant size varies by species, usually growing 2 to 5 feet (0.6 meters to 1.5meters) tall. Some varieties spread aggressively by runners, while others grow in clumps that expand outward each year.

Toxic Look-Alikes: Goldenrod has many look-alikes and some of them are deadly. Groundsel, life root, staggerweed, and ragwort are regional names for deadly look-alike plants in the Senecio genus. Ragwort and groundsels usually have fewer and smaller flower heads and bloom earlier in the season.

These are not hard rules, however, so it can be difficult to identify the plants and distinguish them from other local varieties. You should be very sure of your plant identification before harvesting.

Edible Use: Goldenrod flowers are edible and can be eaten lightly fried or in a salad. It is also used as a flavoring for alcoholic beverages such as cordials and mead, and in fermented homemade soda. Leaves can be cooked and eaten like spinach.

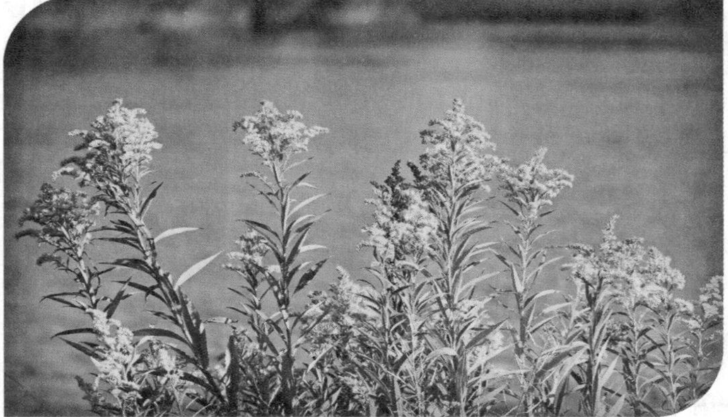

Medicinal Use: I use the leaves and flowers in my medicinal preparations; however, the roots are also used. I use goldenrod to made medicinal tea and tinctures. For children, it can be infused into raw honey or made into a syrup.

Urinary Tract and Kidneys: Goldenrod has astringent and antiseptic properties, that are useful in treating urinary tract infections and bladder infections. It is also effective in restoring balance to the kidneys and in prevention of kidney stones. It is a good choice for chronic conditions and long-term use, though care should be taken as it is a diuretic. Other treatments might be more useful for acute UTI and kidney infections.

Skin, Wounds, and Stopping Bleeding: Goldenrod is an herb of choice to treat and help heal skin wounds, burns, open sores, cuts, boils and other skin irritations. The herb acts as an anti-inflammatory, antibacterial, and antifungal. It helps wounds heal quickly and soothes the irritation. I use goldenrod decoction as a wash, make a poultice, or sometimes use the powdered dried leaves directly on skin wounds. Its common name of "woundwort" came from its ability to stop bleeding when applied to a wound (its dried, powdered form works best as a styptic). You can also use goldenrod to make an ointment or salve. Roots were traditionally used for burns.

Colds, Allergies, and Bronchial Congestion: Goldenrod Tincture is a good choice for treating the symptoms of seasonal allergies and colds. It calms runny eyes and noses, and the sneezes that are triggered by summer and fall allergies.

It is an antiseptic and an expectorant and contains quercetin and rutin, which are natural antihistamines. It also treats sore throats. Goldenrod can also be taken as a tea when needed. For treating a sore throat, try combining it with sage.

Once cooled a bit, the tea can be used as a gargle for laryngitis and pharyngitis (sore throats). Goldenrod helps the body get rid of respiratory congestion caused by allergies, sinus infections, colds and the flu. It works much like Yerba Santa to dry bronchial and respiratory secretions and to expel existing mucous.

Diarrhea: Goldenrod stimulates the digestive systems while calming internal inflammation and irritation that causes diarrhea. It is anti-inflammatory and anti-microbial, so it attacks the symptoms and causes.

Boosts the Cardiovascular System: Goldenrod is a good source of rutin, a powerful antioxidant that improves the cardiovascular and cerebrovascular system. It supports circulation and increases capillary strength. Peoples with this need drink Goldenrod Tea daily, as long as they do not have problems with blood pressure.

Yeast Infections and Anti-Fungal: Goldenrod's antifungal properties make it effective against yeast infections such as *Candida*. Drink the tea or take the decoction daily and use powdered goldenrod, as needed, for external infections. A gargle can be used for oral thrush (Usnea also works well for thrush).

Joint Pain: This herb is anti-inflammatory, and works well to reduce pain and swelling, especially in the joints. It is useful to treat gout, arthritis, and other

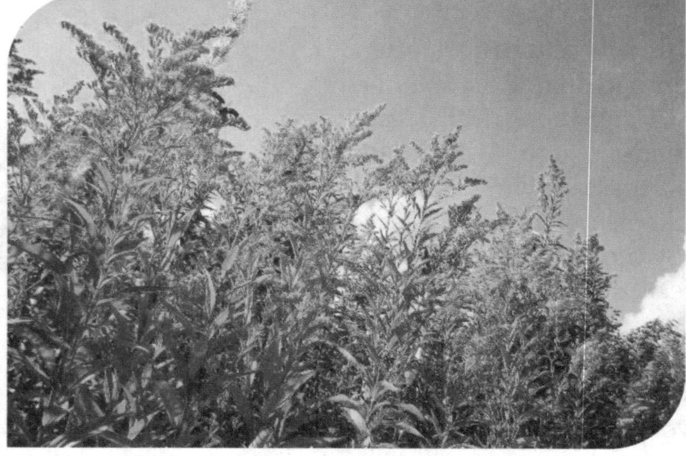

joint pains. Take internally and topically apply a poultice or wash directly to the affected joints.

Harvesting: Harvest healthy leaves and flowers that are free of powdery mildew or other diseases. Pick the leaves throughout the spring and summer and harvest flowers in the late summer or early autumn, just as the flowers open. Leave some flowers on the plant to produce seeds and guarantee a crop the next year. Roots are harvested in early spring or autumn. Hang the plants to dry or use a dehydrator on the lowest setting to dry them for long-term storage.

Warning: Goldenrod is a diuretic and can be overly drying when used long-term as a daily beverage or tea. Do not use goldenrod during pregnancy or when nursing. Consult your doctor if you have a chronic kidney disorder. Do not use goldenrod if you are allergic to any members of the Asteraceae family. Be sure of your plant identification. There are poisonous look-alikes. Goldenrod can increase blood pressure in some people.

Recipes. Goldenrod Tea: You will need 2 cups of boiling water and 1 Tablespoon of fresh goldenrod or 2 teaspoons of dried goldenrod. Bring the water to a boil and pour over the goldenrod. Allow the herbs to infuse for 15 minutes. Strain and serve. Use up to three times a day. This tea is slightly bitter. Adding an equal amount of mint to the herbs improves the flavor.

Goldenrod Decoction: Ingredients: 1-ounce goldenrod herb (leaves or flowers), 1-pint (500ml) of water. Place the herbs in a non-reactive pot with the water over medium heat. Bring the mixture to a boil. Turn the temperature down to a low simmer for 20 minutes. Cool the decoction and strain out the herbs. Store in the refrigerator for up to 3 days. Use 1 to 2 teaspoons per dose, 3 times a day.

Greater Burdock, *Arctium lappa*

Arctium lappa belongs to Asteraceae (Daisy) Family. It is commonly known as greater burdock, edible burdock, lappa, beggar's buttons, thorny burr, or happy major. It is a Eurasian species and is cultivated in gardens for its root, which is used as a vegetable. This plant has become an invasive weed in many places in North America. It is a giant weed with much medicinal potential.

Identification: Greater burdock is a biennial plant. It is tall, and can reach 10 feet (3meters). Its stems are branched, rough and usually sparsely hairy. It flowers from July to September. The fleshy tap-root of this plant can grow up to 3 feet (0.9 meters) deep. Greater Burdock forms a 1.5-inch-wide (3.75 cm) single flower-like flat cluster of small purple flowers surrounded by a rosette of bracts. Leaves of greater burdock are alternate and stalked. They are triangular–broadly oval, usually cordate, and have undulating margins. They have a white-grey-cottony underside and first year growth is in rosettes.

The fruit is flattish, gently curved and is grey-brown in color. It has dark-spotted achene with short yellow hooked hairs on tip. Greater burdock is found almost everywhere, especially in areas soils that are usually rich in nitrogen. Its preferred habitat is in disturbed areas.

Edible Use: The leaves, stems, seeds, and roots are all edible. Young first-year roots and leaves are good raw in salads, but they become too fibrous as they mature and need to be cooked before eating.

The leaves and stalks are also good either raw or cooked. I prefer to remove the outer rind before cooking or eating. The sprouted seeds are also eaten.

Medicinal Use: Greater Burdock is antibacterial and antifungal, helps with digestion and gas, is a diuretic, and regulates blood sugar. It is a powerful

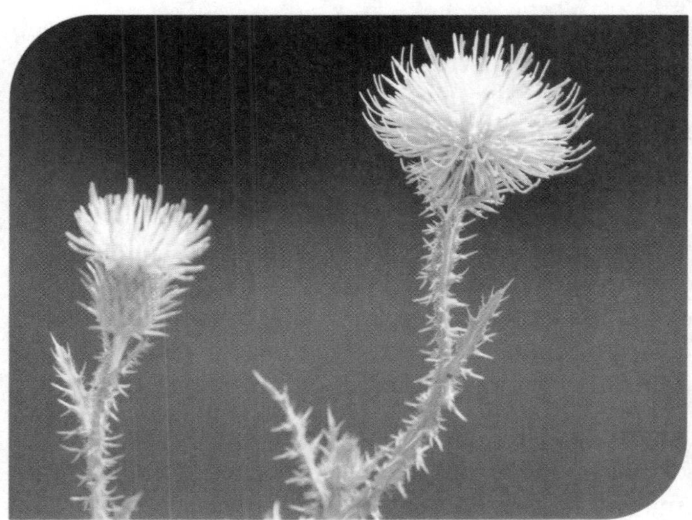

detoxifier. The dried root is most often used for medicine, but the leaves and fruit can also be used.

Detoxing and Liver Cleanser: Its root is particularly good at helping to eliminate heavy metals and other resilient toxins from the body.

It helps with conditions caused by an overload of toxins, such as sore throat and other infections, boils, rashes, and other skin problems.

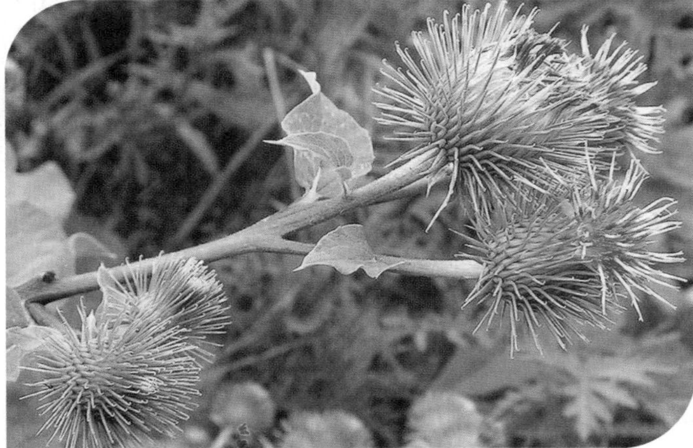

Burdock flowers, Pethan, GNUFL 1.2

Cancer Treatment: Greater burdock is known to kill cancer cells. It flushes away toxins from the body, increases blood circulation to normal cells, protects the organs, and improves the health of the whole body. It is used to treat breast cancers, colon cancer, and even the deadly pancreatic cancer with good results.

I feel confident that it would be effective against other cancers as well. In treating cancer, the greatest success seems to come when herbs are used in combination to kill the cancer cells and support the body.

Try using greater burdock in combination with sheep sorrel and slippery elm to kill the cancer and detox the body during treatment. Remember to also eat a highly nutritious diet with a high concentration of vegetables and fruits and limited meats and fats.

Turkey Tail and Reishi Mushrooms are other cancer go-tos for me. Dosage: Mix 1/4 cup of Anti-Cancer Decoction with 1/4 cup of distilled water. Drink 3 times a day: 2 hours before breakfast, 2 hours after lunch and before bedtime on an empty stomach. Wait at least 2 hours after taking the decoction before eating again.

Anemia: Greater burdock has a high concentration of bioavailable iron. People with iron deficiency anemia are able to increase their iron levels rapidly by taking daily supplements of greater burdock powder or eating greater burdock as a vegetable.

Skin Diseases: Greater burdock is a very soothing herb for the skin. It has mucilaginous properties that enhance its ability to cure skin diseases such as herpes, eczema, psoriasis, acne, impetigo, ringworm, boils, insect bites, burns, and bruises. Use greater burdock tea as a wash and take it internally to clear the body of the toxins that are causing the skin problems. For bruises, burns, and sores, crush the seeds and use as a poultice on the affected skin.

Diabetes: Greater burdock root helps improve digestion and lower blood sugar in diabetics. For this use the fresh root is best, but 1 to 2 grams of dried powdered root can also be taken 3 times daily.

Strengthens the Immune System and Protects the Organs: This herb strengthens the immune system and the lymphatic system, which helps rid the body of toxins and ward off diseases. It also cleans the blood. It cleand and protects the spleen and helps it remove dangerous pathogens from the body. It improves blood quality, liver health, blood circulation, and fights inflammation.

Stimulates the Kidneys, Relieves Fluid Retention: Greater burdock stimulates the kidneys, helping get rid of excess fluids in the body. This reduces swellings, increases urine output, and flushes waste and toxins from the body.

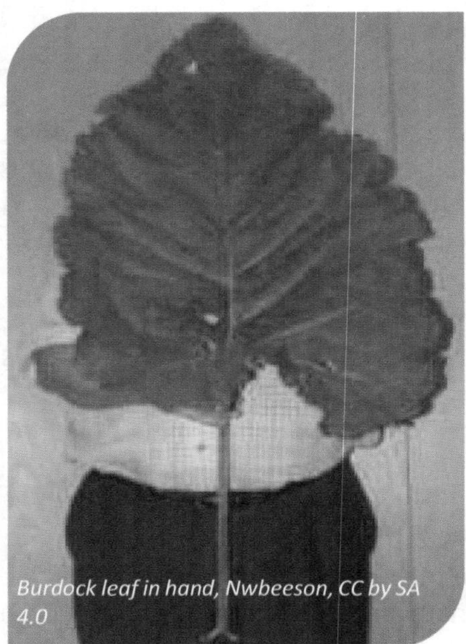

Burdock leaf in hand, Nwbeeson, CC by SA 4.0

Greater Burdock Tea is a natural diuretic.

Osteoarthritis and Degenerative Joint Disease: The anti-inflammatory properties of greater burdock are powerful enough to reduce the inflammation of osteoarthritis. Patients show remarkable improvement when they consume three cups of Greater Burdock Root Tea daily.

Improvement is slow and steady, taking about two months to achieve maximum benefits.

Sore Throats and Tonsillitis: For acute tonsillitis and other sore throats, try Greater Burdock Tea. It relieves pain, inflammation, coughing, and speeds healing. The greater burdock also acts as an antibacterial to kill the harmful bacteria and cure the infection.

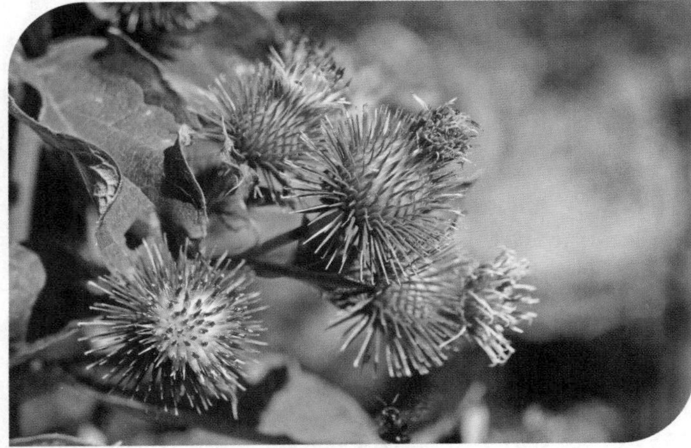

Harvesting: The root must be harvested before it withers at the end of the first year. The best time is after it seeds until late autumn when the roots become very fibrous. Immature flower stalks are harvested in late spring before the flowers appear. Care must be taken when harvesting the seeds. They have tiny, hooked hairs that can latch onto the mucus membranes if inhaled.

Recipes. Anti-Cancer Decoction: To make 1-gallon (4 liters) you need 1-ounce greater burdock root, powdered, 3/4 ounces (21g) sheep sorrel, powdered, 1/4 ounces (7g) slippery elm bark, powdered and 1-gallon (4 liters) distilled water. Equipment: 8-pint (4 Liters) canning jars and lids, sterile, large pot, capable of holding 1 gallon (4 liters) or more, with a tight-fitting lid and boiling water canner.

Bring the greater burdock, sheep sorrel, and slippery elm bark to a boil in 1 gallon (4 liters) of distilled water, tightly covered. Boil the herbs, tightly covered, for 10 minutes, then turn off the heat and stir the mixture.

Cover tightly and let the decoction steep for 12 hours, stirring again after 6 hours. After 12 hours, bring it back to a boil and pour it through a fine mesh strainer or a coffee filter. Pour the decoction into pint (500ml) jars while still hot, leaving ½ inch (1.25 cm) headroom. Cap the jars. Process the jars in a boiling water bath for 10 minutes.

The decoction will keep for 1 year in sealed jars. Store in the refrigerator after opening. Dosage: Mix 1/4 cup of the decoction with 1/4 cup of distilled water. Drink 3 times a day: 2 hours before breakfast, 2 hours after lunch and before bedtime on an empty stomach. Wait at least 2 hours after taking the decoction before eating again.

Henbane, *Hyoscyamus niger*

Henbane is poisonous, so it is advised that you use it with caution. Although native to Europe, it has been cultivated in North America for many years. It's a beautiful plant with a foul smell, and a member of the Solanaceae (Nightshade) family.

Identification: *Hyoscyamus niger* grows from 1 to 3 feet (0.9 meters) tall. A mature henbane plant has leafy, thick, hairy, widely-branched, erect stems. It is an annual and biannual and the biannual growth is used for medicine. Its foul-smelling lobed alternate leaves are grayish-green or yellowish-green in color and have white veins. They spread out like a rosette and are coarsely toothed, large, and wide, growing up

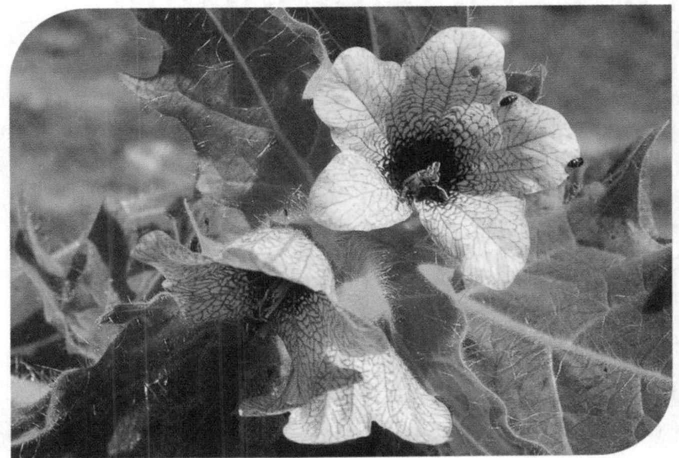

Henbane, photo by K.B. Simoglou - Own work, CC BY-SA 4.0,

to 6 inches (15 cm) wide and 8 inches (20 cm) long. The 5-petaled flowers are a funnel shape and are brownish-yellow in color with dark purple veins. Flowers have a long-spiked inflorescence arrangement in upper leaves with young flowers at the pointed end. Flowers are up to 2 inches (5 cm) across. It flowers from June thru September. The 5-lobed, urn-shaped fruit is 1 inch (2.5 cm). Each fruit is packed with hundreds of tiny black seeds. The roots of henbane are whitish in color. The main taproot is stout and branched. Henbane does not tolerate waterlogged soils. It likes pastures along fencerows and roadsides.

Medicinal Use: Because the plant is poisonous, it is important that all medicines be made precisely and the strength carefully regulated. I prefer to use this plant externally, where there is no danger.

The plant has strong pain-relieving qualities, and is used externally for muscle pains caused by strain or sprain. It has some good applications internally, but I do not recommend using it internally without the close supervision of a medical professional. The above ground parts are used for medicine.

Internal Use: The plant is used to relieve irritable bladders and the pain of cystitis. It is a mild diuretic, hypnotic, and anti-spasmodic. The hypnotic action is the same as belladonna, but with milder effects. Use with great care or find an alternative! Use can be fatal.

Gout, Neuralgia, and Arthritis Pains: External pain from gout, neuralgia, and arthritis are effectively treated with a poultice made from fresh henbane leaves. Crush the leaves and place them directly over the painful area.

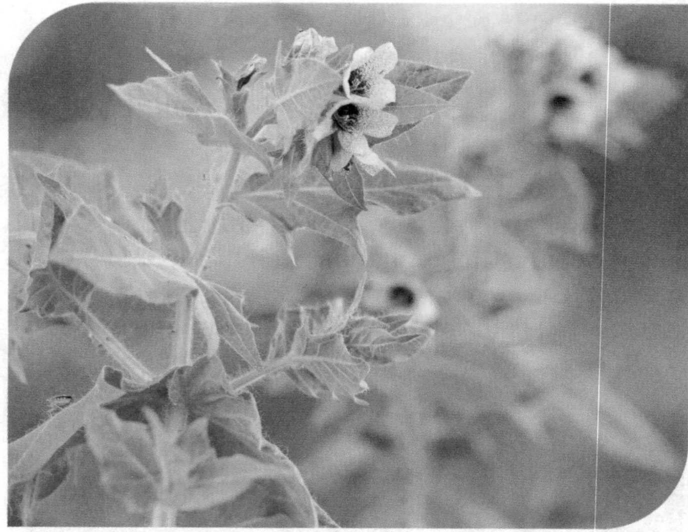

Hemorrhoids: Try a poultice of crushed henbane leaves to reduce the swelling and pain of external hemorrhoids.

Harvesting: Collect the leaves, stems and flowers from the biennial plants when in full flower at the start of summer.

Warning: Henbane is poisonous. Use with great care and do not use internally.

Holy Basil, *Ocimum tenuiflorum/ Ocimum sanctum*

Holy Basil, also known as Tulsi, is a variety of basil in the Lamiaceae (Mint) family. It is a perennial plant often cultivated for religious and medicinal use. It is not the same variety as Thai holy basil or Thai basil.

Holy basil is different from the sweet basil used as a cooking herb. Sweet basil also has medicinal properties but is a different variety of the plant.

Identification: Holy basil grows erect in shrub form up to 1 to 2 feet (0.3m-0.6m). The ovate leaves are green or purple, petioled, and up to 2 inches (5cm) long. The margin is usually, but not always, toothed. The anise scented leaves are strongly aromatic and have a spicy, slightly bitter flavor. They grow in close whorls at the base of reddish or brownish-purple stems. Tiny purple flowers grow on an elongated raceme above the leaves. The flower stems are red and hairy.

Edible Use: Holy basil is edible and can be used as an herb, however its flavor is more bitter than other basils. It is often chewed or used in herbal teas. The dried and ground leaves can be used as a flavoring and stored for later use.

Medicinal Use: Holy basil has many medicinal uses, both internally and externally. It is loaded with vitamins and antioxidants. In addition to treating many diseases, it can prevent disease through its immune system benefits.

Holy basil can be taken as a tea, eaten as a vegetable or flavoring, or taken as a supplement. Dried and crushed holy basil is often placed in capsules for daily supplement use. For preventative use, take 300 to 2,000 mg of dried holy basil daily. For treatment use, take 600 to 1,800 mg two to three times daily.

Inflammation: Holy basil is a powerful anti-inflammatory when taken internally or when rubbed on the skin for swellings and inflammation. Used regularly it leaves the skin soft and treats skin irritations and acne.

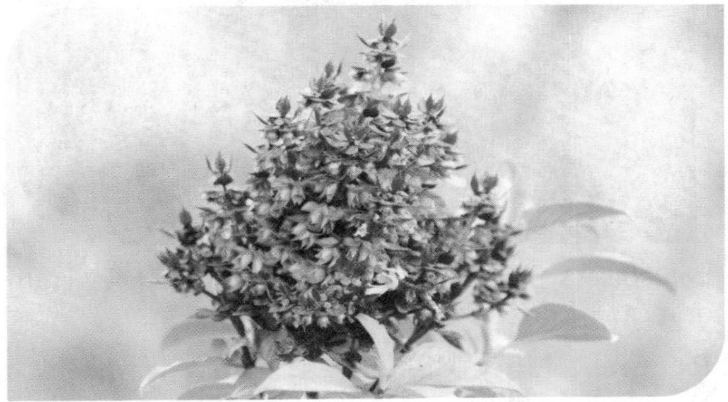

Skin Rashes, Ringworm: Rubbed against the skin, holy basil relieves irritations, soothes rashes, and provides anti-bacterial, anti-fungal, and antibiotic properties. It treats ringworm, poison oak, and other skin conditions.

Holy basil can be brewed in water, then added to your bath water or used as a face wash. A poultice of mashed holy basil leaves, applied directly to infected wounds, is effective in relieving infections and healing wounds. Consuming holy basil as an herb or supplement helps prevent skin problems.

Infections: Essential oils and phytonutrients in holy basil have excellent antibiotic, anti-fungal, and anti-bacterial properties.

Respiratory Disorders: Bronchitis, Asthma: Holy basil relieves congestion in the lungs caused by chronic or acute bronchitis. Additionally, it helps open breathing passages and allows for easier breathing. These benefits to the respiratory system are increased by the presence of healing oils and vitamins in the holy basil essential oil. These healing benefits extend to all damage in the lungs, including damage caused by smoking, environmental factors, or illness.

Stress and Heart Disease: Holy basil contains vitamins and antioxidants that protect the heart from the harmful effects of free radicals. One of these antioxidants, eugenol, is beneficial in reducing blood cholesterol levels. It lowers damaging LDL-cholesterol and raises the beneficial HDL-cholesterol. Users report a reduction in total cholesterol in the circulatory system, kidney, and liver.

In addition, these vitamins and antioxidants reduce the oxidative stress in the body. Holy basil soothes the nerves, reduces inflammation, and lowers blood pressure.

Cancer: Holy basil has anticancer potential, according to recent studies. It inhibits the growth of cancers, including oral cancer, and aids in cell death of cancerous cells.

Type 2 Diabetes: Holy basil works to reduce blood sugar in patients with prediabetes or type 2 diabetes. It helps with weight gain, reduces excess insulin in the blood, decreases insulin resistance, and helps keep blood sugar levels stable over the long term.

Dental Use: Holy basil, used correctly, protects the teeth and kills the bacteria responsible for cavities, plaque, tartar, and bad breath. It also promotes healthy gums. Use holy basil for dental care in moderation. Avoid chewing the leaves and do not keep it in the mouth for long periods. Prolonged contact can damage the teeth.

Detoxifier, Diuretic, and Reduces Risk of Kidney Stones: As a detoxifier and mild diuretic, holy basil reduces the levels of uric acid in the body. Uric acid is mainly responsible for the growth of kidney stones. Other components of holy basil help dissolve the stones, while it also helps relieve the pain from kidney stones as they pass. Holy basil increases urination, flushing toxins from the body and cleansing the kidneys. It helps protect the health of the kidneys and the liver.

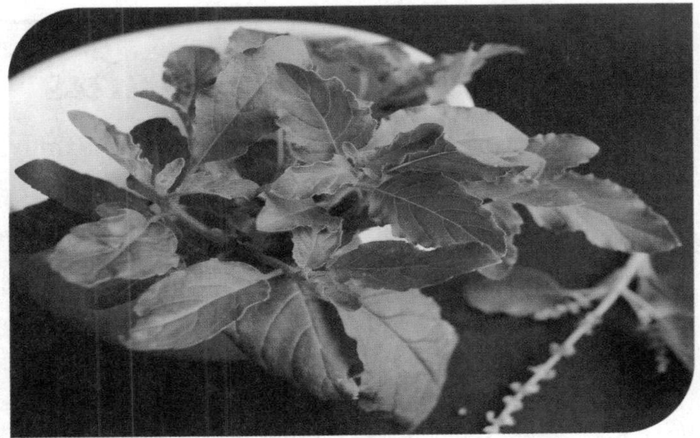

Pain Reliever: Holy basil has pain relieving properties that work well for headaches and minor pains. It helps relieve migraines, sinus headaches, and kidney pain.

Anti-Depressant Effects: Holy basil has known anti-depressant and anti-anxiety properties. It helps users feel less anxious and more relaxed in social situations. Holy basil also relieves stress from physical, mental, and emotional sources.

Eye Inflammations, Cataracts, Macular Degeneration, Glaucoma, Vision: Problems: Taken internally and regularly as a tea or as a supplement, holy basil helps prevent eye problems such as cataracts, macular degeneration, glaucoma, vision problems, and ophthalmia. Boils, conjunctivitis, and other eye inflammations or infections are treated by soaking holy basil in boiled water, then using the water to wash the eye. Holy basil contains high amounts of vitamins A and C, along with high antioxidant content and essential oils that are especially beneficial for the eyes.

Stomach and Digestive System: Holy basil is beneficial to the stomach and digestive system by naturally decreasing stomach acid and increasing mucus secretion. This naturally helps decrease number the effects of peptic ulcers. Eat the whole plant for relief from peptic ulcers, diarrhea, nausea, or vomiting.

Harvesting: Harvest holy basil from a source grown away from pollutants, pesticides, and herbicides. Look for vibrant green leaves without any holes or dark spots. Harvest the young leaves and stems from the top of the plant or cut the stems at ground level. Fresh

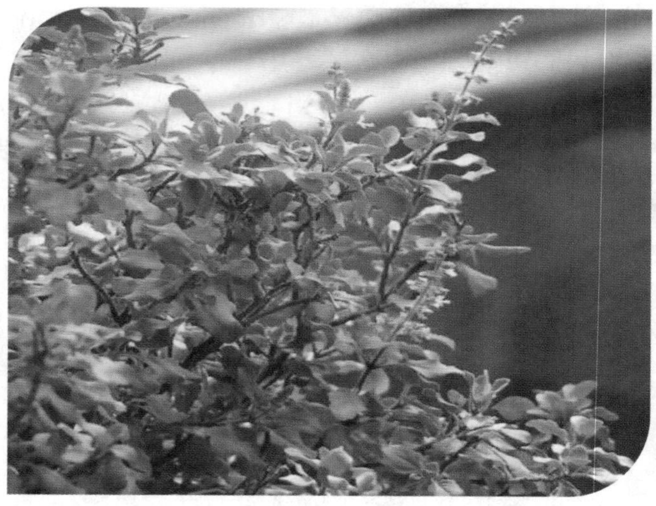

holy. Basil will keep for several days in the refrigerator or it can be dried for future use.

Recipes. Holy Basil Tea: 2 to 3 teaspoons of dried holy basil leaves, 1 cup boiling water. Pour boiling water over dried holy basil leaves and allow the mixture to steep for five to six minutes. Strain and enjoy.

Warning: Holy basil is considered safe for eating and medicinal uses. It should be avoided during pregnancy, when trying to become pregnant, or when breast-feeding because the effects on the child are unknown.

Holy basil can lower blood sugar levels and should be used with care when taking insulin or anti-diabetes drugs. People with hypothyroidism should not use holy basil. It may lower thyroxine levels and worsen the condition. Holy basil can interfere with blood clotting. Stop using holy basil at least 2 weeks before a scheduled surgery.

Hops, *Humulus lupulus*

Wild hops belong to the Cannabaceae (Hemp) Family. Hops are native to Europe, western Asia, and North America. Hops are a bine plant (versus a vine). They have a branching stem with stiff hairs that face downward and provide stability. These allow the plant to climb. Hops grow from 15 to 25 feet (4.5 meters to 7.6 meters) high.

Identification: Hops have green, opposite, lobed leaves. Leaves have 3 to 5 lobes with finely toothed edges and pointed tips. Male and female hops flowers are on separate plants. Male flowers grow in 3 to 5 inches (7.5 cm to 12.5 cm) panicles. The female flower (seed cone) resembles a small pine cone. Flowers are 1½ to 3 inches (3.75 to 7.5 cm) long with overlapping, yellowish-green bracts with a small fruit (achene) at the base. The flowers have a sweet smell.

Edible Use: The female flowers (seed cones or strobiles) are used for tea and for brewing beer. Young leaves and shoots are sometimes used cooked or eaten raw.

Extracts ad oils from hops are used as a flavoring in non-alcoholic beverages and sweets.

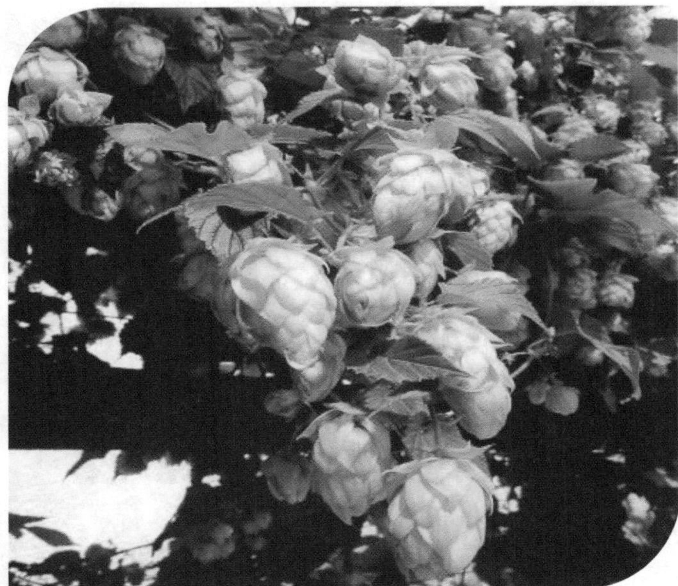

Hops, CCO Creative Commons, own work by moritz320

Medicinal Use: Hops flowers are a sedative and stomachic, so they promote sleep and digestion. When used as a sedative, use fresh hops. For other medicinal uses, you may use dried hops.

Anxiety, Insomnia, and a Sedative: Fresh hops are a strong sedative. For insomnia and anxiety, try a combination of hops and valerian root at bedtime. Use dried hops for the anti-anxiety effects without the strong sedative effects.

Digestion: Hops are a very effective bitter. It is an excellent digestive.

IBS and Irritable Bladder: Hops treat the symptoms of Irritable Bowel Syndrome and irritable bladder. The bitter properties and the sedative qualities reduce spasms of both the bladder and the bowel, relieving the symptoms temporarily without affecting the underlying cause.

Bruises, Boils, and Inflammation: A poultice made of crushed hops helps heal bruises, boils, inflamed tissue, and arthritic joints.

Asthma, PMS, and Muscle Spasms: Hops are an antispasmodic and relieve menstrual cramping, muscle spasms, and bronchial spasms from asthma. It also has phytoestrogenic properties, similar to soy.

Harvesting: Time of harvest varies with the climate. Only the female seed cones are harvested and used in brewing, and both the pollinated and unpollinated hop flowers (strobili) are harvested.

Recipes: Valerian and Hops Infusion: 1-quart (1 Liter) of water, 1 heaping tablespoon of fresh hops, 1 heaping tablespoon of chopped valerian root, raw honey or maple syrup, if desired. Bring a quart (1 Liter) of water to a boil and add the herbs. Cover the pot and turn down the heat to a very low simmer. Simmer the infusion for 5 minutes, then turn the heat off.

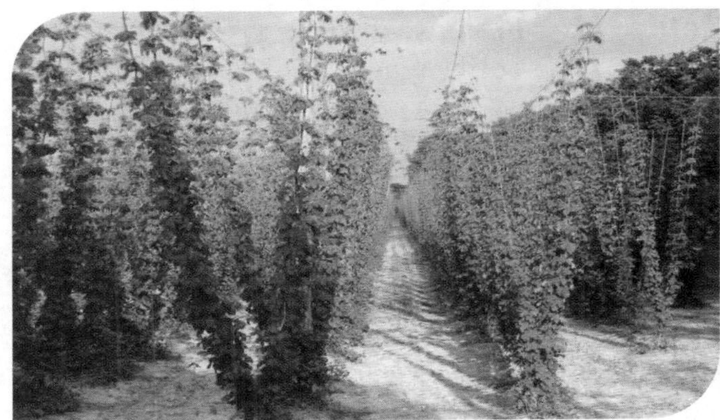

Hops field, Wikipedia Commons

Leave the pot covered and allow the herbs to steep for another 45 minutes. Sweeten the infusion with raw honey or pure maple syrup, if desired. Drink 1 to 1 ½ cups of the infusion at bedtime.

Horseradish, *Armoracia rusticana*

Horseradish is a perennial plant that belongs to Brassicaceae (Mustard) Family. It is a root vegetable that is used as a spice or condiment. It is native to the Southeastern Europe and Western Asia and has naturalized to North America. It is also known as Red Cole. My

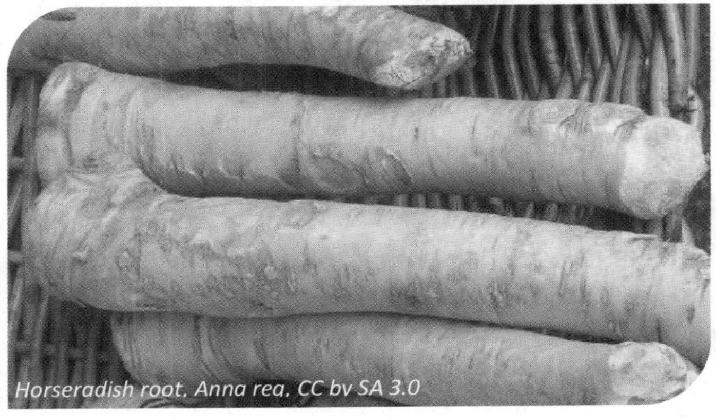

Horseradish root, Anna reg, CC by SA 3.0

favorite edible use for horseradish is as a condiment on meat. It is also one of the many ingredients which I use throughout the wintertime.

Identification: Horseradish is a perennial fast-growing plant that grows from 2 to 3 feet (0.6 m to 0.9 meters). Its flowering season is from May to June. It is self-fertile. The roots are thick and fleshy, a medium brown color on the outside, and smooth to corky on the outside. Roots are pure white on the inside and have a spicy flavor. The flowers of this plant are hermaphroditic (both male and female organs).

Edible Use: The root, leaves, and seeds are all edible, but the root is most often used.

Medicinal Use: The roots of this plant are antiseptic, digestive, diuretic, stimulant, laxative, rubefacient, and expectorant. It is a very powerful stimulant herb that controls bacterial infections, and it can be used both internally and externally.

Colds, Flu, Fevers, and Respiratory Infections: Horseradish infusion is of great value in the treatment of respiratory problems, colds, flu, and fevers. It is an expectorant, anti-bacterial, a weak diuretic, rids the body of excess mucus and fluids, and treats the underlying infection. It is also a key ingredient in my Fire Cider Recipe.

Urinary Tract Infections: The diuretic and anti-bacterial properties work well against urinary tract infections. Horseradish flushes the bacteria and toxins out of the body.

Arthritis, Pleurisy, Chilblains: For arthritis, chilblains, and pleurisy, apply a poultice made from freshly grated horseradish roots or rub the chest with Horseradish Massage Oil, when available.

The herb brings blood to the skin surface and increases blood circulation in the affected area. It warms the skin, decreases inflammation, and promotes healing.

Infected Wounds: The anti-microbial agents found in horseradish are beneficial in treating infected wounds. It acts as an antibiotic against bacteria and pathogenic fungi. Horseradish Vinegar works well for infected wounds.

Harvesting: Harvesting starts in November once the tops are frozen back. Harvesting can be continued through the winter when soils are not frozen. Before

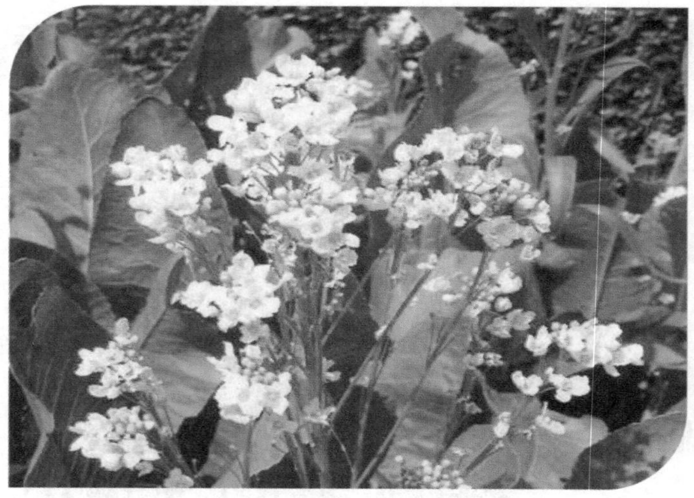

Horseradish plant, Pethan, CC by SA 3.0

digging, mow or cut the dried tops to the ground if still green. Roots are best harvested using a single-row potato digger. Freshly dug roots release valuable volatile oils and begin to lose potency. To avoid this, store them in a box of moist sand in a cool place. Keep the soil moist. Grate it fresh, as needed. Once grated, use it immediately.

Warning: People who have stomach ulcers or thyroid problems should not use this plant internally. Caution should be used when applying horseradish to the skin. It can cause skin irritation and blistering.

Fire Cider or Horseradish Vinegar – alter to your taste buds: Ingredients: ½ cup Grated Horseradish, ½ cup Grated Ginger, ¼ cup Minced Onions, ¼ cup Minced Garlic, 1 Chopped Lemon (rind on), 1 Tbs Black Peppercorns, ¼ tsp Cayenne Pepper and/or 2 Jalapeno Peppers (depends on your spice level), 1 Tbs Turmeric Powder, Raw honey to taste.

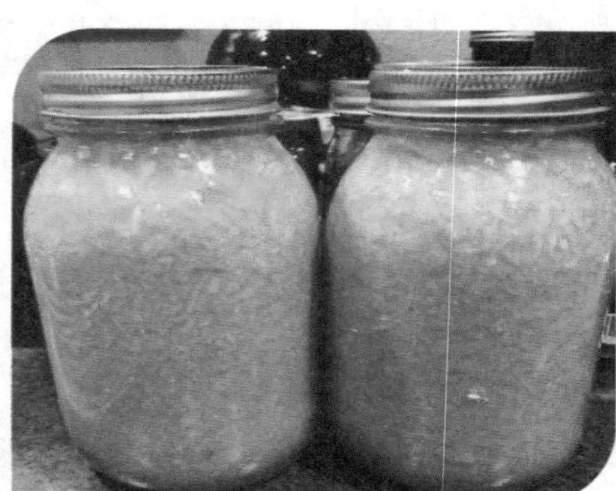

Put all of these into a large quart (liter) glass jar. Fill with organic raw apple cider vinegar. Let sit for 4 to 6 weeks, strain and store. Use within the year. I take it throughout the winter for wellness, usually about an ounce at a time.

Jerusalem Artichoke, *Helianthus tuberosus*

Also called sunroot, sunchoke, and earth apple, the Jerusalem artichoke is a species of sunflower found in Eastern North America. It is easy to cultivate in the garden. It is in the Aster/Daisy Family.

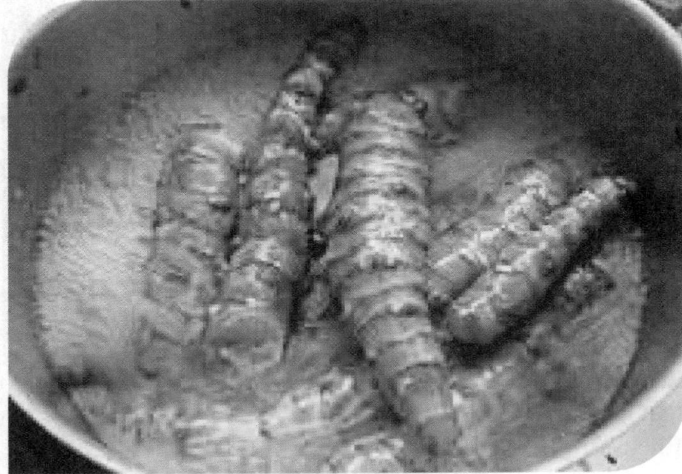

Jerusalem Artichoke, Paul Fenwick, CC SA 3.0

Identification: Jerusalem artichoke grows up to 10 feet (3 meters) tall. Rough, hairy leaves can be found opposing each other on the upper part of the stem, while lower leaves are alternate. The lower leaves are larger, up to a foot long. Higher leaves are smaller and narrow. Yellow flowers are a composite of 60 or more disc florets in the flower head, surrounded by 10 to 20 ray florets. Small sunflower seeds grow on the disc. The flower head grows up to 4 inches (10 cm) in diameter. The edible tubers are elongated, up to 4 inches (10 cm) long and 2 inches (5 cm) in diameter. Their appearance resembles ginger root. However, the color can vary from white to pale brown, or even red or purple.

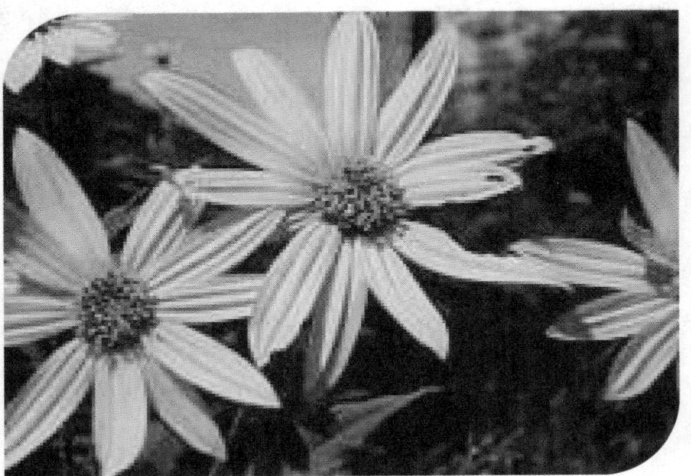

Edible Use: The cooked root tuber is eaten as a vegetable and tastes similar to an artichoke, hence the name. I use the tubers as a substitute for potatoes; they have a sweeter, nuttier flavor.

They can be eaten raw, made into flour, pickled, or cooked. For some people, Jerusalem artichokes cause flatulence and gastric pain, so watch for gastric problems when Jerusalem artichokes are first introduced to the diet.

Medicinal Use: Jerusalem artichoke's medicinal action is due to its high concentration of inulin. It is one of the best sources of this valuable component available. To use Jerusalem artichoke for medicinal purposes, simply include it as a vegetable in the daily diet.

Diabetes: Fresh Jerusalem artichokes are approximately 76% inulin (not to be confused with insulin), which helps regulate blood sugar levels in diabetics. During storage, the inulin is converted to fructose, giving the tuber a sweet taste. Tubers grown in warm weather have higher insulin levels than those in colder regions, but all can be used to help control blood sugar in diabetes.

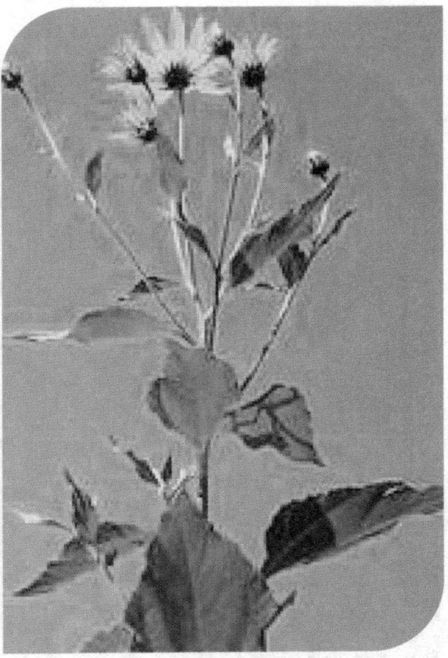

Jerusalem Artichoke Flowers, Paul Fenwick, CC by SA 3.0

Digestive Problems: Jerusalem artichokes are useful as a prebiotic fiber to help increase beneficial gut flora. They also stimulate stomach secretions that help control indigestion, dyspepsia, and slow digestion. However, Jerusalem artichokes do cause gas and intestinal pain in some people.

Enhances the Immune System: Jerusalem artichokes have immune-enhancing properties. They increase the body's defense mechanisms against viruses and bacteria, and they help increase the deployment of white blood cells to areas of infection.

Harvesting: Dig up the roots in autumn or leave them in the ground over the winter to harvest in the spring. Store them in high humidity to prevent them from wilting and softening. Tubers left in the ground will sprout in the spring. The tubers bruise easily and lose moisture quickly, so I usually prefer to leave them in the ground and harvest them when needed.

Warning: Jerusalem Artichokes can cause digestive distress and excessive gas in some people.

Lady's Thumb, *Polygonum persicaria* or *Persicaria maculosa*

Lady's thumb, also known as smartweed, heart's ease, spotted knotweed, or redshank, is a broadleaf weed that is often found growing in large clumps. It grows in disturbed wet soil across North America. It is in the Polygonaceae (Buckwheat/Knotweed) Family.

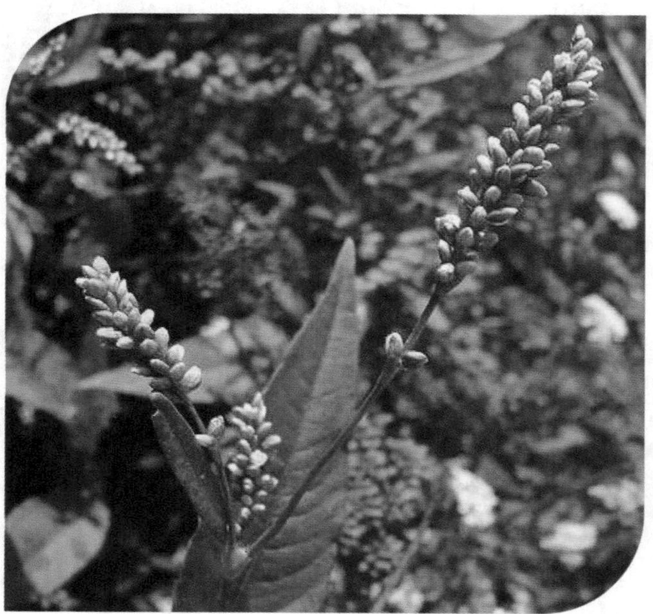

Polygonum persicaria by Bouba at French Wikipedia, photo by Bouba, CC-BY-SA-3.0-migrated

Identification: Lady's thumb grows from 1 to 3 feet tall (0.3 meters to 0.9 meters) and is an erect plant. The 2 to 6-inch-long (5 cm to 17.5 cm) leaves are alternate, narrow, and lance-shaped with wavy edges. They usually, but not always, have a dark green to purple spot in the middle. Leaves may be hairless or covered sparsely with small stiff hairs. Leaf nodes are surrounded by a thin papery membrane that wraps around the stem. The small, dark pink, (rarely white) flowers are densely packed in 1-inch (2.5 cm) spiked terminal clusters. They spike open, while those of the pale look-alike smartweed remain closed (pale smartweed also lacks the purple leaf smudge). Each bloom is approximately 1/8 inch (0.35 cm) across with five petals. Fruits are brown to black and glossy. They have three sides and are egg-shaped. Each fruit contains one tiny seed.

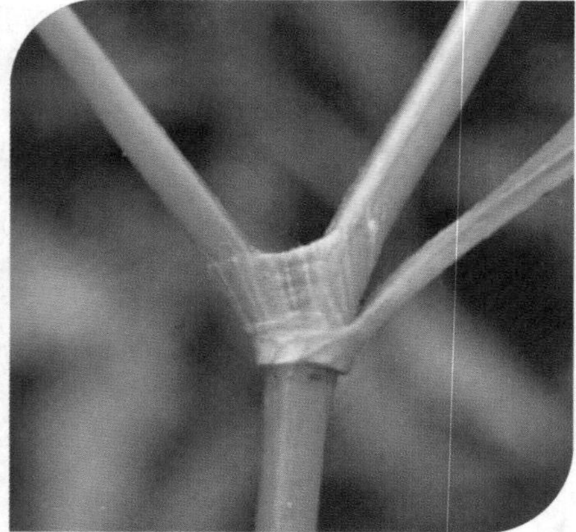

Stem of Lady's Thumb, Martin Olsson, CC by SA 3.0

Edible Use: The leaves and young shoots can be eaten raw or cooked. Gather young leaves and sprouts in the spring to mid-summer. As they mature, they become more peppery and less palatable. The seeds are also edible, but they are rather small and require a lot of work to harvest enough to make a serving.

Medicinal Use: Use as a tea, decoction, or by applying the leaves directly to the skin.

Stomach Pains: For stomach pain and digestive upset, drink a leaf tea.

Skin Ailments: Lady's thumb is a rubefacient, and thus increases blood circulation at the skin's surface, supporting healing. It is also an astringent. Use for poison ivy, poison oak, skin rashes, and other skin ailments. Rub the crushed leaves on the skin or put a poultice on the surface of the skin.

Arthritis: For arthritic pain, soak in a tub of warm water containing a decoction of lady's thumb. The decoction can also be mixed with flour to form a wet poultice to help relieve painful joints.

Lamb's Quarter, Goosefoot, *Chenopodium album*

Lamb's Quarter is also called chualar, pigweed, and also goosefoot from the shape of its leaves. Lamb's quarter likes moist areas and grows near streams, rivers, in open meadows, and wet forest clearings. It is found throughout the world. It is a member of the Amaranthaceae (Amaranth) Family.

Identification: Lamb's quarter looks like a dusty weed from a distance. The alternate toothed leaves are light green on top and whitish on the bottom. They are somewhat diamond-shaped or shaped like a goosefoot.

The leaf surface is waxy and rain and dew rolls right off the leaves. Each leaf grows up to 4 inches (10 cm) long and the entire plant is usually 2 to 4 feet (0.6 to 1.3m) tall. Lamb's quarter produces tiny green flower clusters on top of spikes in summer. The flowers are densely packed together along the main stem and upper branches.

Each flower has five green sepals with no petals. Its seeds are small, round, and flattened. Branches are angular, somewhat ridged, and striped with pink, purple, or yellow. The stems are ribbed and are usually stained with purple or red.

Edible and Other Use: In the USA this plant is considered a weed; however, in some places, it is grown as a food crop. The young shoots, leaves, flowers, and seeds are all edible and can be used like spinach. Lamb's Quarter appears on my plate quite often. I find it a delicious and nutritious addition to my salads and even grow it in my garden.

It has a strong, slightly sweet flavor. The plant does contain oxalic acid so smaller quantities are recommended when eaten raw. The seeds of this herb should be cooked or soaked in water before use. The soaked seeds can also be ground into a powder to use as a flour. Lamb's quarter roots can be crushed to make a mild soap substitute as it contains saponins.

Medicinal Use: The plant is very nutritious and contains a rich source of vitamins A, B-2, C, and Niacin and minerals like calcium, iron, and phosphorus. It has been used as a vegetable to treat scurvy and other nutritional diseases.

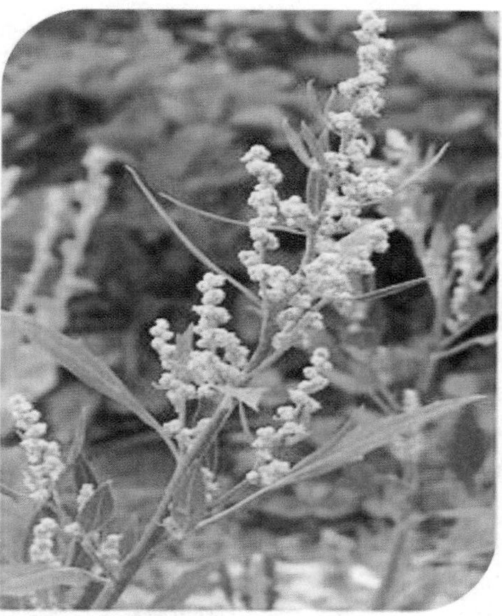

Goosefoot, Photo by Rasbak, CC by SA 3.0

Soothing Burns: Use a poultice made of the leaves to soothe burns. Bruise the leaves and place them on the burned area. Apply a clean cloth over them and leave in place for a few hours.

Skin Irritations, Eczema, Bites, Itching and Swelling: A poultice made from simmered, fresh lamb's quarter leaves can be applied to treat minor skin irritations, itching, rashes, and swelling. It soothes the skin, reduces inflammation (it is an anti-inflammatory), and helps the skin heal. If fresh herbs are not available, use a compress made with Lamb's Quarters Decoction. For internal inflammation, lightly steam the leaves and eat them as a vegetable.

Digestive Issues and as a Mild Laxative: Its leaves are loaded with fiber. This fiber makes it very effective in preventing and treating constipation. Cooked leaves loosen the stools and increase bowel movements.

Taken internally, lamb's quarter relieves stomachaches and digestive complaints, including colic. You can eat the cooked leaves and stems while eating beans to relieve the gas caused by them. Even easier, cook the leaves and stems in the pot with the beans.

Relieves Pain from Arthritis and Gout: Apply a poultice made from fresh, simmered lamb's quarter leaves directly on the skin above the inflammation and pain to treat arthritis and gout. When fresh leaves are not available, use Lamb's Quarters Decoction on the skin as a wash or in a compress.

Dental Health and Tooth Decay: Use a Lamb's Quarter Decoction to treat tooth decay and bad breath. Apply a drop or two of the decoction directly onto the tooth or rinse the mouth with the liquid. It calms inflammation and pain. You can also chew on the raw leaves.

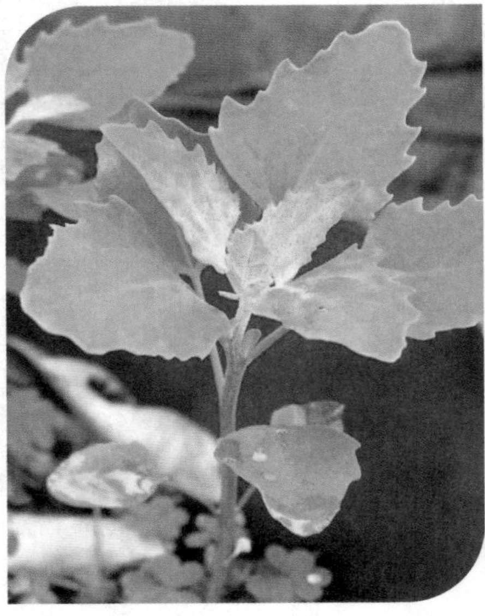

Young goosefoot, 6th Happiness, CC by SA 3.0

Colds, Flu and General Illness: Serve lamb's quarters as a vegetable when people have a cold or flu with respiratory problems. It functions as a mild analgesic to relieve body aches, induces perspiration to bring down fevers, and acts as an expectorant to help the body get rid of excess mucous. It also has anti-asthmatic properties and contains Vitamin C.

Harvesting: Break off or prune the top two inches (5 cm) of shoots. The tops are more tender and less bitter. Choose plants from secluded places, away from roadways, industrial areas, and waste sites where they may pick up high levels of nitrates and other toxins. Wash the leaves before use.

Warning: Lamb's quarter is an edible plant that has very little risk when used in moderate amounts. However, the plant does contain saponins in small quantities. Saponins are broken down by the cooking process. Like many green, leafy vegetables, it also contains oxalate crystals, which are not recommended in large amounts for people susceptible to kidney stones.

Recipes. Lamb's Quarter Decoction: Shred fresh lamb's quarter leaves into small pieces and pack into a cup to measure. Place the leaves in a pot and add an equal measure of water. Bring to a boil and simmer for 10 minutes. Once the herbs are wilted, add more water only if needed to cover the herbs. Cool the decoction and strain out the leaves. Keep in the refrigerator for up to 3 days. (The leaves can be eaten if desired).

Lavender, *Lavandula angustifolia*

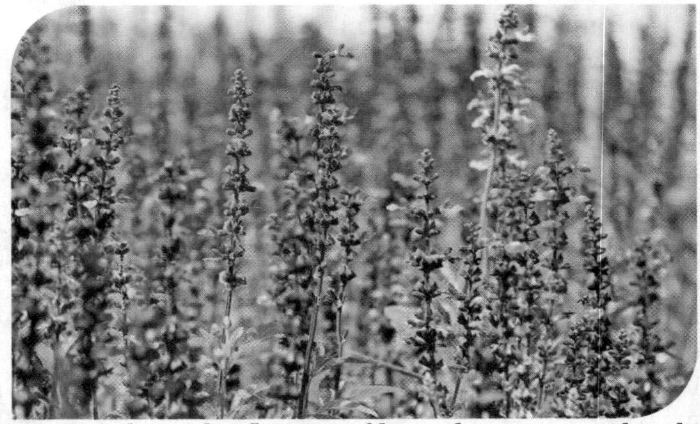

Common lavender belongs to the Lamiaceae (Mint) Family. It is also known as garden lavender, common lavender, narrow-leaved lavender, true lavender, or English lavender.

Identification: Common lavender grows 1 to 3 feet (0.3m to 0.9meters) high in gardens. It has an irregular, erect, bluntly-quadrangular and multi-branched stem that is covered with a yellowish-grey bark, which comes off in flakes. It is covered with fine hairs.

The leaves of lavender are opposite, entire, and linear. When young, they are white with dense hairs on both surfaces. When full grown, leaves are 1 1/2 inch-long (3.75 cm) and green, with scattered hairs on the upper leaf surface. The flowers grow in terminating, blunt spikes from young shoots on long stems. The spikes are composed of whorls of flowers, each having 6 to 10 flowers, and the lower whorls are more distant from one another. The flowers of lavender are very shortly stalked. The calyx of lavender is tubular and ribbed, purple-grey in color, 5-toothed (one tooth is longer than the others) and hairy. The shining oil glands amongst the hairs are visible through a lens. Most of the oil yielded by the flowers is contained in the glands on the calyx. The two-lipped corolla is a beautiful bluish-violet color. It mostly lives and prefers dry grassy slopes amongst rocks, in exposed, usually parched, hot rocky situations often on calcareous soils. While not native to North America, it cultivates easily and spreads wild in many warm, dry areas.

Edible Use: Several parts of lavender are edible including the leaves, flowering tips, and petals. They can be used as a condiment in salads and make a nice tea. Fresh lavender flowers can be added to ice creams, jams, and vinegars as a flavoring. Oil from the flowers is also used as a food flavoring.

Medicinal Use: Medicinal uses are anti-anxiety, antiseptic, antispasmodic, bile-producing, diuretic, nervine, reduces gas, sedative, and stimulant.

Aromatherapy: Lavender is an important relaxing herb, having a soothing and relaxing effect upon the nervous system. In most cases, all that is required is to breathe in the aroma from the oil. This relaxes the body, relieves stress, calms the nervous system, and eases headaches. The same effects can be achieved by adding whole fresh or dried flowers to the bathwater or placing the flowers under the pillowcase at bedtime. I add it to my First Aid Salve so that the aroma is calming to anyone injured who is using the salve.

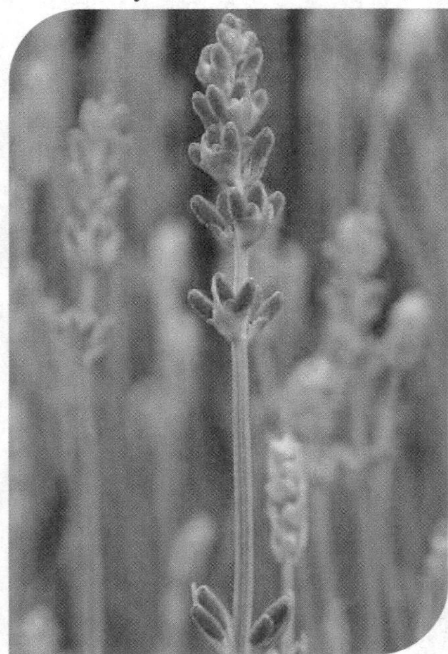

Aches and Pains: Its relaxing effects extend to the muscular system as well. A massage with lavender oil can calm throbbing muscles, relieve arthritis pain, ease and help heal sprains and strains, and relieve backaches and lumbago pain. The oil also contains analgesic compounds that help ease the pain from muscle related stress and injuries.

Kills Lice and Their Nits and Insect Repellent: The essential oil of lavender nourishes the hair, gives it a nice shine, and makes it smell wonderful. It also helps keep the hair free from lice.

Use the essential oil, diluted with a carrier oil such as coconut oil or olive oil, to coat the scalp and hair completely. Give it an hour to soak in and do its magic. Then wash away the oil and use your nit comb. From this point forward, add a drop or two of lavender oil to your shampoo or rinse water to keep lice away. Lavender oil is also an excellent, good-smelling insect repellent.

Respiratory Problems: Lavender essential oil is an excellent treatment for respiratory problems of all kinds. This can include simple, everyday problems like colds, the flu, sore throats, coughs, and sinus congestion. It can also be used for more difficult and chronic respiratory issues like asthma, laryngitis, bronchitis, whooping cough, and tonsillitis.

Apply it topically to the skin on the chest, neck, and under the nose where it will be easily breathed; or add it to a vaporizer or a pot of steaming water. The nicely scented steam opens the air passages and loosens phlegm while it kills the germs that cause the infection.

Urinary Tract Infections, Cystitis and Retained Fluids: The diuretic effects of lavender help it to flush the body from excess fluids and toxins and relieve swellings that may be present. As the fluid is removed, the oil also exerts an antibiotic influence, which kills any underlying infection, and it removes toxins that may also be causing problems.

Lowering Blood Pressure: Removing excess fluids help lower the blood pressure and reduce swellings of all kinds, and the relaxing effects of the lavender help get rid of stresses that may be contributing to the problem.

Harvesting: I usually go out looking for Lavender when the weather is dry and there is no wind. The morning and evening are particularly favorable to gathering flowers because many of the oils are dissipated during the heat of the day. Cut lavender stems are cut at the base of the plant.

Recipes. Lavender Tea: To make lavender tea, start with one teasapoon of dried lavender flowers or one tablespoon of fresh lavender flowers. Place in a tea pot and cover with one cup of boiling water. Cover the tea pot to keep it warm and allow the tea steep for 10 to 15 minutes to absorb the medicinal qualities. Strain it, and drink warm several times daily.

Lavender Tincture: Ingredients: 1½ cups of chopped lavender flowers, stems, and leaves, 1-pint (500 ml)100 proof vodka or brandy. Place the lavender in a glass jar and cover with vodka. Seal the jar tightly and place it in a cool dark place to brew. Allow the tincture to steep for 4 to 6 weeks, shaking the jar daily. Strain the tincture through a coffee filter. Store it in a cool, dark place for up to 3 years.

Lavender Oil Distillation: Distillation equipment: a still OR small pressure cooker, glass tubing, tinned copper tubing, flexible hose, tub of cold water, collection vessel, thermometer. You'll need lavender flowers, stems, and leaves chopped fine or ground, water to cover the herbs. If you have a commercially available still, follow the instructions for steam distillation of essential oil. Otherwise, proceed with my directions to use a pressure cooker for steam distillation. Build a cooling coil out of tin-plated copper tubing. Wrap the tubing around a can or other cylinder to shape it for cooling the oil. Use a small piece of flexible hose to connect the copper tubing to the pressure cooker relief valve.

The steam will rise through the valve and flow into the copper tubing to cool. Bend the copper tubing as needed to place the coil into a pan or a tub of cold water. Cut a small hole in the bottom side of the tub for the copper tubing to exit the tub. Seal the exit hole with a stopper or silicone sealer. The tubing now runs down from the pressure cooker, into the cooling tub, out of the tub into your collection vessel. Place the chopped flowers, stems, and leaves into the pressure cooker. Add water as needed to cover the herbs and fill the pressure cooker to a level of 2 to 3 inches (5 cm to 7.5 cm). Heat the pressure cooker gently and watch for the oil to begin collecting in the collection vessel.

The oil will begin to distill near the boiling point of the water, but before the water boils. Watch for oil production. Monitor the still to make sure it does not boil dry. Collect the distillate until it becomes clear or until most of the water has distilled. The cloudy oil and water mixture indicate oil in the distillate. Once the distillate is clear, it contains only water, and the distillation is finished. Transfer the distilled oil to a dark glass bottle with a tight lid for storage. Lavender Essential Oil is much gentler than most other essential oils and can be safely applied directly to the skin as an antiseptic to help heal wounds and burns.

Leeks, *Allium porrum*

Leeks belong to the Alliaceae (Onion) Family. They are eaten as a vegetable and are quite tasty roasted or in soups. The flavor is mild compared to most members of the onion family.

Identification: Leeks grow from a compressed stem with leaves wrapped in overlapping layers and fanning out at the top. Commercial leeks are white at the base, caused by cultivation methods of piling soil at the base of the stem.

Wild leeks will not exhibit this blanching. Shallow, fibrous roots grow from the stem plate, and the plant grows upward reaching approximately 3 feet (0.9meters). If left in the ground, it produces a large umbel of flowers in the second year. The flowers produce small black, irregular seeds. The flower appears from July to August and has both male and female parts. It is tolerant to frost.

Edible Use: The leek is used extensively around the world as a vegetable and as a flavoring. It contains vitamins, antioxidants, and minerals and is low in calories and high in fiber.

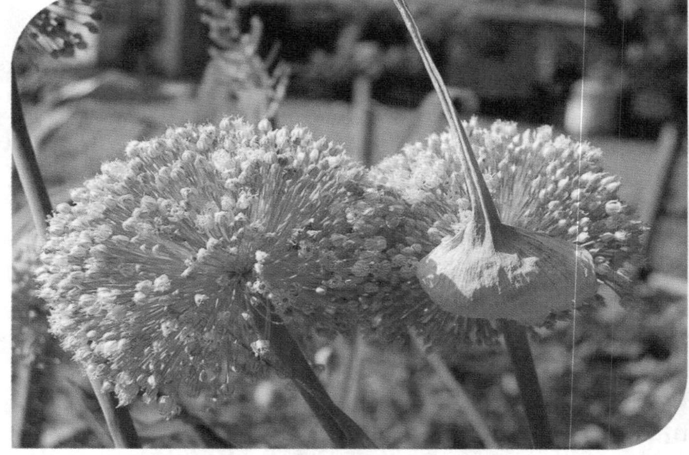

Leek Flower Heads, Photo by Derek Ramsey (Ram-Man) - Own work, CC by SA 2.5

Medicinal Use. Heart Disease, High Blood Pressure, Lowering Cholesterol: Leeks are beneficial to the heart and circulatory system in a number of ways. They contain enzymes that help reduce the harmful cholesterols in the body while increasing the beneficial HDL cholesterols.

They also relax the blood vessels, arteries, and veins, reducing the blood pressure and they reduce the formation of clots and help break down existing clots. In

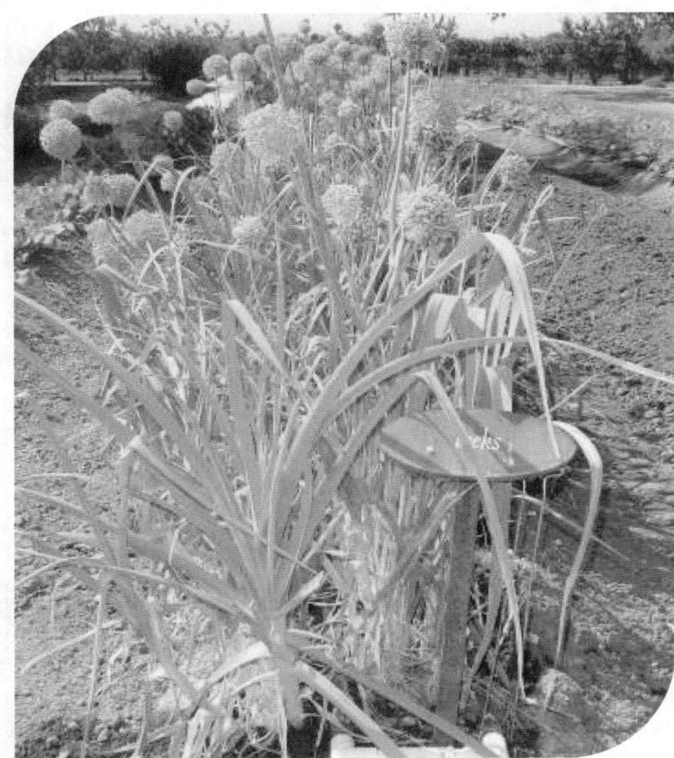

these ways, they reduce the chances of developing coronary heart disease, peripheral vascular diseases, and strokes.

Consuming leeks on a regular basis conveys these beneficial properties.

Stabilize Blood Sugar Levels: Leeks help the body maintain a steady blood sugar level by helping the body metabolize sugars. Leeks also contain nutrients that benefit blood sugar levels. Diabetics and pre-diabetics should eat leeks regularly as part of their healthy diet.

Anti-Bacterial, Anti-Viral, and Anti-Fungal Properties: Eating leeks regularly and often during infections helps your body fight these infections and eliminate them from the body.

Leeks have anti-microbial properties similar to those of garlic and onions that help the body fight internal and external infections.

Eat an extra portion of leeks with meals when fighting infections. For external infections, chop the leeks finely and use them as a poultice on infected tissue.

Prevents Cancer: Plants in the Alliaceae family have multiple cancer-fighting properties, and leeks are included. Eating leeks on a regular basis reduces the chances of prostate and colon cancers. People who eat a lot of leeks also have fewer ovarian cancers.

Eat Leeks During Pregnancy: Leeks contain high levels of folate, which is beneficial for the developing fetus and prevents several different birth defects of the brain and spinal cord.

Anemia: Leeks are also high in iron and therefore beneficial for treating iron deficiency anemia. They also contain significant levels of vitamin C, which helps iron absorption in the body.

Gout, Arthritis, and Urinary Tract Inflammation: Arthritis, gout, and urinary tract problems benefit from the anti-inflammatory and antiseptic properties of leeks to treat these diseases.

High doses of leeks are best, so I recommend eating several servings daily or drinking the juice of the vegetable.

Regular Bowel Movements: The high concentrations of both soluble and insoluble dietary fiber in leeks help the function of the intestinal tract. They facilitate digestion and reduce bloating and associated pain.

Whole Body Cleanse: Drinking leek juice regularly helps cleanse the body of toxins and waste products.

Harvesting: Harvest when the stalks are about an inch (2.5 cm) wide, usually in late summer. In some areas they over-winter and can be harvested in early spring or even year-round.

Warning: Leeks contain oxalates, which may crystalize in the body to cause kidney stones and gravel in the gallbladder.

Lemon Balm, *Melissa officinalis*

Lemon Balm is a perennial member of the Lamiaceae (Mint) Family with valuable healing properties. Sometimes called common balm or balm mint, it is naturalized in North America. I love the lemony scent that is released when I walk through a patch of lemon balm.

Identification: Lemon balm is a mint with shiny bright green leaves and a lemony scent. It may grow to 3 feet (0.9m) in height and is easy to cultivate in the garden. Its appearance is similar to mint or catnip, but the lemon scent is intense when leaves are disturbed or crushed. The leaves are small heart shapes with scalloped edges and a slightly crinkled surface. Small flowers are usually white to yellow but can be pink or purple.

Edible Use: The leaves are edible and often used to make tea and as a flavoring ingredient. It makes a delicious tea for medicinal or culinary use and is enhanced by the use of raw honey to sweeten it.

Medicinal Use: Lemon balm leaves are often used as a tea, extract, tincture, oil, or ointment.

Relieves Anxiety and Insomnia: Lemon balm acts to reduce anxiety and helps people get better sleep. It calms the body and improves mood and intellectual performance in children and adults without negative effects. For reducing the effects of sleep disorders, especially during menopause, try a combination of lemon balm and valerian. Lemon balm helps stop the constant flow of anxious thoughts. It also helps with ADHD and mild depression.

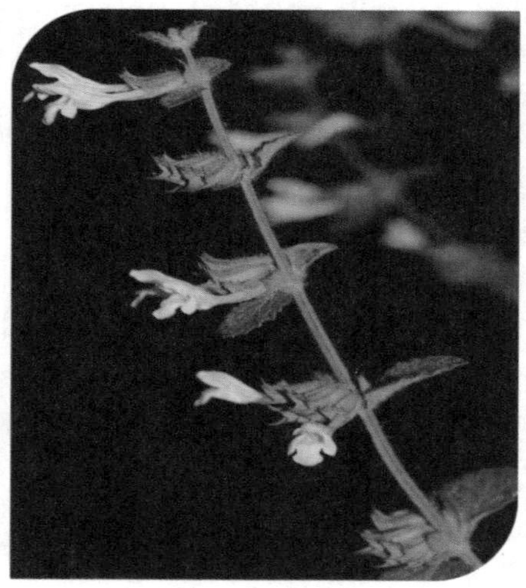

Lemon Balm Flowers, Gideon Pisanty, CC BY 3.0

Mind Calming and Clear Thinking: Lemon balm seems to calm the mind and allows people to think more clearly. It increases mental alertness and promotes a positive attitude.

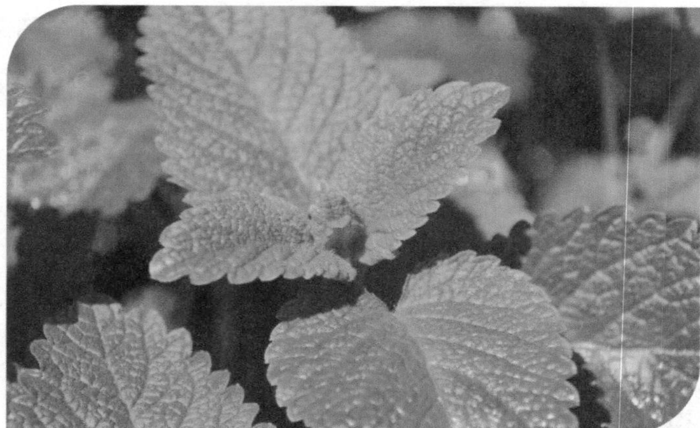

Anti-Viral Effects: Herpes, Cold Sores, and Shingles: Lemon balm is known as an anti-viral and is effective against herpes and cold sores when applied directly to the skin. It acts against the herpes simplex virus and when used regularly, people report fewer outbreaks and fast healing of existing lesions. It also gives relief of symptoms like itching and burning. Try lemon balm essential oil or lemon balm ointment on herpes and cold sores. Apply several times daily or as needed. For shingles take a tincture internally as well as apply topically to the affected area.

PMS Symptoms: Lemon balm reduces symptoms of PMS, including cramping, anxiety, and headaches. It works well for PMS in teenage and adult women. It is an anti-spasmodic.

Protects the Heart: Lemon balm, used regularly, lowers triglycerides and improves cholesterol synthesis. It controls heart palpitations and lowers blood pressure while protecting the heart. It controls the electrical pulses that drive heart palpitations, tachycardia, and arrhythmias.

Protects the Liver: Lemon balm protects the liver from some of the negative effects of the American diet. It supports the liver's production of antioxidants and helps detox the liver.

Antibacterial and Antifungal: Lemon Balm oil has a high level of antibacterial and antifungal activity. It is particularly active against *Candida* yeast infections. Use lemon balm oil, tincture or extract twice a day.

Diabetes: Lemon balm oil, tincture and extract are effective in preventing and treating diabetes. It helps control blood sugar levels and protects the body against the oxidative stress caused by diabetes.

Anti-Inflammatory and Antioxidant: Lemon balm oil acts as an anti-inflammatory and antioxidant. It reduces inflammation in the body, protecting against disease and reducing pain.

Fights Cancer: Lemon balm has been shown to kill some cancer cell lines, including breast cancer, colorectal cancer, and aggressive brain cancers. Lemon balm supports the body in fighting the cancer cells.

Regulates the Thyroid: Hyperthyroidism, or an over-active thyroid benefits from the regular consumption of lemon balm. People with Grave's disease or other over-active thyroid problems find that the oil, tincture or extract helps regulate thyroid-binding problems.

Aids in Digestion: Lemon balm extract has a protective effect on the gastrointestinal system and prevents gastric ulcers. It aids digestion and is useful in treating constipation as well as colic.

Alzheimer's Disease and Dementia: Lemon balm extract is believed to reduce damage from plaque forming proteins in Alzheimer's disease. Regular administration of lemon balm extract increases cognitive function over time and reduces agitation in Alzheimer's patients.

The therapy is not a cure, but is observed to slow progression and help promote mild improvements. As an anti-oxidant it may help protect the brain from neurodegeneration and oxidative damage.

Lemon Balm also improves memory and problem solving in people of all ages and health levels including Alzheimer's patients.

Heals Skin and Reduces Signs of Aging: People who use lemon balm on their skin report that it reduces wrinkles and fine lines giving the skin a more youthful appearance. It is particularly beneficial in supporting the skin against minor blemishes and infections.

Harvesting: Left alone, lemon balm may take over the garden. Several bouts of pruning keep the plant in check. Clip off stems or remove individual leaves for drying on screens, in a dehydrator, or hand them in bunches to dry. I like to harvest just before the plant flowers (early to late summer).

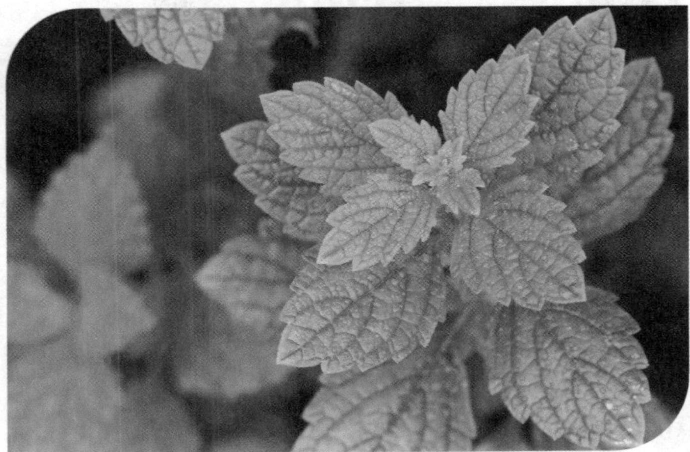

Warning: Lemon balm is considered safe for most people, but should not be used by people on thyroid medication or with underactive thyroids (Hypothyroidism).

Consult a medical profession before using lemon balm regularly if you are pregnant or nursing. Possible side effects include headache, nausea, bloating, gas, indigestion, dizziness, and allergic reactions. Consult a doctor if you are taking other medications or planning surgical treatments.

Recipes. Lemon Balm Tea: You will need: 1 tablespoon fresh lemon balm leaves or 1t dried and 1 cup boiling water. Tear the leaves into small pieces and put into a tea ball, or filter the leaves after brewing.

Pour boiling water over the tea leaves or ball and allow to infuse for 5 minutes. Keep the pot or cup covered while brewing and drinking to retain the beneficial aromatics.

Lemon Balm Extract/Tincture: Ingredients: 1-pint (500ml) jar with a tight-fitting lid, 80 proof or higher vodka or another alcoholic beverage. Wash and dry the leaves and crush them lightly.

Fill the jar 3/4 full with leaves and pour the vodka, filling the jar completely. Cap and store in a cool, dark place, shaking periodically. After 4 to 6 weeks, strain and label.

Lemon Thyme, *Thymus citriodorus*

Lemon thyme is also called citrus thyme. It is easy to recognize lemon thyme by its aroma and flavor, which are both very much like lemon. Even better than the smell are the relaxing benefits and medicinal value of the herb. It is in the Lamiaceae (Mint) Family.

Identification: Lemon thyme is an evergreen perennial that grows as a mat on the ground. It grows to a height of 4 inches (10 cm) and spreads to over a foot away. Its appearance and growth habit is close to that of English thyme.

The leaves are shiny-green with a pale-yellow border around the margins. Some plants have more lemon-yellow leaves or green leaves with pale yellow splotches. The plant produces flowers in mid to late summer. Flowers may vary from pink to lavender and attract butterflies and bees.

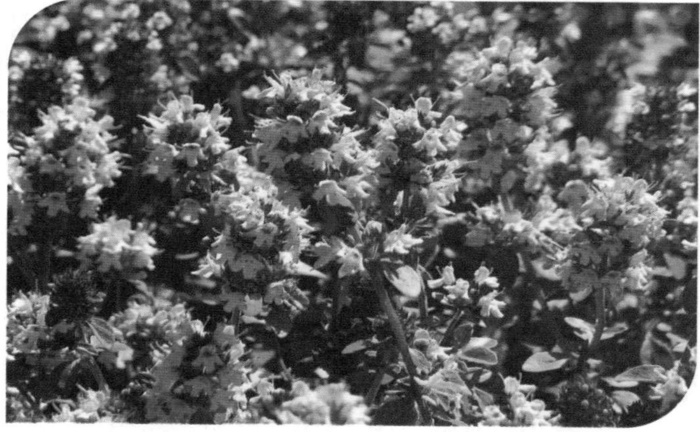

Lemon Thyme flowers, Kor!An (Андрей Корзун), CC by SA 3.0

Edible Use: Lemon thyme is used widely in cooking to flavor chicken, fish, and vegetable dishes and to make a relaxing tea.

Medicinal Use: Immune Function: Lemon Thyme Tea is a relaxing drink that is effective in the treatment of infections and boosting the immune system. It makes a good tonic for regular use.

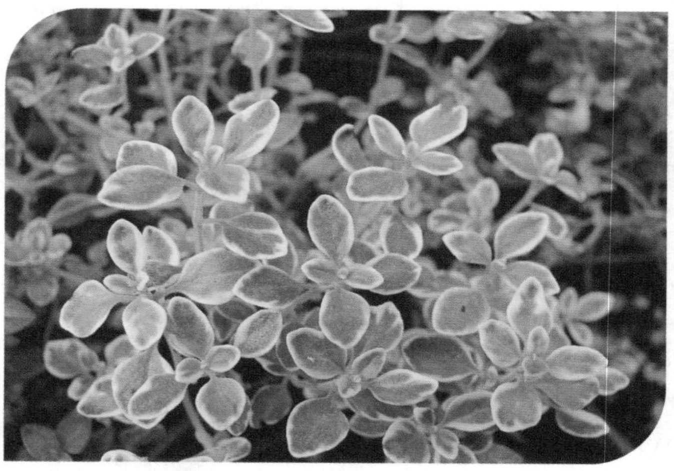

Lemon Thyme, Forest & Kim Starr, CC by SA 3.0

Viral, Bacterial, and Fungal Infections: The anti-microbial properties of lemon thyme make it effective in the fight against most bacterial, fungal, and viral diseases.

Respiratory Problems, Asthma, and Releasing Congestion: Lemon thyme contains many different beneficial compounds for general health and for respiratory health. It is an anti-microbial and a decongestant.

It opens the airways to help asthmatics breathe better and to allow phlegm and other mucous to be released from the body.

Aromatherapy for Asthma: Asthmatics find relief by placing a small pillow filled with dried lemon thyme under their regular pillow. Sleeping on this pillow releases the oils that open the airways and induce better sleep.

Warning: Lemon thyme causes allergic reactions in highly allergic people. Do not give lemon thyme tea during pregnancy or while nursing.

Lemon Thyme Tea: You'll need 1/2 teaspoon of dried lemon thyme or 1 teaspoon of fresh lemon thyme leaves, 1 cup boiling water and honey, optional. Pour the boiling water over the lemon thyme leaves and allow the tea to steep for 5 to 10 minutes.

Strain the tea and drink warm. Add honey as desired for sweetening. Drink two to three cups daily.

Lemon Verbena, *Aloysia triphylla*

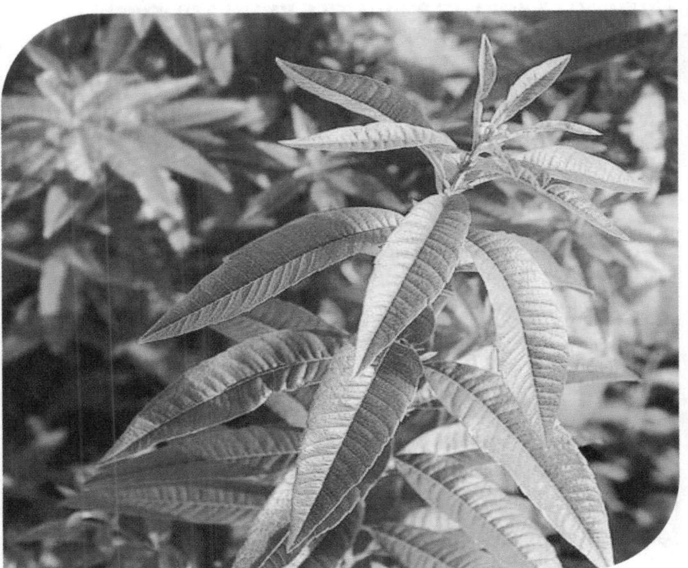

Oh, how I love lemon verbena. I love to crush a stalk in my hand and breathe in the fragrance and flavor. It immediately lifts my mood and soothes away the stresses of the day. The herb is highly aromatic with an herbaceous lemony scent. It is in the Verbenaceae (Verbena) Family. It is not native but is easily cultivated in the garden.

Identification: Lemon verbena is readily identified by its scent and the plant growth. It grows to a height of 6 to 15 feet (1.8m to 4.5m) in good soil. It has thin, pointed leaves that are about 3 to 4 inches (7.5 cm to 10 cm) in length. The leaves are shiny and coarse to the touch. The flowers are light purple and grouped on the stems. They appear throughout the summer.

Edible Use: Lemon verbena leaves are useful as a flavoring or as an addition to salads. It has a mild lemon flavor.

Medicinal Use: Use lemon verbena leaves and flowers internally in the form of an herbal tea and externally as a poultice, oil, or wash.

Bronchial Congestion: Use a tea made from lemon verbena to treat bronchial and nasal congestion. It loosens phlegm, acts as an expectorant, and calms the system. Do not use lemon verbena tea before driving or operating heavy machinery as it has a mild sedative effect.

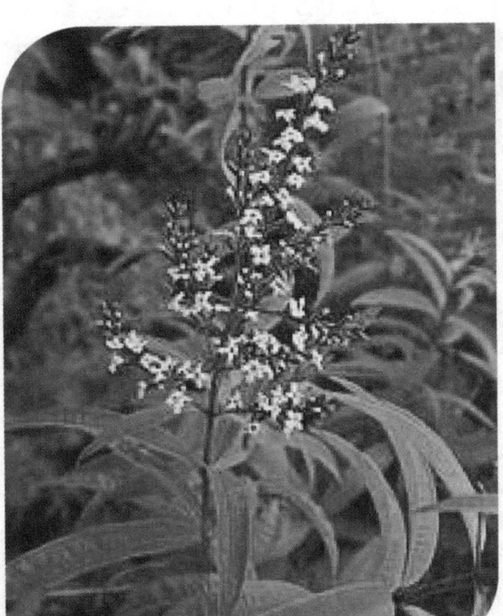

Lemon Verbena, H. Zell, CC by SA 3.0

Staph Infections of the Skin: Staph infections can become serious quickly if left untreated. It prevents the infection from spreading and kills the existing bacteria. For this purpose, use Lemon Verbena Leaf Tincture made with 80 proof alcohol, applied to the skin. When the extraction is not available, a poultice of freshly crushed lemon verbena is applied (note that Usnea also works well on *Staphylococcus*).

Arthritis, Bursitis, and Joint Pain: Peoples with joint pain find significant relief from taking lemon verbena tea. It takes time for the effects to build, but over a period of two to three months of taking the tea twice daily, people report that joint pain is gradually reduced and significant improvement is gained.

Digestive Issues: Try Lemon Verbena Tea for digestive problems as it has a soothing effect on the digestive system. It relieves indigestion and calms the stomach and intestinal spasms to relieve cramping and bloating. Try drinking a cup of tea after meals.

Calms Anxiety: For severe anxiety, try Lemon Verbena Tea. It soothes the nervous system, relieves stress, and lifts the mood.

Harvesting: Lemon verbena likes rich soil and plenty of sunlight. I collect the leaves throughout the year, but I prefer to pick as many as possible before the herb blooms. Extra leaves are dried for future use and are equally beneficial in dried form.

Recipes. Lemon Verbena Tea: 1/4 cup lemon verbena leaves, fresh and crushed, 2 cups boiling water. Pour the boiling water over the herb and allow it to steep for 5 to 8 minutes. Strain and Drink 1 cup.

Lemon Verbena Tincture: Take fresh Lemon Verbena leaves and flowers, chopped, 80 proof vodka or other drinking alcohol and a jar with a tight-fitting lid. Add the lemon verbena to the jar, packing it about three quarters full. Pour the vodka over the leaves and fill the jar, making sure all the leaves are covered. Cap the jar tightly and place it in a cool, dark place, such as a cupboard. Let the tincture steep for 6 to 8 weeks, shaking the jar daily. Pour the alcohol through a fine mesh sieve or a coffee filter to remove all the herb. Store the tincture in a cool, dark cupboard for up to 7 years.

Licorice Root, *Glycyrrhiza glabra*

Licorice root is an adaptogenic herb that thrives in USDA growing zones 6 through 11. It is well known for its strong candy flavor but is a valuable medicinal herb for treating many illnesses.

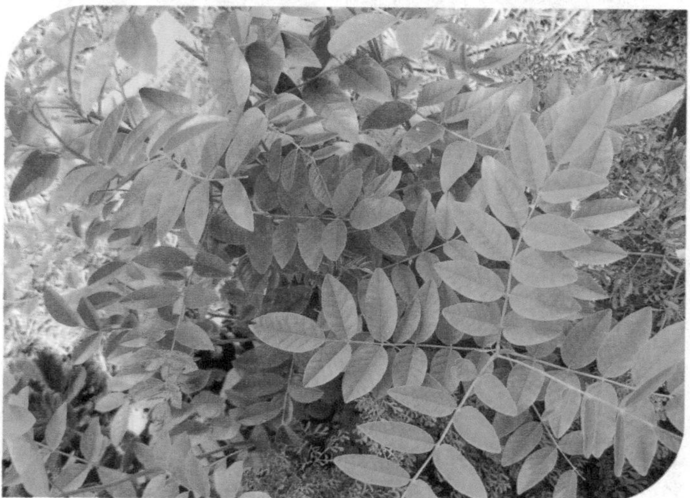

Photo By Gardenology.org, CC by SA 3.0

Glycyrrhiza glabra and Glycyrrhiza uralensis are medicinally similar, but here we are referring to Glycyrrhiza glabra. It is a member of the legume/pea family (Fabaceae).

Identification: Glycyrrhiza glabra grows to approximately 3 feet tall (0.9m). Its pinnate leaves are 3 to 6 inches long (7.5 – 15cm) with 9 to 17 leaflets each. The purple to pale blue flowers are about 1/2 inch long (1.25cm), growing in a loose inflorescence. In the fall the plant produces fruit in the form of an oblong pod, each of which contains several seeds. The root produces runners growing close to the surface.

Medicinal Use: The roots and leaves contain many types of compounds that are medically active: coumarins, triterpenoids, glabrene, and polyphenols. These compounds are antibacterial, antiviral, anti-inflammatory, and include natural steroid compounds.

Glycyrrhizin, one of the components of licorice root, can cause side-effects if overused or taken in large doses. Be aware of all side-effects and interactions before using licorice root.

You can also get deglycyrrhizinated licorice (DGL), which has the glycyrrhizin removed, thus preventing its side effects.

Leaky Gut Syndrome and Inflammation: Leaky gut, or intestinal permeability, is an inflammatory disease of the intestinal tract. Licorice root soothes the intestines and reduces inflammation in the gut and throughout the body.

Peptic Ulcers: Licorice root is effective against the Helicobacter pylori bacteria that cause peptic ulcers. The root kills the bacteria and helps heal the ulcers in most people.

Heartburn, Stomach Problems, and Acid Reflux: Licorice root has shown to be effective against indigestion heartburn, acid reflux, indigestion, stomach pain, and nausea.

Fertility Problems, PMS, and Menopause Symptoms: Licorice root has an estrogen-like effect in women, due to the compound glabrene, which is a phytoestrogen. It has been shown to help menstrual and fertility problems. When used as a hormone replacement therapy, it reduces hot flashes and other symptoms of menopause due to the compounds liquiritigenin and glabrene.

Cancer: Licorice root may aid in the treatment of prostate and breast cancers. Research is still in progress on the use of licorice in cancer treatment, but the early results are promising.

Hepatitis C: Glycyrrhizin is an anti-viral and anti-inflammatory. It may act against the virus causing hepatitis C and helps reduce long-term liver damage from the disease. Herbalists use glycyrrhizin to treat chronic hepatitis C that does not respond to traditional treatments.

Immune System, Antiviral, Antioxidant: Licorice has proven antiviral, antibacterial, and antioxidant effects, boosting the work of the immune system. As an antiviral, it helps prevent diseases such as hepatitis C, HIV, and Influenza.

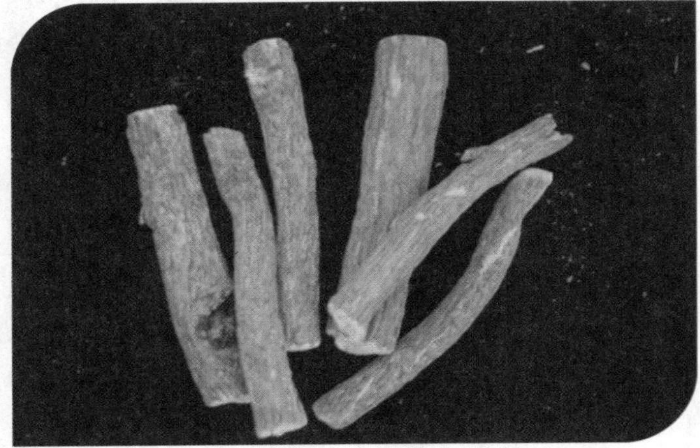

The Common Cold, Cough, and Sore Throats: In addition to its antiviral and anti-bacterial benefits, licorice root also acts as an expectorant, loosening and expelling mucus from the throat and lungs.

It is soothing and anti-inflammatory, which helps relieve the symptoms of sore throats. Use licorice root or leaves in tea, syrups, or to make cough drops for use against sore throats. It can also be used as a gargle.

Respiratory Issues: Licorice is useful in treating respiratory problems. It helps the body produce and expel mucus, which keeps the respiratory system clean and functioning properly. Used for COPD as well.

Treats Eczema, Skin Rashes: Licorice acts as a hydrocortisone to alleviate eczema, cellulitis, and folliculitis. Its anti-inflammatory benefits also help reduce swelling and irritation in skin conditions. Use licorice topically in a cleansing tea or in lotions or gels to relieve itching, redness, scaling, and inflammation caused by eczema or other skin problems.

Harvesting: Licorice is a perennial deciduous plant that requires three to four years to grow roots mature enough for harvest. Harvest the leaves throughout the spring through fall. Wait until the licorice roots are 3 to 4 years old before harvest. Young roots are too small to be of use.

Recipes. Liquid Extract: Licorice extract is a common form of licorice, it is used as a sweetener in candies and some beverages.

Limit your use of licorice extract to 30 mg/ml of glycyrrhizic acid. Higher doses can cause side-effects.

Licorice Root Powder: Licorice root powder is useful as is for treating skin problems or for use in capsules as an oral supplement. Combine it with a gel or lotion base to make a topical ointment or lotion for treating skin problems.

Licorice Leaf Tea: Use dried and crushed licorice leaves as a tea to promote health of the digestive and respiratory tract. Use 1 teaspoon of crushed leaves per 1 cup of boiling water.

DGL Licorice: DGL licorice is a commercial form of licorice with the glycyrrhizin removed. It is considered a safer form of licorice root and is particularly recommended for long term use. DGL is available commercially.

Warning: Long-term use of licorice root or high doses can have serious side effects. Most of the side effects are due to the presence of glycyrrhizin, so using DGL licorice reduces the risks.

Watch for these symptoms: low levels of potassium in the body, hypokalemia, muscle weakness, fluid retention and swelling, metabolism abnormalities, high blood pressure, heart rhythm irregularities, erectile dysfunction, potential drug interactions.

Pregnant or breastfeeding women should avoid licorice in all forms. Patients who are prone to hypertension should also avoid licorice root.

Also avoid use of licorice root if you have heart, liver, or kidney problems. Stop taking licorice root at least two weeks before surgery.

Lovage, *Levisticum officinale*

Lovage is native to Southern Europe, is easy to cultivate in the garden, and has naturalized in Eastern North America. It has a celery-like taste and is in the Apiaceae/ Umbelliferae (Celery/ Parsley /Carrot) Family.

Identification: Lovage grows to a height of 6 feet (1.8m). The plant is erect and its stems and leaves are hairless with a celery scent. Stems are thick and celery-like with additional flat lobed pinnate leaves. Yellow to greenish-yellow flowers, approximately 1 inch (2.5 cm) in diameter, bloom in late spring. Flowers grow in umbels 4 to 6 inches (10 cm to 15 cm) in diameter. Fruit matures in autumn, forming a 2-part seed.

Edible Use: Lovage is edible and a good addition wherever you would normally use celery. The taste is stronger than celery. The leaves can be used as a salad green or brewed into a tea. The seeds are used as a flavoring spice. Lovage is nutritionally healthy, adding B-complex vitamins and vitamin C to the diet.

Medicinal Use: Lovage root and leaves are effectively used in teas, decoctions, infusions, and tinctures. Leaves and roots can be added to bath water and foot soaks. All parts of the plant are medicinally active.

Soothes the Digestive Tract: Lovage seeds are effective in treating digestive problems and relieving intestinal gas. Simply chew the seeds for a quick remedy for digestive upsets, bloating, and gas.

Skin Conditions and Inflammations, Dermatitis, Acne, Psoriasis, Rashes: I prefer lovage root preparations for skin inflammations. The root pieces can be added to bathwater for a long soak or simmered in water to make a decoction for application to the affected areas. Lovage Leaf Oil Extract is also effective for applications to infections, wounds, and treating inflamed skin.

Reduces Inflammation and Irritation in the Body: Lovage is soothing throughout the body. It reduces irritation and inflammation that causes problems such as colitis, inflammatory bowel disease, and other diseases caused by inflammation.

Painful Joints: Painful joints from any cause, especially gout and arthritis, respond to treatment with lovage root both internally and externally. It reduces inflammation and lets the joints heal.

Respiratory Problems: Lovage roots and leaves help increase airflow and oxygen to the body. It loosens phlegm in the lungs and calms irritation.

Anti-Histamine: Lovage is a natural antihistamine that helps fight allergy symptoms. Quercetin, found in lovage, stops the release of histamines and soothes the irritations caused by the allergy. Use Lovage Tea internally and apply a decoction or oil for external relief of skin rashes or irritations.

Prevents Kidney Stones and Helps UTIs: For patients who have a history of kidney stones or urinary tract infections, try Lovage Root Tea or Tincture. It acts as a diuretic and increases the flow of urine without electrolyte loss. This flushing action helps prevent kidney stones from building in the kidneys.

Supports a Healthy Menstrual Cycle: Women can take Lovage Tea a day or two before their menstrual flow begins. It relieves cramping and bloating due to menstruation.

Harvesting: Harvest leaves before the plant flowers and use fresh or dry them for future use. Roots are harvested from plants that are 3 years old or older. Dig up the roots in autumn or early spring.

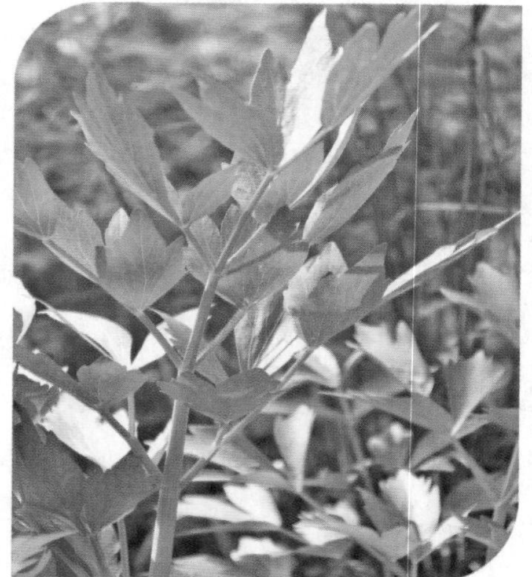

Recipes. **Lovage Tea**: You'll need one teaspoon of dried lovage or 1 tablespoon of fresh lovage leaves and 1 cup of boiling water. Pour the boiling water over the lovage and cover it to keep it warm. Let the tea steep for 10 to 15 minutes to absorb the medicinal qualities. Strain it, and drink warm several times daily.

Lovage Tincture: 1½ cups of chopped lovage root and leaves, 1 pint (500 ml) 80 proof vodka or brandy. Place fresh or dried lovage in a glass jar and cover with vodka. Seal the jar tightly and place it in a cool dark place to brew. Allow the tincture to steep for 4 to 6 weeks, shaking the jar daily. Strain. Label and store it in a cool, dark place for up to 5 years.

Lungwort (Common) Plant, *Pulmonaria officinalis*

Common Lungwort is a beautiful little plant that grows as a groundcover in partial shade on the forest floor, reaching about a foot in height. It has several different names, including Bethlehem Sage, Jerusalem Cowslip, and Pulmonaire. Native to Europe it is easy to cultivate in the garden. It is in the Borage Family. It is different than Lungwort Lichen, also in this book. The leaves look slightly like a diseased lung, giving it the name lungwort and indicating its use in treating lung diseases.

Identification: The bright green leaves come to a point at one end. The leaf top is hairy and rough and leaves are covered with whitish or gray spots. Small bunches of flowers appear in spring. Each flower has 5 pinkish-blue or purple petals. Seeds ripen in late May or June.

Edible Use: The leaves of lungwort are edible both raw and cooked. They have a mucilaginous and hairy texture that makes them less appealing when uncooked.

Medicinal Use: **Bronchitis, Asthma, Whooping Cough:** Lungwort is effective in treating breathing problems such as chronic bronchitis, asthma, and whopping cough. The leaves are soothing and expectorant. Their mucilaginous properties make them useful in treating sore throats. Lungwort relieves bronchial inflammations of the airways and helps the body expel mucus. I like tea made from the leaves and flowers for this purpose. A recipe for Lungwort Tea is below. Alternatively, grind the dried flowers and leaves into a powder to use in capsule form or use a Lungwort Tincture.

Diarrhea and Digestive Complaints: The mucilaginous properties make the leaves effective in treating diarrhea and other digestive problems such as stomach pain, bloating, and indigestion.

Diuretic and Detoxify: Lungwort is a mild diuretic, and thus helps bloating and relieving the body of excess fluids. This is also beneficial for helping remove toxins from the body.

General Tonic for Health and Anti-Aging: Lungwort is rich in antioxidants and other compounds that are beneficial for health, slow down the aging process, and protect the body from free radical damage. It is also an excellent astringent.

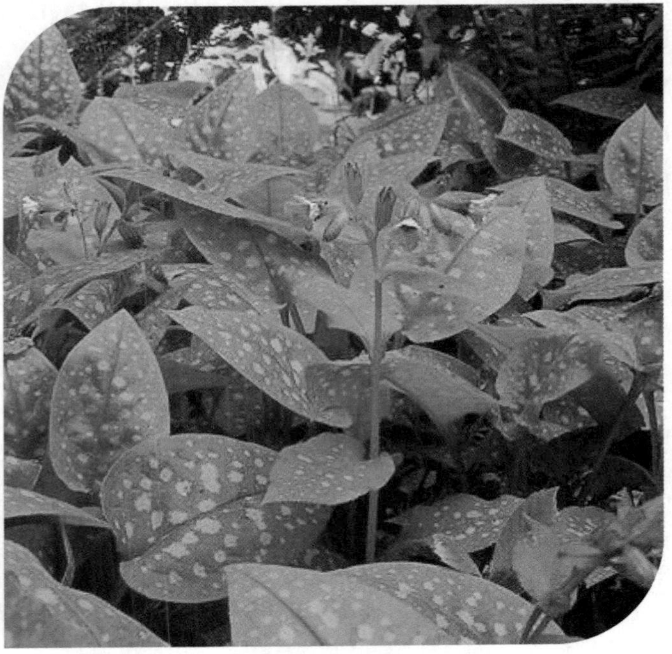

Lungwort with flowers, TeunSpaans, CC by SA 3.0

Wounds, Cuts, Hemorrhoids, and Skin Diseases: Lungwort helps the skin heal from cuts and wounds and contributes to skin health. Apply it directly to the skin as a wash, compress, or poultice as needed for various skin conditions including burns, eczema, rashes, boils and ulcers, and to reduce and heal hemorrhoids. It is anti-inflammatory, anti-bacterial, and astringent.

Urinary Tract Infections, Cystitis, Kidney Problems: Because of its diuretic properties and antibacterial properties, Lungwort is beneficial in helping the body rid itself of excess fluids and aids the kidneys and urinary tract in the process. It treats urinary tract infections like cystitis (bladder infection), and helps expel toxins from the body.

Stops Bleeding: Taken internally as a powder or tea, lungwort is useful in reducing internal bleeding and excess menstrual bleeding. It can be applied directly to external wounds as a powder or whole leaf to bind a wound and stimulate clotting.

Ringworm: A Lungwort Decoction applied several times a day directly onto the skin will help with ringworm.

Harvesting: Harvest the flowers and leaves in the spring when the flowers first appear. Cut off the entire stem with leaves and flowers attached and tie them in bunches for hanging and drying.

Warning: Be cautious taking Lungwort if you are pregnant or breastfeeding. The plant has no known side effects, but caution is always warranted. Lungwort can cause a skin rash in some people. Do not use Lungwort if you experience a rash or any adverse reaction.

Recipes. **Lungwort Tea**: 1 Tablespoon lungwort leaves and flowers, 1 cup boiling water, Raw honey, as desired for sweetness. Pour the boiling water over the leaves and flowers and allow it to steep for 15 minutes. Strain the tea and drink up to three cups daily. Raw honey helps alleviate the bitter flavor for some people.

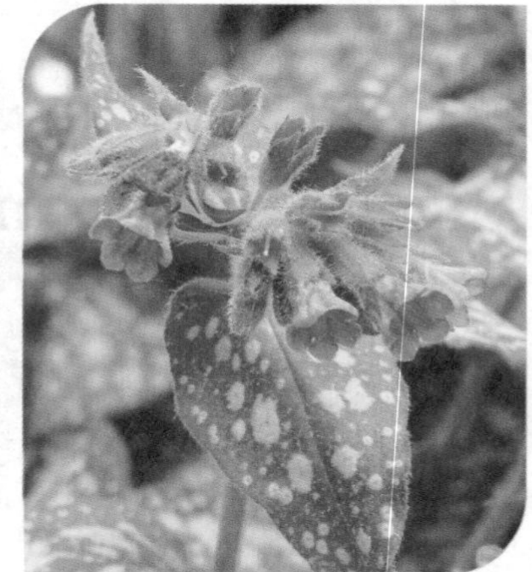

Lungwort Decoction for Wounds: 2 Tablespoons chopped, dried lungwort leaves and 1 cup boiling water. Make a strong tea, infusing the leaves in the boiling water for 20 minutes or until cool. Strain the decoction and use it to wash the skin and affected areas or apply it to a cloth and use as a compress.

Mallow, *Malva sylvestris*

Mallow, also called high mallow, wood mallow, tree mallow, or cheeseweed, is a spreading herb that can be biennial. It is native to Europe and Asia but is naturalized throughout most of North America. This is a different plant than Marshmallow, also in this book. It is in the Malvaceae (Mallow) Family and looks similar to Hibiscus.

Identification: This plant grows from 3 to 10 feet (3m) high. Its branches are bare or covered with fine soft hairs. They have palmately lobed leaves that are dark green in color with long petioles. Leaves are 1 ½ to 2 inches (3.5 cm to 5 cm) across and are creased with 3 to 9 shallow lobes. Leaves on the stem are alternate. The leaves have a course feel but release mucilage when crushed. Purple-pink flowers bloom between May and August. Flowers grow in axillary clusters of 2 to 4 and form

along the main stem. They are about 2 inches (5 cm) in diameter with 5 dark, veined, notched petals. Flowers at the base of the stem open first. The fruit looks like compressed disks or a cheese wheel, leading to the nickname "cheese flower." Ripe seeds are about ¼ inch (0.625 cm) in diameter and are brownish-green to brown in color.

Edible Use: All parts are edible raw or cooked and are mucilagenous. Leaves cook up much like okra. Cooked mallow roots can be beaten and used like egg whites in a meringue.

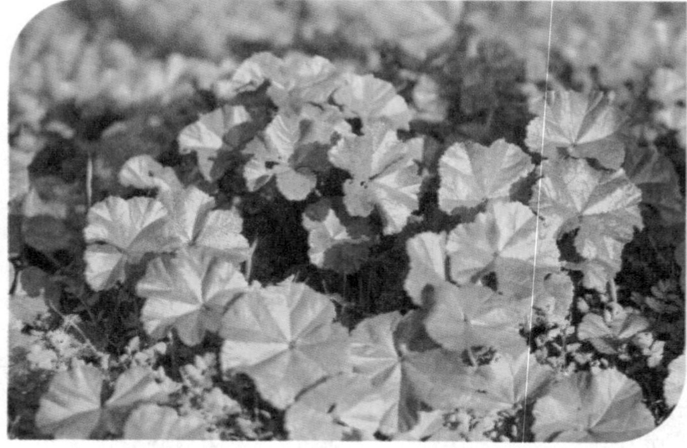

Medicinal Use: Mallow roots, leaves, seeds, and flowers are all used medicinally. The mucilage is very soothing and it is a good anti-inflammatory.

Soothes Irritated Mucous Membranes: Mallow Tea is helpful for cases of irritated mucous membranes. It soothes the lining of the respiratory tract and other mucus membranes for symptom relief of colds, coughs, bronchitis, emphysema, and asthma. It is also anti-inflammatory.

Burns, Bruising, Swelling and Other Topical Use: Mallow soothes inflamed tissue and works well for burns, dermatitis, and any type of swelling. It can be added to a bath or used on the skin.

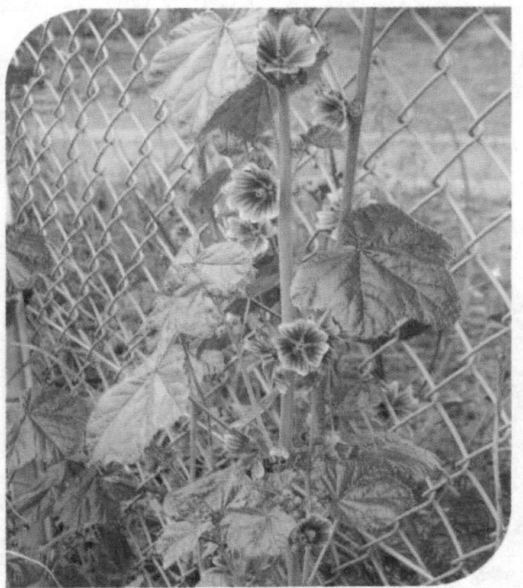

High Mallow, KENPEI, CC by SA 3.0

Anti-bacterial and Urinary Tract Infections: Leaf and flower tincture is antibacterial against *Staphylococcus*, *Streptococcus*, and *Enterococcus*. Best used in conjunction with stronger antibacterial herbs for UTIs and other infections. Mallow relieves the swelling and irritation of the urinary tract and helps promote healing.

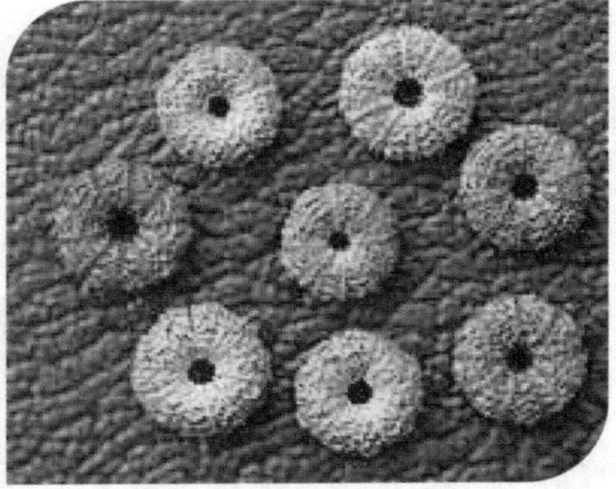

Nutlets or seeds, Qniemiec, CC by SA 3.0

Teething: Mallow Root Tea is safe for use with children and is a good antidote for teething pain and inflammation. Rub the tea onto the gums as often as needed.

Nausea, Stomach and Digestive Upsets: Mallow Leaf or Root Tea relieves nausea. It works well for stomach flu, ulcers, and other stomach upsets, soothing inflammation and promoting normal bowel function.

Recipes: Mallow Root Tea. 1 tablespoon of shredded or powdered mallow root, 1-pint (500 ml) of water. Bring the root and water to a boil and simmer for 5 to 10 minutes. Allow it to cool to drinking temperature and strain out the root. Drink 1 cup, warm or cold.

Marshmallow, *Althaea officinalis*

The common marshmallow plant is grown commercially for medicinal use, but it can be found in many places in the US growing wild. The roots were used to make the original marshmallow candy, unlike today's supermarket version, which are pure sugar. The plant grows in cool, moist places such as the grassy banks of lakes and streams and on the edges of marshes. I have seen it growing wild in many eastern and mid-western states. I grow it in my garden. It is in the Malvaceae (Mallow) Family.

Identification: Marshmallow is a green perennial with large white flowers that bloom from July to September. The plants grow to be from 4 to 6 feet (1.2m to 1.8m) tall and form clumps about 2 1/2 feet (0.8m) in diameter. The leaves vary in shape. Some are spearhead-shaped while others have three or five lobes or may be toothed. They are covered in a fine, velvety fuzz on both sides. The plant has many branchless stems covered in soft white hairs. The stems have saw-toothed projections. The flowers are somewhat trumpet-shaped, about 2 to 3 inches (5 cm to 7.5 cm) across and roughly 3 inches (7.5 cm) deep. The flowers produce seedpods that ripen in August to October, popping open to release small, flat black seeds.

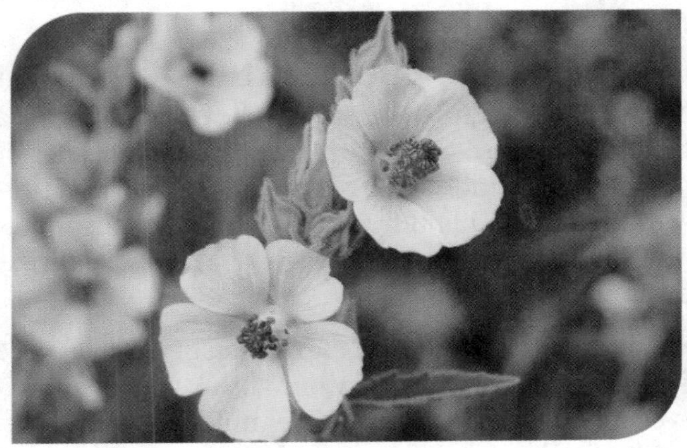

Edible Use: The leaves, flowers, root, and seeds are all edible. The roots contain a mucilage, which is sweet in flavor. Slice and boil the roots for 20 minutes, then remove from the liquid. Boil the remaining liquid again with sugar to taste and whip to make old-fashioned marshmallow candies.

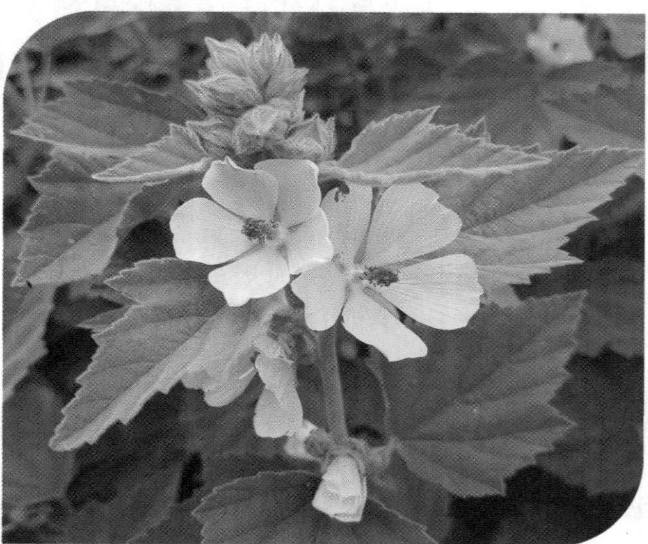

Medicinal Use: The roots, leaves, and flowers are used for medicinal treatments. They are especially valuable for treating problems with the mucous membranes.

Acid Indigestion, Peptic Ulcers, Leaky Gut, and Digestive Issues: I use the root of the marshmallow plant to treat stomach problems caused by excess stomach acid and for Leaky Gut. It is effective in neutralizing the acid and relieving symptoms. The root has a moderate laxative effect, which makes it useful in treating intestinal problems such as colitis, ileitis, irritable bowel syndrome, and diverticulitis. I also use it as an ingredient in my Leaky Gut Blend as it forms a protective layer around perforations in the gut.

Dry Coughs, Bronchitis, Bronchial Asthma, Congestion, and Pleurisy: Because marshmallow is so good at treating the membranes, it makes a good antidote for respiratory problems. It relieves the swelling and irritation of the mucous membrane and calms the respiratory system. It is not an expectorant.

Teething Pain: Young children can be given a piece of peeled fresh roots to chew on. The chewing stick relieves teething pain and has a mildly sweet taste. Watch closely and replace it before it gets so chewed that it could become a choking hazard.

Skin Irritations, Inflammations, and Swellings: For skin irritations, try an ointment or cream prepared from marshmallow root and slippery elm (see recipe below), or make a poultice from the dried and ground root of marshmallow. Simply add a little water to make a paste from the powdered root and water, then apply it to the irritation. Both are equally effective, but the ointment seems to be easier to use and there is no need to worry about it falling off.

Skin Ulcers, Injuries, and Removing Foreign Objects: Marshmallow Root and Slippery Elm Ointment is highly effective in healing skin injuries of all kinds. It also helps in the extraction and healing of foreign objects below the skin such as splinters, and particles imbedded in scrapes and cuts.

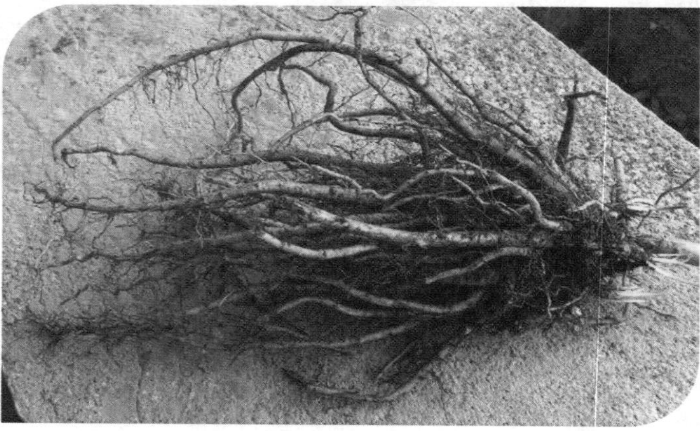

Marshmallow roots, by Victor M. Vicente Selvas, CCO

Urinary Tract Infections and Cystitis: Urinary tract infections and cystitis respond well to a decoction of Marshmallow root. It soothes irritated tissues and relaxes them, which helps with the pain and allows the decoction to work on the infection.

Recipes: Marshmallow Root and Slippery Elm Ointment: Ingredients: 100 g finely ground marshmallow root, 50 g lanolin, 50 g beeswax, 300 g soft paraffin wax, 100 g finely ground slippery elm bark. Heat the marshmallow root, lanolin, beeswax, and paraffin together in a double boiler or in a slow oven using the lowest setting. When cool enough to handle, but not yet set, stir in the slippery elm bark and pour it into a suitable container.

*You can also make this ointment without the slippery elm bark. However, the bark acts as a supplemental medicine and as a preservative to help the ointment keep longer.

Meadow Rue, *Thalictrum occidentale*

Meadow Rue, *Thalictrum occidentale*, is a perennial flowering plant. The herb is in the Ranunculaceae (Buttercup) Family. Despite its name meadow rue, Thalictrum is unrelated to the Rue Family, Rutaceae. Meadow rue is native to the western US, growing from Alaska and western Canada to California, Wyoming, and Colorado. It grows in moist and shady habitats such as meadows and forest understory.

Identification: Meadow rue grows to about 3 feet (0.9m) tall. The leaves of this herb are green in color, bipinnately compound and alternate. Leaves are divided into segments, often with three lobes, and grow on long petioles. The inflorescence is an upright or bent panicle of flowers, with male and female flowers growing on separate plants. The male flower is greenish white or purple, grows no petals, but instead has numerous dangling purple stamens. The female flower grows a cluster of up to 14 immature fruits with purple styles.

Edible Use: The only edible parts of meadow rue are the roots and young leaves. These roots have a bitter flavor and are rarely eaten. Instead they are used as

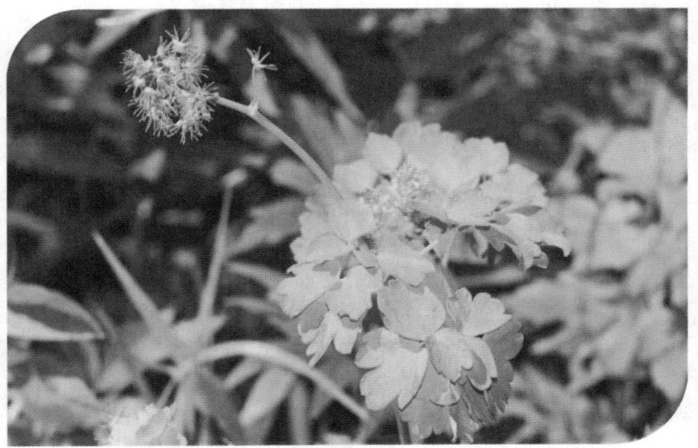

Meadow Rue, By Walter Siegmund, CC by SA 3.0

remedies to treat different ailments. Young leaves of meadow rue can be cooked and consumed as spinach.

Medicinal Use: Urinary Problems. A root decoction of meadow rue treats urinary problems.

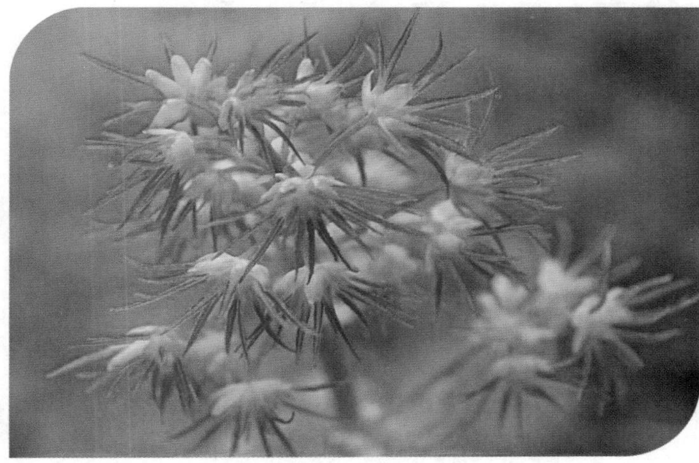

Female Flowers, photo by nordique, CC by SA 2.0

Reducing Fevers: Use a decoction from the roots or an infusion of the leaves to suppress fevers.

Cleans and Purifies the Body: Meadow rue is a general tonic that purifies the blood and cleanses the body.

Sores, Skin Infections, Piles: A poultice of meadow rue can be used to heal sores and skin infections. Crush and mash the root and leaves with a small amount of water for moisture. Apply the macerated herb to the area and cover it with a clean cloth to hold it in position.

Kill Lice and Other Vermin: Wash the hair and other body areas infected with lice, crabs, or other vermin with freshly made and warm Meadow Rue Decoction. Leave it on the skin for 30 minutes, then rinse it well. It should totally eradicate the problem. Follow up with a nit comb after killing lice.

Harvesting: Meadow rue can be harvested year-round. Uproot the plant then pluck off the young leaves and the roots. Wash the roots and the leaves and then dry them in a well-shaded place away from direct sunlight.

Meadow Rue Decoction: You'll need 1-ounce meadow rue roots and 1-pint (500ml) water. Crush or chop finely 1 ounce of meadow rue roots. Boil the root for 15 minutes or more to release the medicinal qualities into the water. Cool the decoction and strain it to remove the root fibers.

Milk Thistle, *Silybum marianum*

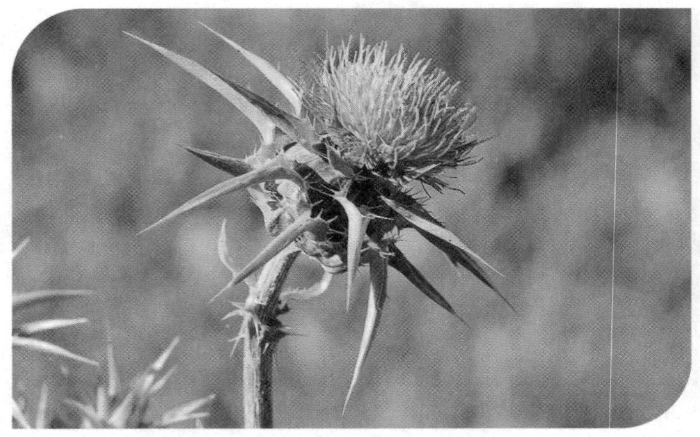

Photo by Fir0002/Flagstaffotos, GNU FDL 1.2,

Milk thistle is known by many names, including blessed milk thistle, blessed thistle, cardus marianus, Mary thistle, Saint Mary's thistle, variegated thistle, Mediterranean milk thistle, and Scotch thistle. It grows in many places in North America and throughout the world. It prefers a warmer climate. It is in the Asteraceae /Compositae (Aster/Daisy) Family.

Identification: Milk thistle is an annual or biennial plant and grows from 2 to 6 feet (0.6 to 1.8meters) tall. The shiny green leaves are oblong or lance-like and can be either lobed or pinnate with distinctive white marbling. They are hairless with spiny margins and white veins. The stem is grooved and hollow in larger plants. Reddish-purple flowers appear from June to August. They are 1 to 5 inches (2.5 cm to 12.5 cm) across.

Edible Use: Eat milk thistle roots raw, boiled, parboiled, or roasted. The young shoots are harvested in the spring and boiled like spinach. Some people peel the bitter stems and soak them overnight before cooking them. Best to trim the leaves and stems to remove the spines before cooking or eating. You can eat the spiny bracts on the flower-head like a globe artichoke. Boil or steam them until tender. Milk Thistle is high in potassium nitrate and is not suitable for cattle or sheep.

Medicinal Use: Both the leaves and the seeds are used medicinally. The seeds can be eaten raw, and both the leaves and seeds can be used as a tincture, extract, or tea. You can grind the milk thistle seeds into a powder and put it into capsules for people who find the flavor disagreeable or need an easy way to take it. I make a tincture of milk thistle seeds and dandelion root for the liver. Silymarin, the most actively medicinal compound in milk thistle, is only found in the seeds.

Supports and Detoxifies the Liver: Milk thistle seeds are excellent at decreasing or even reversing liver damage caused by disease, environmental pollutions, chemotherapy, poisons, and drug or alcohol abuse. Milk thistle dramatically improves liver regeneration in hepatitis, cirrhosis, fatty liver syndrome, and jaundice.

Prevents Gallstones and Kidney Stones: Milk thistle seeds support the endocrine and gastrointestinal systems and helps clean the blood. It works closely with the liver and other digestive organs to purify the body and reduce the risk of gallstones and kidney stones.

Helps Lower High Cholesterol: Milk thistle is a powerful anti-inflammatory with heart-healthy benefits, including lowering high cholesterol by cleaning the blood, decreasing inflammation, and preventing oxidative stress damage within the arteries. Milk thistle is effective in lowering total cholesterol, LDL cholesterol, and triglyceride levels in people with diabetes and heart disease.

Prevent or Control Diabetes: Milk thistle helps control the blood sugar and decreases blood sugar levels in insulin-resistant patients. For best results, use it regularly. The improved blood sugar control is due to the improved health of the liver and its function in releasing insulin and other hormones into the bloodstream.

Antidote for the Ingestion of Poisonous Mushrooms: Milk thistle seed's ability to protect the liver is so strong that it is even able to treat people poisoned by Amanita mushrooms, which destroy the liver. In fact, it is often the only treatment option for these patients and is given intravenously. Always be careful when harvesting and eating mushrooms. If you believe you've ingested poisonous mushrooms, seek medical help immediately.

Estrogen-Like Effects: Milk thistle leaves have some estrogen-like effects that stimulate menstruation and increase the flow of milk in breast-feeding mothers.

Cancer Treatment: Milk thistle seeds are sometimes used as a treatment for prostate, liver, and skin cancer, as silymarin has anticarcinogenic effects and protects the liver and kidneys during chemotherapy.

Acne: Milk thistle is high in anti-oxidants, anti-inflammatories, and flavonoids that reduce the inflammation of acne.

Harvesting: Always wear protective clothing and heavy gloves when harvesting milk thistle, as it is very irritating to the skin. Cut off young flower heads with scissors and young leaves from the stalk. Harvest milk thistle seeds by cutting off the seed-heads and placing them in a paper bag in a cool, dry spot. After the seeds dry, remove them from the seed head, one at a time, and brush away the debris. The cleaned seeds store best in a container with a tight lid.

Warning: Pregnant women should not use milk thistle. Women with estrogen-related conditions such as endometriosis, fibroids, and cancers of the ovaries, breast, or uterus should not use milk thistle. Do not use milk thistle if you are allergic to the Asteraceae/Compositae plant family.

Recipes. Milk Thistle Tea: Crush or grind 1 teaspoon of milk thistle seeds. Add one cup of boiling water and allow the tea to steep until lukewarm.

Milk Thistle Extract: Take 3/4 cup milk thistle seeds, 1 cup vodka or other alcohol, 80 proof or higher. Grind, crush or blend ¾ cups of milk thistle seeds. Place the crushed seeds into a sterile pint-sized (500ml) jar with a tight-fitting lid. Pour 1 cup of vodka over the seed, more if needed to cover the seeds. Stir well to mix the ingredients. Cap the jar tightly and place it in a cool, dark place for 6 to 8 weeks, shaking the jar daily. Add more alcohol, if needed, to keep the seeds covered with liquid. Strain the mixture and reserve the liquid. Discard the seed. Store your extract tightly covered in a cool, dark place.

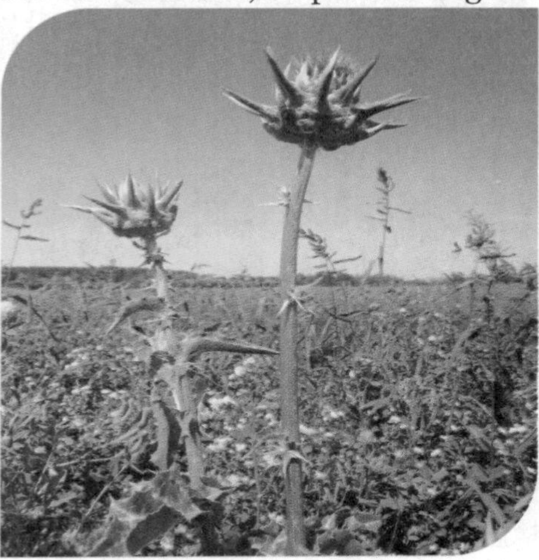

To Use Milk Thistle Extract: This is a highly concentrated extract. Use three drops of Milk Thistle Extract up to three times daily. If this dosage is well tolerated, you can gradually increase the dose.

Mormon Tea, *Ephedra nevadensis*

Ephedra nevadensis belongs to the Ephedraceae Family. It is also known as Mormon Tea, Brigham Tea, Desert Tea and Nevada Ephedra. This herb is said to have gotten its name, Mormon tea, because of its use as a caffeine-free beverage by the Mormons. It is native to dry areas of southwestern North America and Central Mexico.

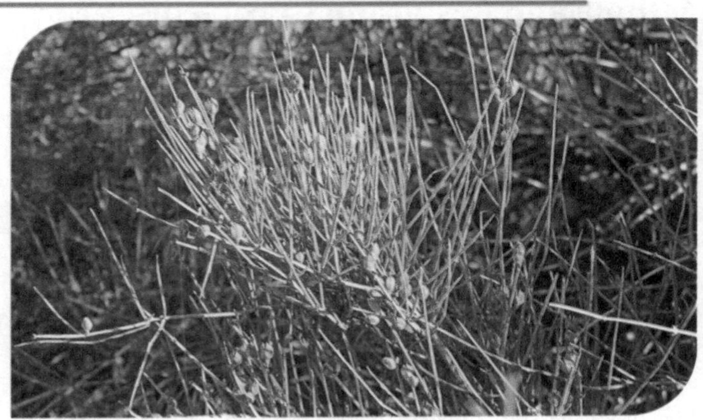

Andrey Zharkikh Wikipedia Commons, cc. 2.0

Identification: This desert shrub has jointed or fluted stems and scale-like leaves. Leaf scales of Mormon tea are in twos, 1 to 2 inches (2.5 cm to 5 cm) long, with sheathing to about the middle. The inflorescence of this plant is cone-like. The ovulate spikes of Mormon tea are distinctly stalked, and the seeds are usually paired. This plant occurs naturally on flats and slopes in all the creosote bush deserts at mostly 1,000 to 4,000 feet (1219 meters) in elevation and sometimes it is found in desert grasslands up to 5,000 feet (1524 meters). The characteristic species that grow with this plant are Joshua tree, white bursage, black-brush, catclaw, burro-bush, black grama, bush muhly, and desert needle-grass.

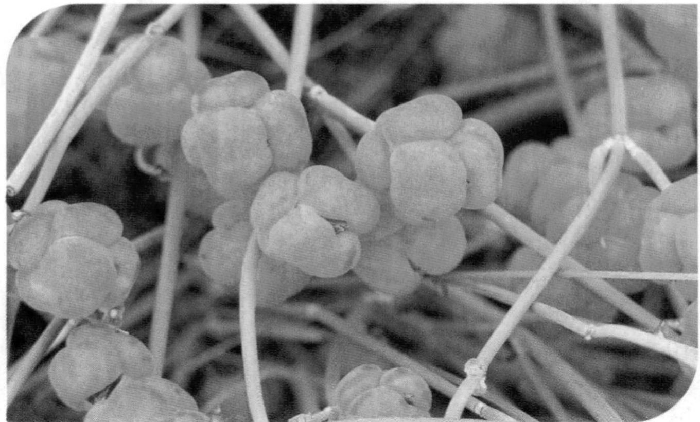

Ripe Female cones with seeds. Photo by Le.Loup.Gris, CC by SA 3.0

Edible Use: Both the fruit and seeds are edible. The fruit is sweet with a mild flavor, while the seed has a bitter taste and can be used cooked. It is sometimes roasted and ground to make bread. However, this plant is famous for its tea. Steep the green or dried twigs in boiling water until the tea turns an amber or pink color.

Medicinal Use: Mormon tea foliage is considered toxic but is used for medicinal purposes. It is a blood purifier, diuretic, fever-reducer, poultice, and tonic.

Urogenital Complaints: Use the stems for urogenital complaints including kidney problems, gonorrhea, and syphilis, if caught in its early stages.

Asthma and Respiratory Problems: Mormon tea and other members of the ephedra family are valuable for the treatment of asthma and respiratory system complaints. It does not cure asthma, but it opens the airways and relieves the symptoms of an attack. It is also useful for allergies and hay fever.

Heart Stimulant (Caution): Members of the ephedra family are known to contain ephedrine, which stimulates the heart and central nervous system. However, *Ephedra nevadensis* has little to none of the stimulant effects of ephedrine. However, drug potency varies from plant to plant, use it with care and do not use it on people with known arrhythmias or other problems where ephedrine is contraindicated.

Sores and Skin Infections: A poultice made from the powdered stems can be applied to sores for effective treatment.

Warning: Pregnant women and breastfeeding mothers should never use Mormon Tea.

Harvesting: Harvest the seeds of this plant by hand from native stands. On good years abundant collections of ephedra seeds can be obtained by flailing the fruiting branches over an open tray. Its stems can be harvested at any time of the year - dry them for future use.

Recipes: Mormon Tea Infusion. Break the stems into small pieces and wash them well. Add them to water and bring to a boil. Reduce the heat and simmer the twigs for 10 to 15 minutes. Once cooled, strain the liquid.

Mormon Tea: To make Mormon Tea, follow the instructions for Mormon Tea Infusion, then dilute the infusion with water until it is the strength you like. I dilute it to the color of tea. You can sweeten it with raw honey, if desired.

Mormon Tea Powder: Dry and powder the branches and twigs of the Mormon Tea Shrub. Moisten the powder to make a paste and use to make a poultice for sores and burns.

Motherwort, *Leonurus cardiaca*

Motherwort is a perennial member of the mint family that is often found at the edges of woodlands and in disturbed soils. It is widely distributed throughout North America and Europe and is sometimes considered invasive.

Identification: Motherwort is an upright bush that can grow to 6 1/2 feet tall (2m) and 3 feet (0.9m) or more wide. Motherwort leaves vary in size and shape along the stem. They are dark green on top and pale below. Lower leaves are deeply lobed with large teeth and can resemble maple or oak leaves.

They can reach five inches long and wide, and are hairy. Moving up the plant, the leaves become smaller with smaller lobes and teeth. At the top of the plant, leaves are usually small, narrow, and unlobed.

The stems are square, hairy, and branch only at the upper part of the plant.

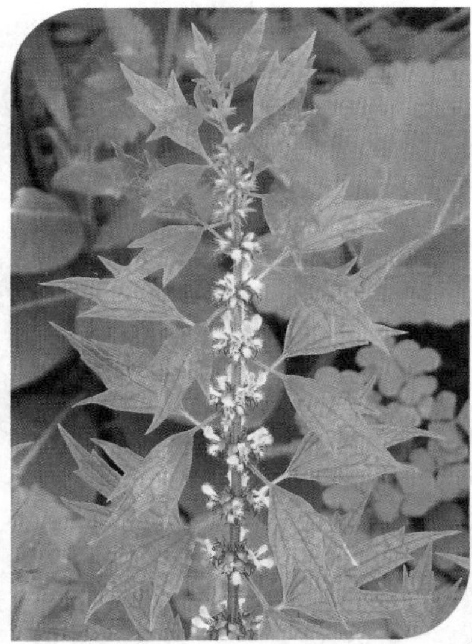

Photo by D. Gordon, Own Work, CC BY-SA 3.0

Hairy pale pink to lavender flowers grow in whorls alternating up the stem at the leaf nodes on the upper part of the plant. They bloom June through early September. The calyx remains on the plant through the winter, becoming brown and stiff when dry. Inside the lobes are 4 nutlets.

Edible Use: The flowers are edible and is used as a flavoring in pea soups, beer, or for making tea. The flavor is very bitter, so the leaves are rarely eaten.

Medicinal Use: Motherwort is best known for its benefits to the heart and for treating women's complaints. The leaves and flowers are the parts of the plant usually used for medicine.

Heart Health: Motherwort has a reputation for treating a wide variety of heart conditions. It is used to prevent calcification of the arteries, treating high cholesterol, hypertension, and other heart conditions.

Motherwort regulates the heart rate, treating rapid heartbeats and improves blood circulation in the body.

Prevents Strokes: This herb reduces the risk of blood clots forming in the body, thereby reducing the risk of strokes from blood clots.

Women's Health Issues (Birth, Delayed Menstruation, PMS): Expectant mothers use motherwort to reduce stress and tension at delivery time (do not take while pregnant). During delivery, it strengthens uterine contractions. It is believed that motherwort can also help the uterus recover after birth.

The herb is also effective at treating menstrual issues and regulating female hormones. It is an emmenagogue (stimulates menstrual flow) and thus helps with delayed menstruation. Herbalists use it to tone the uterus when menstruation is scant or to relieve cramps associated with delayed menstruation and PMS.

ADHD: Motherwort, along with Lemon Balm, Valerian, and Wild Oats, (Avena sativa), is often used to help people with ADHD.

Anxiety and Depression: Motherwort is believed to have a calming effect on the central nervous system and reduces stress, anxiety, worry, and panic attacks. It lifts the mood and reduces depression. For best results in reducing anxiety and depression, use motherwort regularly.

Hyperthyroidism: Motherwort relieves many of the symptoms of an over-active thyroid (hyperthyroidism). It regulates the metabolism, the nervous system, and relieves heart palpitations and anxiety caused by an over-active thyroid. It also helps increase the appetite and improves the overall thyroid health.

Insomnia and Sleep Problems: The calming effects of motherwort help improve sleep problems such as insomnia and restlessness.

Warning: Pregnant women should use the herb under the supervision of a medical professional. It can expedite labor and increase contractions.

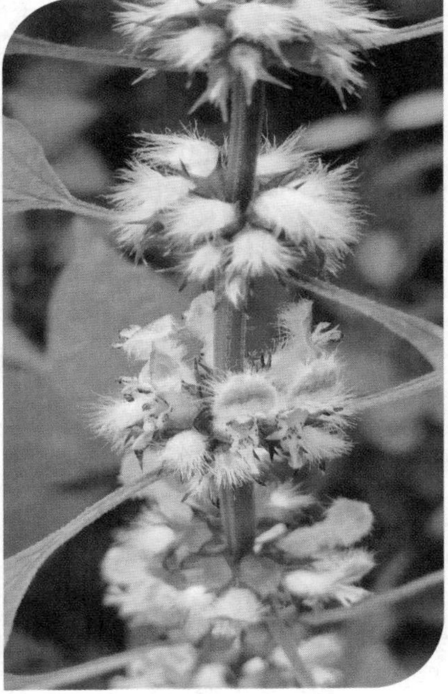

Consult a medical professional before taking the herb is you are taking heart medications or have heart problems.

Add the dried leaves to boiling water and allow it to steep for 10 minutes. Strain and enjoy. Sweeten the tea with honey or lemon if desired to improve the flavor.

Recipes. Motherwort Tea: 1 teaspoon of dried leaves, 1 cup of boiling water.

Motherwort Tincture: Motherwort leaves, stems, and flowers, roughly chopped, 80 proof vodka or similar drinking alcohol.

Glass jar, Sterilize a glass jar and tight-fitting lid. Fill the jar with chopped leaves, stems, and flowers to about 1/2 full. Fill the jar to within 1/4 (0.6cm) inch of the top, completely covering the herbs.

Cap the jar tightly and store it in a cool, dark place. Shake the jar once a day for six weeks. Check the alcohol levels regularly and add more alcohol as necessary to keep the jar full. Strain out the herbs and store the tincture in a sterile jar in a cool, dark place.

Mullein, *Verbascum thapsus*

Mullein belongs to the Scrophulariaceae (Figwort/Snapdragon) family. It is most commonly known as great mullein or common mullein. Its other names include Flannel Plant, Aaron's rod, Hag Taper, Torches, and Velvet Plant.

Mullein is a widely distributed plant in North America and is exceedingly abundant as a naturalized weed in the eastern States. It grows in meadows, by roadsides, and on waste ground, especially on gravel, sand or chalky soil. This plant grows in a vast range of habitats but prefers disturbed ground.

Mullein is widely used for herbal remedies, with well-established emollient and astringent properties. This plant has also been used to make dyes and torches and is a lovely bush toilet paper.

Identification: Mullein is a velvety, soft, biennial plant. When in its second year, Mullein has an erect tall flowering spike that can reach nearly 8 feet (2.4 meters) in height. Its basal rosette, tall flowering stem, and velvety leaves make it easily recognizable.

Each mullein flower is about 3/4 inch (1.875 cm) across and consists of five pale petals, 5 hairy-green sepals, five stamens, and one pistil. In its first growth year, mullein leaves form a basal rosette. They have, very large, long, oval velvety, gray-green leaves that can grow up to 20 inches (50 cm) in length. In their second year, they send up a single tall flowering spike with alternately arranged leaves.

This plant produces small, ovoid capsules approximately 1/4 inch (0.625 cm) in length that contain many minute, brown seeds that are less than 0.04 inches (0.1 cm) in size.

Edible Use: The leaves and flowers are edible, although most people prefer them as a tea.

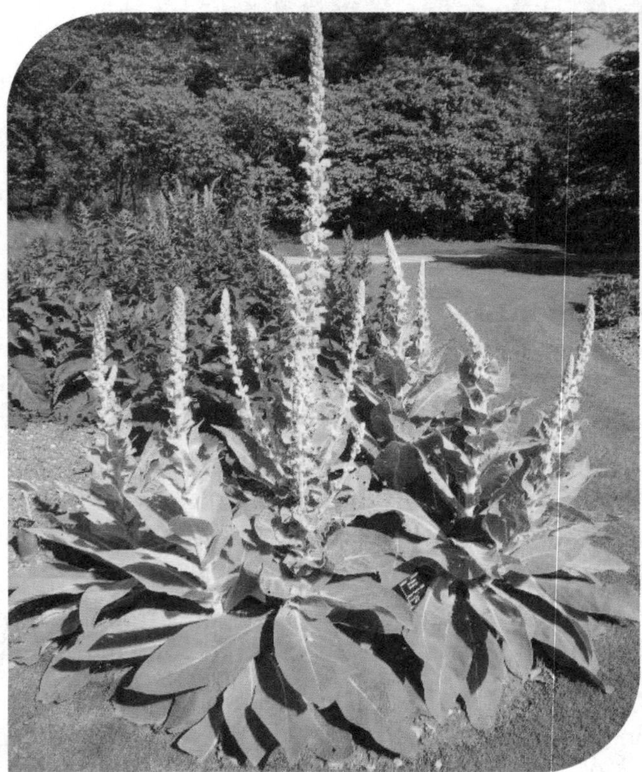

Medicinal Use: The leaves and the flowers of mullein are anti-inflammatory, antiseptic, antispasmodic, astringent, demulcent, diuretic, emollient, expectorant, anodyne (pain-killing) and vulnerary (wound-healing). I make an effective bronchitis tincture using Mullein, Lungwort Lichen and Yerba Santa for both symptomatic treatment and as a curative.

Bronchitis, Emphysema, Laryngitis, Tracheitis, Asthma, and Tuberculosis: Mullein is a commonly used herbal remedy. I value it for its efficacy in the treatment of chest complaints such as bronchitis, tuberculosis, and asthma. It reduces the formation of mucus and stimulates the expulsion of phlegm. It is a specific treatment for tracheitis and bronchitis. For emphysema, try mullein infusion with some coltsfoot. The mixture of herbs acts well as an expectorant for emphysema patients and helps them breathe easier. It also relieves the coughing spasms and wheezing. People improve with long term use.

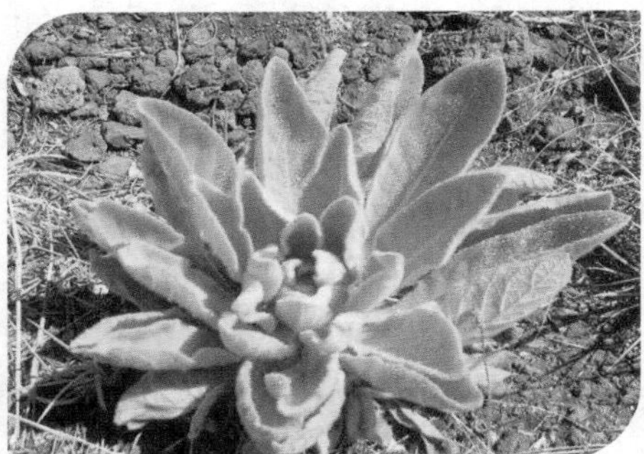

For asthma, mullein can also be inhaled. Mullein can be rolled into a rolling paper and smoked or, for children, the leaves can be burned and the smoke inhaled so as not to introduce them to smoking.

Skin Wounds, Snake Bite, Ulcers, Tumors, and Hemorrhoids: Externally, use a poultice prepared from mullein leaves to heal wounds, ulcers, tumors, and hemorrhoids. Mash the leaves, apply them directly to the skin, and cover them with a clean cloth. Mullein Infused Oil (recipe below) also works well on hemorrhoids. Mullein in a poultice form is drawing and may help draw out snake bite toxins if Plantain (*Plantago*) is not available – I would couple it with internal use. It also works to draw out splinters and the like.

Earaches and Ear Infections: I use an infusion prepared from its flowers infused in olive oil as earache drops. The flowers are strongly bactericidal. I usually mix mullein with garlic and yarrow infused in olive oil for ear infections. I put a few drops into the ear canal with a dropper and plug the ear with a cotton plug. I prefer to treat both ears, even if only one is affected, since the sinuses are connected. Do not use mullein (or any other oil in the ears) for punctured eardrums.

Sunburn, and Inflammatory Skin Conditions: Mullein is anti-inflammatory, which helps it to calm inflammatory skin conditions, especially those of the mucus membranes. For this purpose, I use a few drops of Mullein Infused Oil applied directly to the affected area. The oil also is anti-bacterial which helps prevent infection and speed healing. I often pair St. John's Wort with mullein for sunburns.

Warts: Powdered mullein roots rubbed onto warts helps to kill the virus to the roots and remove the wart. Rub it in several times a day until the wart is completely gone and the skin is healed. The juice of the plant can also be used.

Cramps and Muscle Spasms: For cramping and muscle spasms, try an internal Mullein Infusion. For muscle spasms, Mullein Infused Oil can also be rubbed into the affected muscle.

Gastrointestinal Issues: Mullein Infusion made from the roots is very good for getting rid of intestinal worms and other gastrointestinal issues.

Harvesting: Mullein leaves are best harvested during the second year when the plant is growing a stalk. Harvest when the flowers are in bloom, usually between July and September. The flowers can be used either fresh or dried, although I prefer using them fresh when I can. To dry, bundle the leaves and hang them upside-down to dry.

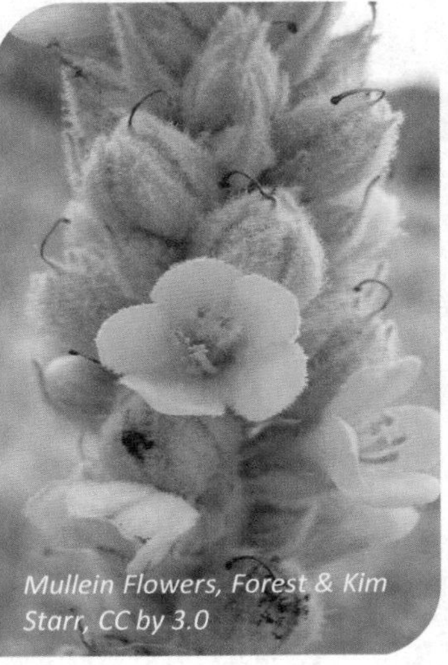
Mullein Flowers, Forest & Kim Starr, CC by 3.0

Warning: Do not use mullein if you are pregnant or breast feeding. In some people, it can cause skin irritations, stomach pain, and breathing difficulties. These are allergic reactions, so discontinue use if these symptoms occur.

Recipes. Mullein Infusion. Ingredients: 1/2 teaspoon powdered mullein root, and 1 cup water. Bring the water and powdered mullein root to a boil and reduce the heat to a simmer. Simmer for 10 minutes.

Mullein Infused Oil: Take 2 cups sweet almond oil or organic olive oil and 1 1/2 cups of mullein flowers, fresh or dried. Place 1 ½ cups of mullein flowers into a pint (500ml) jar with a tight-fitting lid. Pour the oil over the flowers and allow them to infuse for 3-4 weeks. Filter the oil and store it in a dark bottle in a cool, dry place.

Oregano, *Origanum vulgare*

There are many different varieties of oregano; all are medicinal but vary in the amounts of beneficial compounds. The most potent oregano is said to come from Greece and I find that plants grown in the summer heat seem to be more potent. It is in the *Lamiaceae* (Mint) Family.

Identification: You'll find oregano growing in most herb gardens and you may already use it in cooking.

If you are unfamiliar with it, look for bright-green, opposite oval leaves that are slightly hairy. It is a sprawling perennial plant that, like its relative mint, can take over an area. The plant grows close to the ground, reaching 8 to 32 inches (80 cm) tall. Each leaf is 1/2 to 1 1/2 inches long. The flowers are purple and tiny, growing on erect spikes above the leaves.

Edible Use: Oregano is used as a culinary herb to flavor many types of foods, especially in Mediterranean dishes.

Medicinal Use: For medicinal use, oregano can be used as an herb in food, used as a tea, as a tincture, or as an essential oil. The essential oil is very concentrated and should be diluted in a carrier oil before use. It is antiviral, antibacterial, and antifungal. Oregano is used internally to treat infections and externally to treat skin problems and fungal infections.

Boosts the Immune System and Antiviral: Oregano contains a wide range of antioxidants, anti-inflammatory, and anti-infectious properties that help the immune system heal the body faster. It contains vitamins A and C, as well as other compounds that are beneficial in boosting the immune system.

It helps relieve stresses on the body and stimulates the immune system to produce white blood cells, which defend the body against bacteria, viruses, fungi, and cancerous cells.

Yeast and Other Fungal Infections: Oregano oil is a powerful antibacterial, antiviral, and antifungal. It is also an anti-inflammatory, which helps in healing. It inhibits the growth of *Candida*, the yeast that most often causes yeast infections. Carvacrol and thymol are the main components that treat yeast infections and preventing them from spreading.

Use Oregano Tea or Tincture once or twice daily to treat internal yeast infections and for external use, use a tea wash or use well-diluted oregano oil. The diluted essential oil is effective against toenail fungus, athlete's foot, other fungal infections, and ringworm.

Skin Problems: Oregano contains antioxidants and anti-inflammatories that are beneficial to healing, reduce the signs of aging, heal blemishes, and reduce the appearance of scars. They neutralize the free radicals in the skin that cause wrinkles and age spots and they improve skin elasticity.

Cancer: In addition to the beneficial anti-inflammatory benefits and immune boosting effects of oregano for fighting cancer, the carvacrol in oregano has antitumor properties that slow the growth and reproduction of cancer cells and promotes cancer cell death.

Heart Healthy: Oregano Tea contains omega-3 fatty acids and helps improve cholesterol levels. It is also beneficial for the heart in other ways, helping prevent atherosclerosis, heart attacks, and stroke.

Stimulates Metabolism and Weight Loss: Oregano stimulates the metabolism causing the body to burn more calories. It can increase energy levels in some people and can help you lose weight.

Prevent Illness or Speed Recovery: When household members are sick, I often use Oregano Tea or Oil of Oregano to prevent the spread of the illness and to speed recovery of those who are ill. Best to use at the first sign of illness.

Bronchial Infections, Asthma, and Coughs: Add oregano oil to water and create a facial steam for loosening congestion and treating bronchial infections, asthma, and coughing. It relieves the inflammation in the airways.

Harvesting: You can usually find a starter plant at your local garden store. Harvest the leaves and stems before the plant blooms for best flavor. It is still potent after blooming, but the flavor is more bitter.

Warning: Do not take Oil of Oregano when pregnant. It is concentrated and has not been proven safe for pregnancy.

Recipes. Oregano Tea. I prefer to use fresh oregano leaves to make tea, though dried leaves can also be used. Dried leaves will lose the valuable oils and nutrients over time, so make sure your supply is fresh.

You need: 1 Tablespoon fresh oregano leaves or 1 teaspoon dried, 1 cup boiling water, raw honey or maple syrup to taste.

Crush or bruise the oregano leaves in the bottom of a cup or mug. Pour 1 cup of boiling water over the leaves and cover the cup to hold in the heat. Allow the tea to steep for 5 to 10 minutes. Add honey or maple syrup to sweeten the tea and make it palatable.

*To use as a wash, leave the tea unsweetened and allow it to cool before using it.

Oil of Oregano. The essential oil of oregano can be made by steam extraction. If you have the equipment for a steam extraction, it makes a stronger oil that must be diluted before use. See page 37 for instructions. The method below is easier, but it produces an oil that is less potent; no dilution is needed.

Oil of Oregano Infusion. Fresh oregano leaves and stems. Carrier oil such as organic olive oil, grapeseed oil, jojoba oil, or any other suitable oil. Gather several large handfuls of fresh oregano. Wash and air-dry. Chop the sprigs and leaves, bruising them to release the oils. Place the oregano into a clean glass jar, packed, but not overflowing. Heat the carrier oil on a very low heat and pour it over the oregano. Stir the oil gently to coat the oregano and release any air bubbles.

Cover the oil lightly (not sealed) and allow it to cool completely. Allow to steep for 1 week. Warm the oil again to release any moisture. Strain the oil, cover it tightly, and store it in a cool, dark place.

Oxeye Daisy, *Leucanthemum vulgare*

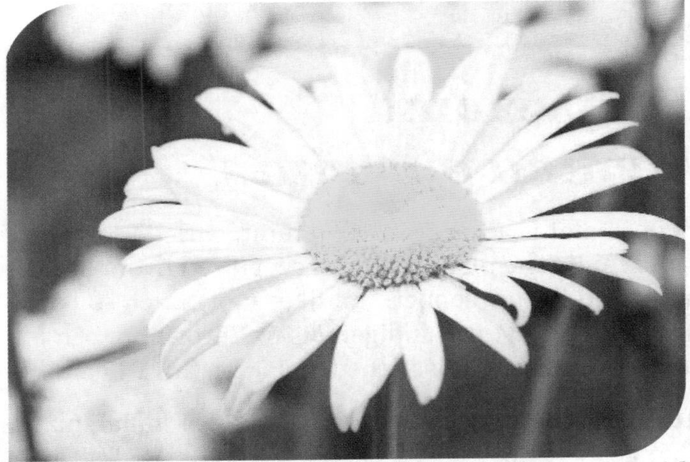

Also known as dog daisy, oxeye daisy is in the Daisy/Aster Family. It is often found in disturbed areas, fields, and roadsides throughout temperate North America, Europe, and Asia. It is an introduced species to North America.

Identification: Oxeye daisy is easily recognized by its white ray flowers with yellow center florets. Each erect plant grows 1 to 3 feet (0.3m to 0.9m) tall from well-developed shallow rhizomes. You'll often find them in groupings, spread by the reach of its rhizome underground. The leaves are long, lobed, irregular, alternate, and coarsely toothed. Leaves become progressively smaller as you go up the stem. Each stem holds one flower that blooms From May to October. It is often confused with Shasta Daisy (also edible), which is much taller.

Edible Use: The leaves, young shoots, flowers, and roots are edible. Young shoots and leaves are good chopped and added to salads. The flavor is strong, so I use them sparingly. The pungent flavor increases with age, so older leaves are best cooked, changing the water during cooking. They are good added to soups and stews. The roots can be eaten raw and are best in the spring.

Medicinal Use: The entire aerial part is medicinally active, but the flowers are most potent. The plant acts as an anti-inflammatory, antispasmodic, diuretic, and tonic. It induces sweating, relieves coughs, and heals wounds.

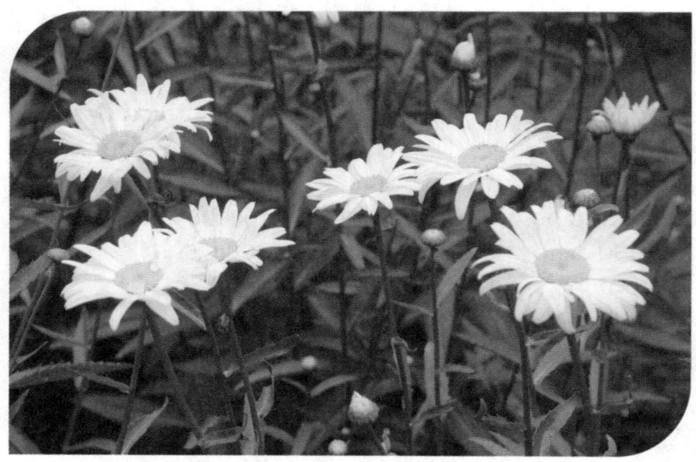

Chest Congestion and Coughing: Oxeye daisy is effective in relieving the coughing spasms of whooping cough and colds, and helping relieve congestion and mucous in the lungs. Try Oxeye Flower Tea or Tincture for this purpose.

Asthma: Oxeye daisy is an antispasmodic and helps relieve spasms in the airway, helping people with asthma breathe easier.

Tonic: Oxeye daisy is a mild tonic for the body, soothing irritation and inflammation in the body.

Wounds, Bruises, Rashes, Fungal Infections, and Other Skin Diseases: Oxeye daisy acts to soothe inflammation and irritations of the skin and is a good ingredient for lotions and salves. Used on the skin, it helps heal cuts, scrapes, bruises, insect bites and stings, and fungal infections. The tea or decoction can be used as a wash.

Eye Infections, Conjunctivitis: Boil the flowers in distilled water and strain through a fine mesh or coffee filter. Cool and use the sterile wash as an eye drop in the treatment of eye infections.

Detoxing, Diuretic Properties: Oxeye daisy is a mild diuretic and promotes sweating. It helps the body remove toxins through the urine and skin.

Insecticide and Flea Control: Dried flower heads, pounded or ground into a powder, are useful as a flea powder and as an insecticide.

Harvesting: Harvest the leaves, flowers, and stems while the plant is in bloom. Dry for future use.

Recipes. Oxeye Daisy Flower Tea: Boil oxeye daisy flowers, leaves, and stalks together, reduce heat and steep for 5 to 10 minutes. Strain and flavor with raw honey.

Peppermint, *Mentha piperita*

Peppermint is also called balm mint, curled mint, and lamb mint. The plant is easily recognized by its classic scent and flavor. Peppermint likes moist, rich soil and spreads quickly. It is indigenous to Europe but can be found worldwide. It is in the Lamiaceae (Mint) Family.

Identification: Peppermint is a perennial plant that grows from 1 to 3 feet (0.3m to 0,9m) tall. It has smooth, square stems and dark green opposite leaves with reddish veins.

The leaves are 1 to 3 inches (2.5 cm to 7.5 cm) long and about half as wide. Leaves have coarsely toothed margins, a pointed tip, and are covered in short hairs. Purple flowers bloom from mid to late summer and are about 1/4 inch (0.6 cm) in length.

The flowers do not produce viable seeds and the plant spreads by underground roots and rooting stems.

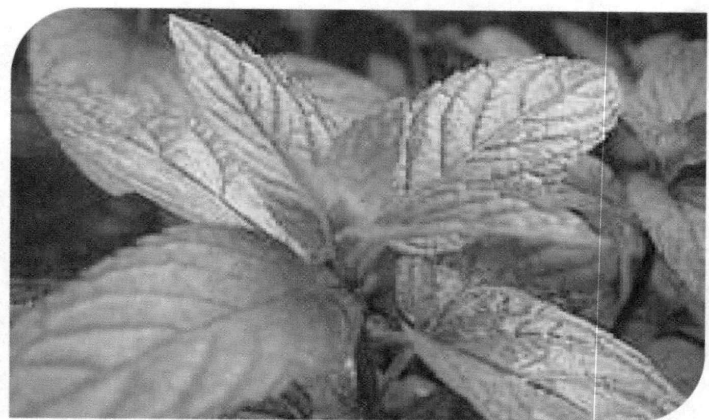

Peppermint, Aleksa Lukic - Own work, CC by 3.0

Edible Use: Peppermint is edible and often used as a tea.

Medicinal Use: **Gastroenteritis, Indigestion, Flatulence, Stomach, Intestinal, and Liver Problems:** Peppermint leaves and tea are well known as a treatment for indigestion, excess gas, nausea, and other stomach upsets.

Peppermint oil stimulates the flow of bile in the body and aids digestion. It is useful for treating problems of the stomach, intestines, and liver. Peppermint oil also contains anti-bacterial and anti-viral components that treat the causes of gastroenteritis while also calming the symptoms.

Menstrual Cramping: Peppermint oil relaxes uterine muscle spasms and relieves menstrual cramping. Women with menstrual cramping can drink peppermint tea or take peppermint oil. The oil is very strong, so only a drop or two is needed.

Appetite Suppression and Stimulation: Peppermint temporarily inhibits hunger, but when the effect wears off the feeling of hunger returns more powerfully. It can be used as an appetite stimulate in this way, just be aware that it takes time to work. Good for children who are failing to thrive due to a lack of appetite.

Headaches and Migraines: The oil also relieves the spasms that cause some types of headaches. For this purpose, use a drop of distilled peppermint oil mixed into a tablespoon of a carrier oil like organic olive oil. Rub the oil onto the forehead or on the scalp over the affected area to relieve the headache. You may also use a peppermint oil infusion, though the distilled oil is stronger.

Diarrhea, Spastic Colon, Irritable Bowel Syndrome, and Crohn's Disease: Peppermint calms the stomach and intestinal tract, relaxes the muscles, and soothes the mucous membranes. It helps treat diarrhea, spastic colon, and irritable bowel syndrome by alleviating the spasms of the intestines and colon.

Itchy Skin: Peppermint oil slightly numbs the skin surface to relieve pain from insect stings, itchy skin, and mild skin irritations. It also has an anti-bacterial component, and it works to bring an increased blood supply to the skin to speed up healing.

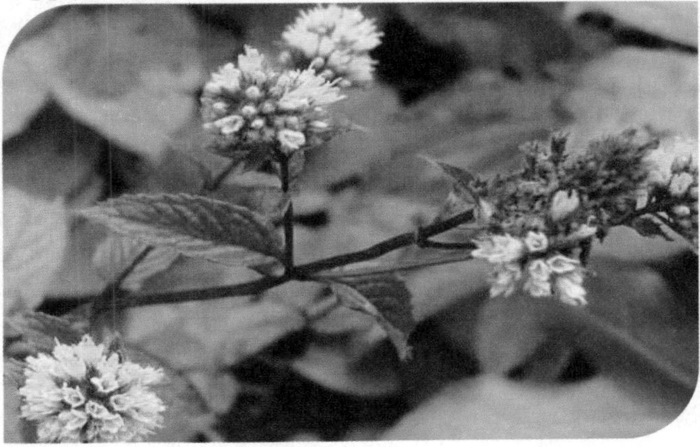

Peppermint Flowers, Sten Porse, CC by SA 3.0

Arthritis, Gout, Neuralgia, Sciatica: These same numbing qualities make it an effective treatment for muscle aches, joint pain, and nerve pain coming from near the surface. Massage the area with Infused Peppermint Oil (recipe below) to relieve the pain. It does not treat the underlying causes, but it gives quick relief from the pain.

Recipes. Peppermint Tea: 1 teaspoon peppermint leaves, 1 cup boiling water. Pour the boiling water over the peppermint leaves and allow the tea to steep for 10 to 15 minutes. Strain and drink.

Infused (Extracted) Peppermint Oil: 3/4 cup dried peppermint leaves, 1 cup organic olive oil. Combine the peppermint leaves and organic olive oil in a glass jar with a tight-fitting lid. Shake daily. Allow the oil and peppermint to steep in a dark cupboard for 4 to 6 weeks. Strain out the peppermint leaves and store the oil in a cool dark place for up to 1 year. Use as a topical relief for headaches, muscle cramps, or as a massage oil for muscle pain.

Plantain, *Plantago major*

Plantago major is a small perennial, often called a weed, and is not the banana-like fruit called plantain found in the grocery store. It is found growing wild in gardens, lawns, backyards, and along paths. It is in the Plantaginaceae Family.

Identification: The distinctive leaves have a ruffled texture. The leaves are oval or almost round and have a chunky footstalk. The leaves grow in a rosette at the base of the plant. Each leaf is 2 to 8 inches (5 cm to 20 cm) long. It has a wavy or smooth margin and five to nine parallel elastic veins. When you break the leaf in half and pull these elastic-like veins can easily be seen. The greenish-white flowers have purple stamens and grow on densely packed stems to a height of 6 to 18 inches (15 cm to 45 cm). The flowers are tiny and mostly eclipsed by the greenish-brown sepals and bracts. The flowering stalks rise high above the foliage. The plants produce many tiny, bitter-tasting seeds. *Plantago lanceolata*, narrow-leafed plantain, can be used like *P. major*.

Edible Use: The leaves and seeds are edible. I enjoy the leaves in a salad and gather them while they are still very young and tender and I love to strip the seeds and pop them in my mouth. As they age, they become tough and fibrous, but they can be cooked in soups and stews. The seeds are sometimes ground into a flour extender or substitute, but they are so tiny that it takes a lot of time and energy to gather enough to make it worthwhile.

Medicinal Use: The plantain herb has many medicinal qualities. It is anti-inflammatory, analgesic, antioxidant, demulcent, diuretic, expectorant, hepatoprotective, immune modulating, and a weak antibiotic.

Healing Wounds, Sores, Insect Bites, and Rashes: A poultice made from crushed plantain leaves is a good choice to promote healing in minor wounds, sores, and insect bites or stings. It will ward off infection, help stop bleeding, and reduce inflammation, taking away the sting or itch. A spit poultice is easily made when you are bitten. Plantain has an excellent drawing effect, and can remove venom or a stinger. My kids know that if they get bitten or stung to chew some plantain and apply it for almost immediate relief. If a wound is infected, I combine plantain with an herb with more antibiotic action such as yarrow. To make a poultice, crush, chew, or bruise fresh plantain leaves and apply them directly to the affected skin. Cover the leaves with a gauze wrapping to hold it in place. Change the poultice as needed.

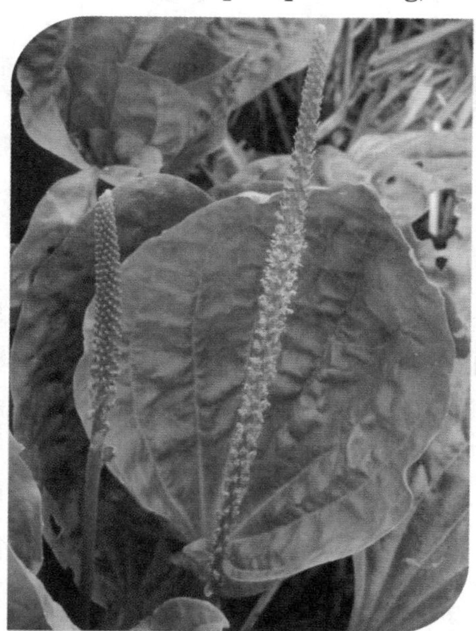

Snake Bite: For snakebite, use plantain both internally and externally. Apply a poultice of fresh plantain leaves directly to the bite to draw out the venom and take 2 tablespoons of freshly pressed plantain juice or 1 teaspoon of Plantain Tincture. The tincture can also be used as a poultice if fresh leaves are not readily available. For snakebite, much depends on the kind of snake and the quick administration of remedies.

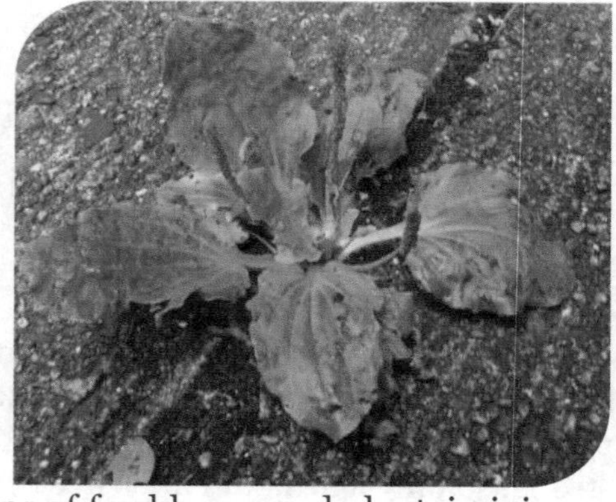

Cystitis, Diarrhea, Respiratory Tract Infections, Ulcers, and Colitis: The juice of common plantain leaves is beneficial for calming inflammation of the mucous membranes, including the membranes of the respiratory tract, digestive tract, and urinary tract.

Plantain for Autoimmune Diseases and Leaky Gut: For autoimmune conditions and other chronic diseases, try drinking Plantain Tea twice daily or take it in tincture form. The benefits build up over time. Just like Plantain works on your skin it also provides healing inside your gut. For Leaky Gut eat fresh leaves and drink it juiced or as a tea daily. Tincture is also effective but supplementing with fresh plantain or tea helps the plantain reach the gut lining for direct healing.

Toothache: The direct application of plantain on a toothache or dental infection is very effective in relieving swelling, infection, and pain. I like to combine it with the application of clove oil. Both can be soaked on cotton and packed into the infected area. Dried leaves can be used if fresh are not available.

Sore Throats and Swelling of the Gums: Add a tablespoon of pressed plantain juice to a half cup of water and use as a gargle at the first sign of a sore throat. It also reduces the inflammation in gum tissue.

Constipation, Intestinal Worms and Inflammatory Bowel Disease: Plantain seeds are excellent at relieving constipation and intestinal worms because of the fiber and mucilage released in the infusion. To relieve constipation, try drinking 1 cup of Plantain Seed Infusion (see recipe below) at bedtime. Be sure to consume the liquid and seeds for its full laxative effect.

Recipes. **Plantain Seed Infusion**: Take 1 teaspoon plantain seeds and 1 cup boiling water. Pour the boiling water over the seeds and allow it to steep while it cools. Drink the mucilage tea and the seeds. **Plantain Tincture**: You'll need plantain leaves, 80 proof vodka or other drinking alcohol and a glass jar with a tight-fitting lid. Fill the jar with fresh plantain leaves that have been chopped into small pieces or half a jar of dried plantain. Pour vodka over the leaves and fill the jar, making sure all the leaves are covered. Cap the jar tightly. Let the tincture marinate for 6 to 8 weeks, shaking the jar occasionally. Pour the alcohol through a fine mesh sieve, cheesecloth, or a coffee filter to remove all of the herbs. Store the tincture in a cool, dark cupboard for up to 5 years. Dosage: 1/2 to 1 teaspoon. To infuse Plantain Oil substitute organic olive oil for the vodka and follow the same instructions.

Plantain Tea: Place 1 teaspoon dried plantain leaves or 1 tablespoon of fresh plantain leaves into a cup of boiling water. Let steep for 10 minutes. Strain out the leaves and drink.

Prickly Pear Cactus, *Opuntia ficus-indica*

The prickly pear cactus is in the Cactaceae (Cactus) Family. It is also known as Indian Fig, Barbary Fig, Cactus Pear, and Mission Cactus. It grows in the Southern United States and Mexico.

Identification: Prickly pear cactus grows up to 16 feet (4.8meters) tall with flat, rounded leaf pads that branch off. The flower and, later, the fruit, grow directly on the leaf pad. The entire cactus, including the fruit, is covered with two different kinds of spines. There are large, fixed spines that are easily seen and small, hair-like spines that are more difficult to see and easily detached. It is these smaller spines that can embed in your skin if you are not careful. The solitary flowers are large, bisexual, and yellow to orange in color. The fruit, called a tuna, is a berry covering numerous hard seeds. Prickly pear cacti are found in semi-arid and desert-like conditions and are easily cultivated in containers. They grow in bushy clusters.

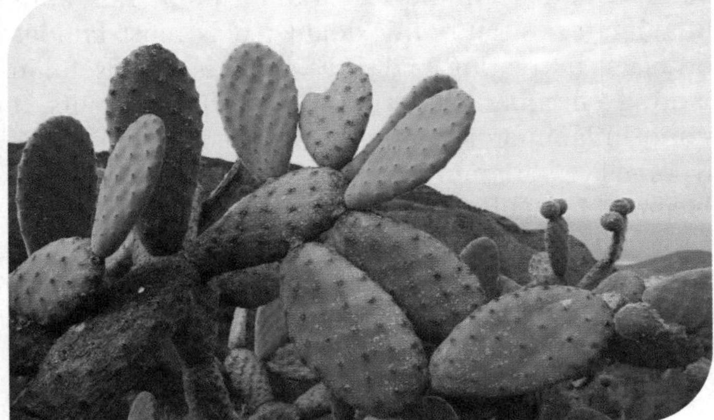

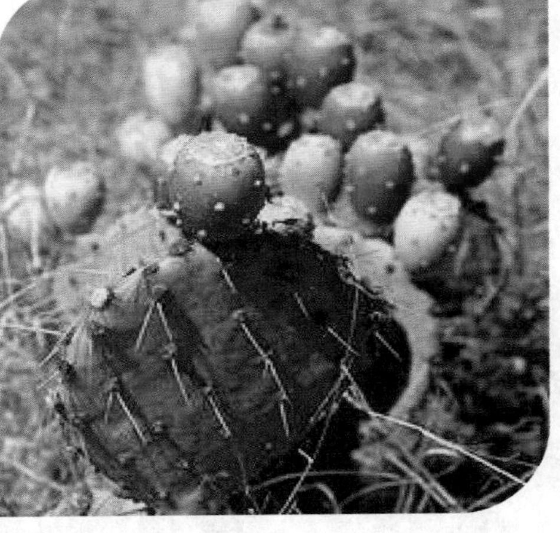

Edible Use: Both the leaf pads and the fruit are edible. Peel them carefully before use (see Harvesting). Drink the juice of the tunas and use the pads in salads, tacos, stir-fries, and soups. The fruit is highly nutritious.

Medicinal Use: The anti-inflammatory effects of the prickly pear fruit are exceptional. Keep a supply of the dried fruit for travel, but the fresh juice is best. For maximum benefits, drink at least 2 ounces (60ml) of juice every day. There are no known health risks with long term use.

Arthritis and Joint Pain: Arthritic joint pain caused by inflammation is greatly helped by the regular consumption of prickly pear juice every day. Relief takes time (one to two months) and increases with use.

Snake Bite and as a Drawing Poultice: The prickly pear leaf is excellent as a drawing plant for toxins. Cut off the outer pad of the prickly pear leaf and mash the inner part and put on a snake bite as soon as possible.

Use it along with *Plantago* and *Echinacea*, if they are available.

Diabetes: Prickly pear cactus is beneficial to the pancreas, which is vital to insulin production. By restoring pancreal health, it helps balance blood sugar.

Heart Disease, Cholesterol and Circulation: The anti-inflammatory benefits assist in the reduction of plaques in the arteries and veins, reducing the chances of heart disease. Pickly pear juice also reduces cholesterol and enhances blood circulation to all parts of the body.

Muscle Soreness and Fatigue: The high vitamin and other nutrient levels combined with the health properties of prickly pear make it an excellent choice for the treatment of fatigue and muscle soreness caused by injury or over use.

All Inflammatory Diseases: The juice is indicated for all inflammatory diseases including skin diseases like psoriasis, eczema, and hives.

Harvesting: Harvesting prickly pear must be done carefully due to their small, hairy spines. Dress in thick long sleeves, long pants, boots, and gloves. I use tongs to pick the ripe fruit and leaves and place them carefully into a basket for processing.

After collection, I hold the fruit or leaf pad over a flame and burn the spines off completely, charring the skin. When they cool, I peel off the skin. Some people use sandpaper to remove the spines, but I prefer charring.

Prunella vulgaris, Self-Heal

Self-heal, *Prunella vulgaris*, is also known as wound root, woundwort, and heal-all. This low-growing plant attracts butterflies and bees. It belongs to the Lamiaceae (Mint) Family. I often find self-heal along roadsides and waste-places, but I prefer to harvest it from the edges of woodlands or grow my own in my garden.

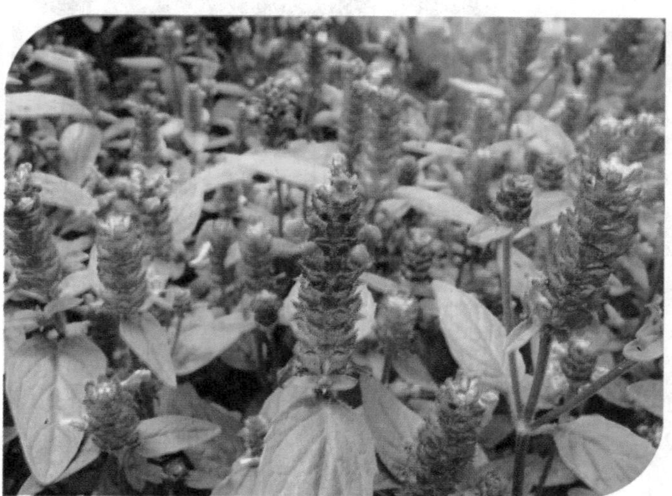

Identification: Self-heal is a perennial plant that grows 4 to 20 inches (10 cm to 50 cm) tall and produces small flowers from April to June and fruit from June to August. Each flower has a light purple upper lip and a whitish, fringed lower lip and a light green or reddish calyx that is hairy on the edges. Its fruit has 4 tiny seeds. Opposite leaves are lance-shaped and 1 to 3 inches (2.5 cm to 7.5 cm) long, growing on a single or a cluster of upright stems. The leaves have white hairs on the underside along the center vein. The leaf margins may be smooth or edged with blunt teeth. The root is a fibrous rhizome with a root crown and spreads through creeping stems that take root.

Edible Use: The young leaves and stems of self-heal are edible. They make a good addition to salads or can be boiled and eaten as a potherb. The aerial parts of the plant can be dried, powdered, and brewed into a cold tea.

Medicinal Use: The plant is nutritional and medicinal. It contains a number of vitamins, minerals, anti-inflammatories, and antioxidants. It is most famous for its use in treating cold sores, but it is also useful in treating a number of internal and external ailments. It is anti-inflammatory, antiviral, astringent, demulcent, hypotensive, immunomodulating, and vulnerary (healing). I usually use it as a complementary herb, using it in conjunction with other more powerful herbs. The entire plant is medicinal but the flowers, stems, and leaves are most commonly used.

Cold Sores and Genital Herpes: Self-heal treats both herpes simplex virus 1 (HSV-1 causes cold sores) and herpes simplex virus 2 (HSV-2 causes genital herpes). This herb has anti-viral properties. It prevents the virus from infecting host cells as well as reducing outbreaks.

Diabetes: Self-heal works to reduce insulin sensitivity in diabetes and pre-diabetes. It helps normalize blood sugar levels and prevents the development of diabetes related health conditions such as atherosclerosis.

Cancer: Research indicates that self-heal induces cell death in cancer cells. Cancerous tumor growth slows or stops with the use of the herb. Try the cold-water Self-Heal Tea or powdered herb in capsules for cancer alongside traditional treatments. Consult your doctor about your treatment.

Stimulates the Immune System: Regular use of self-heal herbs or Self-Heal Tea stimulates the immune system to help the body fight infections and even cancer. It also helps reduce swollen glands and helps clear toxins from the body.

Heals Wounds and Skin Infections: Self-heal's vulnerary, demulcent, and astringent properties stabilize wounded tissues and protects the skin. I use self-heal to treat cuts, burns, and skin wounds of all kinds. Internal wounds on the throat as well as mouth ulcers can be treated with self-heal. I treat surface skin problems, including infections and boils, with a poultice made from the herb and deeper inflammation with Self-Heal Tea.

Insect Bites and Stings, Rashes, and Poison Ivy: Juice from the stem of the plant, applied directly to the irritated tissue, is effective in calming the inflammation, burn, and itch of bites, stings, and rashes of all kinds. A poultice can be made from the plant for larger areas.

Viral Infections Including HIV: Self-heal's anti-viral properties are able to inhibit the growth of viruses in the body and prevent outbreaks. It prevents replication of the virus and helps stop the disease.

Respiratory Infections: Self-heal strengthens the immune system and helps the body fight off upper respiratory infections. It also treats sore throats and abscessed tonsils. Use Self-Heal Tea to treat respiratory infections and to soothe sore throats.

Allergies and Chronic Inflammation: Self-heal is an immunomodulator that regulates the immune system response and reduces chronic inflammation and seasonal allergies. It does not cure allergies but helps modulate the severity of the problem.

Kidney Problems and Hypertension: Self-heal strengthens the kidneys and promotes proper function. It also acts as a diuretic to help remove excess fluids from the body and lowers high blood pressure.

Heart Problems: Self-heal reduces high blood pressure and acts as a tonic for cardiovascular tissues. Regular use of Self-Heal Tea is said to strengthen the heart.

Liver Problems: Self-heal is useful in treating liver problems including hepatitis, jaundice, and a weak liver. It helps detoxify the liver and boosts its function. Use Self-Heal Tea regularly to treat liver problems.

Hemorrhage and Bleeding Caused by Extreme Menstruation: Self-heal stops internal bleeding, including excessive bleeding from menstruation. Take the herb as a tea or in capsule form for internal bleeding, as well as treating the underlying causes.

Digestive Problems, Colic, Crohn's Disease, Gastroenteritis, Ulcers, and Ulcerative Colitis: Self-heal helps to soothe the inflamed gastro-intestinal tissues, stop bleeding, heal ulcers and wounded tissues and fight bacteria, fungus, and viral infections, which contribute to the underlying causes of problems in the gastro-intestinal tract. It is also effective against the bacteria that cause ulcers and helps them heal. Try the herb in capsule form or a soothing Self-Heal Tea for treating digestive problems.

Self-heal also treats flatulence, diarrhea, gastritis, and intestinal parasites.

Hemorrhoids: Self-heal is useful topically to reduce the inflammation and irritation of hemorrhoids. Use a strong tea as a wash on the infected area or to make a compress for the area.

Harvesting: Harvest self-heal flowers when the blooms are open. Removing all flowers encourages the plant to flower again, but some flowers should be left at the end of the season to develop seeds. Dry the flowers and store in a cool, dry, and dark location until needed.

Warning: Self-heal should be used in moderation and is effective at low doses. Long-term use at high doses affects the internal organs, including the liver and kidneys. Self-heal can cause allergic reactions such as a skin rash, nausea, itching, and vomiting. Side effects can include dizziness, constipation, and weakness. The safety of self-heal in pregnancy has not been determined.

Recipes. **Self-Heal Tea (Cold Water Infusion)**. 1-ounce dried self-heal herb, 1-quart (liter) of cold water, 1-quart (1 Liter) jar and lid. A cold infusion extracts some components that are destroyed by heat. Tie the herbs up in muslin or cheese cloth and dampen the bag and herbs. Fill the jar with cold water and place the tied muslin bag into the water. Secure the string so that the herbs will float in the upper third of the water. Cold steep the herbs for one to two days or until the tea is to your taste. Remove the tea bag and store the remaining tea in the refrigerator until needed.

Pulsatilla, *Anemone pulsatilla* and *A. occidentalis*

This lovely flower is also known as anemone, Easter flower, Wild Crocus, Windflower, Pasqueflower, and Prairie Smoke. It is in the Ranunculaceae (Buttercup) Family.

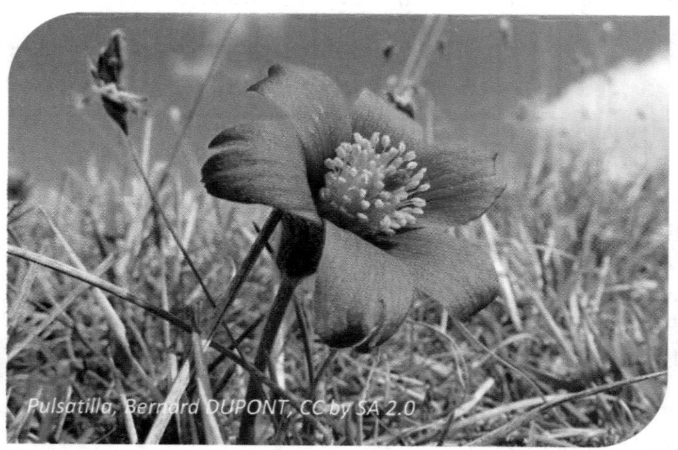
Pulsatilla, Bernard DUPONT, CC by SA 2.0

Identification: Pulsatilla is a perennial that grows 6 to 24 inches (15 cm to 60 cm) tall. The leaves are feathery, delicately divided, and covered with silky hairs. Each plant produces a single light purple or white flower with yellow stamens. The stamens produce feathery, hair-like seeds. These are one the first flowers to arrive in the spring, sometimes pushing through snow to make an appearance. The taproots run 3 feet (0.9m) or more into the ground. When the fruit head matures, the hair-like threads blow in the wind, giving the impression of smoke in the wind.

Medicinal Use: Use Pulsatilla leaves and flowers as either an infusion or a tincture. Pulsatilla must be used carefully and in small doses. In large amounts, it can be harmful or deadly. Avoid touching the fresh plant and only use dried flower heads and leaves in medicinal preparations. There are better options for most of the maladies below. Use with great care.

Skin Problems: For skin diseases, try a blended wash of Pulsatilla and Echinacea. Echinacea is an antibiotic and antiviral, and it stimulates the immune system. It works well with Pulsatilla to relieve skin problems related to inflammation and infection.

Menstrual Problems: Pulsatilla is very effective for menstrual pain, premenstrual tension, restarting menstruation, and menstrual cramping. It also relieves symptoms of menopause such as headaches, hot flashes, and moodiness.

Childbirth and Postpartum Depression: Pulsatilla stimulates the uterus and makes childbirth easier. It also has analgesic properties, which help with labor pain. It is also given after childbirth to relieve symptoms of depression. Either the tea or the tincture is used. Do not take earlier in pregnancy.

Headaches and Sleep Problems: Pulsatilla relaxes an overstimulated nervous system and treats headaches and insomnia. It calms the body and spirit allowing people to sleep soundly when taken in small doses. Note that Lemon Balm also accomplishes this without the dosing risks of Pulsatilla.

Mental Disorders and Panic Attacks: Because of its actions on the nerves, Pulsatilla is useful

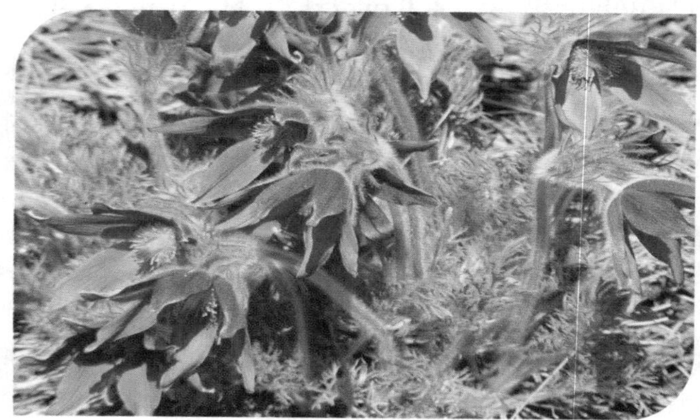

for treating nervous conditions including: hyperactivity, senile dementia, panic, and schizophrenia.

Eye and Ear Problems: Pulsatilla possesses many properties that are beneficial to the eyes and ears. The tea is useful in treating cataracts, conjunctivitis, glaucoma, and tics. The tea is also used to treat earaches, hearing loss and inflammations of the ear.

Heart Health: Pulsatilla is beneficial to the heart in numerous ways. It is used to cure thickening of the heart muscle and clear venous congestion. It relieves inflammation in the circulatory system and helps restore normal function. However, it should not be used for people with slow heart rates (bradycardia).

Drug Withdrawal: Pulsatilla is useful to help with withdrawal from sedatives, hypnotic drugs, anticonvulsants, and muscle relaxants. Be careful to give only the prescribed dosages of Pulsatilla Infusion or tincture.

Harvesting: Pick Pulsatilla flowering stalks and leaves when the plant is in full bloom, usually in the early spring near Easter.

Warning: Pulsatilla should never be used internally for pregnant women.

Given in large doses, Pulsatilla can be harmful and may cause coma, seizures, asphyxiation, and death. It can also cause a slowing of the heart rate. Wear gloves when harvesting Pulsatilla flower heads. Use only the dried flower heads and dried leaves in herbal preparations. The fresh herb is an irritant.

Recipes. Pulsatilla and Echinacea Tea: 1/2 teaspoon dried Pulsatilla flowers, 1 teaspoon dried Echinacea root and leaves and 1 cup boiling water. Pour the boiling water over the herbs and allow them to steep for 10 minutes. Strain and drink.

Purslane, *Portulaca oleracea*

Purslane is another of those backyard weeds that is under appreciated. While it is usually considered a weed, it is an excellent groundcover, vegetable, and medicine. I love to eat it in a salad. It has a salty, sour flavor that adds variety with its taste and texture. It is in the Portulacaceae (Purslane) Family and is also called common purslane, pigweed, little hogweed, verdolaga, or red root.

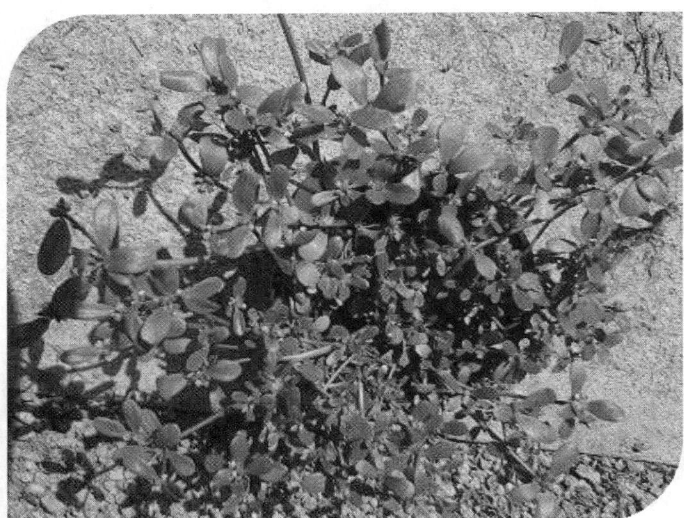

Purslane by JeffSKleinman, CC SA 4.0

Identification: *Portulaca oleracea* is a succulent that sprawls along the ground. It grows about 6 inches tall (15 cm) in a wide mat. Purslane stems are smooth and reddish or pink. The deep green thick leaves grow in groups at the stem joints and ends. Leaves can be alternate or opposite. Small yellow flowers, growing in clusters of two or three, appear in late summer and open for a few hours on sunny mornings.

Each flower has five parts and is up to 1/4 inch (0.6 cm) wide. Seeds form in tiny pods that open when the seeds are mature. The plant has a deep taproot and fibrous secondary roots. These help it survive poor soils and periods of drought. It prefers a sunny spot with dry soil.

Edible Use: Purslane has a sour, salty flavor and can be a little bitter when leaves are mature. Purslane leaves, stems, and flowers are edible raw, cooked, and pickled. When cooked like spinach, it can be a bit slimy.

Cooked purslane does not shrink as much as most greens, so a small patch can provide vegetables for an entire family. The leaves can be pickled to provide purslane during the winter months. Seeds can be collected and ground into a flour.

Medicinal Use. Uterine Bleeding: Purslane seeds are used for abnormal uterine bleeding. It helps decrease the volume and the duration of bleeding.

Asthma and Bronchial Complaints: People who eat purslane in vegetable portions or take purslane extract show improvement in overall pulmonary function.

Purslane helps with shortness of breath and opens bronchial tubes to increase oxygen reaching the lungs. For asthma attacks and other bronchial conditions, try a Purslane & Mullein Mix (recipe below). Therapeutic effects of purslane for respiratory diseases are indicated in ancient Iranian medical books. The bronchodilatory effect of the extract of *Portulaca oleracea* in the airways of asthmatic patients was examined. The results of the study showed that purslane has a relatively potent but transient bronchodilatory effect on asthmatic airways.

Diabetes: Purslane seeds or their extracts are effective in improving serum insulin levels and reduce triglycerides with long-term, daily use. People report lower blood sugar readings and better management.

Fungal Infections: Purslane has antifungal properties against the most common causes of athlete's foot, jock itch, and ringworm. Apply purslane extract to affected areas several times a day, until the infection is gone.

Lower Cholesterol: Purslane naturally lowers cholesterol due it its high pectin content. Take 1 teaspoon of purslane tincture or 2 teaspoons of fresh purslane juice daily.

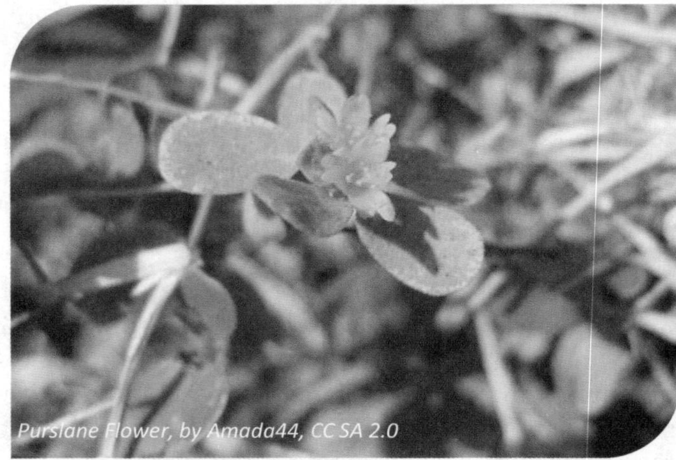
Purslane Flower, by Amada44, CC SA 2.0

Cancer: Gastric Carcinoma and Colon Adenoma. Purslane leaves and seeds have been shown to be an anti-cancer medicine for certain cancers. It also has a high Omega 3 and gamma-linoleic acid content. It is an excellent anti-oxidant.

Warning: Purslane is considered safe to eat in large portions without any side effects.

Recipes. Purslane & Mullein Mixture for Asthma: 3 droppers of Purslane tincture, 1 1/2 droppers Mullein tincture, 1/4 cup water. Add the Purslane and Mullein tinctures to the water. Note that when measuring with a dropper, the dropper will not fill up; this is fine. Drink the mixture in part or in full as needed.

Red Clover, *Trifolium pretense*

Red clover is a member of the Fabaceae (Pea) Family. I often find it growing along roadsides and fields. It is a biennial or short-lived perennial that grows to 18 inches (45 cm) tall.

Identification: The plant grows from a long, deep taproot and slender, hairy, hollow stems. The leaves are alternate, divided into three leaflets, and green with a pale crescent in the outer half of the leaf. Leaflets are 1/2 to 1 1/5 inches (0.25 cm to 3.125 cm) long and 1/2-inch (0.25 cm) wide and fine-toothed with prominent "V" marks. Pink to red flowers appear in rounded heads from May to September.

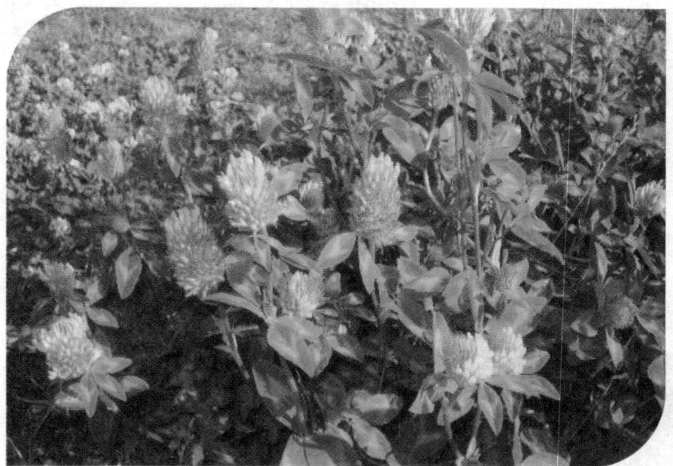
By Sanja565658 - Own work, CC BY-SA 3.0

Edible Use: I eat the leaves and young flowering heads both raw and cooked. The flowers make a sweet herbal tea and the ground seed pods and flowers can be used as a flour substitute. The taproot is edible when cooked.

Medicinal Use. How to Use Red Clover: Red clover can be taken as a dried herb, tincture, or as a tea made from the blossoms.

Relieves Symptoms of Menopause: Because of its phytoestrogen isoflavone content, red clover flowers work as a natural alternative to hormone replacement for women. It relieves symptoms of menopause, including reducing the frequency of hot flashes and night sweats. I usually pair it with Black Cohash for menopause symptom relief.

Osteoporosis: By acting as a natural hormone replacement, red clover may slow bone loss and even boost bone density in pre- and peri-menopausal women.

Cardiovascular Health: Red clover helps protect against heart disease by increasing HDL (good) cholesterol in pre- and post-menopausal women. It also has blood-thinning properties, which improve blood flow and prevent clotting.

Skin Conditions Including Eczema, Psoriasis, and Other Skin Irritations: Red clover flower tea, supported with yellow dock and nettles, is an excellent internal remedy for skin irritations. Use an external poultice made from chopped red clover flower and water applied directly to skin lesions.

Harvesting: Harvest red clover from fields, away from heavy pollution areas such as roadsides. Unlike most herbs, red clover needs to be harvested in the early morning while there is still some dew present on the flower.

Pick the blossoms one to two weeks after blooming. Snip the blossom head off and leave the rest of the plant alone.

Use the blossoms fresh or place them on a drying rack in a warm dark, ventilated, and dry place. Turn them frequently until the blossoms are dried through. Store the dried herb in a cool, dry, and dark place. When harvesting young leaves, try to get them before the plant flowers.

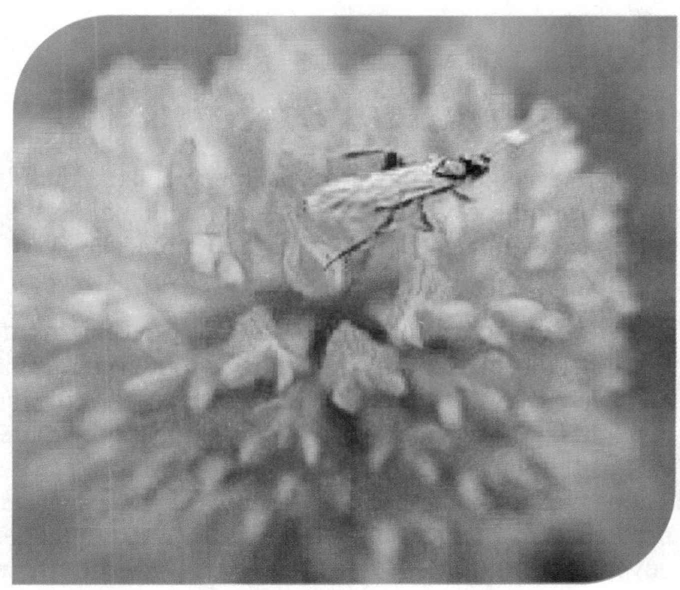

Guttorm Raknes, Own work, CC by SA 4.0

Use them cooked as a green, in soups, and salads. The leaves can also be dried and powdered for use as a flavoring on foods. They tend to be more bitter after the flowers appear.

Warning: In general, red clover is very safe, with few side effects, except for occasional gas. The anticoagulant effect and hormonal effects may be undesirable for some people.

Due to its hormonal activity, don't use red clover for women with a history of endometriosis, breast cancer, uterine cancer, fibroids, or other estrogen-sensitive conditions.

Red clover contains coumarin derivatives and must be used with caution in individuals taking anticoagulation therapy. Also, do not take red clover before surgery or childbirth. It can inhibit blood clotting and healing.

Recipes. Red Clover Tea (hot): Red clover blossoms, fresh or dried, and 1 cup boiling water. Steep three fresh red clover blossoms or 2 to 3 teaspoons of dried flowers in 1 cup boiling water.

Allow the tea to steep while cooling for 15 minutes. Drink warm or allow to cool for external use. Drink up to three times daily for maximum benefits.

Red Clover Tea (Cold): Add one-half cup of red clover blossoms to a quart (a liter) of water and allow it to steep in the refrigerator for 24 hours.

Rosemary, *Rosmarinus officinalis*

I love the scent and flavor of rosemary. I use it mainly to flavor potatoes and lamb and as a medicinal herb. It grows easily in a garden. It is in the Lamiaceae (Mint) Family.

Identification: Rosemary, is a woody herb with fragrant needle-like leaves and a fibrous root system. It is an evergreen shrub that can withstand extreme droughts. Most bushes are upright reaching 5 feet (1.5m) tall, but some can develop into trailing plants. The leaves look like hemlock needles. They are green on the top and white on the underside, with both sides covered with short, dense, wooly hair. White, pink, purple, or blue flowers appear in the spring and in the summer in cooler climates and year-round in warmer climates.

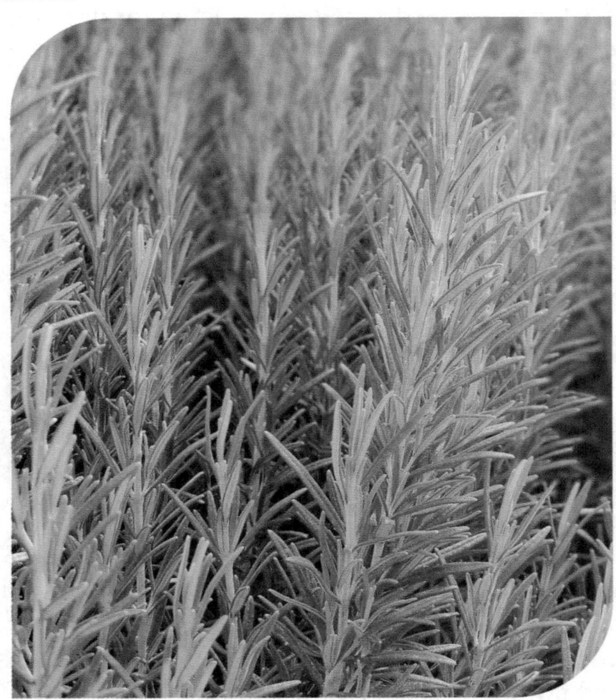

Edible Use: Rosemary is often used in cooking. The leaves and the flower petals are edible and nutritious.

Medicinal Use: Rosemary contains caffeic acid, carnosic acid, carnosol, and rosemarinic acid, anti-inflammatories, and anti-oxidants.

Stimulates Digestion: The stimulant properties of rosemary bring circulation to the digestive organs and help relieve digestive problems, especially indigestion. You may use rosemary in your food and/or use a tincture or infused oil before a large meal.

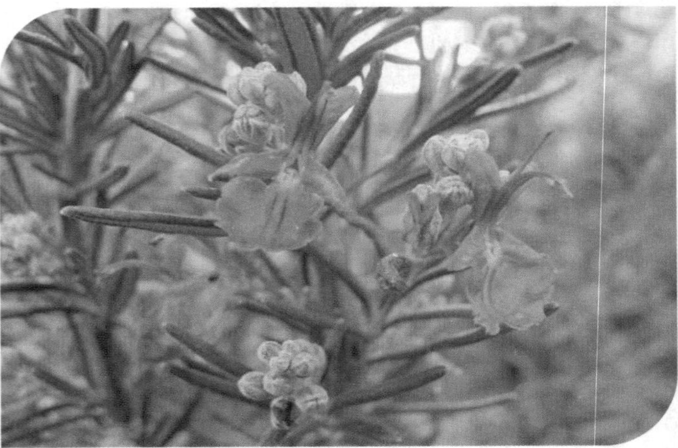

Rosemary in bloom, Margalob, CC by SA 4.0

Improves Concentration and Memory, Neuroprotective: Rosemary is known as a brain tonic. It seems to improve concentration and memory. It stimulates the circulatory system, bringing more oxygen to the brain. It is used for elderly dementia patients. It also has a neuroprotective effect due to the carnosic acid found in rosemary.

Circulatory Problems and Headaches: Rosemary is a mild stimulant, well-known for increasing circulation. Use it for problems with the cardiovascular system, poor circulation, and low blood pressure. These same stimulant properties make it a good choice for alleviating headaches, especially migraines. Rosemary has a mild analgesic effect, but the main relief comes from opening up the blood flow to the brain.

Inflammation, Colitis, Arthritis: The analgesic properties and anti-inflammatory properties help reduce the pain and swelling of joints inflamed from arthritis. People report that it helps their pain and swelling but does not completely alleviate it, so it usually used in combination with other herbs. It also reduces gut inflammation.

Antifungal: Rosemary is a good antifungal and I often add rosemary essential oil to an external antifungal salve.

Antibacterial: *Pseudomonas* and Staph: Rosemary essential oil inhibits the bacterium *Pseudomonas*. It also works to kill *Staphylococcus*, as does oregano oil.

Anti-cancer and Hepatoprotective: Rosemary has been researched for a variety of cancers and it has many properties, such as caffeic acid, carnosic acid, carnosol, and rosemarinic acid that help fight cancer. It also protects the liver.

Hair Loss: Rosemary essential oil has been shown to be as effective as the prescription hair growth drug Minoxidil. Apply in a carrier oil on the scalp (I prefer coconut oil) and keep using long-term.

Halitosis: Rosemary makes an extremely effective mouthwash. It can get rid of bad breath very quickly. Gargle and rinse with Rosemary Mouthwash every morning and night, more often if needed. A mouthwash recipe is below.

Recipes. Rosemary Mouthwash: Bring 2 cups of water to a boil and remove it from the heat. Steep 1 heaping tablespoon of dried rosemary flowers and/or leaves in the water for 30 minutes. Store the mouthwash tightly covered in the refrigerator for up to 3 days.

Queen Anne's Lace, *Daucus carota*

Queen Anne's lace is often used as an ornamental. It is also known as wild carrot because of its carrot scent and because it is a member of the Apiaceae (Carrot) Family. Be careful with identification as there are look-alikes, like the deadly hemlock plant. My favorite story to tell them apart is about Queen Anne sewing a piece of lace. She pricked her finger and a single drop of blood fell into the center of the flowers, symbolizing the single red or purple flower in the center of each umbel. The presence of this blood colored flower is a positive identification for Queen Anne's Lace. As a rule, if you are unsure don't pick it.

Identification: Queen Anne's Lace grows to 1 to 4 feet (0.3m to 1.2m) tall. The flower stems are green, hairy, and may have long red stripes. They are thin and have a thin hollow space in the center. Clusters of flowers, called umbels, are arranged in a tight pattern gathered into a larger umbrella shaped cluster. The umbels are flat across the top and 3 to 4 inches (7.25 cm to 10 cm) wide. Blooms may be pink in bud and white when in full bloom. In the center there is a single reddish or purple flower. Seeing this red or purple flower is a definitive marker for Queen Anne's lace, but not all varieties have the color.

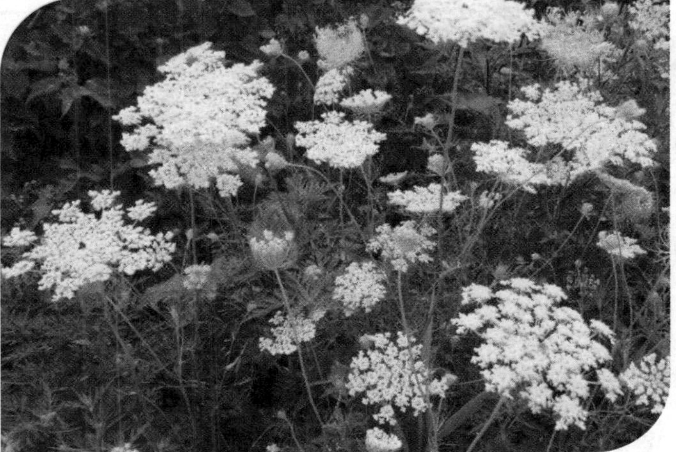

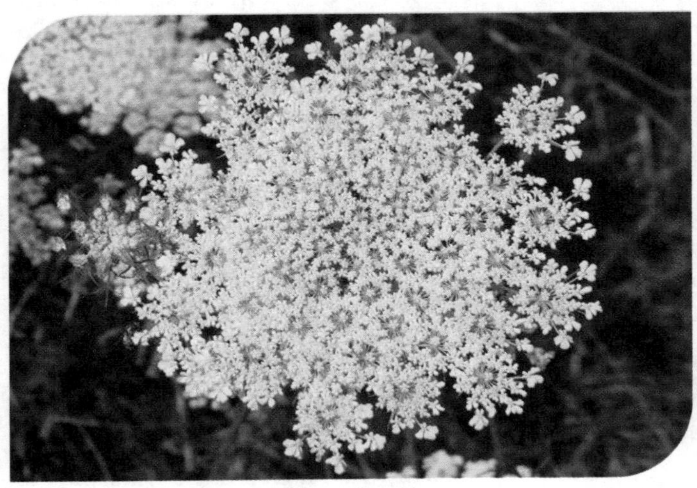

Queen Anne's Lace, Jrosenberry1, CC 4.0

When the flowers die, Queen Anne's lace flowers curl into a bird's nest shape as they dry. Leaves on Queen Anne's lace are lance-shaped serrated leaflets. Each leaf is 2 to 4 inches (5 cm to 10 cm) in length and slightly hairy on the underside. The plant has a single thin taproot that is shaped like a carrot.

Edible Use: The thin taproot from Queen Anne's lace is edible cooked, however it quickly becomes very fibrous and woody as growth progresses. For eating purposes, only young roots are tender enough to cook and eat. The flowers are edible and are good battered and fried. The first-year leaves are edible in small portions. Caution is necessary when handling or eating the plant because of its close resemblance to poison hemlock. Make sure of your identification before consuming any herb! Remember: Queen Anne has hairy legs.

Gallstones, Kidney Stones, Chronic Kidney Problems, Bladder Problems, and Gout: Queen Anne's lace seeds and roots are used for treating gall bladder problems and kidney problems. It acts to remove excess water from the body and reduce inflammation.

Colic, Upset Stomach, and Flatulence: The soothing and diuretic properties of the root are helpful for treating stomach and intestinal upsets.

Skin Problems: For itchy dermatitis, a poultice made from the grated root helps relieve an itchy rash. The seed oil is also good for soothing and lubricating the skin. It is also anti-inflammatory.

Birth Control and Conception: Queen Anne's Lace seeds have been used to prepare the womb for pregnancy when used before ovulation. If taken after ovulation or as an emergency contraceptive seeds should be used for 3 days. Use with care. Do not use during pregnancy!

Warning: Do not use while pregnant or nursing. There are a lot of poisonous look-alikes so be careful with proper identification.

Sage, *Salvia officinalis*

There are many different varieties of sage, and many of them have medicinal properties. Here we are discussing common sage. I try to use it in cooking so that I get the beneficial compounds often. It is in the Lamiaceae (Mint) Family and is easy to cultivate in the garden.

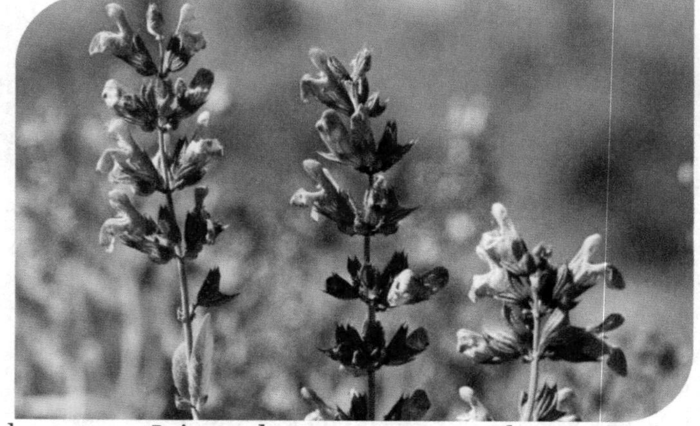

Identification: Common sage grows to approximately 2 feet (0.6m) tall and wide. It flowers in late spring or summer, producing lavender, purple, pink or white flowers. Leaves are oblong, approximately 2 1/2 inches (3.75 cm) long and 1 inch (2.5 cm) wide. The leaves are grey-green colored and wrinkled on the top, while the underside is white and covered in short, soft hairs.

Edible Use: Sage is commonly used as a cooking herb.

Medicinal Use: Sage is an antiseptic, antimicrobial, anti-mutagenic, antibacterial, helps stop neuropathic pain, improves memory, lowers blood glucose levels, and alleviated menopause symptoms. It is an excellent all-around herb.

Digestion Aid: Sage help in the digestion of rich, fatty meats, which perhaps is why it is used so often in sausage recipes. Its stimulant properties work to move fats through the digestive system efficiently and prevent indigestion.

Balances Hormones for Men and Women: Sage is effective in balancing hormones. It is used to promote normal menstruation and to treat menopausal symptoms such as hot flashes, night sweats, headaches, and mental fog. It is also useful in treating premature ejaculation in men.

Sore Throats: The most effective remedy is a gargle, but many people object to the flavor. Thus we have added a recipe below for a better-tasting throat spray that is almost as effective. Both remedies contain several herbs that fight infection and calm the inflammation of a sore throat.

Speed Healing in Wounds: For slow-healing wounds, make a compress by soaking a cotton pad in sage infusion. Apply the cotton pad to the wound and hold in place with tape or a clean piece of cloth or gauze. The sage infusion relieves the pain almost immediately, fights infection, and brings more blood to the area to speed healing.

Hair Growth: Sage essential oil improves blood circulation to the scalp and roots of the hair. This encourages thick hair growth and is often paired with rosemary essential oil.

Warning: Sage can significantly reduce the amount of milk produced in nursing mothers. Avoid its use when breastfeeding.

Recipes. Sage Throat Spray: 3 tablespoons dried or fresh sage leaves, 3/4 cup boiling water, 1/4 cup Echinacea Extract, 1 tablespoon raw honey. Pour the boiling water over the sage leaves and allow it to steep for 30 minutes. Strain out the leaves. Add the Echinacea extract and raw honey. Store in a bottle with a spray top, preferably with a fine mist. Spray in the back of the throat as often as needed.

Sage Gargle for a Sore Throat: This gargle doesn't taste great, but it works! 1 tablespoon dried sage leaves, 1 cup boiling water, 1 teaspoon goldenseal root powder, 5 drops Cayenne Infusion, 1/2 cup apple cider vinegar, with live culture.

Pour the boiling water over the dried sage and allow it to steep for 45 minutes. Strain out the leaves and add the goldenseal root powder, cayenne infusion, and vinegar. Gargle with this mixture every hour for as long as you can stand it. Spit out the gargle.

Sheep Sorrel, *Rumex acetosella*

Sheep sorrel is one of the most useful medicinal herbs, and yet many people pull them out or spray them to rid their yard or field of it. Sheep sorrel is also known as red sorrel, narrow-leafed dock, spinach dock, sour weed, and field sorrel. It is a member of the Polygonaceae (Buckwheat) Family. The plant grows as a common perennial in most areas.

Identification: Sheep sorrel has small green leaves shaped like arrowheads and deeply ridged, upright red stems that are branched at the top. The plant grows to 18 inches (45 cm) tall at most. It grows from an aggressively spreading rhizome.

Sheep sorrel blooms from March to November and are either all male or all female. Yellowish-green male flowers or maroon colored female flowers grow on a tall, upright stem. The maroon female flowers develop into red achenes. It is one of the first species to appear when an area has been disturbed.

Edible Use: Sheep sorrel is edible raw as a salad green or as a garnish. The flavor is tart and lemony. It can be used as a curdling agent during the cheese-making process and can be cooked like spinach.

Livestock will eat the plant, but it is not very nutritious and can cause problems if too much is consumed because of its high concentration of oxalates.

Medicinal Use: Use sheep sorrel leaves as a juice, tea, and powder or capsules.

Detoxification: Sheep sorrel is useful for detoxification. It has a diuretic effect and flushes the body when ample water is consumed. It also has laxative effects. For detoxification, use freshly juiced leaves or Sheep Sorrel Tea, though the tea and powder are less effective than the fresh juice.

Gastro-Intestinal Problems, Kidney, and Urinary Tract Diseases, Cysts, Swellings, and Skin Cancers: For tumors, swellings, cysts, and cancers close to the skin surface, use a leaf poultice. Apply the macerated leaf poultice directly over the affected area several times daily until the problem is resolved.

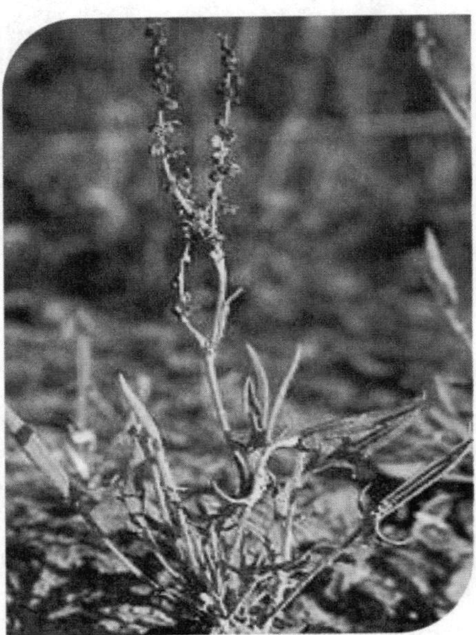

Henripekka Kallio, CC by SA 3.0, Female flowers Sheep Sorrel,

Intestinal Parasites and Worms: Use the tea internally to kill and flush worms and intestinal parasites out of the system. One cup of tea, taken twice daily for two weeks does the job.

Colds, Flu, and Sinusitis: Sheep sorrel is an excellent treatment for reducing the inflammation and pain that accompanies colds, flu, and sinusitis. The tannins help reduce the production of mucus and its anti-microbial action helps kill bacterial infections. Use sheep sorrel as soon as the illness begins to reduce the severity of the disease.

Warning: Because of its high oxalate content, people with kidney stones, arthritis, or hyperacidity should not use sheep sorrel.

Sheep Sorrel Tea: You'll need 1 teaspoon dried sheep sorrel leaves and 1 cup water.

Bring the water to a boil and pour over the dried sheep sorrel leaves. Cover and let the tea steep for 5 to 10 minutes. Drink warm.

Skullcap, *Scutellaria lateriflora*

Skullcap is also called blue skullcap, side-flowering skullcap, Quaker bonnet, hoodwort, mad dog skullcap, helmet flower, and blue pimpernel. It is a calming herb, useful for anxiety and nervous disorders of all kinds. It is in the Lamiaceae (Mint) Family. It likes moist areas throughout much of North America, where it is native, and is cultivated in much of Europe. North American skullcaps can be used interchangeably for medicine. Note that they are used differently than Chinese Skullcap (S. baicalensis), another useful herb.

Identification: The plant has smooth, square erect stems that reach 1 to 4 feet (0.3m to 1.2m) tall. The stems are leafy and branched, with oblong, opposite toothed leaves. Each leaf is 1 to 3 inches (2.5 cm to 7.5 cm) long, with smaller leaves at the top of the stems. The 2-lobed helmeted flowers are blue-violet to whitish. Each flower is about 1 inch (2.5 cm) long and grows in short spike-like racemes or singularly in the axils of the upper leaves. The flowers are tubular and the upper hooded lip gives it its name of "skullcap". Each flower produces 4 nut-like fruits. It blooms from July through September.

Medicinal Use: Skullcap is usually used as a hot tea or tincture, but some people prefer to use powdered skullcap in capsule form. Tinctures should be made with fresh herbs for optimal potency. Skullcap seems to act upon benzodiazepine GABA receptors in the brain. GABA is a neurotransmitter that helps prevent overstimulation of the nervous system. If it gets too low you can have seizures, epilepsy, anxiety, depression, insomnia and more.

American skullcap interacts with these GABA receptors, binding to the benzodiazepine site, as does Valerian and California Poppy, both in this book. The leaves, stems, and flowers are used medicinally, though many people only use the leaves. The plant is rich in vitamins, minerals, and tannins. The plant is relaxing and acts as a natural tranquilizer and sleep aid. It is similar to valerian root in properties and activity.

Anxiety, Tension, Depression, and Insomnia: Skullcap relaxes the nervous system, reduces stress, and relieves anxiety. It reduces body tension and allows the body to relax into sleep. It calms people who are overly nervous, hysterical, or unable to relax.

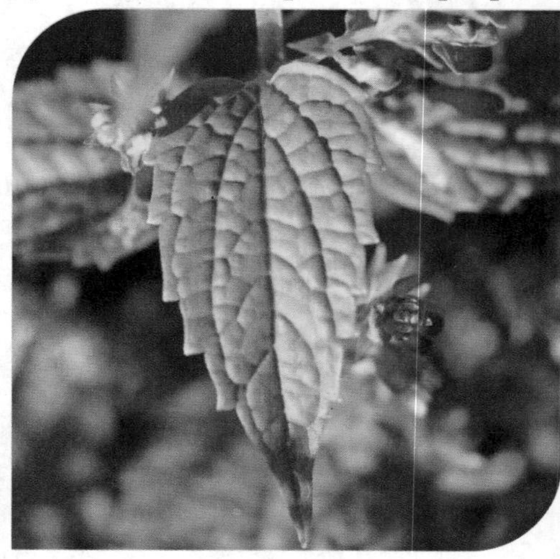
Millspaugh, C.F(1854-1923) Commons Wikipedia

Its antioxidant properties help with oxidative stress, which is associated with depression and anxiety disorders, and it binds to benzodiazepine GABA receptors in the brain.

Antioxidant and Neuroprotective: Skullcap is an excellent antioxidant and functions as a neuroprotective for diseases such as Alzheimer's and Parkinson's.

Muscle Spasms and Tension, Muscle, Seizures, Twitches, Calms the Nervous System: Skullcap is an antispasmodic. It eases muscle twitches, spasms, and seizures by relaxing the muscles, relieving involuntary muscle movements, and calming the nervous system.

Tension Headaches and Perhaps Migraines: People taking skullcap report that it helps relieve tension headaches. It may also help migraines.

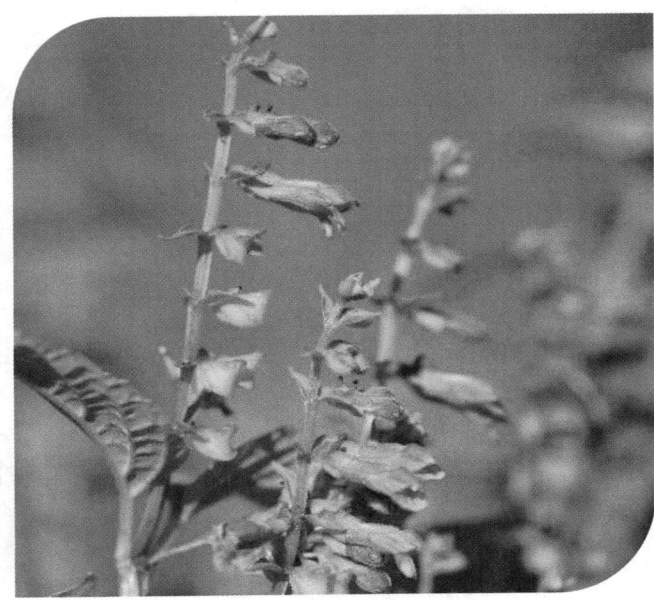

Drug Withdrawal, Smoking Withdrawal, Alcohol Withdrawal: Skullcap helps with withdrawal from drugs, especially benzodiazepines like Valium and Xanax. It also assists with withdrawal from alcohol and smoking by calming the body, relieving tremors, relaxing the mind, and relieving anxiety and depression.

Exhaustion and Depression: Skullcap is calming and allows the body and mind to rest. This is essential in treating exhaustion and depression. With good sleep and a calm mind, the body is able to put itself back in order and heal mentally and physically.

Harvesting: Wait to harvest skullcap until the plant is in full bloom. Remove stems, leaves, and flowers by pruning off the top of the plant, leaving approximately 3 to 4 inches (7.5 cm to 10 cm) to regrow. The herb is most potent when freshly harvested, but can be used dried.

Warning: Do not take skullcap while pregnant or breastfeeding. Safety is unknown. Use skullcap sparingly in small doses. Large doses may be harmful or could cause liver damage.

Recipes. **Skullcap Tea:** 1 Tablespoon fresh skullcap leaves or 1 teaspoon dried, 1 cup boiling water, raw honey or Maple Syrup, if desired. Crush the herbs and place them in a tea ball. Pour 1 cup of boiling water over the herbs and steep for 5 to 10 minutes. Remove the teaball and sweeten the tea, if desired.

St. John's Wort, *Hypericum perforatum*

St. John's Wort, also called Klamath Weed, is recognized as an invasive weed in most parts of North America. It gets its name from its uncanny ability to bloom on June 24, the birthday of St. John the Baptist. It is in the Hypericaceae (St. John's Wort) Family.

Identification: St. John's Wort is an herbaceous perennial with creeping rhizomes. The stems are erect and grow up to 3 feet (0.9m) tall. The stems branch in the upper section and produce narrow, yellow-green leaves that are less than 1 inch (2.5 cm) long. The leaves have tiny oil glands that look like small windows when the plant is held to the light. Bright yellow flowers, measuring 1 inch (2.5 cm) across, appear on the upper branches from late spring to mid-summer. The flowers have five petals with pointed sepals. The sepals have noticeable black dots. The large stamens are grouped into three bundles and the flower buds have a red resin when squeezed. The plant is widespread. It likes dry soil and sunny locations.

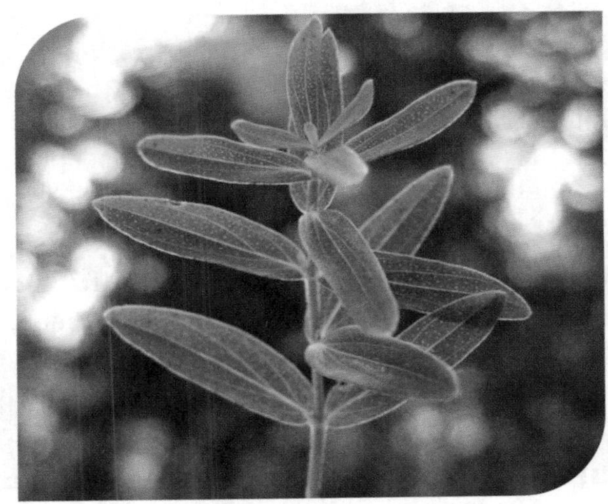

Medicinal Use: The flowers and leaves are used for medicine. They are best used fresh if available.

Depression, Anxiety, SAD and OCD: St John's Wort is most commonly used for treating depression, restlessness, anxiety, and insomnia without adverse effects. People with bipolar disorder should not take it, as it seems to increase the risk of mania. It should also not be taken by people already on an SSRI medication. It is very effective for SAD (Seasonal Affective Disorder) and OCD and is often paired with Lemon Balm.

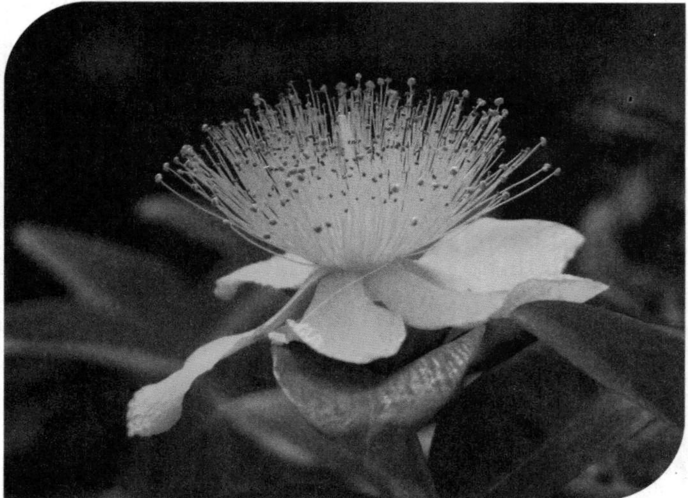

Menopause, PMS and Menstrual Cramping: St John's Wort reduces the symptoms of hormonal imbalances in menopause including depression and fatigue. It helps balance the hormones and stimulates the organs, increasing the tone of the uterus. It is also beneficial for relieving cramping, bloating, and mood symptoms of PMS.

Opiate Withdrawal and Quitting Smoking: St John's Wort helps with the symptoms of mild opiate withdrawal and aids people trying to quit smoking. It calms the nervous system and alleviates the physical symptoms of withdrawal from opiate-based drugs and helps relieve anxiety and depression for people quitting smoking. Use an internal St John's Wort Tincture for this.

Cuts, Bruises, Burns, Sunburns, and Other Injuries: Extracted St John's Oil is an excellent antiseptic and anti-viral and contains tannins that facilitate healing. Apply topically to heal burns, sunburns, injuries, wounds, and infections.

Neuralgia, Bell's Palsy and Nerve Pain: Nerve pain and neuralgia benefit from topically applied oil and internal tincture or tea. You can also use it for sharp and convulsive trigeminal neuralgia and sciatica. Apply the oil or salve on the affected areas 3x/day.

Muscle Pains: For back pain, muscle pain, and general body aches, use St John's Wort Oil or salve. It is useful taken internally and when massaged externally into the muscles.

Peptic Ulcers, Gastric Problems: St John's Wort attacks ulcers and gastric problems by calming the digestive organs and by attacking the bacteria and viruses that are causing the problem. It is effective against infective digestive problems such as gastroenteritis, dysentery, and diarrhea.

Hemorrhoids: The oil of St John's Wort is almost a miracle cure for hemorrhoids. It effectively reduces the inflammation, relieves the pain, and speeds the healing process. Use the recipe below and apply topical to the affected area 3x/day.

Epstein Barr Virus, Shingles, Hepatitis and Herpes Virus: The healing properties of hypericin, found in the petals and stems of St. John's Wort, may work as an anti-viral. It can also be applied externally for herpes and shingles outbreaks.

Removing Fluids and Toxins: The diuretic properties of St John's wort help to remove fluids from the body and flush away toxins through urination.

Bedwetting in Childhood: Giving 5 to 10 drops of St John's wort tincture in the late afternoon can help children with bedwetting problems. Flushing the excess fluids out of the system before bedtime helps prevent the buildup of fluids in the bladder.

Arthritis and Gout: St John's Wort reduces inflammation and pain, relieving the symptoms of these joint diseases. For best results, use it daily as the benefits increase over time as the inflamed joints heal.

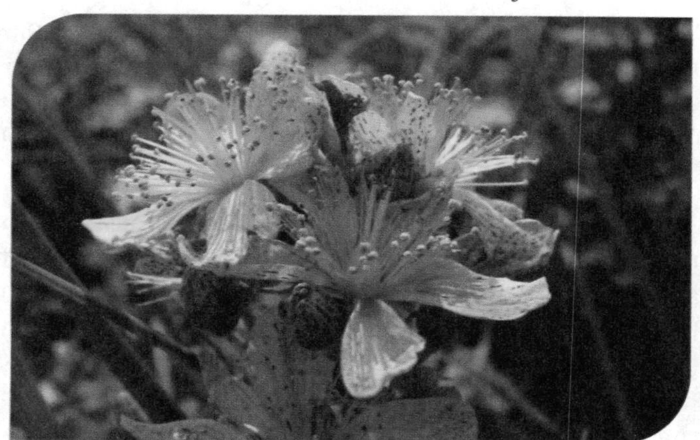

Chest Colds, Congestion, and Respiratory Disease: In addition to the anti-inflammatory and anti-microbial benefits of St John's wort, it is also an effective expectorant that helps clear chest congestion and phlegm. It speeds healing of infections and common coughs and colds. It is also used against influenza.

Warning: St John's Wort interacts with a lot of modern medicines. It should not be taken by people already on an SSRI medication and may cause sun sensitivity to very fair-skinned people. It may interact with Warfarin, Digitoxin, and HIV medications. Do not take for 2 weeks prior to surgery. Check with your physician before using.

Recipes. St John's Wort Tincture: Ingredients: St John's Wort flowers and leaves, 80 proof grain alcohol or vodka, a clean jar with a tight-fitting lid.

Loosely pack the flowers and leaves into the glass jar, filling it to the top. Add the alcohol to the jar, covering the flowers and leaves. Cap the jar tightly. Label. Add more alcohol as needed to replace evaporation. Shake the jar daily and allow it to steep for 4 to 6 weeks. Strain the herbs out. Cap the jar and keep it in a cool, dark cupboard. Take the tincture for a prolonged period as needed to cure chronic conditions.

St John's Wort Infused Oil: Four ounces(112g) of fresh St. John's Wort flowers and 2 cups organic olive oil. Mix the herbs and olive oil in a double boiler and place them over very low heat.

Steep the oil and herbs for 2 to 3 hours, keeping the oil at a low simmer. Strain the oil and remove the herbs. Store your infused oil in a cool, dark cupboard.

*St John's wort oil works well on its own, however, it can be even more healing when mixed with other herbs.

Stinging Nettle, *Urtica dioica*

I love stinging nettle, though I know many who don't due to its sting. It is nutritious, medicinal, and makes beautiful fiber. I even have a nettle shirt! Dock usually grows near it and can be used to take away the sting. It is in the Lamiaceae (Mint) Family.

Identification: Stinging nettle is a perennial, growing from 3 to 8 feet (0.9m to 2.4m) tall. It is dioecious and herbaceous, dying back in the winter.

The leaves are mostly oval or occasionally heart-shaped. The soft, green leaves are 1 to 4 inches (2.5 cm to 10 cm) long and are arranged oppositely on a square erect stem. The leaves have a serrated margin and cordate base. Both the leaves and stems are very hairy with non-stinging hairs and many stinging hairs. Numerous flowers appear June to September in dense inflorescences. They are greenish or brownish, growing in branched clusters. Male and female flowers grow on separate plants or branches. Stinging nettle is widely distributed, especially where the average annual rainfall is high. I find it in places with moist soil.

Edible Use: The leaves are edible. Stinging nettles have a flavor similar to mild spinach when cooked. I eat them raw by folding over the leaves but most people blanch them in water to remove the sting before cooking and eating. Only eat stinging nettle leaves before the flowers appear. Beyond that time, they can cause internal irritation, especially of the urinary tract. The seeds are also edible. Dried nettle leaves and flowers make a nice herbal tea.

Medicinal Use: Nettle can be taken as a tea or tincture and is my number one go to for allergies.

Allergies (including Hay Fever): Stinging nettle tincture is my first recommendation for allergies as it usually completely alleviates the problem. I often recommend coupling it with local raw honey. It is an excellent anti-inflammatory.

Arthritis, Gout Pain, and Inflammation: Stinging nettle treats arthritis, gout, and other inflammatory conditions. It suppresses inflammation, flushes toxins from the body, and helps reduce the pain of these conditions.

It is used in Germany as a treatment for Rheumatoid Arthritis and is thought to inhibit the cascade of inflammation. Externally, a compress made by soaking a cotton pad in nettle tincture and placing it over the painful joint is helpful. Stinging an area can also help restore and repair joint injuries and reestablish nerve communication. I have used it successfully to treat shoulder injuries.

Eczema and Skin Inflammations: Both the internal tincture and infusion of stinging nettle are useful for treating eczema and other skin inflammations.

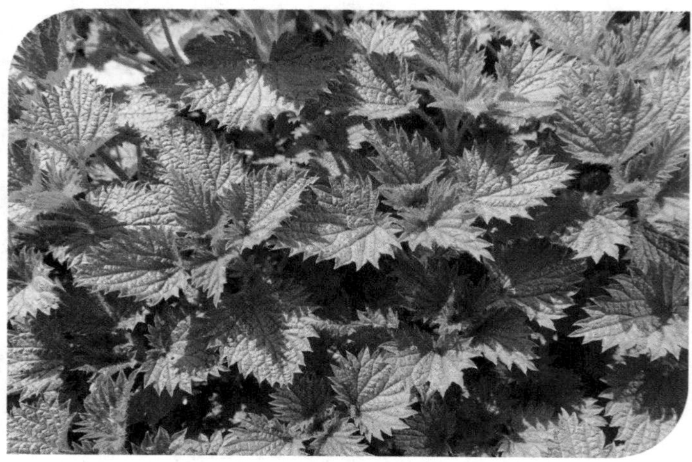

Burns, Insect Bites, and Wounds: Use a double strength Nettle Infusion as a wash to treat burned skin, sunburns, insect bites, wounds, and other skin irritations. Stinging nettle has combudoron, which has been shown to help with burn treatment. Make the Nettle Infusion recipe using 2 tablespoons of dried or fresh nettle leaves. Use the cooled liquid to wash and treat these conditions, allowing it to dry on the skin.

Menstrual Problems: Women with heavy uterine bleeding and other menstrual problems benefit from stinging nettle.

Sprains, Cramps, Tendonitis, and Sciatica: Muscle cramping, injuries and nerve pain benefit from the application of a compress made by soaking a cotton pad in Nettle Tincture and applying it over the affected area. Fasten it in place for best results.

Stimulates Blood Flow: Stinging nettle stimulates the circulatory system and blood flow. To stimulate blood flow and improve circulation, use a Nettle Infusion or Tea. It can also be used externally as the sting brings healing and blood flow to the area.

Anemia, Cardiac Insufficiency, Swellings, Enlarged Spleen and as a Whole-Body Tonic: For serious conditions such as these, use fresh nettle juice prepared by soaking and blending the whole fresh plant.

Hair Rinse: Use Nettle Tea as a hair rinse to increase shine. Couple it with Horsetail and Rosemary for maximum results.

Recipes. Nettle Infusion: You will need 1 tablespoon dried and crushed nettle leaves and 1 cup boiling water. Pour the boiling water over the nettle leaves and allow it to steep for 10 to 15 minutes. Strain and drink twice daily.

Nettle Tincture. Ingredients: stinging nettle leaves, fresh or crushed and dried (fresh is best), 80 proof vodka or other drinking alcohol of same strength, a glass jar with a tight-fitting lid.

Fill the jar with fresh nettle leaves that have been sliced into thin pieces and crushed. Pour vodka over the leaves and fill the jar, making sure all the leaves are covered. Cap the jar tightly. Label it. Let the tincture infuse for 4 to 6 weeks, shaking the jar daily. Add more alcohol if needed to keep the jar full. Pour the alcohol through a fine mesh sieve or a coffee filter to remove all of the herbs. Store the tincture in a cool, dark cupboard for up to 5 years. Dosage: 1/2 to 1 teaspoon, twice daily.

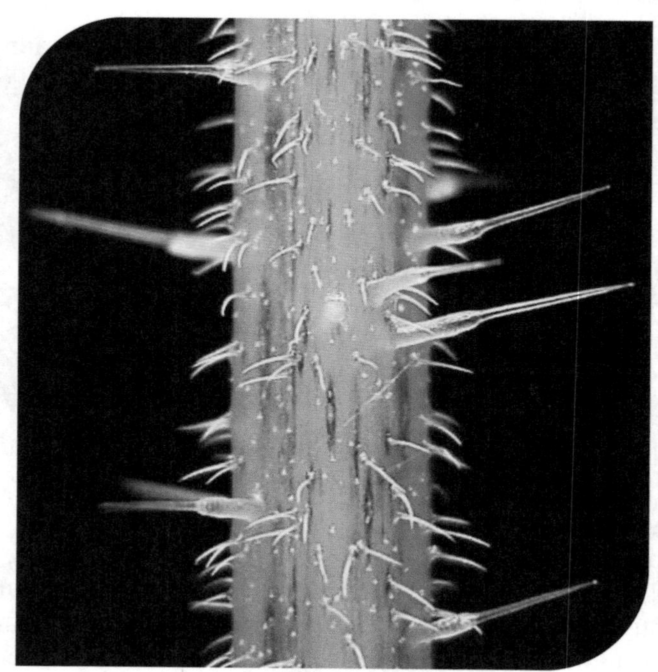

Stinging nettle, Frank Vincentz - Own work, CC by SA 3.0

Sweet Grass, *Hierochloe odorata* or *Anthoxanthum nitens*

This fragrant grass is also known as vanilla grass and holy grass, and is considered a sacred plant and is used ceremonially by many. It is native to Northern Eurasia and much of North America. It is in the Poaceae (Grass) Family. It is also used for weaving.

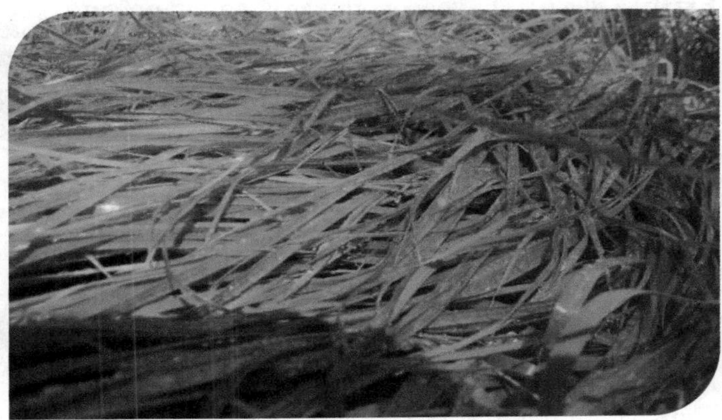

Sweet Grass, Kodemizer, CC by SA 3.0

Identification: Sweet grass is a perennial grass that is hardy in extreme cold. The fragrant grass blades are not stiff and after it reaches about 8 inches (20 cm) tall it leans over and grows horizontally until the end of summer, reaching about 3 feet (0.9m) in length. Its blades are shiny and smooth and, if you look under the soil, you can see a broad smooth leaf base. The undersides are light in color.

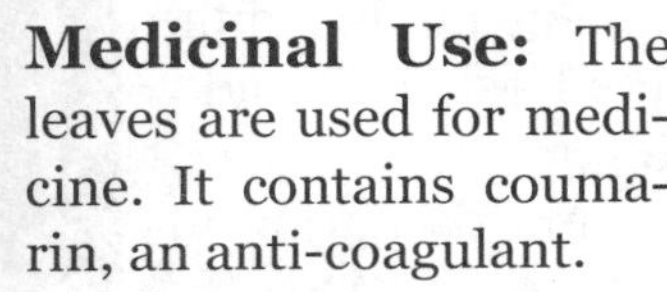

Medicinal Use: The leaves are used for medicine. It contains coumarin, an anti-coagulant.

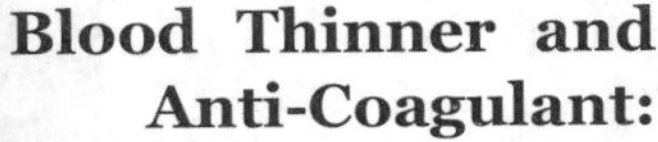

Blood Thinner and Anti-Coagulant: Sweet grass contains coumarin, which transforms in the body into an anti-coagulant. Coumarin also gives sweet grass its sweet smell. Do not use on people with bleeding issues. Use carefully; excess can be toxic.

Common Colds, Bronchial Congestion: Inhale the smoke from burning sweet grass to treat common colds and congestion or drink the leaves as a tea for colds.

Insect Repellent: Two compounds found in sweet grass, phytol and coumarin, work as well as DEET in repelling mosquitoes.

Sore Throats, Coughs, Fever, Venereal Disease: Sweet grass leaf tea is used to treat sore throats, coughs, and fevers as well as venereal diseases. Use internally with care.

Harvesting: Harvest sweet grass throughout the summer, cutting it above the ground in the amounts needed. Best used fresh throughout the summer and dry a supply at the end of summer for winter use.

Warning: Be careful with internal use. Large doses can be carcinogenic and toxic. Use with great care.

Sweet Marjoram, *Origanum majorana*

Sweet marjoram, also called pot marjoram, is a tender perennial herb with a piney-citrus flavor. It is related to oregano and has some similar uses and a milder flavor. The plant is widely cultivated in herb gardens and can be found growing wild where it has escaped cultivation. I grow it in my garden for easy access. It is in the Lamiaceae (Mint) Family.

Identification: Sweet marjoram has smooth narrow opposite leaves approximately 1/5 to 3/5 inches long that are oval in shape with a slight point. The margin is smooth and the base is tapered. The leaf has numerous hairs that give it a smooth, velvety texture. The grey-green leaves are aromatic and flavorful. It grows to a height of 10 to 24 inches (60 cm) on several thin boughs. The stems are square and purple. The plant produces delicate white or pink blossoms on spikes at the end of the branches during late summer and early autumn.

Edible Use: The leaves, flowers, and stems are all edible.

Medicinal Use: The leaves of this herb have many medicinal uses and can be taken in food, or the distilled oil can be used.

Digestive and Respiratory Tonic: Sweet marjoram is an effective tonic for the digestive and respiratory tracts. It is an excellent treatment for problems related to these areas.

Menstrual Aid: The herb is capable of inducing menstruation and should never be used in significant amounts by pregnant women. Used in medicinal quantities, it calms the uterus and relieves pain and cramping. It balances the hormones and relieves the symptoms of menopause and pre-menstrual syndrome. It helps bring on menstruation when delayed.

Polycystic Ovarian Syndrome: People with PCOS and its related fertility problems may find relief with sweet marjoram. By balancing the hormones, it is able to relieve the symptoms of this disease and is said to help women to conceive.

Promotes Breast Milk Production: Nursing mothers report an increase in breast milk production when eating marjoram daily.

Diabetes: People with type II diabetes can add sweet marjoram and rosemary to their daily diet. The combination aids the use of insulin in the body and improves blood sugar management.

Muscle Spasms, Tension Headaches, and Over-Used Muscles: Marjoram essential oil has a calming effect on muscles and tension headaches. Some people say that simply breathing in the oil is enough to relieve a tension headache. Two or three drops added to a vaporizer or bath water is enough. It is also very effective for relieving muscle spasms and pain when diluted and used as a massage oil.

Lowers Blood Pressure: Sweet marjoram essential oil lowers blood pressure through breathing in the scent of marjoram essential oil. The relaxation of the body and release of stress helps lower the blood pressure naturally.

How to Use Marjoram Medicinally: As little as one tablespoon of dried marjoram, sprinkled on food, taken in capsules or used as a tea is enough to derive health benefits. For fresh herbs, add a quarter cup of chopped marjoram on your salads or other foods. Both the fresh and dried herb are beneficial.

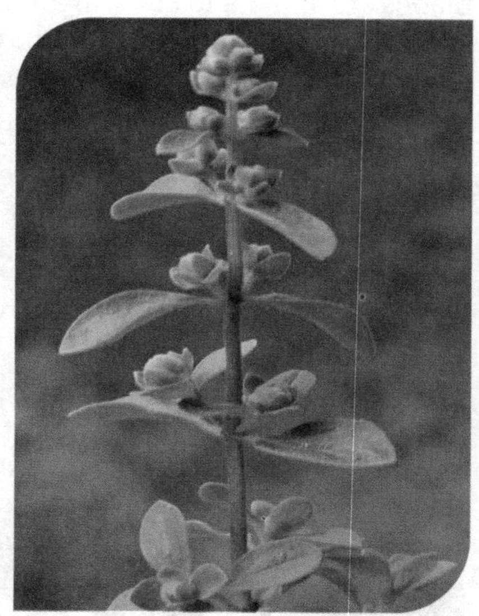

Warning: Do not use in high doses if pregnant, as it can bring on menstruation.

Thorn Apple, *Datura stramonium*

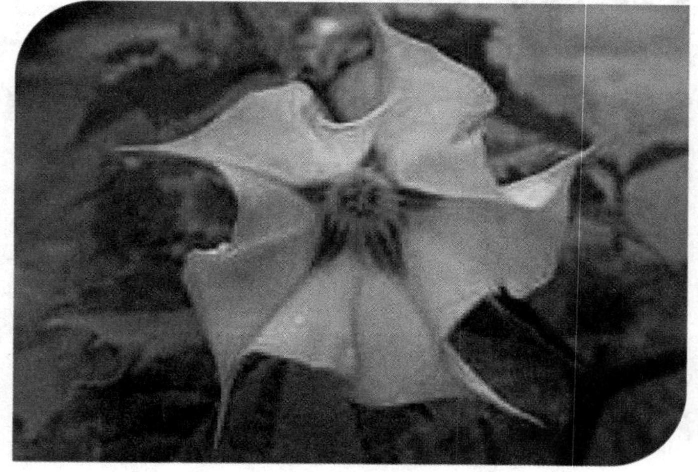

Thorn Apple is a member of the Solanaceae (Nightshade) Family and must be used with care. Like other family members, it can be highly beneficial for medicinal purposes when used carefully in very small doses, and it can be deadly when used improperly.

It is also called jimsonweed, moon flower, and devil's snare. It grows wild across the warmer parts of the United States. It is often found in farm yards and along roadsides.

Identification: These 2 to 5-foot-tall annual bushes are foul-smelling, freely branching, and erect. The plant grows from a long, thick, and fibrous root. Stems are stout, leafy, smooth, and pale yellow-green. They form many forks and branches, with a leaf and flower at each fork. Leaves are 3 to 8 inches (7.5 cm to 20 cm) long, soft, irregularly undulated and toothed. The surface is smooth, with a darker green upper surface and a light green underside.

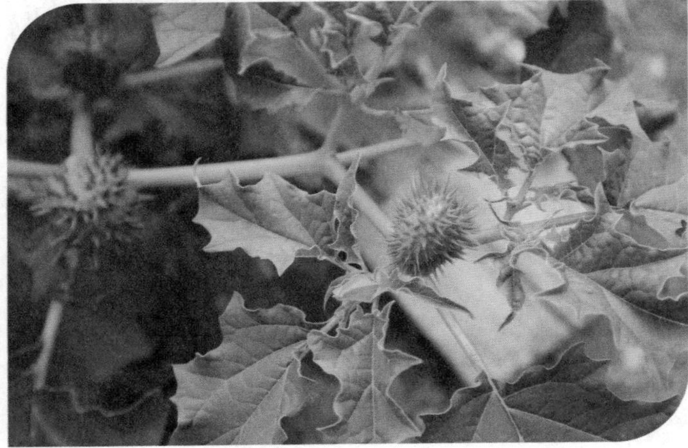

White, creamy, or violet trumpet-shaped flowers appear throughout the summer. Flowers are approximately 2 to 4 inches (5 cm to 10 cm) long on short stems growing from the branch forks or the leaf axils. The calyx is swollen at the base, long and tubular and surrounded with five sharp teeth. The corolla is only partially open and has prominent ribs. The flowers open at night.

Seeds are egg-shaped capsules, approximately 1 to 3 inches (2.5 cm to 7.5 cm) in diameter and either bald or covered with spines. When mature, it splits into four chambers, each containing many small black seeds.

Medicinal Use: The leaves and seeds are used in medicine. Traditionally the leaves are smoked. Today, some people use a Thorn Apple Seed Salve for external use and have discontinued using the herb as a smoke or extract because of its toxic effects. It is similar to Belladonna (deadly nightshade) in its constituents.

Asthma: Thorn apple leaves have long been smoked in cigarette or pipe form, mixed with tobacco, for the treatment of asthma.

I do not recommend this method since over-consumption causes delirium and hallucinations and even death. Mullein is a much better choice.

Burns, Wounds, Boils, and Skin Inflammations: A salve made with thorn apple seeds reduces inflammations in burns and other skin wounds and inflammations. The seeds have pain-relieving and narcotic properties.

Whooping Cough and Other Coughs: The narcotic and anti-spasmatic properties of thorn apple seeds are potent and useful in severe cases of whooping cough and muscle spasms.

Muscle Spasms and Parkinson's Disease: The tremors of Parkinson's disease and other muscle spasms respond to the anti-spasmatic properties of the seed extract. Start with the minimum dose and increase it only if necessary.

Warning: The plant contains dangerous levels of toxins and has a significant risk of overdose when used without medical supervision. Toxicity can also vary from plant to plant and with the maturity of the plant, so a safe dose one year might be toxic the next year as the plant matures. Use thorn apple only under the supervision of a highly skilled medical professional.

Recipes. Thorn Apple Seed Extract: 1/4 teaspoon thorn apple seeds, 1/4 cup 80 proof alcohol. Mix the alcohol and crushed seeds together in a small bottle and cover tightly. Allow the mixture to steep for 2 to 4 weeks. Strain out the seeds and store the extract in a cool, dark place for up to 3 years. Keep out of reach of children and mark it clearly as a poison.

Dosing: It is impossible to accurately recommend a dosage since the strength of seeds from each individual plant varies. Start with 1 drop and increase the dosage only as needed to get the desired effects. Watch carefully for symptoms of toxicity. Use only under medical supervision.

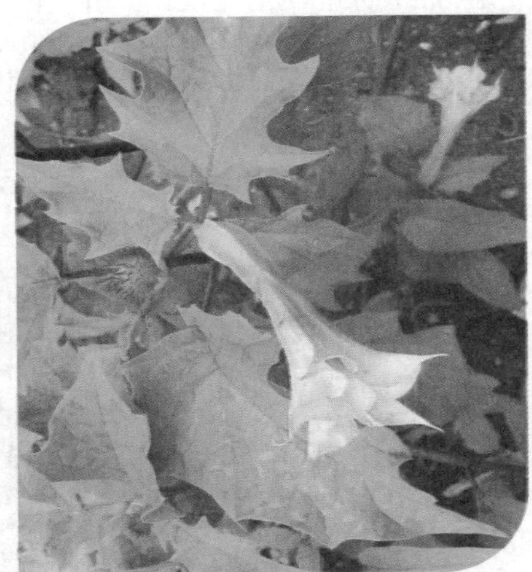

Thorn Apple, Skäpperöd, CC by SA 3.0

Thorn Apple Oil or Salve (For external use only): You will need 1/4 teaspoon thorn apple seeds, 1/2 cup coconut oil or olive oil (coconut oil is preferred if you want a solid salve). Place the coconut oil and crushed thorn apple seeds together in a small glass jar. Place the jar and its contents into a pot of barely simmering water. Keep the water level so that the jar stands upright and does not float. Maintain a very low simmer for 2 hours. Turn off the heat and allow the oil to cool. Strain the seeds out of the oil and discard them. Use the cooled oil as a rub or salve on painful joints.

Thyme, *Thymus vulgaris*

Thymus vulgaris is the same evergreen herb that we use for cooking. It is a member of the Lamiaceae (Mint) Family. This fragrant plant grows in hot, sunny locations.

Identification: Thyme is a perennial shrub with square stems growing from a thin woody base. It grows 6 to 12 inches (15 cm to 30 cm) tall. The leaves are small, light-green, and slightly curved. Small purple or white flowers appear in the summer.

Edible Use: I use it as a cooking herb for its intense flavor and as an herbal tea.

Medicinal Use: The Romans used thyme to purify their rooms and to flavor cheese and liqueurs. It has been placed under pillows to aid sleep and prevent nightmares. Thyme is an antiseptic, anti-viral, anti-parasitic, and anti-fungal. I prefer to use fresh thyme whenever possible. However, I also dry thyme sprigs for future use.

Sore Throat, Coughs, and Bronchitis: The anti-bacterial components of thyme are valuable in combatting bronchitis and coughs. Infuse the whole herb in water and use it for gargling and as a weak thyme tea.

Mouthwash, Dental Cavities and Gum Disease: Weak thyme tea is a valuable mouthwash. It has

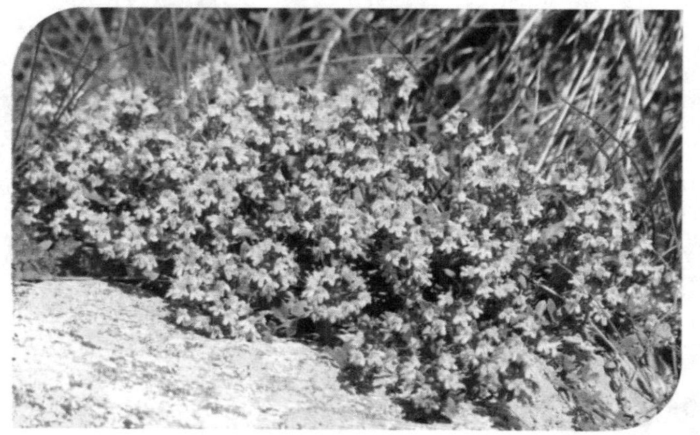

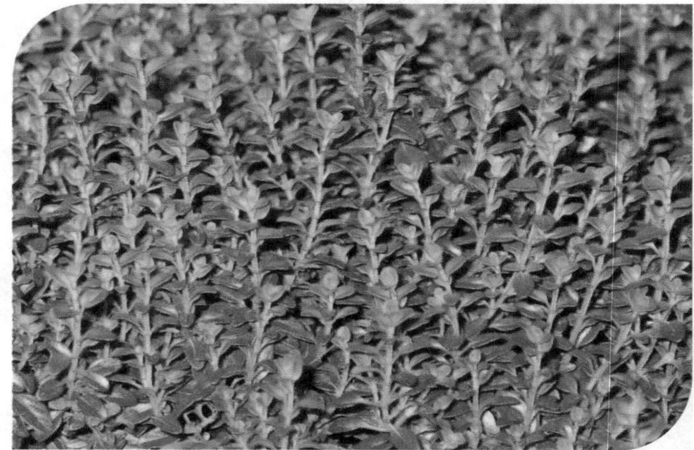

antiseptic properties, which help prevent cavities and treat gingivitis.

Acne: Try Thyme Tincture for treating acne. Dab a drop of thyme tincture onto blemishes once or twice daily. It dries up acne and kills the bacteria that cause them.

Boosts the Immune System: The many vitamins, minerals, and antioxidants in thyme give the immune system a boost. Also, thyme encourages white blood cell formation and increases the body's resistance to bacteria and viruses. Thyme based formulas, Thyme Tea, and Thyme essential oil are all good formulas for boosting the immune system.

Digestive Upsets and Worms: Thyme is effective against digestive problems caused by bacteria and viruses, including stomach flus and diarrhea. It is also used for intestinal problems, including worms.

Seizures and Antispasmodic: Thyme has antispasmodic properties and prevents and treats epileptic seizures in some people. Oil of Thyme or Thyme Tincture are the best products to use for this purpose.

Lice, Scabies, and Crabs: The anti-parasitic properties of thyme oil make it a good treatment for lice, scabies, and crabs. Add a few drops of Oil of Thyme to olive oil or coconut oil and coat the affected area. Cover the coated areas and leave on for 1 hour, then wash away. Follow up with nit removal and repeat as needed.

Skin Inflammations: Try a Thyme Leaf Poultice for skin inflammations and sores. Mash the leaves into a paste, place it on the skin over the affected areas and cover it with a clean cloth.

Warts: Mix one drop of Essential Oil of Thyme with a tablespoon of olive oil or coconut oil, or mix it full strength into a pre-made salve. Place on warts daily until the wart is gone.

Harvesting: Harvest thyme leaves often during the summer. Frequent trimming keeps the bushes from becoming woody and increases yield. Use fresh leaves whenever possible and freeze or dry leaves for future use.

Warning: Thyme is safe for use in adults and children. The essential oil is very strong and sometimes causes skin irritations if used full strength. Always dilute the essential oil in a carrier oil before use.

Valerian Root, *Valeriana officinalis*

Valerian is in the Caprifoliaceae (Honeysuckle) Family. There are many species of Valerian, most medicinal, but this is the species most commonly used medicinally. I grow it in my garden and it is my go-to occasional herbal sleep aid. It is also called garden heliotrope and nature's Valium.

Identification: Valerian usually grows from 1 to 5 feet (0.3m to 1.5m) tall depending on the location and the soil conditions. It has a straight round stem that is topped by an umbrella-like flowerhead.

Its opposite dark green leaves have a pinnate blade with 6 to 11 pairs of terminal leaflets. These leaflets have prickly margins and are hairy underneath.

Valerian flowers are in branched batches and each flower is about 1/5 inch long. They are tiny white to pink blossoms. The flower has three stamens and a distinctive scent.

Edible Use: The seeds are edible when lightly roasted.

Medicinal Use: The root is most commonly used but the leaves may also be used for medicine (though they are less potent than the roots).

Insomnia: I use Valerian as a sleep aid with excellent results. People, including myself, report that they get to sleep faster and can sleep longer without waking. They also report that they awaken refreshed without residual drowsiness. It can become habit forming so only use when needed.

Anxiety and Panic Attacks: Valerian root has a calming effect that is beneficial to people with panic and anxiety disorders.

Depression and Obsessive-Compulsive Behavior: Valerian root improves symptoms of depression and obsessive-compulsive disorder (OCD) when used in small doses. In larger doses, it can have the opposite effect.

Epilepsy: Valerian has a relaxing effect on the muscles of the body. For regular use (to prevent attacks), usual dosage is between 100 mg to 1 gram of dried and powdered root.

Start with a low dose, depending on the person's size and the severity of the disease, and increase it gradually until you find a level that works. It can also be used for acute attacks.

Menstrual Cramps: Because of its analgesic properties and its ability to relax the smooth muscles, this herb makes a good treatment for pain and cramping during menstruation.

Lowers Blood Pressure and Pulse Rate: Valerian relaxes the blood vessels to naturally reduce blood pressure and pulse rate.

Quitting Smoking: Valerian root is calming and helps lessen the effects of nicotine withdrawal.

It especially helps with the irritability people often experience when quitting. Use in tincture form.

Harvesting: Cut the flowering tops off as they appear. This enables a better development of the root. In the first year, many of the young plants do not flower but produce a luxuriant crop of leaves. Harvest the roots in autumn. Dig deeply to get the entire root system, planting some back for future harvests. Slice the roots into small sections and dry for future use.

Warning: In ordinary doses, Valerian exerts a quieting and soothing influence upon the brain and nervous system. However, in large repeated doses it can produce pain in the head, heaviness, and stupor. It can become addictive, only use when needed.

Do not use during pregnancy, as its effects are unknown.

Violets, *Viola* spp. including *Viola sororia* (common violet) and *Viola odorata* (sweet violet)

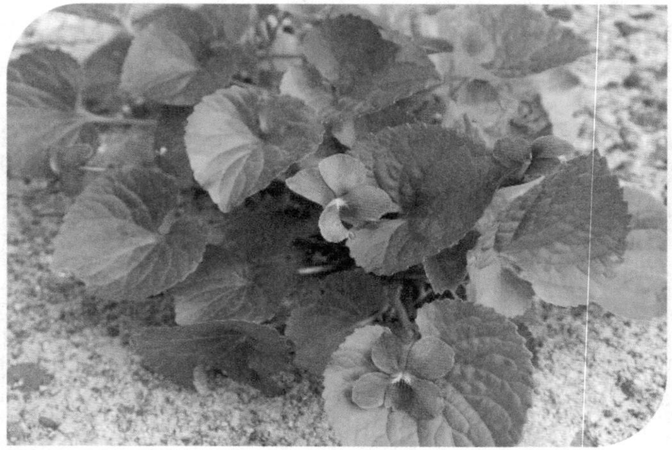

Wild violets are beautiful little plants that are both edible and medicinal. Pansies are also edible. They are in the Violaceae (Violet) Family.

Identification: Wild violets are short plants, usually only 4 to 6 inches (10 cm to 15 cm) high. They grow in clumps with purple, blue, yellow, or white flowers growing on a leafless stalk. Each flower has 5 parts of unequal size. The flowers bloom from early spring into the early summer. Heart-shaped basal leaves grow from its underground root. The leaf margin is toothed but rounded.

These low-growing, perennial plants prefer shady areas, but can grow in sunny locations. The native wildflower favors woods, thickets, and stream banks.

Edible Use: Both the flowers and leaves are edible. Younger leaves and flowers are tender for fresh eating. Older leaves need to be cooked in soups or stews to tenderize them and relieve some of their bitterness. The leaves have a mucilaginous texture that can thicken liquids. Use sweet violets in sweet dishes. The roots and seeds are not eaten and may cause nausea and vomiting.

Freshly picked flowers are beautiful as a garnish in salads, on cakes or pastries, or other foods. Flowers and leaves are rich in vitamins A and C, as well as antioxidants and phytochemicals.

Medicinal Use: Wild violets are an excellent tonic for helping the body detoxify. They strengthen the immune system and stimulate the lymphatic system. They help the body eliminate waste and toxins in the body. Violets are cooling, moistening and relieve pain. They work as a blood cleanser and are safe for elders and children. I use the flowers and leaves internally as a tea or tincture and externally for skin conditions.

Sore Throats, Colds, Sinus Infections, and Other Respiratory Conditions: Wild violets strengthen the immune system and reduce inflammation in the respiratory system. Its mucilaginous properties are useful in soothing the bronchial passages and works as an expectorant to remove mucous from the body. The herb is useful to treat sore throats, colds, sinus infections and other respiratory and bronchial conditions. I like to use Wild Violet Tea for these conditions, but eating the herb is also effective.

Whooping Cough and Dry Hacking Cough: Wild violet has been used for centuries as a bronchial remedy for dry coughs and other bronchial conditions. As a tonic for the lymphatic system and immune system, it helps relieve the underlying problems causing these conditions. Try Wild Violet Tea for coughs.

Anti-inflammatory, Arthritis, and Joint Pain: Wild violets are anti-inflammatory and contain a variety of phytochemicals that are antioxidants and free radical scavengers. Violets can be eaten or taken in tea as an effective anti-inflammatory. The anti-inflammatory effects of wild violet flowers are useful in treating joint pains of all kinds, including the neck and back.

Pound the leaves and flowers to a paste made with a little water, then apply the paste to the skin directly above the painful area. You can cover the poultice with cloth to hold it in place. Use wild violet internally as well as externally for joint pains.

Minor Scrapes and Bruises: Wild violets have antiseptic properties and analgesic properties that relieve the pain while preventing or treating infections and helping the area heal quickly. Use the tea as a wash for areas of skin or apply the flowers as a poultice.

Mild Laxative: Violets have a mild laxative effect and are deemed safe for children.

Lowering Cholesterol and Blood Thinning: The mucilage in violet leaves is helpful in lowering cholesterol levels and in balancing the intestinal flora. The leaves are also high in vitamins A, C, and rutin. Rutin is an antioxidant and anti-inflammatory and has blood thinning properties.

For lowering cholesterol and use as a blood thinner, try eating the leaves, taking leaf powder in capsule form, or using a tea or tincture.

Hemorrhoids and Varicose Veins: The rutin contained in violet leaves is helpful in reducing the inflammation that causes hemorrhoids and varicose veins.

Its mild laxative effect helps prevent straining. You can use a poultice directly on the hemorrhoids or veins or you can apply a salve or infused violet oil.

Skin Conditions, Abrasions, Dermatitis, Insect Bites, Eczema: As an anti-inflammatory and a cooling and soothing herb, wild violet is useful for treating minor skin problems including eczema and other rashes, insect bites and abrasions. Use Wild Violet Tea as a wash on the skin or make a salve or infused oil with the herb for skin use.

Harvesting: I begin harvesting wild violets in April, May, and June when the flowers are freshly opening. The exact time depends on the weather. Once they begin to open, I go back daily to pick what I need.

Gather the petals in the morning while the blooms are fresh. They tend to wilt in the afternoon or in heat. Dry some flowers for use year-round.

Be careful where you gather. Roadsides and parks are often sprayed with pesticides. Look for flowers in pristine areas away from industrial areas, waste areas, and roadsides. Also remember, African Violets are not wild violets and cannot be used.

Warning: Some people get a skin rash on contact with the wild violet leaf. There is no known internal toxicity, but allergies are always possible. Large doses of the roots or seeds can cause severe stomach upset, vomiting, high blood pressure and breathing problems.

Be sure about your identification (if it is in bloom identification is much easier) as there are poisonous look-alikes.

Recipes. Wild Violet Tea: *You can make this tea with all flowers, if you have enough, but 1-part flower to 2 parts leaves works as well. An all-flower recipe makes a milder tasting tea. Ingredients: 2 teaspoons of dried wild violet leaves (or flowers, if desired), 1 teaspoon of dried flowers, 1 cup boiling water, raw honey, optional. Pour the boiling water over the flowers and leaves and allow it to steep for about 5 minutes. Strain the tea and drink. Sweeten with honey, if desired.

NOTE: Do not sweeten the tea if you are using it as a wash on injured skin or for other external use.

White Mustard, *Sinapis alba*

White mustard belongs to the Brassicaceae (Mustard) family. It is mostly grown for its seeds or as fodder crop and is widespread. White mustard seeds are yellow in color and are also called yellow mustard. Brown and black mustards are different but also have medicinal uses.

Identification: White mustard is an annual herb, growing from 1 to 2 feet (0.3m to 0.6m) tall. It flowers from July to September. The white mustard flower has a yellow corolla, just over 1/2 inch (1.25 cm) in diameter with four petals that are 1/4 to 1/2 inch (0.75 cm to 1.25 cm) long. It contains four spreading sepals and six stamens (4 long and two short). The alternate leaves are stalked with a coarsely hairy leaflet. Its stems are branched and also hairy. Each leaf is irregularly pinnately lobed, with irregular sawtooth edges. The terminal leaflets are large and clearly lobed. The fruit of white mustard has many tiny round pale-yellow seeds.

Edible Use: The seeds, flowers, leaves and extracted oil are edible. I like to eat the young leaves in salads, and I sometimes cook the older leaves as a vegetable or potherb. The seeds make a spicy condiment or flavoring when finely ground.

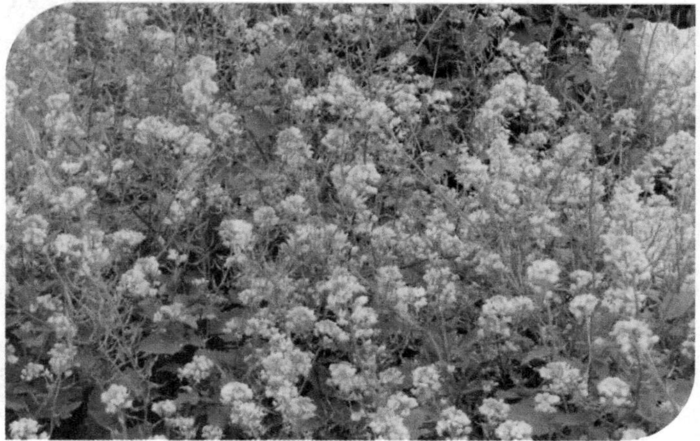

SuperJew, own work, White Mustard near Abu Ghosh.CC 3.0

Medicinal Use: White mustard is antibacterial and antifungal, digestive, diuretic, emetic, expectorant, rubefacient, and stimulant. It is used internally and externally.

Pneumonia, Bronchitis, Respiratory Diseases: The seeds of white mustard, powdered and made into a poultice, are good for treating respiratory diseases. They act as an irritant to loosen phlegm and help expel mucus from the body. The poultice is applied to the chest and left in place until the skin reddens, then promptly removed. The mustard is an irritant and can cause blistering if left in place too long.

Poison Ingestion: Ground mustard seed, taken by mouth in quantity, can cause vomiting. You can use it to bring up poisons and other undesirable substances that have been ingested.

Preventing Infection: To prevent infection in a wound, or anywhere in the body, white mustard is a good ally. It has abundant sulfur compounds, which help prevent infection and fight any invading infection. Often used in combination with garlic. For best effects, use fresh mustard seeds, ground into a paste. When using dried mustard seeds, soak them in water before grinding them.

Prevents Cancer: Mustard seeds contain beneficial substances that reduce the risk and the reoccurrence of cancer. It does not cure cancer, but seems to prevent the spread or the return of it. One tablespoon of crushed or ground white mustard seed daily is enough to provide these powerful benefits.

Arthritis: White mustard applied to the skin is an irritant. The skin irritation brings an increased blood supply to the area. The skin and joints are warmed, and pain is reduced. You must be careful to wash the mustard away once the skin reddens to prevent blisters and other damage to the skin.

To treat arthritis and other joint pain, mix ground white mustard seeds with enough vinegar to make a paste. Apply to the skin over the affected area. White mustard seed powder (1 tablespoon) added to the bath water is also beneficial for arthritic pain.

Sore Throats: Mustard Seed Tea made from the leaves of the white mustard plant has a beneficial effect on sore throats. The increased blood circulation and sulfur content help the throat to heal. Gargle Mustard Seed Tea several times daily, beginning at the first sign of throat irritation. Its action is similar to that of a cayenne gargle.

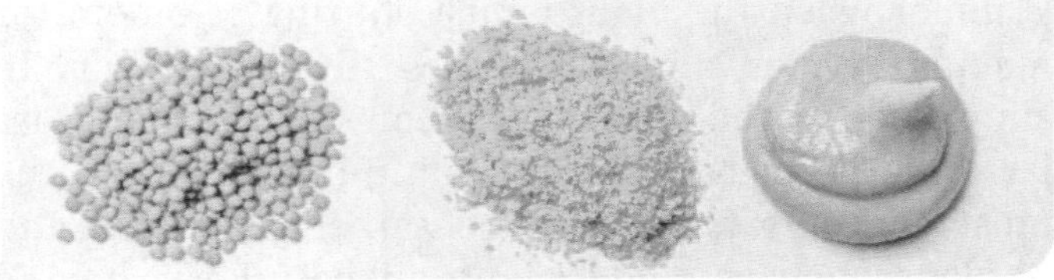

Chilblains (Chill Burns): Chilblains benefit from the warming power of white mustard. Mix one-part white mustard seed powder and four parts ground flax seeds together to make a paste. Use this mixture as a poultice to get rid of chilblains.

Recipes: Mustard Seed Tea. You need 1 teaspoon crushed mustard seeds and 1 cup boiling water. Pour the water over the mustard seeds and let it steep covered for 2 to 4 minutes.

Yellow Mustard Poultice. You'll need: one tablespoon ground white mustard seeds, 1/2 cup flour, 1 egg white, 8 ounces (250ml) of hot water. Mix the mustard and flour together, then add the egg white and water to form a loose paste. Apply immediately to the body over the affected area.

Wild Lettuce, *Lactuca canadensis, L. virosa* and *L. serriola*

This member of the Daisy/Aster Family is very widespread. Its sap is well known for pain relief. Most *Lactuca* species of wild lettuce contain these pain-relieving lactones in their milky latex. It is also known as prickly lettuce and opium lettuce (although it does not actually contain opium).

Identification: Wild lettuce grows to be 3 to 5 feet (0.9m to 1.5m) tall, usually on a single stem, and has a milky sap throughout the root, leaves, and stems. The central stem is light-green to reddish-green, occasionally with purple streaks. Its green alternating leaves sometimes have purple edges or a yellowish color.

The lance-shaped leaves can grow up to 3 inches (7.5 cm) across and 10 inches (25 cm) long. Leaves are usually, but not always, lobed and look similar to a dandelion leaf. Some species have spines/prickly hairs along the midrib on the underside of the leaf and some have teeth on their leaf margins that are very prickly.

The white milky sap turns tan after exposure to air. This is an important diagnostic feature. Wild lettuce blooms in the late summer to early autumn. Its flowers are small and are similar to dandelions with yellow or slightly reddish - orange petals. Flower heads are much smaller than those of dandelion - about 1/3 inch (0.8 cm) across with 12 to 25 rays – and they are well above the leaves on a tall stem, unlike dandelion, whose flowers are low to the ground. After 3 to 4 weeks, the flowers are replaced with dark brown, dry fruits with white hairs. The taproot is thick and deep.

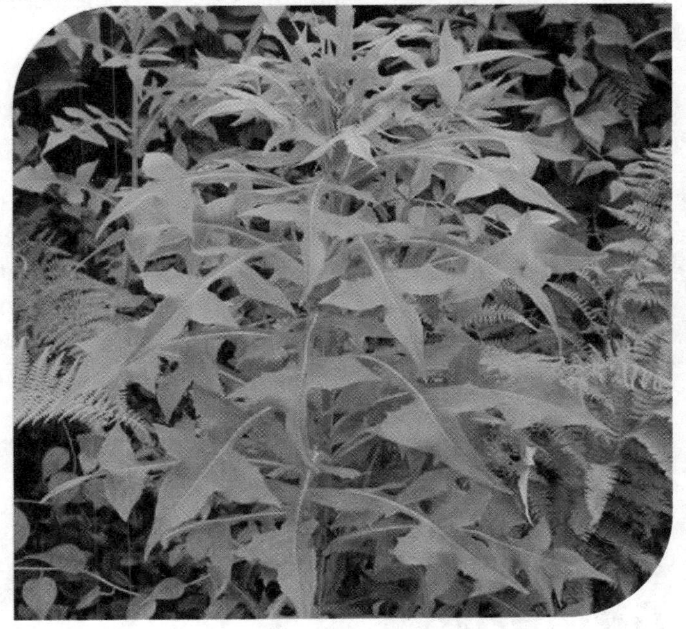

Photo:http://extension.umass.edu/landscape/weeds/lactuca-canadensis

Edible Use: This slightly bitter lettuce is good to eat when the leaves are cooked like spinach. Boiling removes some of its bitterness. It can be eaten raw, but is usually too bitter for most people's tastes.

Medicinal Use: The white latex sap that runs through the plant contains sesquiterpene lactones,

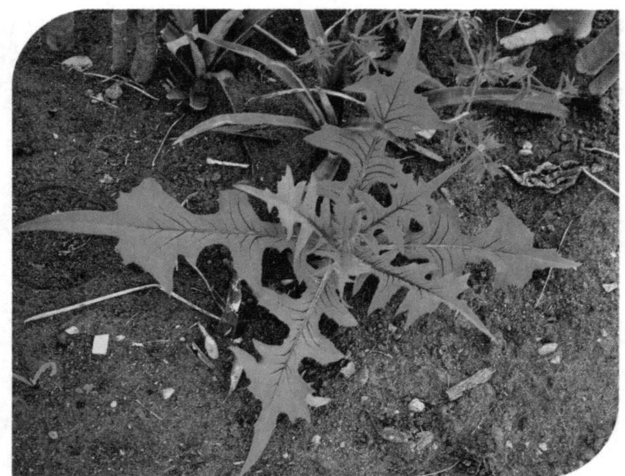

which are its primary medicinal components, similar to Chicory (also in this book). Older plants have higher concentrations of sap, especially while the plant is just beginning to bloom. Best to use the sap after it dries or use a tincture form to make full use of its medicinal compounds.

Insomnia and Sedative: The sedative properties of wild lettuce come from the milky sap that runs through the stems and leaves. It calms restlessness and anxiety and induces sleep without being addictive.

Pain Relief and Shock: Wild lettuce has also been called opium lettuce because of its weak opium-like effects. Used in small doses, it has a sedative and pain-relieving effect without causing the stomach upset and high of a true opium. It is also helpful in the treatment of shock, menstrual pain, muscular pain, joints pain, and colic.

Warts: Apply the white sap to the skin as a treatment for external warts. Cover the wart with sap once or twice a day until the wart is gone.

Warning: Use with caution as it has a sedative effect. Do not overdose.

Harvesting: Collect the leaves and stems in the summer when the plant is just starting to bloom for maximum medicinal properties. Even better is to simply collect the milky sap directly into a small glass jar. This is more time-consuming but gives you the most concentrated dose. The sap turns brown and hardens when dry. Older plants are best. Leave behind enough of the plant so that it will recover.

Recipes. Wild Lettuce Tincture: You will need: vodka, brandy or other 80 proof alcohol, fresh or dried wild lettuce leaves. Fill a clean, sterile, glass jar with chopped fresh milky leaves or use 2 ounces (56g) of dried wild lettuce per cup of alcohol. You may also use the sap. Cover the herbs with vodka or other drinkable alcohol. Stir the herbs to remove air bubbles. Move the container to a cool, dark place and allow the tincture to steep for 3 to 4 weeks, shaking daily. Strain out the herbs and discard. Store in a cool, dark place for up to 5 years.

Wild Teasel, *Dipsacus sylvestris/ fullonum*

Also known as Fuller's Teasel, Wild Teasel, or Common Teasel, this plant grows throughout most of the United States and coastal Canada. It is listed as a noxious weed in many states, but it has many good uses. Teasel grows in large patches, crowding out other plants once established. In the fall, it attracts large flocks of birds, who use the seeds as a winter food source. It likes to grow along stream banks, roadsides, pastureland, prairies, meadows, savannas, and woodland borders. It is a water loving plant that grows in a variety of soils including sandy soils in moist areas and heavy clay in poorly drained areas. It is in the Caprifoliaceae, the honeysuckle family.

Identification: Teasel is a biennial herbaceous plant. It has lance shaped leaves and grows from 3 to 8 feet in height. The first-year leaves form a rosette at the base of the stem with the flower stem emerging from the center in the second year. Each leaf is 8 to 16 inches (20 cm-40 cm) long and 1 to 2.5 inches (2.5 cm to 6 cm) across. The underside of the leaf has a row of spines along the midrib and the stems are also covered in small spines. The plant has a two-year

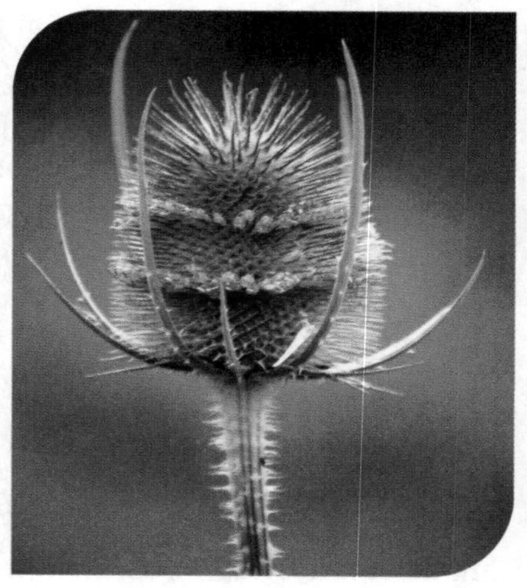

lifecycle, growing leaves and stems in the first year and producing flowers in the second year. It has erect hollow pale green to reddish-green stems. Its stems are hairless with longitudinal ridges and white spines.

Teasel flowers June through August. It has a cylindrical inflorescence of dark pink, purple, or lavender flowers on the top of the flower stem. The inflorescence is ovoid or conical, up to 4 inches long (10cm) and 2 inches (5cm) across. When the flowers drop, the flower cylinder dries into spiny hard bracts with small seeds maturing mid-autumn.

The plant has a deep taproot with fibrous secondary roots that can grow up to 2 feet long (0.6m) and up to an inch (2.5cm) in diameter.

Edible Use: The young leaves are edible, but the short hairs make them unappetizing. They can be eaten cooked or raw. The roots are used medicinally but are not eaten.

Non-Edible Use: A water-soluble blue dye, used as an indigo substitute, is obtained from the plant. When the plant is mixed with alum, a yellow dye is obtained.

The stalks work as a spindle for friction fire, and can be paired with a clematis fireboard.

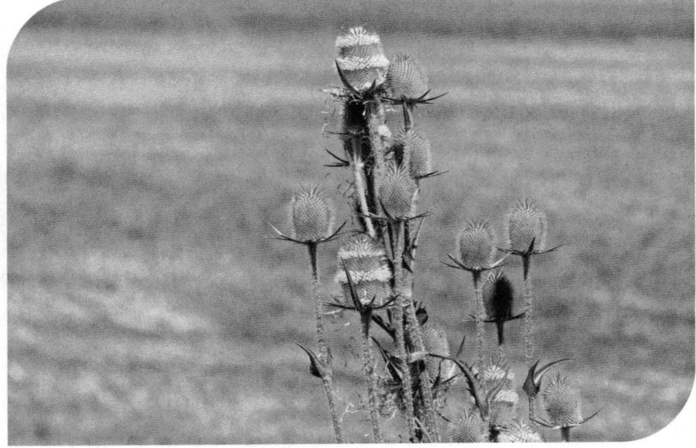

Medicinal Use: Teasel root can be taken internally and externally, but you must be very careful with internal dosing, especially if you have, or suspect you have, Lyme Disease. For Lyme, I prefer to use teasel in a tincture form with a maximum dose of 9 drops split into 3 drops each in the morning, afternoon, and evening. Begin by taking 1 drop in the morning of the first day. On the second day, take one drop in the morning and one in the evening. On the third day, take one drop in the morning, afternoon, and evening. Continue adding one drop each day until you reach the maximum of 9 drops total each day (three in the morning, three in the afternoon, and three in the evening.) Note that you may have a Jarisch-Herxheimer ("herx")" reaction if you have Lyme. A "herx" reaction is an adverse response to the cytokines that are released as the Lyme bacteria are killed. Once the bacterial waste and dead bacteria are expelled this reaction goes away. This does mean that the spirochaetes that cause Lyme are dying, which is good news, but you may feel worse before you feel better.

Personally, I use teasel tincture in larger amounts as a Lyme preventative when I am in an area with Lyme-carrying deer ticks (see "Lyme Prevention" below).

Treats Chronic Lyme Disease: Lyme disease is a bacterial infection of the spirochete Borrelia burgdorferi and is transmitted by infected deer/black-legged (Ixodes spp.) ticks. The spirochaetes drill into human tissue and, in time, seal themselves in by creating a biofilm, which acts as a barrier to antibiotics.

Teasel is not an antibiotic, but it acts to boost the effectiveness of antibiotics, dumping the bacteria back into the blood stream where antibiotics can more easily attack and clear the infection. In most cases, antibiotics given soon after infection work well for Lyme, but in the case of Chronic Lyme Disease, where antibiotics are not working well enough, adding teasel to the cure can make all the difference. It may still take 6 months or longer to clear the infection, but the teasel is thought to draw the spirochaetes out of the tissue, thus exposing them to the antibiotics. Please see suggested dosing instructions above.

Lyme Prevention: I use teasel tincture as a Lyme preventative when I am in an area with Lyme-carrying ticks. I take a dropperful 2x/day if I am in the woods in a known Lyme area. I know many other people who work in the woods who also use teasel in this way. It keeps Borrelia from burrowing into my tissues in case of an infection. If you do get a tick bite save the tick to get it tested for Lyme. If antibiotics are taken early Lyme can be prevented.

Osteoporosis, Osteopenia, and Bone Fractures: Teasel root increases blood circulation so that the body can rebuild and repair tendons and bones. It stimulates new bone growth and helps increase bone mass. It is an effective treatment for both Osteoporosis and Osteopenia and for bone fractures once the bone has been properly set.

Natural Diuretic: Teasel root is excellent at ridding the body of excess water and encouraging urine flow. Teasel rids the body of unnecessary water weight, salt, and toxins.

It helps reduce inflammation and swelling and can be useful in reducing a fever by stimulating sweating.

Candida and Yeast Infections: Teasel root works to purge excess yeast and Candida from the body into the bloodstream where it dies and is eliminated. Teasel is useful in keeping yeast infections and Candida under control.

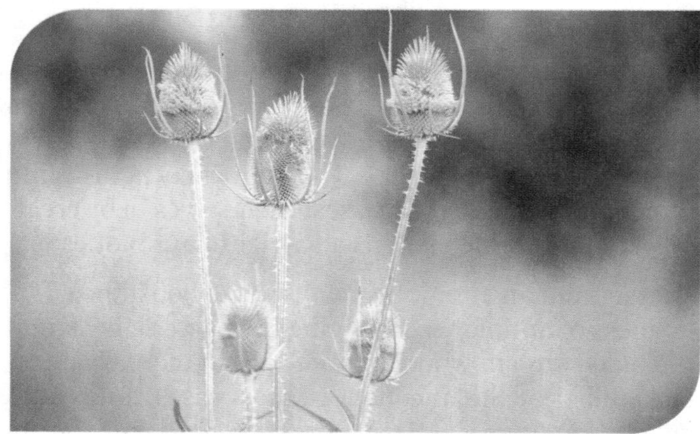

Arthritis: Teasel root is an anti-inflammatory and helps repair damaged joints that cause arthritis. It gives some short-term pain relief, but it takes long-term use for effective arthritis relief.

Jaundice and Liver Problems: Teasel is a liver tonic, and is helpful in treating liver problems of many types, including jaundice.

The diuretic properties of teasel root support the liver and help clear the body of the toxins that cause jaundice. It supports the liver and helps reduce inflammation and infections, but it does not cure the underlying cause.

Wounds and Inflammation – External Application: For skin wounds and inflammation, teasel root powder can be sprinkled directly on the affected site. To use, grind dried teasel root into a fine powder and apply or add water to make a poultice.

Harvesting Teasel: I recommend wearing gloves and protective clothing to protect your skin from the teasel spines. Harvest the roots after the end of the first year's growth between early autumn and early spring. Once they have flower stalks it is too late, as the roots become woody.

Dig up the plant with a spading fork, pushing deeply into the soil next to the plant. The taproot is deep with additional secondary roots. Wiggle the fork to loosen the soil and push it as deep as possible. Grab the plant with a gloved hand and pull the plant up, loosening more with the spading fork as needed.

Take enough teasel root to make a year's supply of tincture at once. Wash them, slice them and cut away the brown parts, tough roots, or soft roots. You want to use the center of the root. Use fresh root to make tincture or place them in the dehydrator to dry for powder or future use. Make sure to cut them before they dry out, as they are very difficult to cut once they are dry.

Warning: Take care in dosing teasel root tincture, starting with one drop only and slowly increasing it as tolerated.

Teasel root can cause a "herx" reaction in some people (see "Lyme" section above). These side effects subside over time.

Fresh Teasel Root Tincture Recipe: Fresh teasel root, sliced and chopped into small pieces, 100 proof vodka or similar proof drinking alcohol, 2 clean jars with tight-fitting lids, Strainer. Use the center of the fresh root for this recipe. Place the chopped root in a clean jar, filling it to within one inch of the top. Cover it with 100 proof alcohol, completely filling the jar to the rim.

Cap it tightly and label /date the jar. Shake the jar weekly. Refill with 100 proof alcohol if needed. Allow the tincture to macerate for 6 to 8 weeks, then strain and move it to a clean jar. Store Teasel Tincture in a cool, dark place for up to 5 years.

Dose Teasel Tincture carefully, starting with 1 drop and increasing by 1 drop daily to a maximum of 9 drops total daily if using for Lyme. Divide the doses into morning, afternoon, and night doses, never giving more than 3 drops per dose.

Wooly Lamb's Ear, *Stachys byzantina*

Wooly Lamb's Ear was used in WWII as a field dressing for wounds on the battlefield. It is easy to cultivate in the garden in full sun. It is also known as wooly wound wort, wooly betony and silver carpet. It is in the Lamiaceae (Mint) Family.

Identification: This perennial plant has soft, fuzzy leaves that are densely covered with silver-white or gray hairs with the texture of velvet. Leaves have a curved shape and are 2 to 4 inches (5 cm to 10 cm) long with a rounded point. The undersides are more silvery-white in color than the tops. Flowering stems grow erect, with square stems, and are usually 1 to 2 feet (0.3 meters to 0.6 meters) tall. The flowering spikes are 4 to 10 inches (10 cm to 15 cm) long with many purple flowers crowded together on the stem. Small leaves appear on the flowering stems as well. The crushed plant has a pleasant scent, mildly like apple or pineapple.

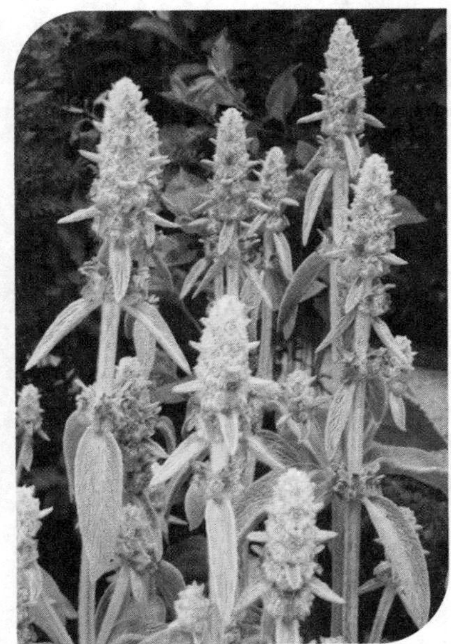

Wolly Lamb's Ear, Jean-Pol ANDMONT, CC by SA 3.0

Edible and Other Use: The leaves are edible and best when young and tender. Eat them fresh in salads or steam them as a green vegetable. Wooly Lamb's Ear is soft and very absorbent, which makes it a good substitute for toilet paper. The highly absorbent properties of the leaves make it useful as a feminine hygiene product too.

Medicinal Use: Lamb's Ear is antibacterial, antiseptic, antispasmodic, and astringent. It is also a diuretic, febrifuge, good for digestion, styptic, tonic, vermifuge, and wound-healing.

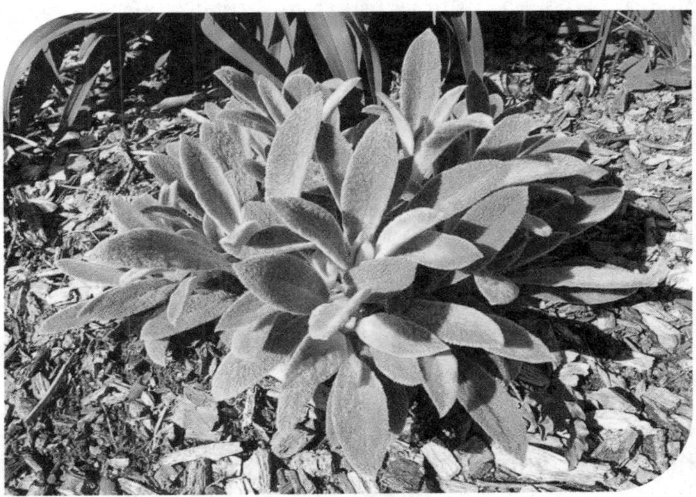

Wound Dressing: The soft, fuzzy leaves of Lamb's Ear make an excellent dressing for wounds of all kinds. They are antibacterial, antiseptic, and anti-inflammatory and are said to combat MRSA. The leaves absorb blood and encourage clotting. Place several whole leaves on the wound and cover it with a soft cloth or gauze. Leave in place until it is time to change the dressing.

Wound Wash, Eye Wash, Conjunctivitis, and Sties: Make a medicinal tea to use as an eyewash. When cool, the tea makes an excellent antibacterial wash for wounds of all kinds. When using it as an eyewash or to treat pinkeye, make the tea with distilled water and bring it to a full boil. Then strain it twice to make sure no fine particles remain.

Diarrhea, Fevers, and Internal Bleeding: Wooly Lamb's Ear works for internal bleeding, for diarrhea, and for reducing fevers. For these purposes, drink Wooly Lamb's Ear Tea (recipe found below).

Sore Mouth and Sore Throat: The same tea, used as a gargle, is effective for treating a sore throat or mouth. Swish the tea around in the mouth or gargle with it several times a day. It relieves the pain and the antibiotic properties help cure the underlying infection.

Liver and Heart Tonic: The healthful benefits of Wooly Lamb's Ear make it a good general tonic, especially for the liver and heart. Take the tea daily or consume the leaves as an herb or vegetable.

Insect Bites and Hemorrhoids: The anti-inflammatory benefits of lamb's ear make it effective in dealing with painful bee stings and insect bites. It also has some analgesic properties, which help with pain.

Recipes. Wooly Lamb's Ear Tea: You will only need fresh leaves of Wooly Lamb's Ear and water. Bruise the fresh leaves by pounding then add them to a pot of simmering water. Simmer the leaves for a 5 to 10 minutes and cool. Strain the liquid through a fine sieve or coffee filter to remove all leaf particles. Drink or use as a wash.

Yarrow, *Achillea millefolium*

I always keep yarrow in my medicine bag, as it has many uses. It is also called nosebleed plant, squirrel's tale, plumajillo, and soldier's woundwort. I recognize it by its feathery leaf shape, texture, and scent. It is in the Aster/Daisy Family. It is found in temperate zones throughout the world.

Identification: Yarrow is an erect plant that grows from a spreading rhizome. The plant has finely divided feathery leaves that grow along the stem. Plants grow 1 to 3 feet (0.3m to 0.9 meters) in full sun to partial shade. Its bipinnate or tripinnate leaves are 2 to 8 inches (5 cm to 20 cm) long, and can be hairy. Leaves are arranged spirally on the stem in groups of 2 to 3. Each leaf is divided into many leaflets, which are further divided into smaller leaflets. The silvery-green leaves are fern-like and feathery.

Flowers bloom from May to July. Each inflorescence is a cluster of 15 to 40 tiny disk flowers surrounded by 3 to 8 ray flowers. The scent of yarrow is similar to chrysanthemums, and the flowers are very long lasting. Colors range from white to yellow, pink, and red. Yarrow is a good companion plant in a garden, as it repels many garden pests while attracting beneficial insects.

Edible Use: You can eat the leaves raw or cooked. They are bitter and are best eaten young. The plant is very nutritious; however, I don't recommend eating a lot of it because of its blood clotting ability.

The flowers and leaves are used to make tea, but the leaf tea is bitter. A little raw honey helps.

Medicinal Use: All parts of the plant are used medicinally.

Stopping Internal & External Bleeding: Yarrow quickly stops bleeding by contracting the blood vessels and encouraging clotting. Yarrow contains anti-inflammatory and antibacterial compounds that ease swelling and promote healing. It also helps disinfect wounds. If it is possible, clean the wound before applying yarrow. Yarrow will quickly stop bleeding and bind any dirt or infectious materials into the wound, so best to clean first if possible.

To use yarrow leaves on a wound or abscess, chop or rip the leaves finely and apply to the wound. I often carry dried powdered yarrow with me for this purpose. Cover the wound with a soft cloth and leave it in place. Repeat 2 to 3 times daily until the wound is healed over and the swelling is gone. Yarrow oil or tincture can be used to treat nosebleeds and other minor injuries, as can yarrow powder. Place a few drops of oil or tincture on the affected area or apply it to a tissue or cloth and place it on the wound.

Bruises, Sprains, Swelling, and Hemorrhoids: For bruises, sprains, hemorrhoids, and other swellings, use a poultice of yarrow leaves or stems pounded into a paste and applied to the injured area and cover. Infused yarrow oil or salve works well for bruises, sprains, swelling, and hemorrhoids.

Antibacterial and Antifungal: Yarrow is a strong antibacterial and antifungal. It will heal a wound quickly. Do not use on deep puncture wounds as it will heal it too quickly and you want the wound to heal from the inside out. It is a great addition to a first aid salve. It is also a strong antifungal.

Fevers, Colds, and Measles: Yarrow reduces the duration of the measles virus, colds, and fevers. It is quick to bring down a fever. Either chew raw yarrow or drink yarrow tea to induce sweating and reduce fevers.

An easier (and more palatable) method is to take yarrow in tincture form. It opens the pores, encouraging perspiration, and purifies and moves the blood.

Menstrual Problems: Yarrow tea or tincture treats menstrual problems ranging from a lack of menstruation to excessive bleeding and cramping. It tones the uterine muscles after childbirth, reduces cramping by relaxing the smooth muscles, and prevents hemorrhage. It also helps to bring on menses.

Dental Pain: To reduce inflammation and relieve dental pain, chew on a piece of fresh yarrow root or yarrow leaves. In addition to its anti-inflammatory and anti-infection benefits, yarrow contains salicylic acid, a pain reliever that acts quickly.

Mastitis: As an antibacterial and an anti-inflammatory yarrow works well for mastitis. A leaf poultice seems to work the best while alternating between warm and cold compresses (cabbage leaves also work well for mastitis).

Anxiety and Relaxation without Sedation: Yarrow seems to reduce anxiety without sedative effects. It has a calming effect on the central nervous system.

Harvesting: Yarrow is best when young, picked in the spring or early summer before the flowers have been pollinated. Dry the leaves, stems, and flowers for later use. Once the herb is dry, store it in a capped jar in a cool, dark, and dry location.

Warning: Do not eat yarrow or take yarrow tea during pregnancy. Some people are allergic to yarrow. Do not use it if you are allergic to plants in the Aster/Daisy family, if you develop a rash, or if any irritation occurs. Do not use before surgery.

Recipes. Yarrow Tea: One teaspoon dried yarrow flowers and/or leaves, one cup boiling water, sweetener, if desired. Pour one cup of boiling water over one teaspoon of dried yarrow flowers or leaves. Cover and allow the tea to steep for 5 minutes. Sweeten with raw honey or maple syrup.

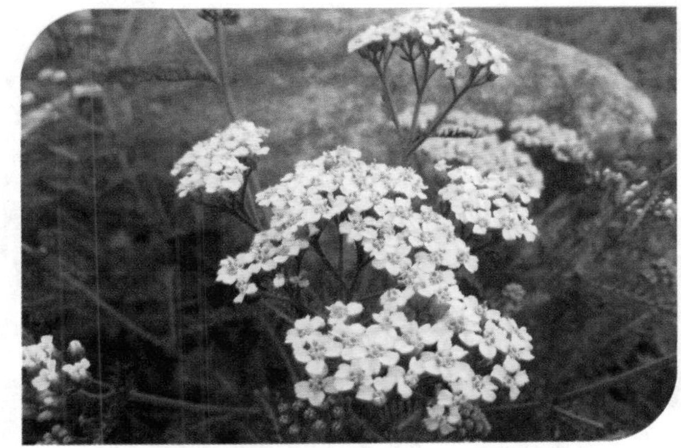

Yarrow Tincture: Ingredients: fresh yarrow leaves and flowers, vodka, brandy, or other alcohol, 80 proof or higher. Chop yarrow into small pieces and pack it tightly to fill a glass jar. Fill the jar with alcohol and cover it tightly. Check the jar every few days and add more alcohol as needed to keep the jar full. Allow the tincture to steep for 6 to 8 weeks. Strain the alcohol through a few layers of cheesecloth and squeeze out all the liquid. Discard the herbs, label the jar and store your tincture in a cool, dark place.

Yarrow Oil: Fresh or dried yarrow leaves, organic olive oil or another carrier oil. If using fresh yarrow, cut the leaves into one-inch (2.5 cm) pieces and allow them to dry. Place the herbs into a jar or heatproof container and add oil just to cover the herbs. Fill a small pot about 1/3 full of water and bring to a boil. Turn the heat down to a simmer before using. Place the jar of oil and herbs into the water, preventing the water from getting into the oil container. Use the water like a double-boiler to gently heat the herbs and oil for 2 to 3 hours. Do not overheat! Allow the oil to cool, then filter it through a couple of layers of cheesecloth. Squeeze the cheesecloth to get all the oil. Discard the herb and use the oil for medicinal purposes.

Yarrow Salve: Ingredients: ½ cup (4 oz or 125ml)) Infused Yarrow Oil, 1-ounce Beeswax. Using a double boiler, mix the beeswax and the infused oil until the beeswax has melted. Check the consistency by dipping a spoon in and putting it in the fridge to harden. If it is not hard enough, add more beeswax. If too hard add more oil. Pour into your jar or tins and let harden. Label and date.

Forest, Scrublands, and Woodlands

Amaranthus caudatus

Amaranthus caudatus is a brilliantly beautiful plant. Its tails of bright red flowers make it easy to locate, even at a distance. It is also called loves-lies-bleeding, tassel flower, velvet flower, foxtail amaranth, pendant amaranth, and quilete. It is in the Amaranthaceae (Amaranth) Family. *Amaranthus caudatus* is widespread throughout North America. It often grows in disturbed ground.

Identification: *Amaranthus caudatus* is an annual flowering plant. It grows from 3 to 8 feet (0.9m to 2.4m) tall in full sun with a spread of 1 to 3 feet (0.3m to 0.9m). It blooms from July until the first frost. The red flowers are very small and have no petals. They bloom in drooping terminal tassel-like panicles that are 1 to 2 feet (0.3m to 0.6m) long. The seeds ripen in September.

Edible Use: The leaves and seeds of *Amaranthus caudatus* are edible. Amaranth leaves can be eaten raw or cooked. The seeds are used as a grain. They do not need to be cooked, but are good toasted in a little oil. The seeds are also good when sprouted.

Medicinal Use: The plant is astringent, anti-parasitic, and diuretic.

Diabetes: People with diabetes can substitute Amaranthus for rice and also eat the seeds and leaves as often as possible. It has anti-diabetic properties that help regulate blood sugar and brings it down significantly.

Lowers Cholesterol: Amaranthus seeds and oil are a healthy choice for those with hypertension, cardiovascular disease, and high cholesterol.

Sore Throats, Mouth Sores, and Canker Sores: A gargle made from dried and powdered Amaranthus leaves is an effective treatment for sore throats and canker sores. To make a gargle, boil 2 tablespoons of powdered amaranth leaves in 1 cup of water for 10 minutes. Let it cool and gargle and swish with it three or more times a day.

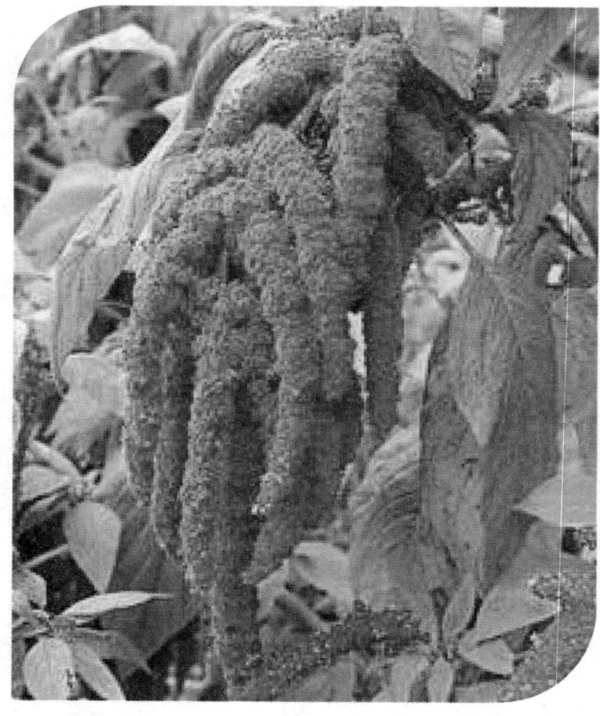

Amaranthus caudatus, Tubifex, CC by SA 3.0

Heavy Menstrual Bleeding and Stopping Bleeding: *Amaranthus caudatus* is a powerful blood clotting agent and works to stop excess menstrual bleeding. Boil 1 tablespoon of root powder in 1 cup of water. Let it cool, then consume. For external bleeding, dust the affected area with the root powder. It quickly stops nosebleeds and bleeding from other small wounds.

Vaginal Infections: Use an Amaranthus leaf and root powder decoction internally, and use externally as a douche to treat vaginal discharge.

Warning: *Amaranthus caudatus* should not be used by people who have gout, rheumatoid arthritis, or kidney disorders. It should not be given to pregnant women, nursing mothers, or babies.

American Ginseng, *Panax quinquefolius*

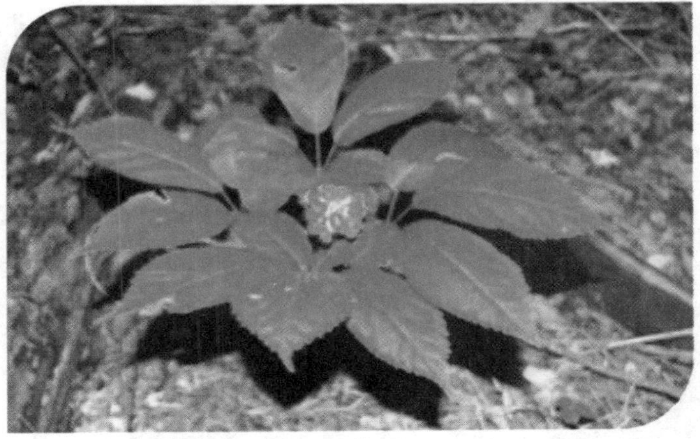

Photo by John Carl Jacobs, CC by SA 4.0

American ginseng, also known as *Panax ginseng*, is in the Araliaceae (Ginseng/Ivy) Family. It is native to eastern North America and cultivated widely elsewhere. Its aromatic root forks as it matures.

Identification: Plants grow 6 to 18 inches (15 cm to 45 cm) tall. Its leaves are palmate and divided into 3 to 7 (usually 4 or 5) lance-shaped, sharp-toothed leaflets. The flowers are whitish-greenish, and fruits are pea-sized red berries with two seeds each.

The neck of the rhizome shows scars left by each year's growth. Counting the leaf scars ages the root. Its medicinal compounds, called ginsenosides, increase in concentration as the root ages. In general, harvest roots 4 years or older.

Medicinal Use: *Panax* species have a well-deserved reputation as powerful adaptogens. They help the body recover from the effects of stress and adrenal fatigue, much like Reishi or Ashwagandha. It is also used as an aphrodisiac and for erectile disfunction. American ginseng is a relaxant, while the Asian version, *P. ginseng*, is said to be more stimulating. The mature root and leaves can be chewed, powdered and put into capsules, extracted in alcohol as a tincture, or made into a tea.

Diabetes: Ginseng has many benefits for diabetics. American ginseng helps regulate blood sugar. Taking take 2 to 5 drops of American Ginseng tincture before each meal helps prevent post-meal spikes in blood sugar levels. It is recommended starting with 2 drops and monitoring blood sugar levels. Increase the dosage one drop at a time, as needed, up to 5 drops per meal, depending on the potency of your tincture. American ginseng contains a class of compounds called ginsenosides, which possess antioxidant and anti-inflammatory properties, two important factors in the progression of diabetes. American ginseng also promotes the secretion of insulin, necessary for regulation of blood sugar levels.

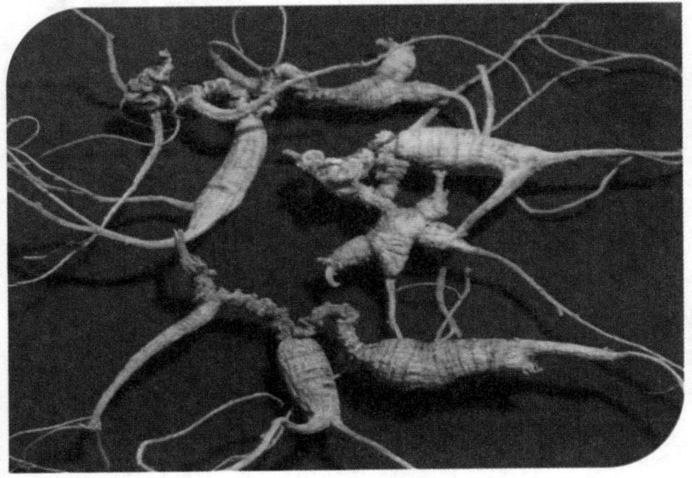

Ginseng helps lower high blood pressure in diabetics. Regular use gives some protection to the heart and retina from diabetes-induced damage.

Cold and Flu: American Ginseng helps fight the common cold and flu when taken regularly. People who take ginseng daily report fewer colds and less severe cold and flu symptoms.

Tonic for Fatigue, Stress, Memory, and Concentration: American ginseng has properties that boost energy and stamina and reduces fatigue caused by failing health and everyday stresses. It also betters cognitive performance, and enhances memory.

Erectile Dysfunction: American ginseng is an effective treatment for erectile dysfunction when taken on a regular basis. Favorable results are only seen when the herb is taken daily over the long term. It seems to work by opening up necessary blood vessels for improved blood flow.

Other Uses for American Ginseng: Since *Panax* is a tonic and reduces the stress on the body, it is effective for use in many different diseases and conditions. It is said to raise the spirits and to improve sleep, mood, and general outlook on life. It is also an antispasmodic.

Harvesting: Like all plants, the ginseng root needs to be treated with great respect. Do not harvest the roots before the berries ripen and the seeds set, in late summer or early autumn. When uncovering the neck of the root, look for four or more leaf scars, one scar for each year of age. Roots less than four years old do not contain enough beneficial properties to be effective. Note the location of younger roots and leave them in the ground or dig them up for relocation. The root branches underground, so dig carefully, and excavate a large area. Use the root fresh and dry some for future use.

Warning: Avoid American Ginseng if taking warfarin or other blood thinning therapies. Not recommended for pregnant or breastfeeding women. Ginseng should not be taken if someone has a hormone-related condition such as endometriosis, fibroids, or cancers of the breast, ovaries, uterus, or prostate. Do not use ginseng for people with heart disease except under the close supervision of a healthcare professional. Ginseng may decrease the rate and force of heartbeats.

Occasional side effects include headaches, anxiety, upset stomach, and sometimes trouble sleeping.

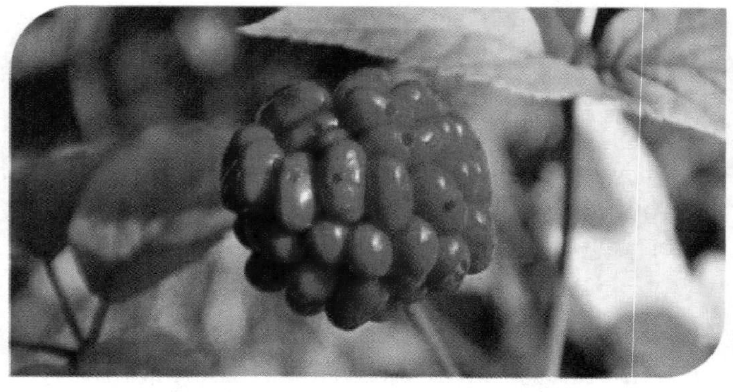

Photo by Drginseng, CC by SA 3.0

Recipes. American Ginseng Tea: Here is a simple ginseng tea with cooling properties. It keeps the body balanced and improves mental alertness. Avoid taking ginseng tea close to bedtime. You'll need 1/2 ounce of American Ginseng root fibers, 3 cups of water, a few grains of salt (optional). Bring the water to a boil. Add ginseng and simmer for 5 to 10 minutes. Season with salt, if desired. Strain the tea and allow it to cool. Serve at room temperature or cold.

American Ginseng Extract: See Section on Tinctures and Extracts. Use 8 ounces (230g) of American ginseng root, pounded into fibers or ground, with 1-quart (1 Liter) of 80 proof or better alcohol and infuse it for 6 to 8 weeks.

Angelica, *Angelica archangelica*

According to legend, an angel revealed in a dream how to use angelica to cure the plague. It was reverently called "The Root of the Holy Ghost" and was believed to ward off witchcraft and evil spirits. It is also called Wild Celery.

Angelica is a useful medicinal plant, but care must be taken to identify the plant correctly before using it. It is similar in appearance to other poisonous plants like water hemlock and giant hogweed. Please note the distinguishing features listed below and be sure you have the correct plant before harvesting.

The plant is found in the North Eastern parts of North America and in Northern Europe and grows in moist, cool woodlands, along stream banks, and in shady places. It is widely cultivated as an ornamental and medicinal plant. There are many varieties, but it is the *Angelica archangelica* that is used medicinally. It is in the Apiaceae/Umbelliferae (Carrot/Celery) Family.

Identification: Angelica is a biennial plant that dies after it sets its seed in its second year. During the first

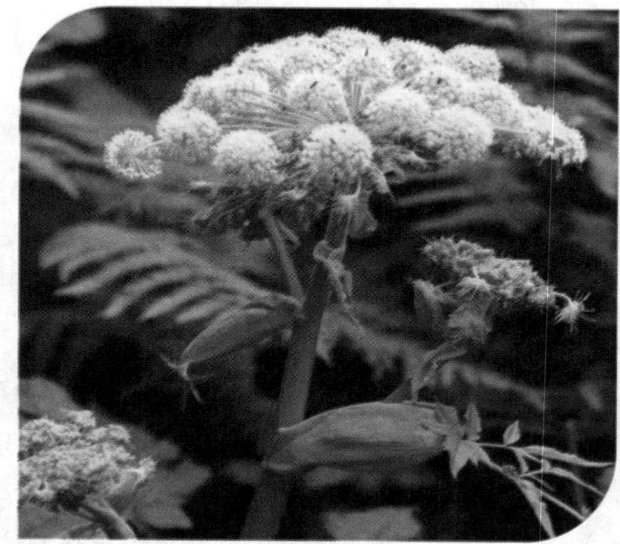

Photo By H. Zell, CC by SA 3.0

year, the plant puts out leaves, but most of its growth and its flowering stage occurs in the second year. It grows from 4 to 6 feet (1.2m – 1.8m) tall and occasionally up to 10 feet tall (3m), with large dark green bipinnate leaves. Each leaf contains many leaflets, divided into three main groups.

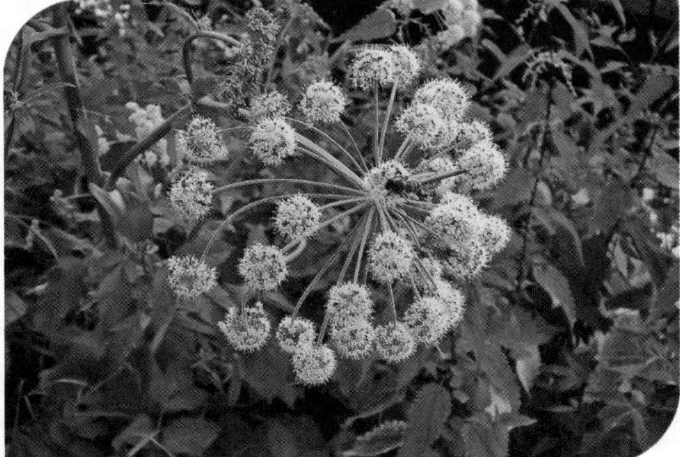

Photo By Franz Xaver, CC by SA 3.0

Each subdivision is further divided into three groups. The leaves are finely serrated. The lower leaves are the largest, up to 2 feet wide (0.6m). The leaf stalks are flattened and fluted. Stems are curved inward with sheathing that forms an elongated bowl that holds water. Stems are dark purple, round, smooth and hollow and are 1 to 2 inches (2.5cm-5cm) across.

The small, plentiful white, yellowish, or greenish-white flowers grow in large, compound umbels, up to 6 inches wide (15cm). The star-shaped flowers appear in July after the second year.

The fruit are small, oblong and pale yellow. Each is 1/6 to 1/4 inch (0.4cm – 0.6cm) in length when ripe and they reside in round heads that are up to 8 to 10 inches (20cm – 25cm) in diameter.

The root is branched, thick, and fleshy with small rootlets. The root is 3 to 6 inches (7.5cm – 15 cm) long.

Edible Use: The fresh root is rumored to be poisonous, but cooked and crystalized pieces of root and stem are used as decorative pieces for cakes and are used for flavoring in alcoholic beverages.

Young shoots and leaves are edible raw or cooked. The flavor is sweet and similar to celery with a slight licorice taste. Use the shoots in salads or boil them like a pot herb. Use angelica stems when young and tender. Preserve them in sugar or candy them for use as a decoration on sweet treats.

Angelica root must be dried and preserved for later use. Do not use it fresh.

Medicinal Use: The entire plant is used medicinally. Leaves, stems, and flowers are crushed and used in a bath or as a poultice. The medicine from the roots is best extracted using alcoholic tinctures. Roots can be dried and powdered for medicinal use.

Respiratory Issues: The herb is well known as an expectorant and is used to treat bronchitis, asthma, colic, coughs, and the common cold. The root is best used for respiratory ailments, but stems and seeds are also usable when necessary. A tincture or a tea will work as an expectorant.

Digestive Aid, Stimulates Appetite, and Intestinal Infections: Angelica stimulates the appetite, improves digestion, soothes colic, and reduces the production of intestinal gas. It also increases the production of stomach acid. It has been used as a cure for the plague, dysentery, cholera and intestinal infections. The herb is anti-bacterial and kills the bacteria that cause many gastric illnesses, like E. coli.

Nerve Pain: Rub angelica directly on the skin to treat neuralgia or nerve pain. It acts as an anesthetic.

Joint Pain: The anti-inflammatory properties of Angelica are useful for treating arthritis, gout, swelling, and for broken bones. For joint pain, a poultice made from crushed leaves is effective.

Anti-Seizure Effects: Recent studies show that Angelica archangelica protects the body against chemically induced seizures. Angelica essential oil exhibits

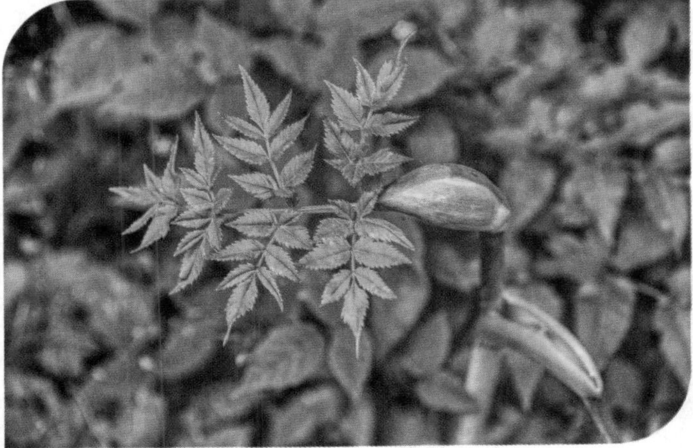

anti-seizure effects, probably due to the presence of terpenes in the oil.

Sore Throats and Mouth Sores: The antibacterial and anti-inflammatory properties of the root is useful in treating sore throats and mouth sores. Use an Angelica Infusion as a gargle or wash several times a day.

Menstrual Problems: Angelica regulates female hormones, regulates the menstrual cycle, and controls menstrual discharge.

Acne: Anti-bacterial and anti-inflammatory compounds in angelica help prevent and control acne. Use an angelica decoction or angelica tea as a face wash.

Anxiety: Recent studies showed that angelica has an antidepressant and anti-anxiety effect. It reduces stress and improves relaxation.

Cancer: Angelica archangelica has been shown to be effective against breast cancer cells. It reduces proliferation of the cancer cells and reduces tumor growth. Research is ongoing into its anti-tumor properties.

Anti-Fungal: Powdered angelica root is used to treat athlete's foot and other fungal infections.

Improves Circulation: Angelica strengthens the heart and improves blood circulation throughout the body.

Harvesting: While all the parts of the herb are useable for culinary and medicinal purposes, they are useable only during certain parts of the year. The roots are best harvested in the fall or winter of the first year. The stem and leaves are best in the spring or early summer of the second year, before the flowers appear. Dry the roots at or below 95 F and store in an airtight container.

Warning: Some people are allergic to Angelica. Avoid using angelica with anti-coagulant drugs. Do not use during pregnancy or breastfeeding. People with Diabetes should not use Angelica

Recipes. Angelica Tea or Decoction: Add 1/2 teaspoon of powdered angelica root to one cup of boiling water. Simmer for 10 to 15 minutes. Turn off the heat and let the tea steep for another 8 to 10 minutes. Strain out the root and store the decoction in a glass jar for later use. Use as a wash for skin problems or drink a cup after meals.

Candied Angelica: Trim angelica shoots and cut into strips. Blanch the strips in boiling water, then cook them in sugar syrup, gradually increasing the amount of sugar. Dry them and store in a sealed container. Keep the syrup for other uses.

Arnica cordifolia, Heartleaf Arnica and *A. montana*

Heartleaf arnica, also known as mountain tobacco, is one of the many Arnica species used for medicine. It is a member of the Daisy/Aster Family. It grows in high meadows, coniferous forests, and the western mountains at elevations from 3500 to 10,000 feet. It is native to western North American from Alaska to California and New Mexico, and east to Michigan. It is relatively easy to cultivate in the garden.

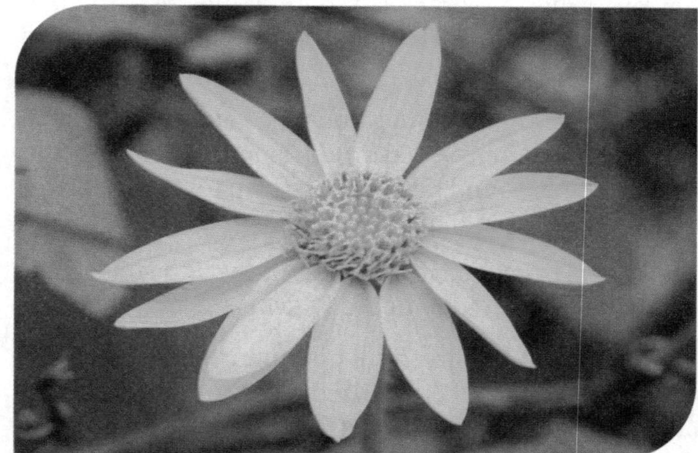

Arnica cordifolia, Pellaea, CC by 2.0

Identification: Arnica is a rhizomatous perennial growing from one or more erect stems. It grows between 12 and 20 inches (30 cm to 50 cm) tall.

The stems are hairy with two to four pairs of heart-shaped to arrowhead-shaped leaves. Cordate leaves are often produced on separate short shoots, are coarsely toothed and wither when the plant flowers. The leaves on the upper part of the plant are hairy, like the stalk. Lower leaves have rounded tips. The flowers are small and yellow, forming 1 to 5 daisy-like flowering heads per plant, and each flower head has a golden yellow disc with 10 to 15 yellow rays. The rays are pointed and about 1 inch (2.5 cm) long. The entire flower head is about 2 1/2 inches (3.7 cm) in diameter. The seeds form in a small, hairy achene, about 1/2-inch (1.25 cm)-long. Flowers appear from May to August.

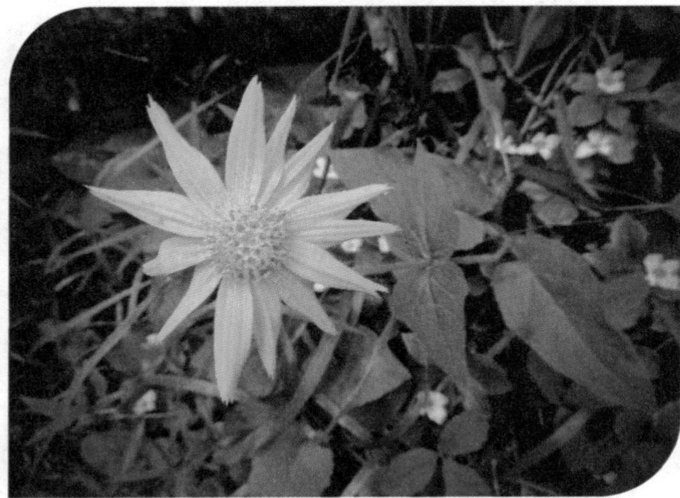

Heartleaf Arnica, Walter Siegmund, CC by SA 3.0

Medicinal Use: Use the flowers externally to reduce inflammation, reduce bruising, and for pain. It is antimicrobial and antiseptic. It can be used in small doses internally with great care.

How to Use Arnica on Skin: I often use Arnica externally on the skin as a salve or oil to promote healing in sprains, muscle pulls, contusions, and bruises. Use a diluted oil or salve on areas that need tissue stimulation and healing. Arnica treats common skin problems like infections, itching, and eczema.

Arthritis: Arnica is excellent at relieving arthritis pain, especially in cold weather. It warms the area and stimulates blood flow, and is anti-inflammatory. Rub arnica salve into the painful joint, or apply it as a poultice of bruised leaves or flowers.

Frostbite and Chilblains: Because it is warming and stimulates blood flow to an area, Arnica is used for the treatment of frostbite and chilblains. Use a poultice of leaves or flowers, or a salve or oil made with Arnica.

Bruises, Black Eyes, Muscle Aches, Inflammation, Sprains, Phlebitis, Carpal Tunnel, and Swelling: Arnica applied topically is useful in the treatment of a wide variety of external conditions. It reduces inflammation, warms the skin and muscle, relieves pain, and promotes healing. It is excellent for any strains, sprains, swellings, carpal tunnel, muscle soreness, and to reduce bruising.

Sore Throat and Toothache: For a sore throat or a toothache, try chewing the root. If the mouth is too sore for chewing, mash it and apply it to the swollen area. Gargling Arnica Tea is also effective for some people.

Other Uses of Arnica: Some people use Arnica to make homemade cigarettes, known as mountain tobacco.

Harvesting: When harvesting from the wild, pick flowers sparingly, never harvest rhizomes or roots; this destroys the plant. The plant will grow back as long as the rhizome survives in place.

I prefer the flowers for medicinal use but leaves and stems also contain beneficial properties. Pick flowers in the early afternoon, after the morning dew has evaporated.

Warning: Arnica can be highly toxic if taken internally. I do not recommend internal use, except homeopathically.

Avoid using undiluted Arnica preparations topically on open wounds, as it can cause inflammation and irritation. Dilute the oil and extracts with a carrier solution or oil if using on broken skin.

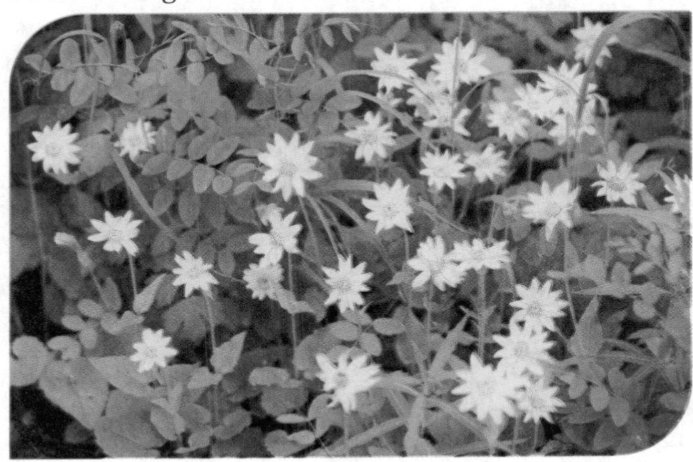

Arrowleaf Balsamroot, *Balsamorhiza sagittata*

Arrowleaf balsamroot, also known locally as the Oregon Sunflower, is a tough plant. It grows in grasslands, steppe, and scrubland areas, often on hillsides, in the western part of North America. It is in the Aster/Sunflower/Daisy Family.

Identification: Arrowleaf Balsamroot grows 1 to 2 feet (0.3 to 0.6 meters) tall. Its basal silver-green leaves grow up to 2 feet (0.6 meters) long and are arrow-shaped. Larger leaves are at the base of the plant and the leaves get smaller toward the top of the stem. Leaves are "wooly" and covered in fine white hairs.

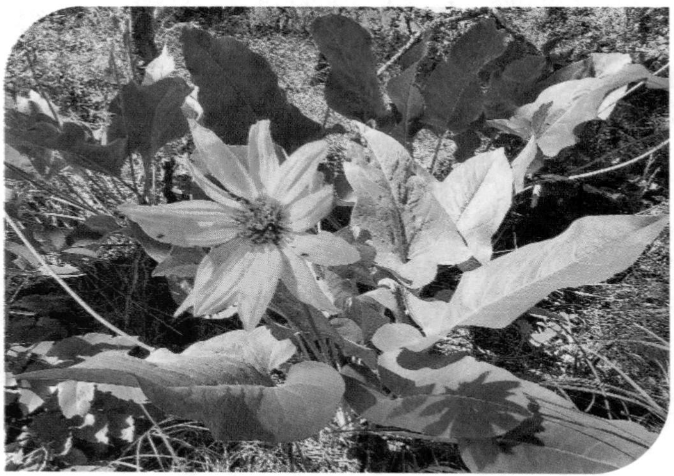

Flower stems grow from the root crown to 6 to 30 inches (15 cm to 75 cm) tall. Each flower stem has one flower head that resembles a sunflower with 8 to 25 yellow rays surrounding a disc. This plant grows from a deep taproot reaching 8 feet (2.4 meters) into the ground. It also has deep lateral roots that extend up to 3 feet (0.9 meters) around the plant.

Edible Use: This plant is an excellent food source. Its leaves can be eaten raw or cooked. Peel the stems before eating to get rid of the tough exterior. The seeds are nutritious and can be roasted like sunflower seeds. The root is eaten steamed or can be dried and pounded into a flour. The root can also be used as a coffee substitute.

Medicinal Use: The leaves, stems and roots contain medicinally active compounds. It acts internally as a disinfectant and expectorant.

Stimulates the Immune System: Taken internally, arrowleaf balsamroot roots enhance the action of the immune system, works as an antimicrobial, and stimulates the activity of white blood cells.

Toothaches, Sore Mouths, and Body Aches: Traditionally used to treat toothache pain and sore mouths by chewing on the root. Inhaling root smoke is said to treat body aches.

Sore Throat, Bronchial Congestion, Coughs, and TB: Balsamroot Tincture made from the dried or fresh root treats sore throats and loosens phlegm. Try putting your tincture into warm water and drink as a tea. You can also make cough syrup by simmering the root in raw honey (recipe below). Chew on the root to ease sore throat pain. Root infusions are used traditionally to treat tuberculosis and whooping cough.

Soothes Skin Burns, Wounds, Eczema, and Bruises: Use the balsamroot leaves as a compress on the skin to relieve pain and help heal burns, wounds, bruises, and rashes. Dry and powder the leaves or bruise and mash fresh leaves and place them on the skin or infuse them in oil for a salve.

Fungal Infections, Ringworm, Jock Itch, and Athlete's Foot: Use the dried and powdered root as an antifungal to heal common fungal infections. Apply the powder and leave in place to heal ringworm, jock itch, and athlete's foot.

Stomach Problems: The root, leaves, and stems are soothing for the digestive tract. Try a tea made from the entire plant.

Harvesting: Leaves and stems are easily harvested by cutting the stem and leaf from the plant. The root is more difficult because there is a very deep taproot as

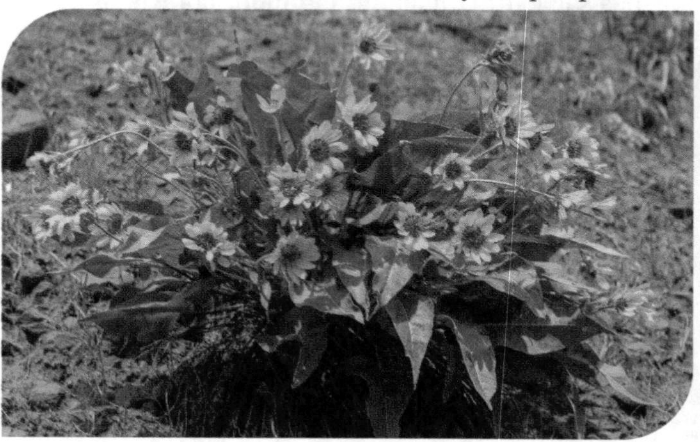

well as lateral roots and it often grows in rocky soil. Harvest the root in mid-spring to mid-August. You'll probably need to dig out a large area to get most of the root. Bring good tools and only take what you need from this slow-growing plant.

Recipes. Balsamroot and Raw Honey Cough Syrup: You'll need 3 to 4 Tablespoons of fresh Arrowleaf Balsamroot root, chopped into small pieces, and 1 cup raw honey. Bring the honey to a simmer and add the chopped balsamroot. Keep the heat at a low simmer for 2 to 3 hours. Strain the warm honey to remove the root pieces. Place in a clean jar and label and date. Use 1 to 2 teaspoons every 2 to 4 hours or as needed.

Bearberry, *Arctostaphylos uva ursi*, or *Arbutus uva ursi*

Also called kinnikinnik, uva ursi, hog cranberry, mountain cranberry, upland cranberry, bear's grape, and red bearberry, this herb is a small evergreen shrub that grows in northern North America and in higher elevations throughout the Appalachian Mountains. It likes acidic dry soils, especially sandy and gravel rich soils. It is in the Ericaceae (Heath) Family. It is commonly used in smoking mixtures.

Identification: The alternate paddle-shaped leaves are small and shiny with a thick, stiff feel. The underside is lighter in color than the green topside. Leaves are up to an inch (2.5 cm) long and have rounded tips. The leaves are evergreen, changing from dark green to

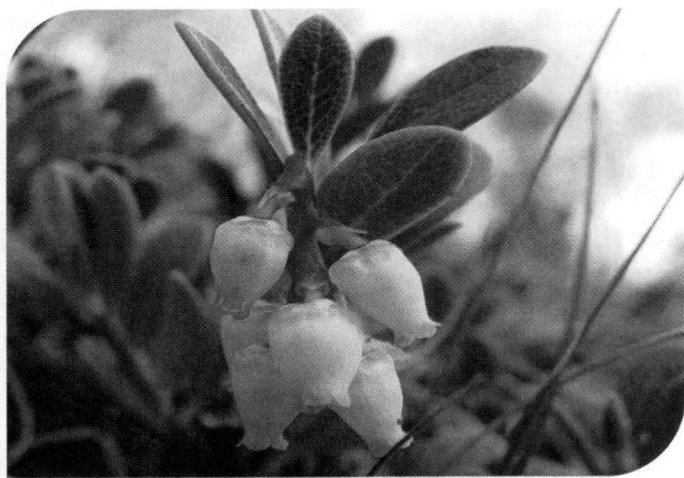

Bearberry, Jesse Taylor - Own work, CC by SA 3.0

a reddish-green and then to purple in autumn. The small dark brown buds have three scales.

Bearberry has small white or pink, urn-shaped flowers that appear in terminal clusters from May to June. They mature into pink to bright red fleshy drupes. The fruit is 1/4 to 1/2 inch (0.75 cm to 1.25 cm) in diameter and can remain on the plant until winter. Each mealy fruit contains up to five tiny hard seeds.

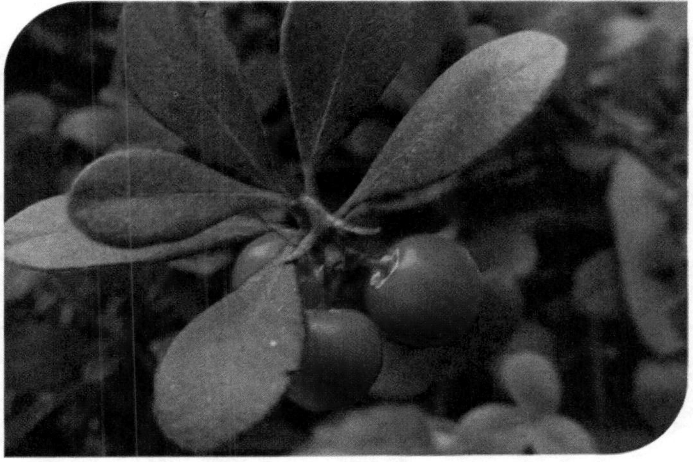

Bearberry Flowers, By Yvonne Zimmermann - Own work, CC BY-SA 3.0

The root system has a fibrous main root with buried stems that give rise to the stems of the herb. These trailing stems form layered mats with small roots and have stems growing up 6 inches (15 cm) tall when mature, with a reddish- brown bark. Younger branches are white to pale green.

Edible Use: Bearberry fruits are edible, but they are not tasty, so they are rarely eaten or used in cooking. They are sometimes used in pemmican.

Medicinal Use: The leaves and berries are used for medicine. I usually use it in tincture form for internal use.

Urinary Tract Infections, Nephritis, Kidney Stones, Cystitis, and Gout: Bearberry leaves treat kidney (nephritis), bladder (cystitis), and urinary tract infections extremely well. It is a diuretic, increasing the urine volume, and it has antiseptic properties that reduce bacteria populations in the kidneys, bladder, and urinary tract. It relieves bladder inflammation and helps relieves the pain of kidney

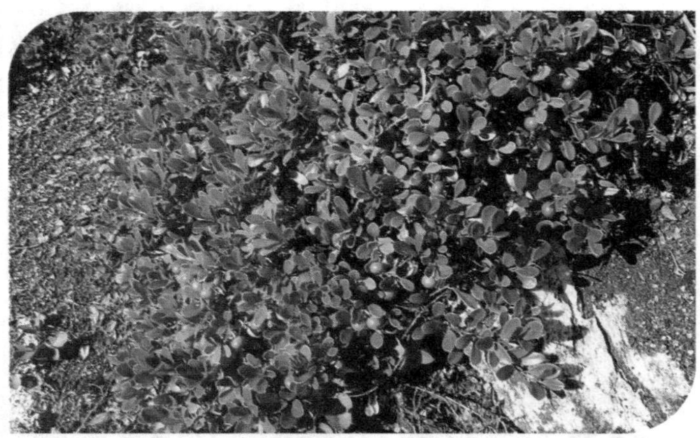

Bearberry, Walter Siegmund - Own work, CC by 2.5

stones. It also reduces uric acid in the body, and thus is useful in treating gout.

Bearberry leaves work best for urinary tract problems when the urine is less acidic or even slightly alkaline. Use at the first sign of infection. I often use it for UTIs as a blended tincture with Usnea, Goldenrod, and Oregon Grape Root, and also drink unsweetened cranberry juice or take a concentrated cranberry supplement. To decrease acidity, follow a vegetable-based diet, eliminating meat and milk products from the diet until the problem is eliminated.

Painful Sex in Women and the Urinogenital System: Bearberry tea or tincture treats long-term inflammation of the urethra in women. The tannins in the berries and leaves have a strong astringent action and reduce inflammation in the urinogenital system.

Vaginal Infections: Bearberry is an effective internal treatment against vaginal infections, including yeast infections. It has astringent and anti-inflammatory effects that help soothe the vaginal region. You can also use the leaf and berry tea as a douche or sitz bath twice a day.

Post-Partum Use and Uterine Hemorrhage: Drinking Bearberry Tea soon after giving birth helps increase uterine contractions and prevents hemorrhages. It helps prevent post-partum infections and helps incisions heal. It can also be used as a douche or sitz bath due to its astringent and tightening effects. Not for longer-term internal use if the mother is breast-feeding.

Prevents Scurvy: Bearberry berries and leaves are rich in vitamin C, which is necessary to prevent Scurvy. In winter months it can be difficult to find adequate sources of vitamin C. Drinking bearberry tea or eating its berries adds vitamin C to the diet.

Stomach and Intestinal Cramping: Bearberry has muscle relaxant properties that soothe stomach and intestinal cramping. It also has antiseptic properties that are effective against the most common causes of diarrhea and stomach upsets.

Harvesting: Bearberry leaves can be picked from mid-spring to mid-autumn. Pick the mature berries before the first frost.

Warning: Bearberry should not be used by people with high blood pressure, by pregnant women, or women who are nursing. Bearberry can induce nausea in some people and can cause stomach irritation. Soaking the bearberry leaves overnight before use may help. Not for continued long term use. Best used for acute treatment.

Recipes. Bearberry Leaf and Berry Tea: *Soaking the leaves and berries before brewing the tea removes some of the tannins and helps reduce digestive discomfort if using internally. You can also use the leaf only.

3 Tablespoons of dried leaves and berries, chopped, 1-quart (1 Liter) water. Soak the dried leaves and berries in cold water overnight or for up to one day. Drain. Bring a quart (liter) of water to a boil. Add dried leaves and berries. Reduce the heat to a simmer and cover tightly. Simmer the tea for about five minutes. Turn off the heat. Allow the tea to steep, tightly covered for 30 minutes. Strain. Drink one cup, two to three times daily, lukewarm on an empty stomach.

Bee Balm, Oswego Tea, *Monarda didyma*

Bee Balm is also known as Oswego Tea, horse mint, Indian nettle, Red Bergamot and Scarlet Bergamot. It gets the name Oswego tea because of its use by the Oswego Tribe. It is in the Lamiaceae (Mint) Family and is easily cultivated in the garden. This is a great herb to plant to attract hummingbirds, bees, and butterflies. It is a perennial and grows naturally in much of North America, Europe, and Asia.

Identification: Bee balm has straight, ridged, square stems and grows to 3 feet (0.9 meters) tall. Its course opposite leaves can be smooth or have a thin coating of fine hairs. The leaves have a strong fragrance and are 3 to 6 inches (7.5 cm to 15 cm) long. Their showy flowers range in color from deep pink to bright red to purple. They are approximately 1 ½ inches (3.75 cm) long and are grouped in dense heads of many flowers. They bloom in mid to late summer. The plant spreads on underground shoots, increasing the size of the plant every autumn. The plant in the center will begin to die back after three to four years.

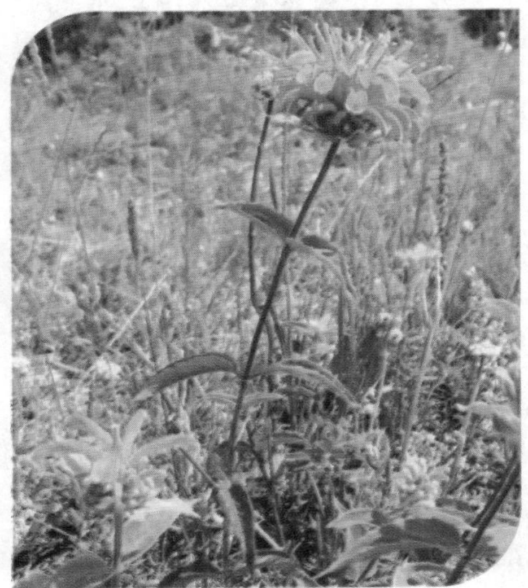

Edible Use: Oswego tea is made from dried leaves of the bee balm plant. The leaves and flowers are edible. Bee balm flowers are lovely as a garnish in salads, and dried leaves can be used like sage to flavor meats.

Medicinal Use: Leaves and flowers are used medicinally.

Menstrual Problems: Bee balm is an anti-spasmodic, and large doses of bee balm tea cause the uterus to contract, bringing on the menstrual period. However, it can also cause miscarriage and thus should be avoided during pregnancy

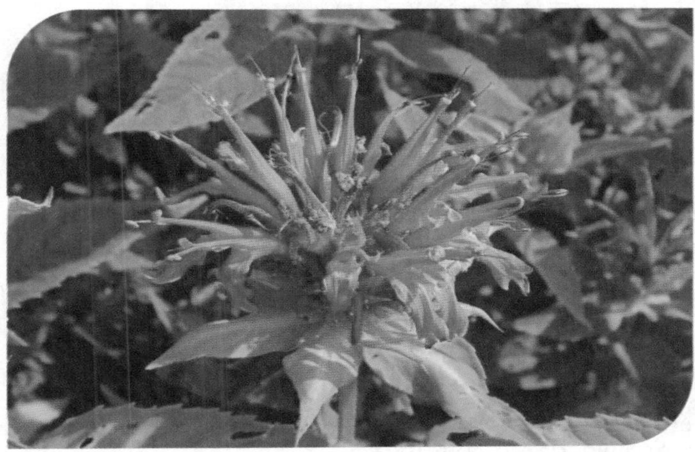

H. Zell, own work, CC 3.0

Colds, Sore Throats, and Congestion: Bee balm leaves are useful for treating colds, sore throats, and nasal and chest congestion in the form of a tea or in a steam vaporizer. Breathe in the vapors to open sinuses and clear congestion from the lungs.

Fevers: Oswego/Bee Balm tea is a mild diuretic, expelling water from the body through both sweat and urination. Sweating helps cool the body and reduce fevers.

Nausea, Vomiting, Flatulence, and Stomach Problems: Like most mints, bee balm has a soothing effect on the stomach and can calm flatulence, nausea, and vomiting. However, it is not appropriate for use with nausea caused by pregnancy. Large doses can cause miscarriage.

Nervine for Calm: Bee balm works similarly to Lemon Balm as a nervine, though it is less powerful than Lemon Balm for this use.

Stings, Scrapes, and Rashes: Bee balm is wonderful in a healing salve and helps soothe bites, stings, and rashes.

Harvesting: Pick the leaves in the mid to late morning after the morning dew has dried. Pick your yearly supply during the summer and dry them for future use. Collect the flowers when they are beginning to fully open. Dry them and store them in a sealed jar in a dark place.

Recipes. Oswego Tea: You'll need 1 teaspoon Oswego Tea/Bee Balm Leaves and 1 cup boiling water. Pour the boiling water over the tea leaves and allow the tea to steep for 5 to 10 minutes. Strain out the leaves and drink.

Black Cohosh, *Actaea racemosa*

I find black cohosh to be a very valuable herb for menopause, and I rarely use it for other uses, except as a supplementary herb. It balances hormones, which helps many conditions without curing them. Black cohosh is in the Ranunculaceae (Buttercup) Family. Black cohosh is native to eastern North America. It is found as far south as Georgia and west to Missouri/Arkansas and the Great Lakes region. It grows wild in small woodland openings.

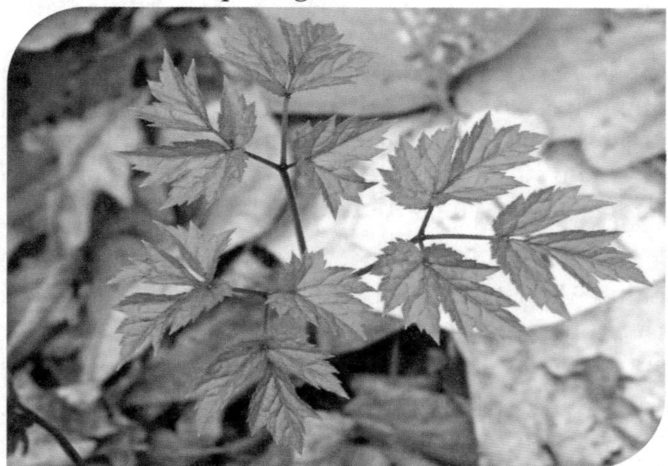

Identification: Black cohosh is a perennial with large compound leaves that grow from its rhizome. It grows up to 2 feet (0.6m) in height with distinctive serrated basal leaves that can be 3 feet (0.9m) long, growing in sets of 3 leaflets. Flowers bloom from June to September on an 8-foot tall stem, with racemes (flower clusters) up to 20 inches (50 cm) long. These white flowers occur in tight clusters with a white stigma surrounded by long stamens.

The flowers have no petals or sepals. A distinguishing feature is the sweet, putrid smell of the flowers that attracts flies, gnats, and beetles. The fruit is a 1/4-inch to 1/2-inch (0.74 cm to 1.25 cm) long dry follicle containing several seeds.

Medicinal Use: I mainly use black cohosh root for menstrual problems and menopause, although it is also useful for digestive problems and as a sedative. The best benefits are achieved when black cohosh is taken regularly long-term. Often it takes a month or more before benefits are noticed. The root is used medicinally.

Menopause, Menstrual Problems, Improved Ovulation, and PCOS: Black Cohosh works to balance hormones in women, helping to relieve menopausal symptoms such as hot flashes, moodiness, night sweats, headaches, heart palpitations, vaginal dryness, and mental fog.

It is also used for menstrual problems, painful intercourse, decreased sex drive, and Polycystic Ovary Syndrome (PCOS) and has been shown to improve ovulation in women.

Osteoporosis: By balancing hormones, black cohosh reduces bone loss caused by osteoporosis in women.

Reducing Anxiety and Aiding Sleep: Black cohosh has a sedative effect that calms the nervous system and reduces anxiety. It promotes restful sleep.

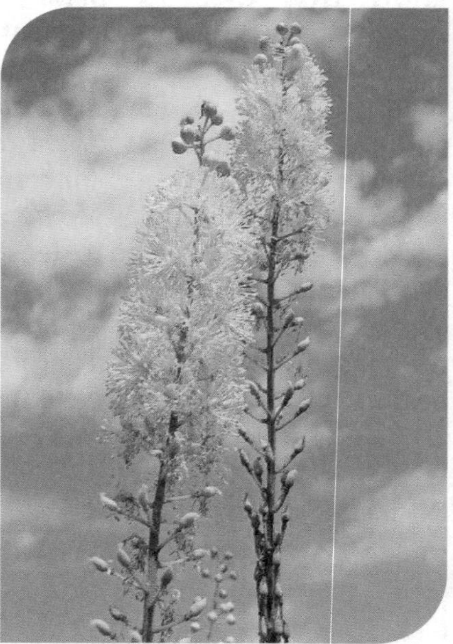

Black Cohosh Inflorescence, H. Zell, CC by SA 3.0

Digestive Problems: For digestive problems, crush a small piece of black cohosh root and boil it in a small amount of water. Drink the water to relieve stomach pain and intestinal problems. It helps improve digestion and elimination and prevents gastric ulcers. Black cohosh is only moderately effective for other digestive problems. There are better remedies out there.

Warning: People who are allergic to aspirin, have liver problems, have issues with seizures, or have a high risk of blood clots or stroke should not use black cohosh.

Pregnant and breastfeeding women, women with endometriosis, uterine cancer, or breast cancer should not take black cohosh.

Bleeding Heart, *Dicentra formosa*

Bleeding heart is a calming herb and is useful for the nervous system after a shock or an accident. It is also known as Pacific Bleeding Heart and Western Bleeding Heart. It is in the Papaveraceae (Poppy) Family and grows in moist areas of coniferous forests in the Pacific Northwest.

Identification: Bleeding heart is a perennial with fern-like, lacy, divided leaves. It grows from a rhizome and reaches 18 to 24 inches (45 cm to 60 cm) tall when mature. Heart-shaped dangling pink flowers bloom in clusters from mid-spring through autumn. Flower stems reach above the leaves, each with 5 to 15 blooms. Seeds form in pointed, pea-like pods. Depending on the weather, the plant may go dormant during the hot summer months. They have shallow rhizomes that are easy to harvest but are also sensitive to foot traffic.

Medicinal Use: Use bleeding-heart with great care and in small doses as it is a very potent narcotic and is toxic in higher doses. The root is mostly used, though the flowers and leaves also have medicinal properties.

Toothache: The root is good for relieving toothache pain. Chew the root and place it on the painful tooth.

Bruises, Sprains, Joint Pain, Nerve Pain: A compress made with Bleeding Heart Decoction or by heating root pieces in water and applying them as a poultice is effective in relieving nerve and muscle pain and helping bruises and sprains to heal.

Shocks to the Nervous System, Anxiety, and Nervous Disorders: Bleeding heart root decoction and tincture are both effective in relieving anxiety and nerves. It is effective in calming people after a

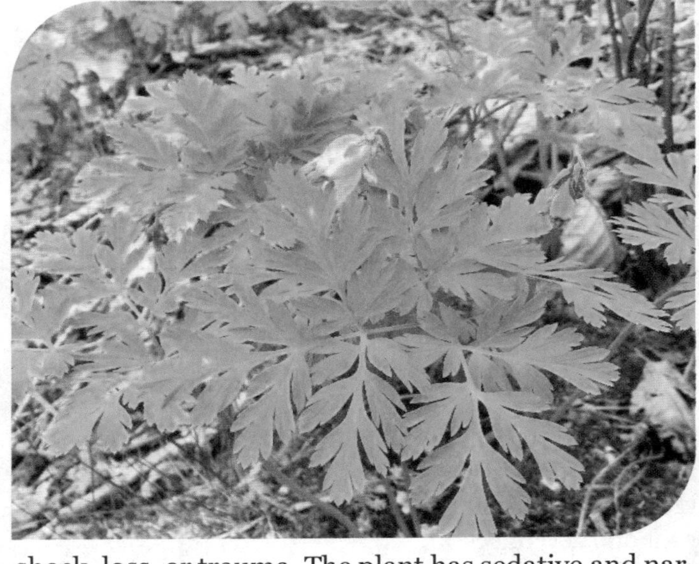

shock, loss, or trauma. The plant has sedative and narcotic properties.

Muscle Tremors: Compounds in bleeding heart are calming and relaxing for the nervous system. They relax the muscles and suppress muscle tremors exhibited in some nervous system disorders.

Diuretic: This diuretic herb helps flush toxins and other poisons from the blood, liver, and kidneys. However, there are safer herbs for this use.

Increases Metabolism and Stimulates Appetite: Bleeding heart calms the nervous system while increasing the metabolic process, often giving you more energy and an increased appetite.

Cancer and Swollen Lymph Nodes: Bleeding heart tincture has been used traditionally for the treatment of cancer, swollen lymph nodes, and enlarged glands.

Harvesting: Bleeding heart is a rare plant and is becoming endangered in some areas. Check the status in your area before collecting and do not overharvest. Use it sparingly because it is rare in the wild, or, even better, grow your own supply so that you do not disturb the plants growing in the wild. Gather the roots of bleeding heart in the summer, if the plant goes dormant, or in the autumn when the leaves begin to change and after the seed pods have matured.

Warning: Avoid using bleeding heart during pregnancy or breast-feeding. Use bleeding heart sparingly, a little goes a long way. Do not use if you have liver disease. Do not use in combinations with other sedatives and note that it can cause a false positive for opiate use on a drug test. Consult a medical professional before use.

Recipes. Bleeding Heart Tincture: Finely chopped fresh or dried bleeding-heart rhizome to fill ½ a jar, 80 proof or better alcohol such as vodka or brandy.

Place the rhizome pieces into a clean jar with a tight-fitting lid. Cover the herb completely, filling the jar with alcohol. Cap and label and place it in a cool, dark cupboard. Shake the jar daily for 6 to 8 weeks while the tincture steeps. Strain, label, and store. Usual dosage is 10 to 20 drops of fresh tincture, and 15 to 30 drops if using dried roots. Use with care.

Bloodroot, *Sanguinaria canadensis*

Bloodroot is mainly for the treatment of skin cancers, ulcers, and wounds that won't heal. I have always known the herb as bloodroot, but it is also called red-root and red puccoon.

The juice is red and quickly dyes the skin and has been used by the Algonquin Tribe to paint the skin for ritual. It is in the Papaveraceae (Poppy) Family.

Use with great caution! This herb grows in eastern North America in moist thickets and dry woods and on floodplains and near streams.

Identification: Bloodroot is a stemless, rhizomatous wildflower that blooms in early spring. The herb grows from 6 to 10 inches (15 cm to 25 cm) tall. The leaves go dormant in mid to late summer. When the bloodroot flower is sprouting, it's usually wrapped by one deeply-scalloped, grayish-green, palmate basal leaf. Bloodroot has a hermaphroditic flower that has 8 to 12 fragile white petals, yellow stamens, and two sepals positioned below the leaves, which fall off after the flowers open. The root is a blood-red rhizome that will branch out and grow new rhizomes.

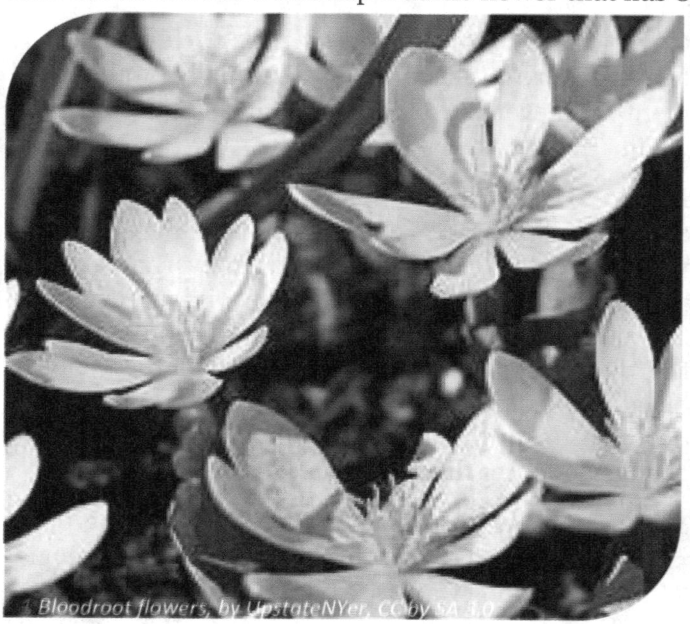

Bloodroot flowers, by UpstateNYer, CC by SA 3.0

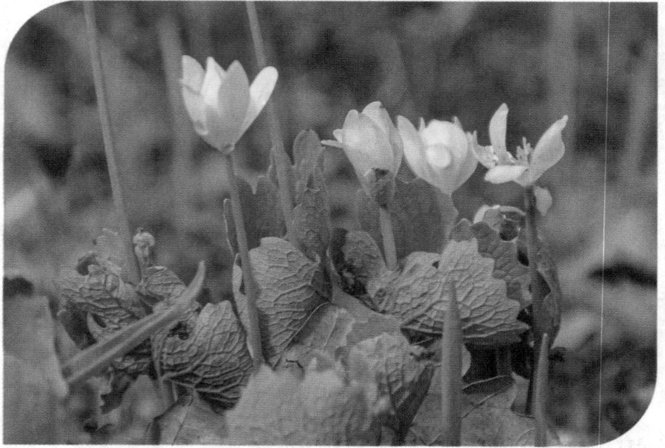

Medicinal Use: Caution is advised. Bloodroot is a toxic plant, and serious problems can arise. Use small doses only as advised by a medical professional or find an alternative plant. The root is used medicinally.

Skin Cancers, Ulcers, Moles, Skin Tags, Warts, Eczema and Other Skin Conditions: Treating skin problems is what bloodroot does best. However, use with great caution and in moderate amounts as it will also kill healthy cells and can cause permanent scarring and sloughing of the skin. Traditionally, people made and applied a salve from bloodroot to the affected area.

They covered it with a bandage and left it in place for a week or so. Usually, only one application is required, but extensive areas, deep lesions, or other tough cases may require repeated application.

The bloodroot kills the cancerous or damaged cells and covers the area with a scab.

Leave it alone to heal, and check the area to be sure that all of the cancer is removed so that it doesn't return. The bloodroot also has anti-inflammatory, anti-bacterial, anti-fungal, and anesthetic properties that help the skin to heal while relieving pain. The salve can be used to remove skin tags, warts, moles and other unwanted skin lesions. Apply the salve directly to the lesion, keeping it well away from the healthy skin. If you decide to use this plant do so with great caution and in small doses. I use a facial mask once a month with a very small amount of bloodroot in it (along with other ingredients). This is a good example of my utilizing it in small and infrequent doses.

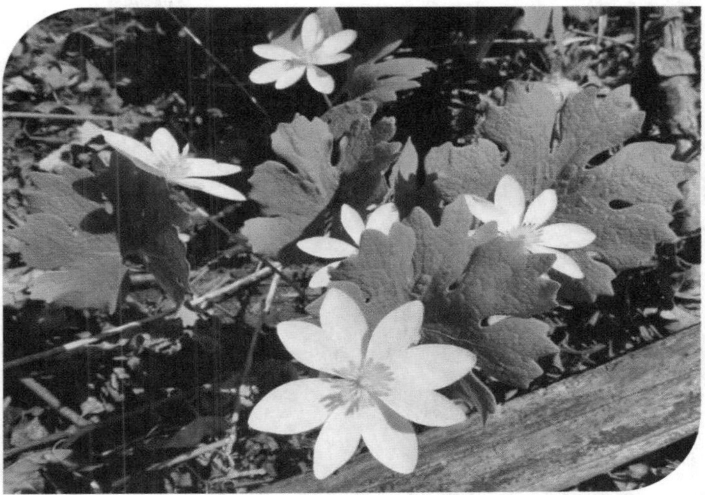

Treating Respiratory Problems: Bloodroot is a bronchial muscle relaxant used to treat asthma, whooping cough, influenza, and as a treatment for croup.

Gastrointestinal Problems: Bloodroot powder treats gastrointestinal bleeding, abdominal cramps, nausea, and vomiting. In large doses, it acts as an emetic, causing the very problems it treats. Use with great care or find an alternative herb.

Diphtheria, Tuberculosis, and Respiratory Illnesses: Small doses of bloodroot decoction are an antibacterial agent useful for the treatment of bacterial diseases such as diphtheria, tuberculosis, asthma, bronchitis, and pneumonia. For respiratory illnesses, it has the added benefit of cleaning out the mucus and congestion and suppressing coughs. However, I prefer other, safer remedies. For sore throats, you can dilute the decoction in a glass of water and use it as a gargle.

Menstrual Problems: Small doses of Bloodroot Decoction are beneficial for treating menstrual problems including excessive bleeding and cramping. Again, I prefer other plants for this purpose.

Dental Care: Extracts from bloodroot help fight infections like gingivitis and prevent the formation cavities, tartar, and plaque. Add a drop of bloodroot decoction to your toothpaste for this purpose or use a diluted tea as a rinse.

Harvesting: Wear protective gloves to protect your hands from staining red and to avoid the medicine being absorbed through your skin. Best harvested in autumn when the strength of the plant is returning to the root and the tops are dying back. Dig up the root and the surrounding area, removing the rhizomes. Leave a few behind for next year's plants. Dry for future use.

Warning: Great caution is advised. Bloodroot is a toxic plant that can cause tunnel vision, nausea, and death. Do not use bloodroot if you may be pregnant or if you are nursing. It may also cause permanent scarring or disfiguration when used topically.

Blue Cohosh, *Caulophyllum thalictroides*

Blue cohosh is also known as squaw root or papoose root for its use to induce labor. It is a perennial member of the Berberidaceae (Barberry) Family.

Do not confuse it with Black Cohosh. They are very different. It is found on the floor of hardwood forests in eastern North America. It prefers moist soil, hillsides, and shady locations with rich soil.

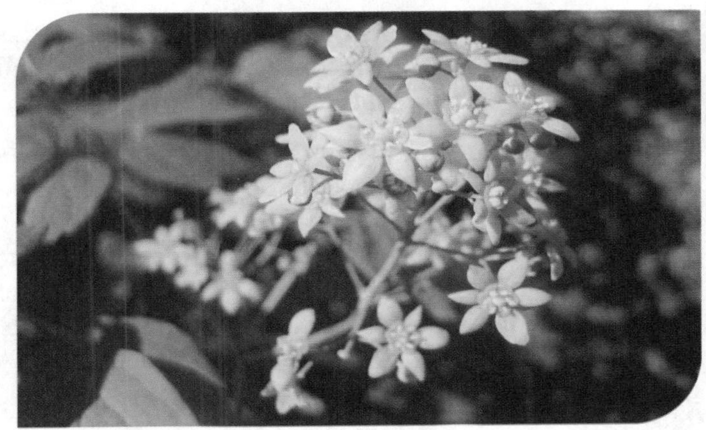

Blue Cohosh, Biosthmors - Own work, CC by SA 4.0

Identification: A single smooth stalk, 1 to 3 feet (0.3m to 0.9m) tall, grows from the rhizome, and contains a single three-lobed leaf and a fruiting stalk. Its leaflets are serrated at the tip and the leaves turn a bluish-green hue when mature. It has deep blue fruits.

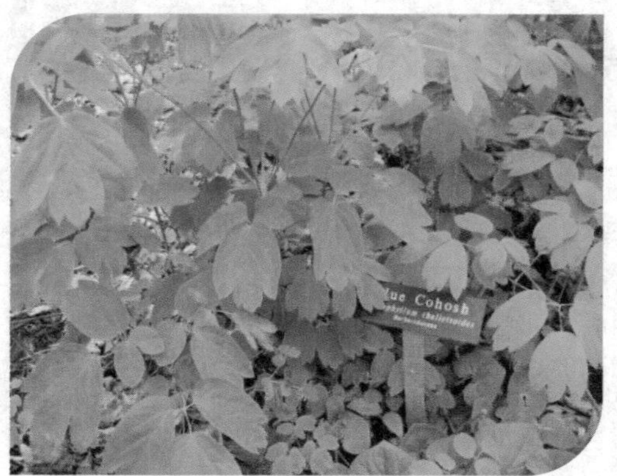

Blue Cohosh, by Carol, CC by SA 3.0

Medicinal Use. Childbirth: The root has oxytocic properties that promote childbirth. Do not take during pregnancy until 1 to 2 weeks before the due date and only under a doctor's care. It causes powerful uterine contractions that are regular and productive, encouraging a quick and easy birth. It also has a calming effect, helping the mother relax between contractions and reducing pain.

Menstrual Problems: Blue cohosh root is used for menstrual problems, including delayed menstruation, cramping, and profuse hemorrhage.

Harvesting: Harvest blue cohosh root in late autumn, when it stores its strength. You can also harvest the rhizomes in the spring, just as the new growth begins, if needed. Dry and store the roots for future use.

Warning: Do not use during pregnancy. Do not use for estrogen-sensitive diseases such as endometriosis, fibroids, and certain cancers. Blue cohosh can elevate blood pressure so careful using for heart patients and people with high blood pressure. Excessive dosage can cause nausea, vomiting, and a lack of muscle coordination.

Butterbur, Arctic Sweet Coltsfoot, *Petasites frigidus*

Butterbur, or Sweet Coltsfoot, is a plant that grows in moist areas throughout the Northern Hemisphere. The name butterbur reportedly came about because the leaves were used to wrap butter for keeping. It is also called bog rhubarb. It is in the Aster/Daisy Family. Note that Arrowleaf coltsfoot (*P. frigidus* var. *sagittatus*) has the same medicinal properties as butterbur; it has arrow-shaped leaves.

Butterbur or Sweet Coltsfoot is not the same plant as *Tussilago farfara*, known commonly as coltsfoot and also in this book, though they are closely related.

Identification: Butterbur or sweet coltsfoot flowers appear in February and March, before the larger basal leaves that arrive in late spring. The flowers have a sweet scent, and are often the first flowers seen in the new year in the cold wetlands in the North. A cluster of white to purple-pink flower heads appears on the tip of a fleshy stalk, which is covered with sheathed leaves.

The flowers give way to silver-white seed heads and its large basal, rhubarb-like leaves arise near the flowering stalk directly from an underground rhizome. The basal leaves are palmately divided and their underside is "wooly" with white hairs.

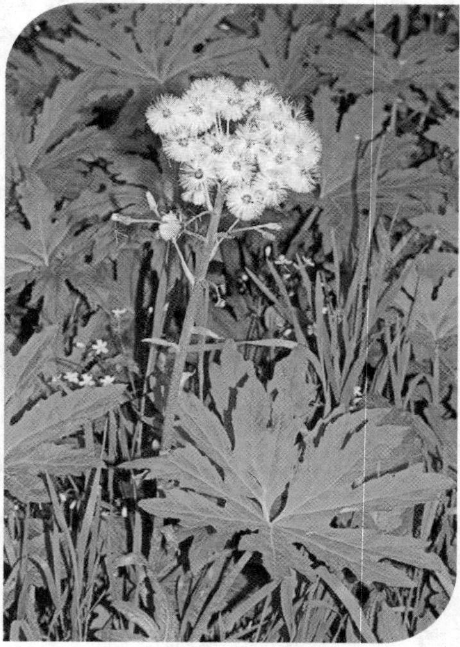

Petasites frigidus by Walter Siegmund (talk), Own work, CC-BY-SA-3.0

Edible Use: The flowers, flower stalks, and leaf stalks are edible cooked in limited amounts. The ash (after burning the aerial part) is a good salt substitute.

Medicinal Use: The roots, mature leaves, and stems are all used medicinally. It is antispasmodic, anti-inflammatory, a vasodilator, and mucilaginous. I use it as a tea or a tincture. Only collect mature leaves, as young leaves contain small amounts of pyrrolizidine alkaloids, which are hepatotoxic.

Allergies: Butterbur leaf is very effective for allergies, including hay fever, reducing histamine and leukotriene release. It has been shown to be as effective as many prescription allergy medications without causing drowsiness.

Bronchial Spasms, Chronic Coughs, and Spasmodic Airways and Asthma: Butterbur leaf is useful against asthma and restricted bronchial passages. It reduces the sensitivity and the frequency of attacks. As an antispasmodic, it reduces spasms of the bronchial tract while also relieving inflammation, and is excellent for any chronic cough like those caused by emphysema or bronchitis.

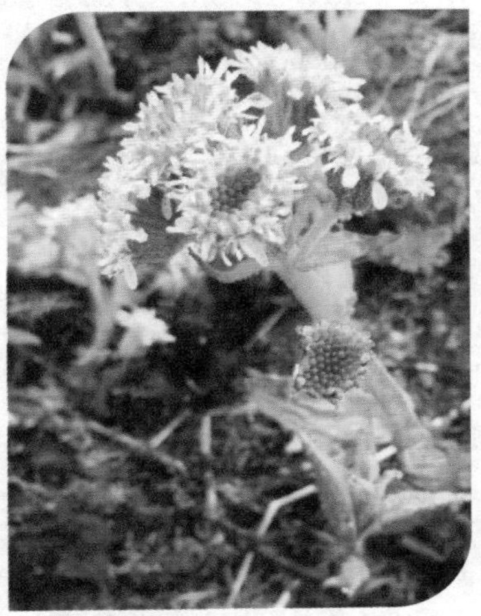

Migraine Headaches: The herb relaxes vasoconstriction and relieves inflammation that can trigger migraine headaches. Like feverfew, it is best taken daily as a preventative rather than as a rescue treatment, though it works as a cure as well. I often pair it with Feverfew in tincture form. Taken daily, butterbur leaf reduces the incidents of migraines.

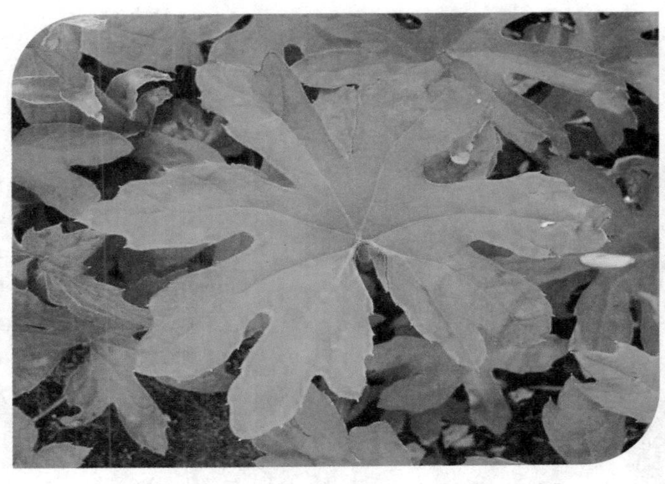

Petasites frigidus by Stan Shebs, Own work, CC-BY-SA-2.5

Inflammation and Muscle Sprains: The plant is a strong anti-inflammatory and antispasmodic. Externally a root poultice can be used to treat inflammation and pain due to a muscle sprain or strain.

Harvesting: Harvest roots in spring. Harvest the leaves and stems throughout the summer once they are fully grown. Young leaves contain small amounts of pyrrolizidine alkaloids, which are hepatotoxic.

Warning: Avoid using butterbur if you have liver problems. Do not use if you are pregnant or breastfeeding, or for children under age 7. Adverse reactions can include GI symptoms, nausea, flatulence, and gassy stomach. Allergies are possible.

California Buckwheat, *Eriogonum fasciculatum*

California Buckwheat is in the Polygonaceae (Buckwheat) Family. It is a wild buckwheat species and is commonly known as eastern Mojave buckwheat. This shrub is a native to the Southwestern United States and Northwestern Mexico. It grows on dry slopes, canyons, and washes in scrubland and coastal areas.

Identification: *Eriogonum fasciculatum* is varied in appearance. Sometimes it is a compact bramble and sometimes it is a spreading bush approaching 6 feet (1.8m) in height and 10 feet (3.0m) wide. It has numerous flexible slim branches.

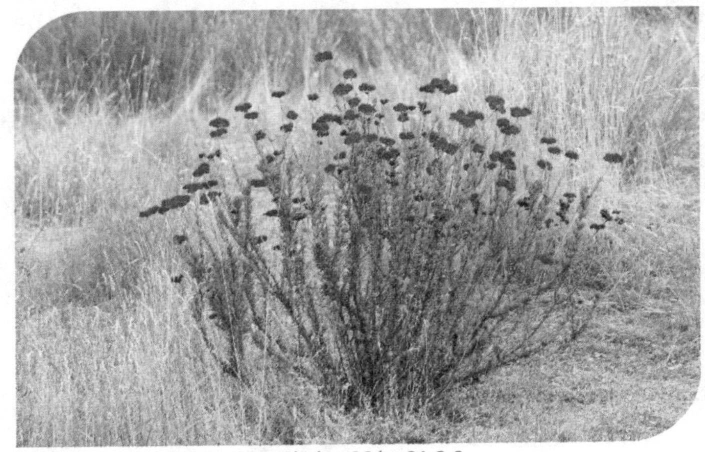

California Buckwheat, Stan Shebs, CC by SA 3.0

Its leaves and are 1 1/2 to 2 inches (3.75 cm to 5 cm) long and less than 1/2 inch (1.25 cm) wide. Leaves grow in a whorled cluster at nodes along the branches. They are wooly and leathery on the undersides and roll under along the edges.

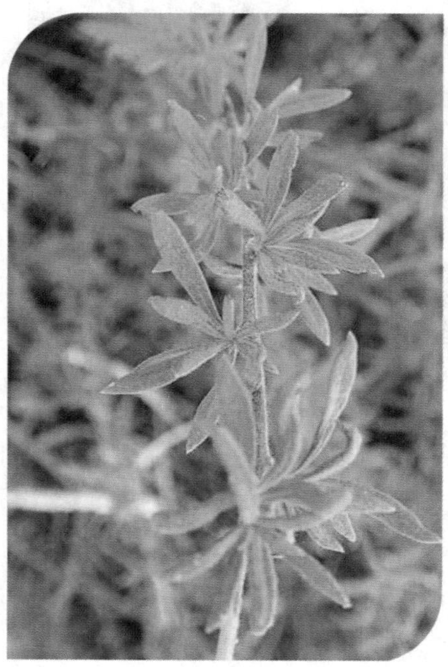

Photo by Krzysztof Ziarnek, Kenraiz, Own work,

Its flowers are dense clusters that are 1 to 6 inches wide (2.5 cm to 15 cm). Each distinct flower is white and pink and only a few millimeters across. It blooms from May to October. It has light brown small seeds.

Edible Use: The seeds are eaten raw or dried for later use. Seeds can be ground into a powder and used as a flour. Young sprouts can also be consumed, and the seeds can be sprouted to eat.

Medicinal Use: The seeds, leaves, flowers, and roots are all used for medicine. Older, mature plants are more potent. The roots are dried and ground for medicine and a strong, thick tea is made from the leaves or the roots.

Wound Care: The leaves, flowers, and roots are used for skin wounds. Fresh leaves or flowers can be applied as a poultice. Ground leaves and ground roots are mixed with water or oil and applied as a poultice. California Buckwheat Tea can be used as a wash.

Colds, Coughs, and Sore Throats: A mild leaf tea works for colds, coughs, and sore throats. The hot root tea can also be used for colds and laryngitis.

Diarrhea and Stomach Illnesses: For diarrhea and other stomach troubles, use a strong decoction made from the roots of California Buckwheat. It cleans out the system and gets rid of irritants.

Oral Care: For sore gums or for use as a mouthwash, use a weak leaf tea. It is a mild pain reliever and calms inflammation. Swish a mouthful of tea around for a few minutes, then spit it out.

Headaches: For headaches and other aches and pains, use a strong tea made from the leaves. It relieves the immediate pain and flushes toxins from the system.

Heart Health: A tea made from dried flowers or dried roots helps prevent heart problems.

Harvesting: The seeds mature in early autumn and dry right on the plant. Wait until the seed pods have dried and turned to a rusty brown before harvesting. Once dried, they can easily be hand-stripped from the plants into open tubs or bags. Harvest older roots as they contain more medicine.

Recipes. Strong California Buckwheat Root Tea: 1 tablespoon California buckwheat shredded root, 1 pint (500 ml) of water. Mix the root into the water and bring to a boil. Reduce the heat to a simmer. Cover and simmer the tea for 15 minutes.* Strain and serve warm or cold. *For a weaker tea, reduce the brewing time to 5 minutes

California Buckwheat Leaf Tea. 1 teaspoon California buckwheat leaves, dried or 1 tablespoon fresh, 1 cup boiling water. Pour the boiling water over the leaves and steep for 5 to 10 minutes. Strain.

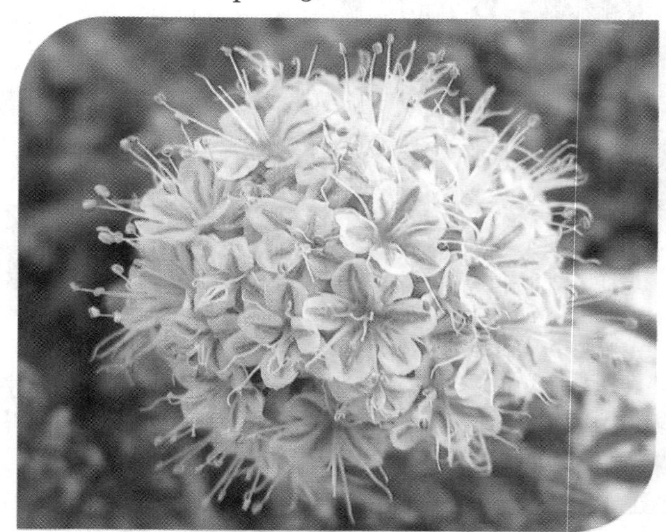

Cardinal Flower, *Lobelia cardinalis*

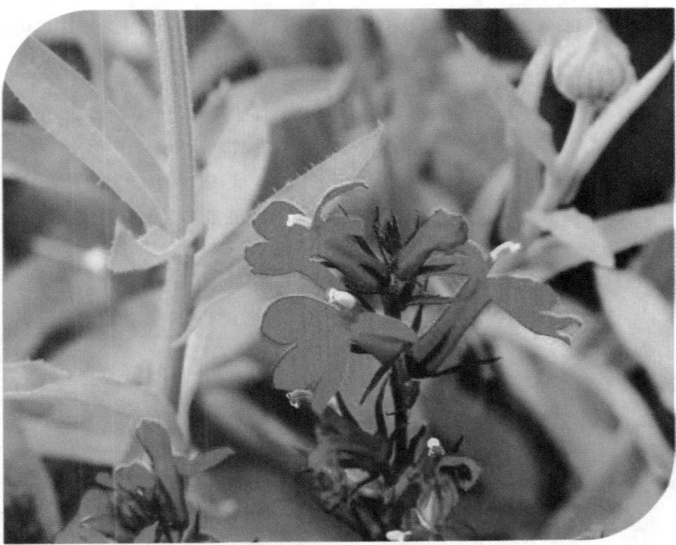

Cardinal flower is a beautiful showy plant with brilliant red flowers. This plant is hard to miss. It is in the Campanulaceae (Bellflower) Family. It grows in wet soil, swamps, stream banks, and along rivers.

Identification: The flowers are a cardinal red color and are 2-lipped with five deep lobes. They grow on an erect raceme approximately 2 to 3 feet (0.6m to 0.9m) tall and flower during the summer and autumn. The toothed lanceolate to oval leaves grow 8 inches (20 cm) long and 2 inches (5 cm) wide.

Medicinal Use: Traditional uses for cardinal flower are below. It isn't used as often as it used to be in herbal medicine but is still an important plant to know. All parts are used medicinally.

Bronchitis: Cardinal flower is used as an expectorant for bronchitis.

Epilepsy, Diphtheria, Tonsillitis: The anti-inflammatory and narcotic properties of the roots help it treat convulsive and inflammatory diseases such as these. It relaxes spasms and allows the body to heal.

Eye Diseases: A weak tea made from 1 teaspoon of root or leaves per cup of boiling water is useful as an eye wash.

Sprains, Bruises, and Skin Irritations: As an external application for relieving pain and encouraging healing in sprains, strains, bruises, and other surface irritations, try Cardinal Flower tea or a Lobelia Seed Vinegar Preparation. It relaxes the muscles and speeds healing though I do prefer other plants for this use.

Warning: Some other plants in the *Lobelia* genus are toxic, so it is wise to be careful in the use of cardinal flower since it could potentially be toxic in larger doses. Symptoms of toxicity would include nausea, vomiting, diarrhea, excessive saliva, weakness, dilation of pupils, convulsions or coma.

Lobelia Vinegar Preparation: Use the fast method only in emergencies. A slower maceration is best. Ingredients: 4 ounces (113g) powdered Lobelia seed and 1-quart (1 Liter) of vinegar. Macerate the vinegar and seed powder for seven days, shaking daily. Filter mixture through a coffee filter to remove the seed powder. Store in a cool, dry place. Fast Method: Place the vinegar and seed powder in the top of a double boiler and cover. Bring water to a simmer in the lower pot. Warm the vinegar mixture this way for 1 hour. Cool and strain.

Cat's Claw, *Uncaria tomentosa*

Cat's Claw, or uña de gato, grows in Central and South America, where it grows profusely in the rainforest. The root and vine bark are imported here for medicinal use. It is a useful plant and I try to keep a supply on hand. It is in the Rubiaceae (Bedstraw/Madder) Family.

Identification: Cat's claw, *Uncaria tomentosa*, is a tropical woody vine whose hooked claw-shaped thorns give it its name. The vine grows to a length of up to 100 feet (30meters), climbing anything in its path.

The bright green elongated leaves grow in opposing pairs. They have a smooth edge that may be rounded or come to a point. The flowers are yellow, trumpet shaped, and have five petals. The barbs are hook-shaped and curled like a cat's claw.

Medicinal Use: The inner bark of the vine or root is used. It is taken as a powder, in capsules, as a tea, or as a double-extracted tincture.

Cancer Treatment and Prevention: Cat's claw prevents and helps treat cancer. It contains anti-inflammatory, anti-oxidant, and anti-tumor properties that prevent cancer cells from developing in the body. It helps the immune system fight existing cancerous cells by enhancing white blood cell function. People in chemotherapy report that it helps relieve pain and other symptoms related to chemotherapy drugs.

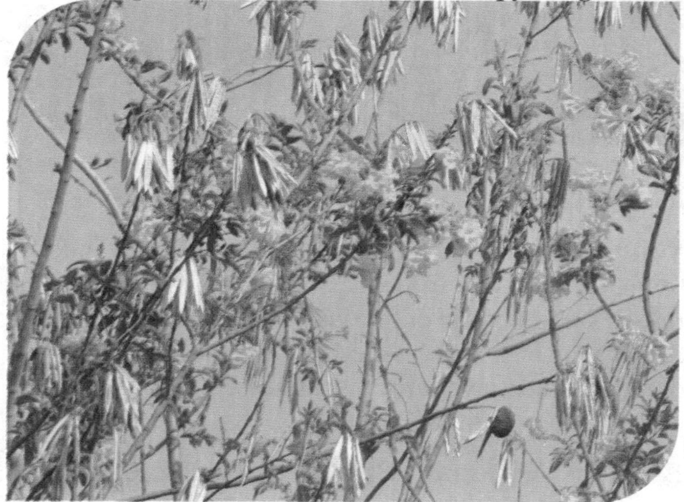

Irritable Bowel Syndrome, Crohn's Disease, Colitis, Ulcers, and Other Gastrointestinal Issues: Cat's Claw helps support the digestive system, relieving inflammation in the stomach and intestines. It has anti-bacterial, anti-fungal, and anti-viral properties that help rid the body of the underlying causes. It fights diseases of the intestines, stomach, and liver while restoring the body's natural flora and healing the digestive system.

Anti-Inflammatory and Autoimmune Conditions: Inflammation is a cause of many body diseases, including autoimmune diseases, arthritis, and heart disease. Reducing swelling in joints, wounds, and bodily organs helps the body heal faster and reduces pain. They are still researching its use in certain autoimmune diseases, and some recommend not taking it if you have an autoimmune issue due to the way it boosts the immune system.

Osteoarthritis and Rheumatoid Arthritis: The anti-inflammatory effects of this herb are very beneficial for osteoarthritis and rheumatoid arthritis. It calms the inflammation, reduces swelling, and relieves the associated pain.

Powerful Anti-Viral: Cat's claw is useful in treating viral diseases due to its quinovic acid glycosides. It is used to treat herpes, Epstein-Barr, hepatitis B and C, HPV, HIV, Dengue Fever, and other viral diseases. I would try it against any of the tropical viral diseases, given the need.

Helps the Body Heal, Chronic Fatigue Syndrome: Its anti-inflammatory and anti-bacterial properties help the body from getting an infection and calm the body's response to the damage, helping it heal. It also helps people with Chronic Fatigue Syndrome.

Lowers Blood Pressure: Cat's claw increases circulation throughout the body and helps lower blood pressure for people with hypertension.

Supports the Immune System and Help for Mold Exposure: Cat's claw contains isopteropodin, which helps increase the body's white blood cell count, eliminates free radicals from the body, and helps fight infection. Its anti-inflammatory and anti-oxidant properties also help with mycotoxin exposure.

Regulates Female Hormones and the Menstrual Cycle: Cat's Claw helps regulate the female hormones that keep the menstrual cycle regular and helps to alleviate bloating, cramping, and mood changes that are associated with it. If you are pregnant or trying to conceive avoid this plant. It can cause miscarriages and may prevent conception.

Detoxification: Cat's claw is beneficial in detoxifying the whole body and cleansing the blood and lymph. It is excellent at removing toxins, drugs, heavy metals, and other foreign substances from the body. It also boosts the effectiveness of the kidneys, spleen, pancreas, and digestive system due to its cleansing effects.

Warning: Do not take cat's claw if you are pregnant, nursing, or trying to get pregnant. Do not take if you have an autoimmune disorder. It may cause a flare-up. Consult your health professional if you are taking blood thinners or any other prescription drugs as it interacts with some of them. Side effects can include nausea, diarrhea, and dizziness.

Cleavers/Bedstraw, *Galium aparine*

Cleavers, also called Bedstraw, catchweed, sticky weed, and goosegrass, is an annual plant that grows in damp, rich soils along riverbanks and fence lines in eastern and western North America and is found worldwide. It is in the Rubiaceae (Bedstraw) Family. You often find the plant and its seeds stuck to your clothing like Velcro after walking through it.

Identification: A climbing hairy, almost sticky, stem grows from a thin taproot to a height of 2 to 6 feet (0.6m to 1.8m). The plant has coarse leaves with a variable shape. The leaves grow in whorls around the stem, and the stem, leaves, and fruit are usually covered with small, spiny hairs. Its leaves may be oblong to lance-like or even linear. Cleavers flowers are small and white or greenish-white in color and flower from early summer until autumn. The flowers have a sweet smell.

Edible Use: Cleavers are edible. I prefer them cooked as their hairs and hooks get stuck in my throat when I eat them raw. Their seeds can be roasted as a coffee substitute. They are a good green to juice and drink.

Medicinal Use: Cleavers are astringent, anti-inflammatory, diuretic, detoxifying, febrifuge and promote sweating. It is effective both internally and externally. I use the leaves for medicine and infuse them cold into oil, water, or a tincture. Do not boil.

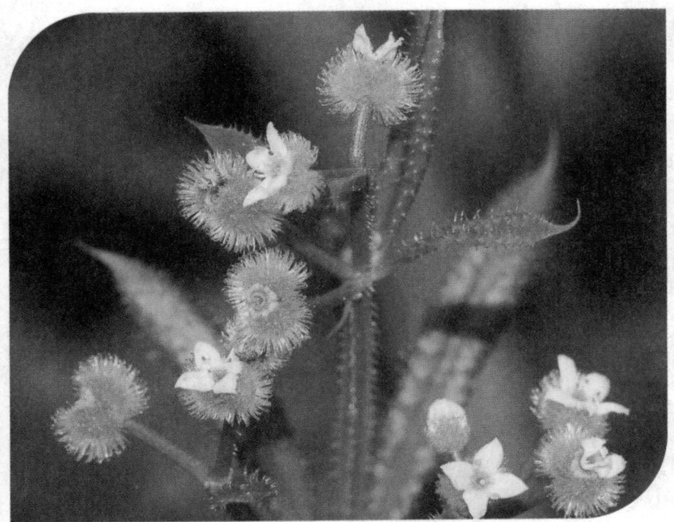

3 Cleavers flowers and fruit, Alvesgaspar, CC by 3.0

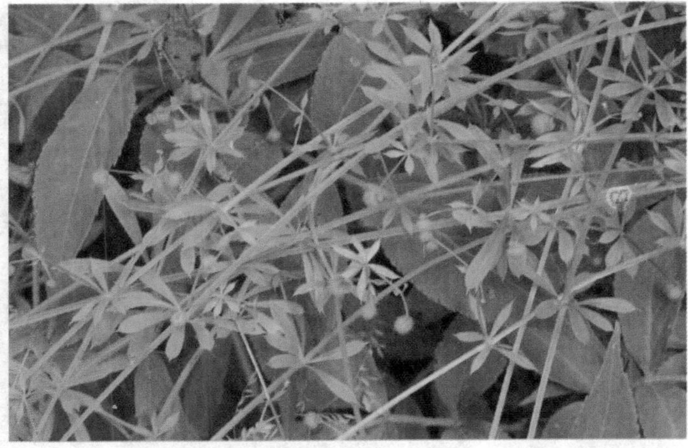

2 Cleavers growing over the tops of other plants, Mike Pennington, CC by SA 2.0

Rejuvenate the Skin, Slow the Signs of Aging: Cleaver tea is said to have a toning effect to tighten skin and smooth out wrinkles when applied externally.

Detoxify the Body, Drain the Lymphatic System, and Swollen Glands: Cleavers are a diuretic. They work well to remove toxins from the body and to clean the lymphatic system.

Skin Disorders, Acne, Psoriasis, Eczema, Abscesses, and Boils: Cleavers works internally and externally to improve the condition of the skin, detoxify the blood and lymph, and reduce inflammation associated with these conditions. They are also antibacterial, which helps treat the underlying infections. Use both internally and externally for these conditions.

Kidney Stones, Bladder and Urinary Tract Infections: Cleavers are very effective at treating bladder infections, urinary tract infections, and kidney stones. It dissolves stones, clears obstructions, and flushes them out of the body. The antibacterial action is effective at curing the underlying infections.

Cancer: Research has been done that supports the use of cleavers to treat tumors, especially those of the breast, skin, head, neck, bladder, cervix, prostate, and lymphatic system.

Chickenpox, Measles, and Fevers: To treat chickenpox and the measles, try cleavers internally to treat the disease and externally on the skin to relieve the itching and general discomfort from the rash. Cleavers also helps bring down the accompanying fever.

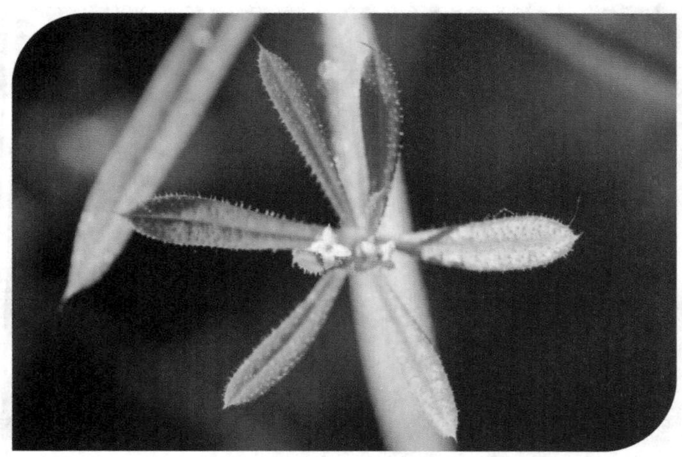

Stop Bleeding, Burns, and Sunburns: Freshly picked cleavers leaves are excellent for stopping bleeding in wounds, cuts, or other surface bleeding. Apply the leaves directly to the wound. It also reduces inflammation and speeds healing. The leaves can be made into a poultice for larger wounds.

Tonsillitis, Sore Throat, Glandular Fever, and Prostate Problems: Cleaver juice works well for glandular problems like tonsillitis, glandular fever, and for prostate problems and prostate cancers. When fresh juice is not available an infusion can be used, although it is not usually as effective as the juice for these issues.

Harvesting: Harvest cleavers in spring to mid-summer and use fresh or dry for later use.

Recipes. Cleaver Juice. Fresh cleavers leaves and water. Wash the fresh leaves thoroughly and place them in a blender with a small amount of water. Use only as much water as needed to blend. Blend the leaves into a pulp and strain out the juice with a fine sieve. I recommend making a large batch of juice and freezing the extra. Most people drink 2 cups daily to treat cancers and tumors.

Club Moss, *Lycopodium clavatum*

Club moss is a vascular spore-bearing plant and propogates via spores. It is in the Club Moss Family, Lycopodiaceae, and is not a true moss but is more closely related to ferns and horsetail. Club Moss is found worldwide and is also called staghorn, ground pine, and running pine,

Identification: The yellow-green leaves are scale-like and short and taper to a fine feathery point. The 3 to 4-foot-long, ground-hugging stem of this plant is highly branched with small, spirally arranged scaly leaves. The stem runs along the ground producing roots at frequent intervals. It resembles the seedling of coniferous trees, though there is no relationship between them. Its spores grow on two or sometimes three yellow-green barrel-shaped cones that are on small, 6-inch (15 cm) stalks.

Medicinal Use: Mostly the spores are used in medicine, but sometimes an extract of the entire plant is used.

Respiratory Problems: Club moss spore decoctions are used to treat ailments like chronic lung, bronchial disorders, and other respiratory issues.

Congestion, Colds, and Flu: Club moss spores act to dry out mucous membranes and relieve congestion. Try a 1/4 teaspoon of the spores mixed into a glass of water three times a day until the congestion clears.

Urinary Tract Disorders: Club moss is a diuretic, increasing the amount of urine expelled and flushing toxins from the body. To treat urinary tract problems, use a decoction of the whole plant. Common usage is 1 to 2 tablespoons of the decoction 3 to 4 times a day.

Skin Conditions: Club moss spores treat many different skin conditions, including allergic reactions, sunburns, psoriasis, eczema, fungal infections, chickenpox, contact dermatitis, hives, and insect bites and stings. Make a salve with the spores of club moss. The spores can also be applied lightly as a

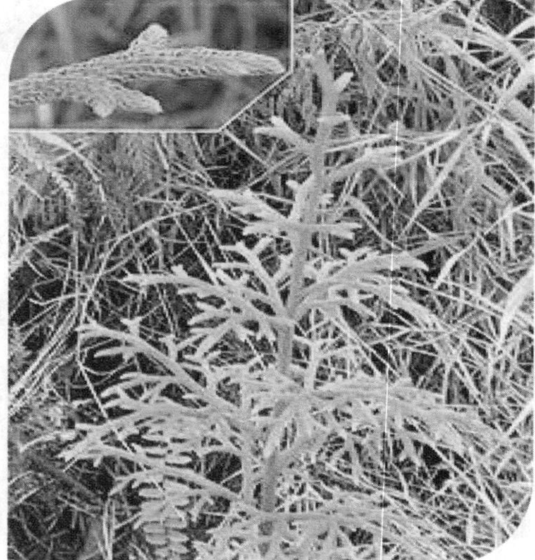

powder and rubbed into wounds, folds of skin, or anywhere that you prefer not to use oil. The powder absorbs moisture and helps heal wounds.

Rheumatoid Arthritis: A decoction of the entire plant is said to help rheumatoid arthritis symptoms.

Flatulence: Both constipation and flatulence can be treated with spores from club moss. As little as 1/4 teaspoon mixed with water eases symptoms and resolves the problem.

Kidney Diseases: Club Moss Decoction made from the whole plant is used to treat kidney disease and related disorders. It works to eliminate kidney stones and cleanse the system.

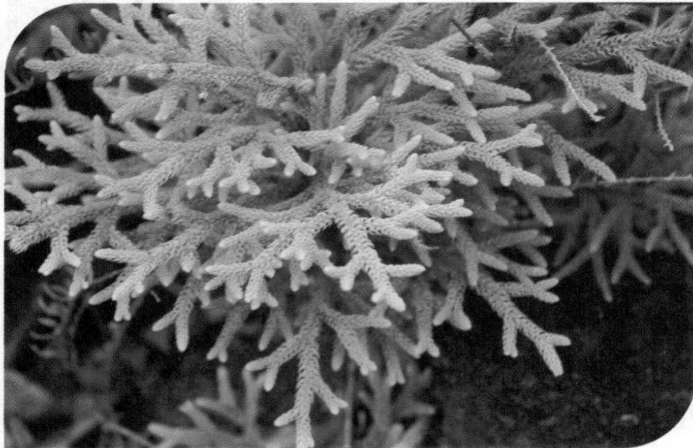

Wound Treatment: Open wounds and sores that refuse to heal are well served by the application of club moss spores. Apply the spores as a powder and rub it into the affected area.

Harvesting: Harvesting of club moss should be done when the spore heads are dry, mature, and ripened, though the spores can also be harvested while still green. For a ripe plant just cut off the plant and spread them on a sheet to dry until the cones open. Shake them and collect the spore powder. To collect the spore heads from green cones, cut off the cones and break them open. Place the cones in a paper bag and place them in a cool, dry place to open. When the cones open, shake out the spores and remove the remaining plant material.

Warning: Club moss contains small amounts of alkaloids, which are a toxic substance and can cause paralysis to the motor nerves if consumed in large amounts.

Recipes. Club Moss Decoction: 1 ounce of ground or finely chopped club moss plant, 2 cups of water. Bring the water to a boil and add the club moss plant. Turn the heat down to a slow simmer and simmer the decoction for 15 minutes. Allow the decoction to cool and strain out the herb. Keep the decoction in the refrigerator and use within 3 days. Use a maximum of one cup daily, split into 4 or more doses.

Club Moss Salve. 5 ounces (150ml) of organic olive oil or other carrier oil, 1 ounce (28g) of shaved beeswax, 1 tablespoon of club moss spore powder. Heat the olive oil gently over very low heat in a double boiler. Add the club moss spore powder. Keep the oil on very low heat for 20 to 30 minutes while the spores release their medicine into the oil. Add the shaved beeswax and stir until the salve is thoroughly mixed. Do not strain out the spores. Pour the salve into a sanitized jar and cover it tightly. Keep the salve refrigerated if in a very hot climate. Apply 2 to 3 times daily, as needed.

Coltsfoot, *Tussilago farfara*

Coltsfoot is in the Aster/Daisy Family, and is closely related to Butterbur. It is native to Eurasia but has naturalized in the US and Canada. It is also known as coughwort, podbel, and son-before-the-father.

Identification: Coltsfoot is a rather unusual perennial. The flowers look like dandelion, but they appear early, in April, and die before the leaves appear. It grows between 4 and 6 inches (10 cm to 15 cm) tall and is usually found in open areas with disturbed soil.

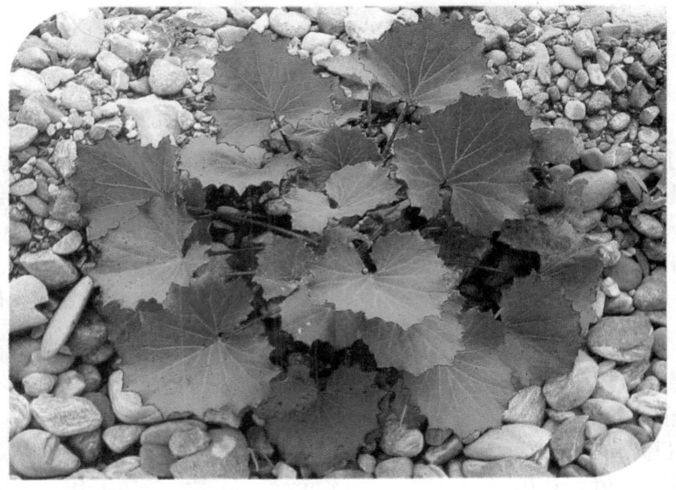

The top of the leaf is smooth, while the underside is covered with white downy hairs. Leaves at the top of the plant are green, while those closer to the ground are white or grayish in color. These basal leaves are 2 to 10 inches (5 cm to 25 cm) long and serrated on the edges. The single bright yellow flowers are a little over a half inch (1.25 cm) across and look like dandelion. Its small white root spreads underground.

Edible Use: Coltsfoot flowers and leaves are edible. They are good in salads (in small amounts only). Young leaves are also used in soups or stews. To use the leaves as a vegetable, wash them after boiling to get rid of the bitterness. Dried or fresh leaves and flowers can be used to make an aromatic tea.

Medicinal Use: Both the leaves and flowers have medicinal value, although the flowers have the highest concentrations of medicinal compounds. People rarely use the roots, but they have medicinal properties as well. This plant has anti-inflammatory and anti-tussive properties, due to it containing mucilage and tannins.

Asthma, Whooping Cough, Laryngitis, Coughs, Emphysema, and Bronchial Congestion: The botanical name *Tussilago* means 'cough dispeller,' and it does the job well. Use it to relieve congestion and expel mucous. It is especially useful for chronic coughs like emphysema and whooping cough. Coltsfoot Decoction, taken throughout the day, is used as a remedy for chronic coughs of all causes.

Eczema, Sores, and Skin Inflammations: The flowers, prepared as a poultice, are helpful applied directly onto skin inflammations, sores, and eczema.

Warning: Coltsfoot leaves contain small amounts of toxic compounds, which are destroyed by cooking. Eat raw leaves sparingly and boil, drain, and rinse leaves when using as a vegetable.

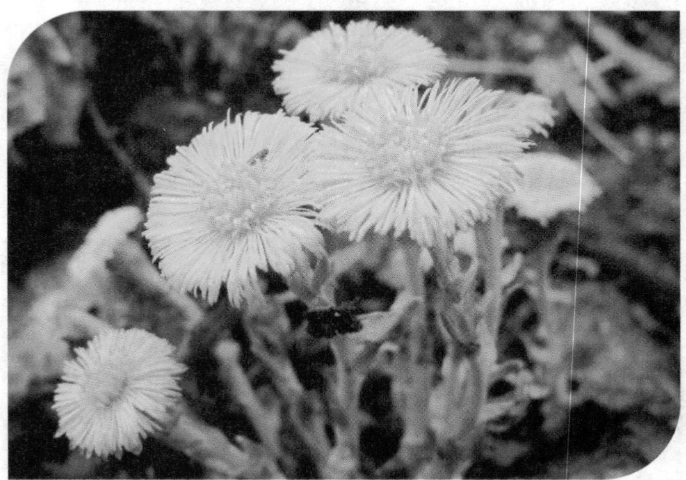

Recipes. Coltsfoot Decoction. 1-ounce coltsfoot leaves, 1-quart (1 Liter) water, raw honey, as desired. Combine the coltsfoot leaves and water over medium-high heat and bring to a boil. Reduce the heat and boil the decoction until the water is reduced by half. Cool and strain the decoction to remove the leaves. Sweeten the decoction with raw honey as desired. It can be bitter, depending on the age of the leaves. Drink 1/4 cup at a time, throughout the day or as needed to provide relief.

False Hellebore, Indian Poke, *Veratrum viride*

There are several plants that go by the name of False Hellebore or Indian Poke. This is *Veratrum viride*, not *Phytolacca acinosa* or other pokeweeds. It is in the Lily Family. It is found in pastures, meadows, open woods, damp soils, and swamps. It grows throughout most of eastern and western North America (not mid).

Identification: False Hellebore is an erect perennial herb that grows 2 to 7 feet (0.6m to 2.1meters) tall. The leaves are broad on the lower part and spirally arranged on the stout stem. Leaves are 4 to 14 inches (10 cm to 35 cm) long and 2 to 8 inches (5 cm to 20 cm) wide. The leaf blade of this plant is widest near the

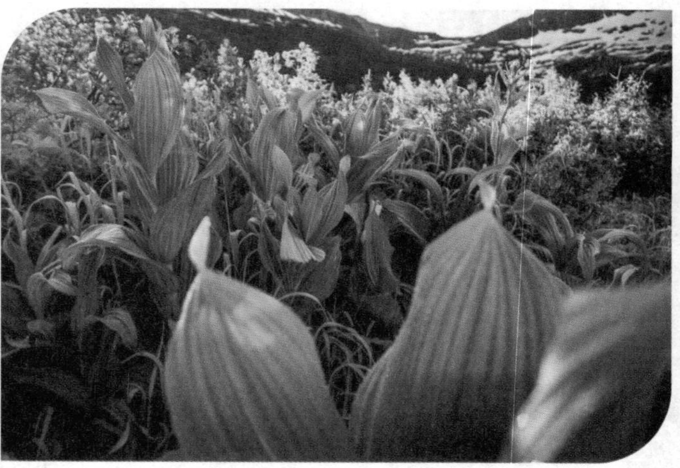

middle and tapering at both ends (ovate). The leaves are feathery on the underside. The flowers are arranged on a large branched inflorescence approximately 1 to 2 1/2 feet (0.7m) long. The flowers are ¼ to ½ inch (0.75 cm to 1.25 cm) long with six green to yellow-green tepals.

The ovary is positioned above the sepal attachment and produces flat, winged seeds. The fruit splits along two or more seams when dry to release seeds. The fruit grows up to 1 1/4 inches (3.2 cm) long.

Medicinal Use. Treating High Blood Pressure and Rapid Heartbeat: False Hellebore Root contains chelidonic acid and other alkaloids. Some of the alkaloids expand peripheral blood vessels and lower blood pressure by slowing the heartbeat. Several pharmaceutical drugs for high blood pressure and rapid heartbeat have been developed from False Hellebore compounds.

This herb is highly effective, so only very small doses should be used since an overdose is potentially deadly. I prefer other home methods than this plant for lowering blood pressure and heart rate, as the strength can vary from plant to plant and in how it is made. If you choose to use False Hellebore for this purpose, start with very small doses of the decoction and have very close medical supervision.

Reducing Fevers in Acute Diseases: In acute disease situations such as peritonitis and acute pneumonia, a decoction of False Hellebore acts as a febrifuge (brings down the fever). However, do not forget the other effects of the decoction and use it sparingly under complete medical supervision. I much prefer Yarrow to bring down a fever.

Body Pain, Arthritis, and Muscle Pains: A decoction of the leaves or roots, diluted with water, works as a wash to reduce or relieve shoulder pains, intense arthritis pain, severe aches of the muscles and body parts, pains at the rear portion of the neck and fast electric shock in all parts of the body. Alternately, use a salve made from False Hellebore as a rub to relieve pain.

Other Uses: The roots of False Hellebore are slightly soapy and can be used to do laundry. Grate the root and add it to water.

Harvesting: Wear gloves when harvesting. Pick individual leaves and leave the plant intact. Dry the leaves for storage. Harvest rhizomes only from mature plants. Collect the roots in autumn and dry them for future use.

Warning: Take precaution and use only small doses, if you use it internally at all. False Hellebore is considered to be very toxic. Veratrum viride contains numerous toxins that may cause vomiting and nausea. If the poison is not evacuated, vertigo and cold sweats start, respiration slows, blood pressure and cardiac rhythm falls, and the heart fails eventually leading to death.

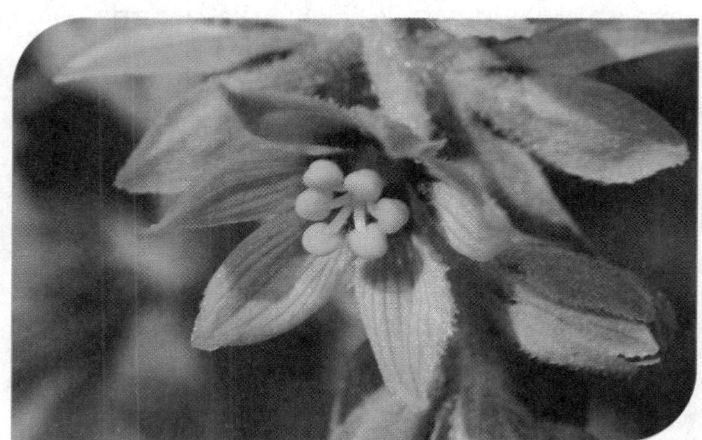

Walter Siegmund - Own work, CC by SA 3.0

Recipes. Indian Poke Leaf Decoction: 1 ounce chopped Indian poke Leaves, 1 pint (500 ml) of water. Cover the chopped leaves with water and bring to a boil.

Turn off the heat and allow the leaves to steep for 10 to 15 minutes. Strain out the leaves and store the decoction in the refrigerator for up to 3 days or freeze.

False Solomon's Seal, *Maianthemum racemosum (Smilacina racemosa)*

False Solomon's Seal, also called Solomon's plume and feathery false lily of the valley, is a flowering plant that grows across continental North America. It is a useful plant, but often gets overlooked in favor of more versatile plants. I recommend you get familiar with this plant since it grows almost everywhere. It has been moved from the Lily Family to the Asparagus Family.

Note that this is a different plant than true Solomon's Seal. You can easily tell them apart when flowering as False Solomon's Seal has terminal feathery flower clusters with red berries while Solomon's Seal carries their bell-shaped flowers and dark blue berries on the underside of their stem. It likes moist forests.

Identification: False Solomon's seal grows up to 3 feet (0.9m) tall from underground rhizomes, producing single unbranched arching stems with large leaves that are up to 6 inches (15 cm) long and half as wide. They have smooth margins and parallel veins. The stem is green, softly hairy and, when in flower, ends in a cluster of feathery white flowers. Each flower has 6 tepals, 6 stamens, a pistil, and short style. Their small star-shaped flowers appear in mid-spring. The flowers produce round, green fruits that turn red or red and purple-striped when mature. Each berry has a few seeds.

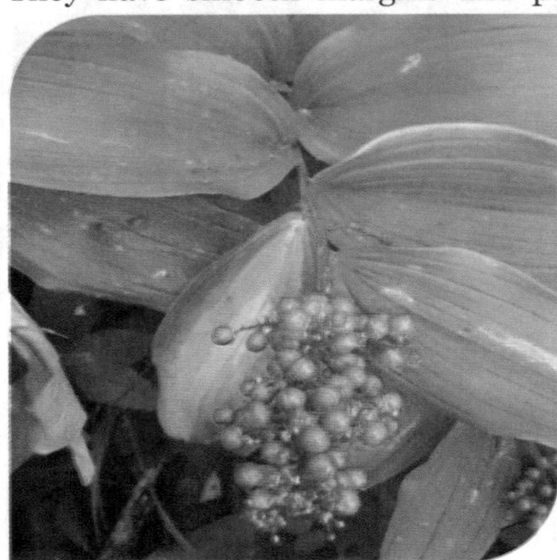

Edible Use: The fruit are eaten raw or cooked. They have a bitter-sweet flavor and are a good source of vitamin C. Eat in small quantities only, larger amounts have a laxative effect. Young shoots are eaten raw or cooked as a green vegetable. The roots are eaten cooked. Soak the root first in water, change the water and cook. Eat like potatoes.

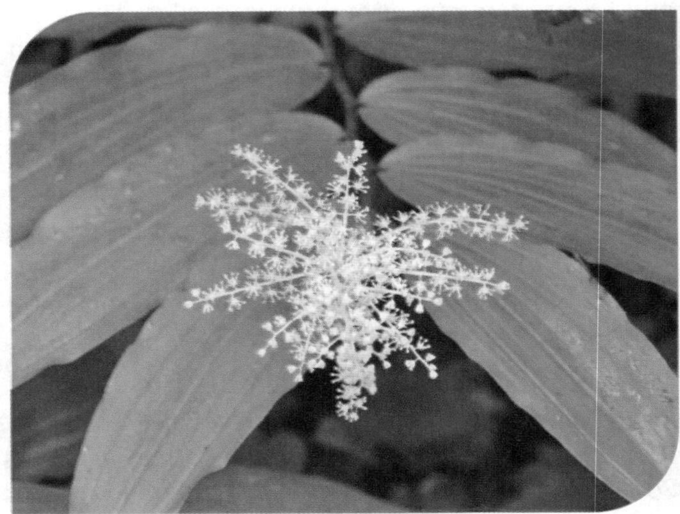

Medical Use: False Solomon's seal root is used medicinally for a variety of problems. The roots and leaves of False Solomon's seal are used to make tincture, salve, tea, or capsules. It is a lubricating plant and the rhizomes contain saponins.

Sore Throats and Oral Irritations: A strong root tea is valuable for sore throats and other mouth irritations. Try the root tea double in strength and use it to gargle several times a day until all irritation is gone.

Coughs: Make an infusion of leaves as a cough remedy. Sweeten with raw honey for extra soothing power.

Congestion: For bronchial congestion, try breathing in the steam while making a root decoction. Then use the decoction internally to treat symptoms.

Regulating the Menstrual Cycle and Hormonal Swings: False Solomon's Seal Root Tea or Root Tincture is used to regulate the menstrual cycle, to relieve symptoms of menstrual disorders, and help with swings in hormone levels.

Stomach Complaints: An infusion of the root is used to relieve stomach pain and soothe the digestive system.

Stop Bleeding and Treat Wounds: Use a poultice from the crushed leaves or root and apply it to wounds, scrapes, rashes, cuts, burns, and insect bites. Its anti-inflammatory nature reduces the irritation in the area and soothes the skin. Dried powdered root stops bleeding in skin wounds. You can also use the tea as an external wash.

Arthritis: To relieve arthritic pain and to reduce swelling in the joints, mix the dried powdered root with water to make a thick paste. Rub the paste on the affected joint. It acts as an analgesic and anti-inflammatory to help heal the joint. Taking an internal decoction of False Solomon's Seal leaves also soothes arthritic joints.

Harvesting: Harvest leaves, stems and berries by plucking them from the plant whenever they are available. Use only healthy leaves. Dig the rhizomes in autumn and slice them before drying for future us

False Unicorn Root, *Chamaelirium luteum*

False unicorn root is a similar plant to true unicorn root (also in this book) and has many of the same uses. The two plants are different with different dosages. It is in the Melanthiaceae (Bunchflower) Family. False unicorn root is also known as fairywant, helionas root, eratrum luteum, blazing star root, devil's bit, and starwort. The name varies with location. This herb grows in swampy areas east of the Mississippi River and in the southern states. In recent years, it has become hard to find and is possibly facing extinction. Take only the plants you need and replant it whenever possible.

Identification: False unicorn root grows low to the ground with stems 1 to 3 feet (0.3 to 0.9meters) long. Stems are smooth and angular and alternate leaves grow in a whorl at the base of the plant. The whorl consists of six leaves, each 3 to 6 inches (7.5 cm to 15 cm) long. The flowers are greenish-white, purple or lavender, formed into a dense terminal and appearing from May to June. The flowers are either male or female, with one sex per plant. The flower stalk of the female plant grows to be approximately 4 feet (1.2meters) tall. Fine, wiry pale roots grow from a bulbous rhizome.

Medicinal Use: False unicorn root can be taken as a tea, tincture, and dried root. Its uses are similar to those of True Unicorn Root, but the dosages are different.

Appropriate dosage for False Unicorn is 1 cup of tea, three times daily, or 2 to 4 ml of tincture three times a day, or 1/4 to 1/2 teaspoon of dried, powdered root, three times daily.

The Female Reproductive System: False Unicorn Root is one of the best tonics for the reproductive system and is equally beneficial for women and men. It regulates the female reproductive system and balances hormones, encouraging normal function and a regular menstrual cycle. It is used to treat missed menstrual periods and to relieve symptoms of menopause. It improves fertility and low sex drive in women. Do not use during pregnancy.

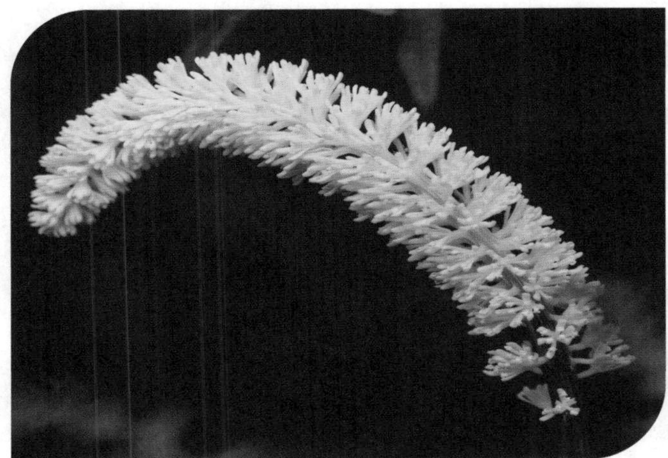

False Unicorn for Men: The hormonal balancing effects extend to men also, and many men report that it is useful in improving the symptoms of erectile dysfunction. For impotence, nocturnal emissions, and erectile dysfunction, the standard dose is 1/4 to 1/2 teaspoon of dried, powdered root, three times daily.

Sexually Transmitted Diseases: False Unicorn is used to treat gonorrhea and other STDs via a vaginal douche. Men can wash with the tea and take the powdered root orally.

Chronic Pelvic Inflammation and Vaginal Infections: False unicorn root combined with Echinacea angustifolia can treat chronic pelvic inflammation. It is used internally as well as externally as a douche to treat vaginal infections with good results.

Sore Throats: False Unicorn Root Tea treats a sore throat. Gargle with the tea hourly when a sore throat is present, though feedback is that you don't really need it that often. The gargle relieves the pain almost immediately, and the relief lasts for a few hours. Young patients can sip the tea, but no more than 3 cups should be taken daily.

Harvesting: Dig up the roots in the autumn as the plant is dying back and after the seeds have been released. This is important because the plant is being over-harvested and is facing extinction. Only take what you need. Clean and dry the root for future use. Store it in a cool, dry place for up to three years. Grind the root when ready to use.

Warning: Take only the recommended dosages; an excess can cause vomiting and nausea. Avoid taking it during pregnancy. False Unicorn Root is a cardiac toxin in large doses.

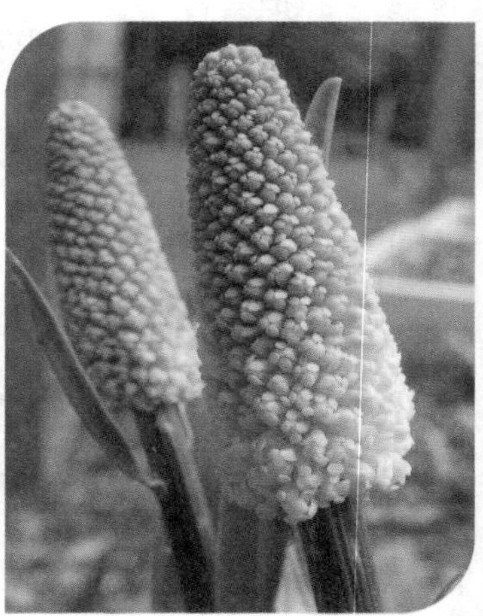

Recipes. False Unicorn Root Tea. 1 to 2 teaspoons of shredded root, 1 cup water. Put the root in the water and bring to a boil. Reduce the heat and simmer gently for 10 to 15 minutes. Drink the tea three times daily.

Fireweed, *Chamaenerion or Chamerion angustifolium; (Epilobium angustifolium)*

Fireweed got its name because it is most often the first plant to return after a fire. Its underground runners are able to withstand the fire and quickly bounce back. Also known as Willow Herb. It is in the Onagraceae (Evening Primrose) Family.

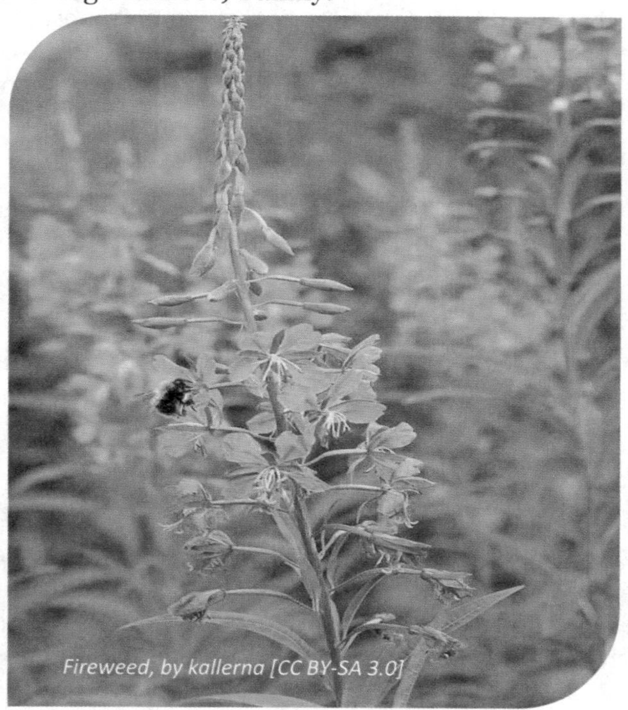

Fireweed, by kallerna [CC BY-SA 3.0]

Identification: The plant is often found in full sun on disturbed land, after a forest fire, or on recently cleared land. Fireweed grows to 8 feet (2.4m) tall and produces gorgeous purple or pink flowers on spikes. Each flower has four petals like its evening primrose relatives. The long, alternate, lance-shaped leaves are green with a silvery underside and a central vein. The purple fruits are long and narrow, opening to release seeds attached to feathery white tufts that carry them on the wind. Fireweed also spreads underground, forming large patches that are connected by underground roots.

Edible Use: Firewood shoots are edible and nutritious eaten raw or cooked. Harvest them in the spring while young and tender or peel the fibrous skin off older shoots. Young leaves can be eaten like spinach and the flowers and fruits can be eaten raw and used as a carbohydrate extender.

Medicinal Use: Fireweed is anti-inflammatory and very astringent. It has antifungal properties and helps build a healthy gut.

Digestive Tract, Colitis, Irritable Bowel Syndrome, *Candida*, Leaky Gut: Fireweed Leaf Tea helps build a healthy intestinal tract. It encourages healthy bacteria colonies while preventing and correcting the overgrowth of fungus and *Candida*. With a healthy intestinal tract comes better food absorption and better digestion. The herb has a mild laxative effect, keeping food moving easily through the system and improving muscle tone in the gut. Its antispasmodic properties treat intestinal spasms and chronic diarrhea. Fireweed leaf tea, decoction, or tincture treats colitis and IBS.

Lung Congestion and Sore Throats: Fireweed is high in mucilage and has anti-spasmodic properties that make it useful for treating lung problems, asthma, coughs, and bronchial spasms. The mucilage soothes a sore throat.

Anti-inflammatory: Fireweed is an anti-inflammatory. It is ideal for long term use where inflammation is chronic.

Migraines: Fireweed Tincture is used for migraines. Take as soon as the headache begins and up to 3 times daily as needed. Butterbur and Feverfew also work well for migraines, as does magnesium.

Skin Problems: Both the leaves and flowers are soothing to the skin and are useful in treating inflammatory skin problems as well as those caused by bacteria or fungal infections. Use a Fireweed Decoction as a wash or compress on psoriasis, eczema, acne, skin rashes, wounds, infections, and burns.

Harvesting: Harvest young shoots in the spring and early summer while the leaves are close to the stem and point upward. Young leaves can be harvested individually for edible use. Flower buds are edible. If you harvest when the plant is in flower simply pinch off leaves that are vibrant green and healthy looking. Air dry the leaves or use a dehydrator on low. Store in a cool, dark, and dry place. Harvest roots in the summer and autumn and mash them to make a soothing poultice.

Recipes: Fireweed Leaf Tea: Add several fireweed leaves to a cup of boiling water and let it steep for about 15 minutes. Remove the leaves and enjoy. Use up to three cups daily.

Fireweed Tincture: You'll need: 4 ounces (113g) fresh fireweed leaves and flowers, 8 ounces (250ml) 80 proof vodka, brandy, or other drinking alcohol and a clean, sterile glass jar and tight-fitting lid. Chop and pound the fireweed herb to a pulp and put into a glass jar. Mix in the alcohol slowly, stirring to spread the herb throughout the alcohol. Cap. Place the jar in a cool, dry place for 5 to 6 weeks, shaking daily. Strain the pulp from the liquid and place the tincture in a clean jar. Cover tightly, label and date. Store the tincture in a cool, dark place for 3 to 5 years.

Fireweed Decoction: Ingredients: 2 ounces (56g) of fireweed leaves, 1-quart (1 Liter) of water. Bring the water and leaves to a boil and turn off the heat. Steep the decoction for 30 minutes. Strain the mixture and store in the refrigerator for up to 3 days. Take 2 ounces (60ml) every four to 6 hours or as needed or use the decoction as a wash or in a compress directly on the skin.

Goldenseal, *Hydrastis canadensis*

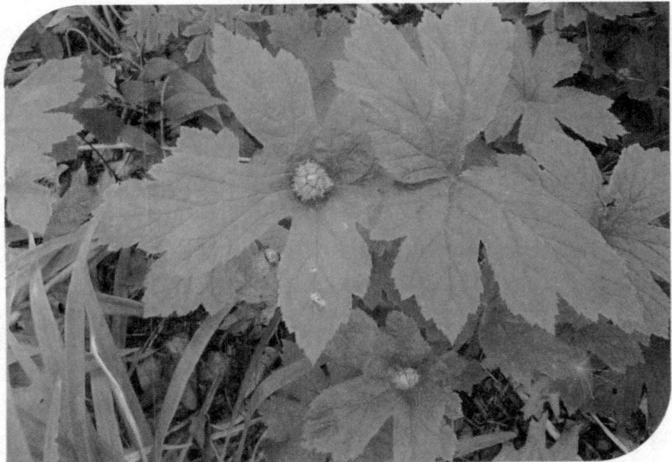

Goldenseal often seems like a cure-all. It is as an anti-inflammatory, an anti-microbial, and an immune booster. *Hydrastis canadensis* is also known as Orangeroot or Yellow Puccoon. Goldenseal is in the Buttercup family, Ranunculaceae, though its leaves and fruit somewhat resemble those of the Raspberry and the *Rubus* genus. Goldenseal is commonly found in rich, moist, shady forests, under hardwood trees. Goldenseal grows across eastern North America.

Identification: Goldenseal has a thick knotty, yellowish-brown rhizome that is approximately 2 inches (5 cm) long and ½ inch (1.25 cm) thick with a lot of rootlets. The plant grows 6 to 12 (15 cm to 30 cm) inches tall. It has a strong odor and bitter taste. It produces a fruit similar to the raspberry in appearance, but the fruit is not edible. The plant is easily distinguished from other Ranunculaceae family members during the flowering period as it has only 2 deeply alternate palmately-lobed leaves on the stem and solitary white flowers that have no petals.

It flowers from approximately late April through early May. Its single flowers have numerous white protruded stamens. The 3 sepals fall as the flower opens. Its basal leaf is usually solitary and quickly falls off leaving just the two cauline leaves. They are toothed, 5-lobed with ridged veins, and are 1 to 4 inches (2.5 cm to 10 cm) when the flower opens, but grow to 12 inches (30 cm). Its fruits first appear green and then ripen into a bright red aggregate of achenes. These are visible from mid to late summer.

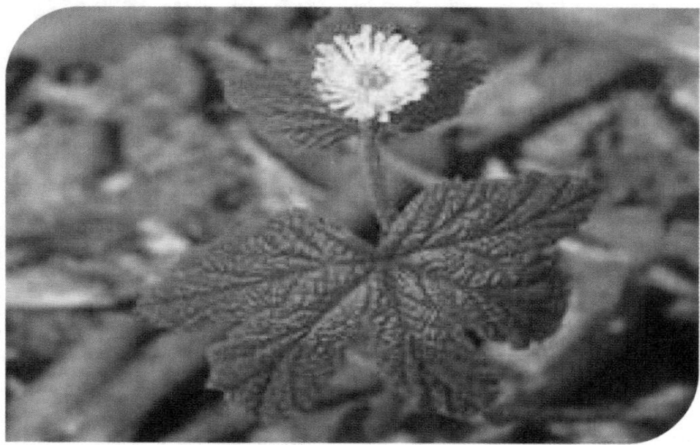

Goldenseal, Luiscoronel, CC by SA 3.0

Medicinal Use: The root is used for medicine. Dosage depends on the size of the person and the degree of illness. Use smaller doses as a preventative. Do not use if you have an autoimmune disorder.

Use Goldenseal in Combination with Other Herbs: Goldenseal is often combined with Echinacea. Goldenseal boosts the effects of many other herbs.

Respiratory Issues, Colds, and Flu: Goldenseal reduces irritation and inflammation of the mucous membranes, making it an ideal addition for the treatment of respiratory problems. It is also anti-microbial and anti-viral. For colds, the flu, and other respiratory problems its efficacy is well established.

Bacterial and Viral Infections: The anti-microbial properties of goldenseal root are effective against many bacterial infections including vaginal infections, infectious diarrhea, colds and flu, eye infections, and urinary tract infections.

Goldenseal root is used for bacterial and viral infections. Goldenseal infusion can be used as a douche. Infections respond well to both internal and external use of goldenseal extract.

Skin Eruptions: Topical application of goldenseal root treats skin ulcers, boils, rashes, and general skin irritations. For extensive skin infections or rashes, add internal goldenseal root powder taken for up to three weeks. Extensive or chronic problems may require multiple rounds of goldenseal, each followed by a week off. Mouth ulcers like canker sores and other irritations to the mucous membranes of the mouth can be treated effectively using this herb.

Cleanse Body Toxins: Goldenseal helps remove toxins from the body and purify the kidneys and urinary tract. Often used in combination with other herbs for this purpose.

Lower Blood Sugar Levels in Diabetics: Goldenseal helps boost the production of insulin in diabetics and lowers blood sugar levels. Monitor diabetics carefully when giving goldenseal because some have had elevated blood pressure as a result of taking goldenseal. When blood pressure is a problem, choose a different treatment.

Goldenseal will not replace injected insulin, but it does encourage the body to produce more insulin so that the Type 2 diabetics may be able to reduce their insulin doses over time.

Yeast and Fungal Infections: Goldenseal treats yeast infections, athlete's foot, and skin irritations caused by fungi and bacteria, such as acne. Treat the affected area by applying goldenseal extract to the problem area.

Bleeding: Goldenseal powder applied to wounds helps stop or control bleeding. It is also used internally for controlling heavy menstrual bleeding and internal bleeding. It tones the blood vessels, reducing bleeding quickly.

Harvesting: Harvest goldenseal in the autumn after the plant has died back. Look for older plants with large rhizomes. Take care when digging roots to keep the rhizomes intact. Leave as many of the fibrous roots behind as possible to reestablish the plants.

Warning: People with autoimmune conditions should not use goldenseal internally as it is an immune-system booster and may lead to a flare-up. Watch blood sugar and blood pressure closely when using goldenseal, because it can lower blood sugars and raise blood pressure.

Goldenseal Extract: 1/2 cup Goldenseal root, ground into a powder, 2 cups of distilled water. Nonreactive pot: stainless steel or enamel. Bring the water to a boil and add the goldenseal powder. Reduce the heat to a low simmer. Simmer the mixture until the water is reduced by one quarter, leaving 1 1/2 cups of liquid in the pot. Allow the mixture to cool to room temperature, then strain out the root. Store the mixture in the refrigerator for up to 3 days or divide into small portions and store in the freezer for longer periods.

Horsetail, *Equisetum arvense*

Horsetail is often considered a weed, one that is particularly hard to exterminate. I rejoice at the sight of this herb. It grows easily and spreads in almost any soil. It spreads by spores rather than seeds. Its high silica content makes its scouring ability useful to gently clean your teeth or wash your dishes. I have used it for both.

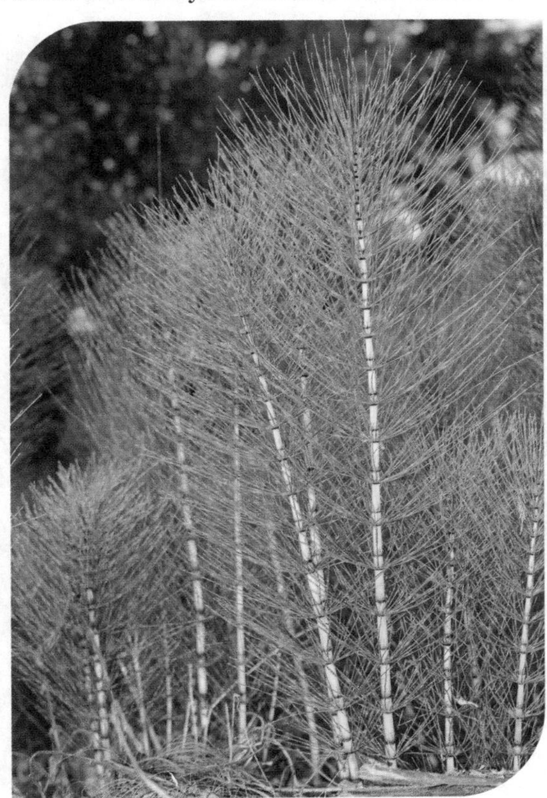

Identification: Also known as snake grass, puzzle grass, bottlebrush, and mare's tale, common horsetail is an unusual looking plant. The leaves are not true leaves and do not conduct photosynthesis. They are arranged in whorls fused into nodal sheaths. Photosynthesis happens in the hollow green stems. The stems are jointed and have 3 to 40 ridges. There may be whorls of branches at the nodes. This perennial plant has no flowers and produces no seeds. It reproduces entirely by spores.

Edible Use: The early spring fertile shoots (tan in color) of both Giant Horsetail (*Equisetum telmateia*) and Common Horsetail can be peeled and eaten raw. The green infertile shoots are cooked and eaten like asparagus. They are bitter, especially as they age. Do not eat them raw. Changing the water three to four times during cooking helps relieve the bitter flavor. The roots can be eaten raw, but they are difficult to collect in quantity, so they usually are eaten only in a starvation situation.

Medicinal Use: The green vegetative stalks of Horsetail are extremely high in silica, which benefits joints and connective tissue. It is a gentle diuretic, astringent, and styptic.

Bleeding and Healing Wounds: The plant's styptic properties make it useful in healing wounds and stopping bleeding. Collect the barren stems or tops and apply directly to the wound. It is also useful to treat excessive menstruation when taken as a supplement.

Promotes Healthy Bones, Hair, and Teeth: Because it contains high amounts of silica, it promotes strong hair, teeth, and bones and increases bone density in people with osteoporosis when used consistently. It can also be made into a strengthening conditioning wash for the hair. A tooth powder of Horsetail helps with cavities and enamel repair.

Kidney Problems and Edema: Horsetail is a diuretic, helping to rid the body of excess fluids and salts. It is useful for treating related kidney problems and edemas but it is not for long-term use. It promotes the elimination of uric acid, preventing or reducing the formation of kidney stones.

Alleviates Signs of Aging: The silica in horsetail stimulates the production of collagen, which is important in the skin aging process. It helps prevent fine lines and wrinkles and promotes healthy hair. It can be used internally, externally as a toner, or added to a topical cream or salve.

Treats Infections: Horsetail has anti-inflammatory, anti-fungal, and antimicrobial properties that help to prevent and treat infections. Treat skin infections with a warm compress or poultice made of the crushed, dried herb. Use two to three times daily.

Foot Fungus and Infections: Soak the feet in water infused with a generous portion of horsetail powder. Soak the feet for 15 minutes daily to treat an infection and every other day to prevent infections.

Nasal Congestion, Bronchitis, and Respiratory Ailments: Boil horsetail tea and inhale the vapors or use horsetail tea in your steam humidifier. Inhaling the herb vapors can help alleviate nasal and bronchial congestion. It acts as an expectorant and strengthens the immune system while relieving the inflammation.

Sore Throat: Make a gargle with salt water, horsetail powder, and lemon juice for a sore throat. Gargle several times a day until symptoms disappear.

Bladder Problems, Urinary Tract Infections, and Frequent Urination: Take a capsule of horsetail powder, up to 2 grams, three times daily to relieve bladder problems and frequent urination caused by urinary tract infections. It is also helpful to soak in a bath containing horsetail powder. Soak for at least 15 minutes, several times weekly.

Boosts Immunity and Relieves Inflammation: The antibacterial and antiseptic properties of horsetail products boost the body's immunity and protects against invasion by pathogens that can infect the body. It also relieves inflammation throughout the body. Take horsetail tea or horsetail powder in capsule form regularly for best effects.

Increases Brain Function and Cognition: The antioxidants in horsetail increase cognitive abilities by increasing the neural pathways. It is said to increase cognitive abilities and is used for people with dementia and Alzheimer's disease. Try horsetail powder in capsule form.

Treats Diabetes: Horsetail supplements and Horsetail Tea act to balance insulin levels in the body, lowering blood sugar and preventing the peaks and valleys common in diabetes. Use horsetail as a temporary diabetes management when necessary. Not for long term use.

Harvesting: For medicine, harvest the green vegetative stalks spring through early summer when the leaves are still "up" and bright green. You can also snip the tops off in summer.

Warning: Use horsetail moderately and for a limited time only. Overuse can have side effects, which tend to occur after two or more months of use. Long-term use can cause side effects including: thiamine deficiency, potassium deficiency, lowered blood sugar levels, nicotine toxicity, and kidney irritation. Do not consume horsetail if you are pregnant or lactating. Avoid using *Equisetum palustre* (Marsh Horsetail), as it has slight toxicity. Be careful where you collect Horsetail as it collects toxins, especially in agricultural areas.

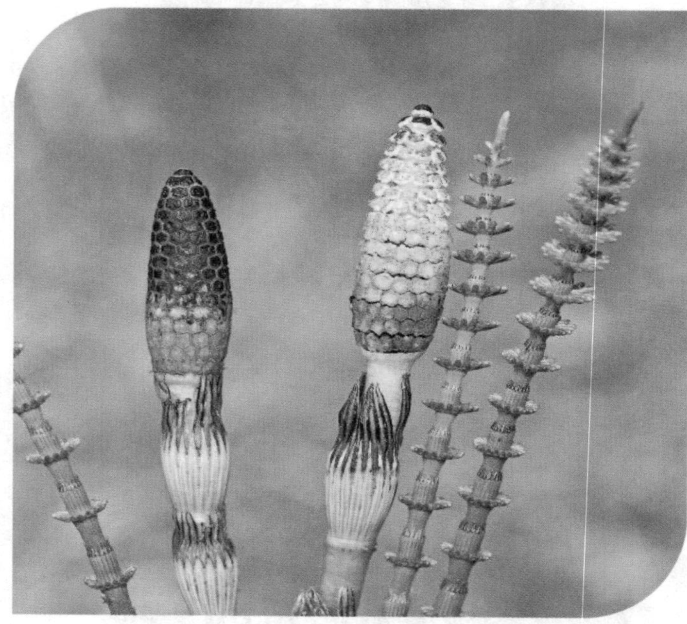

Recipes: Horsetail Tea: Ingredients: 2 to 3 teaspoons of horsetail, 1 cup spring water, raw honey (optional). Pour water over the herb bring to a boil. Boil for 5 minutes, then allow it to infuse for another 15 minutes. For treating bone health problems, allow the tea to boil longer to extract more silica. Strain and sweeten to taste with raw honey.

Kudzu, *Pueraria lobata, P. thunbergiana*

Farmers began importing Kudzu in the 1930's and 40's, hoping that the plant would control soil erosion and provide fodder for cattle. Kudzu grows very fast and was a major agricultural problem in the South in the 1960's, and early 70's. It has been fought back and is no longer as prevalent as it once was. However, many patches still exist. Luckily almost the entire plant is edible. It is a legume in the Fabaceae (Pea) Family.

Identification: Kudzu is a twining and trailing perennial vine that grows quickly and covers everything in its path. Folks in the south joke that if you go on vacation, your house may be completely swallowed by the time you get back. It is a familiar sight to find kudzu covering abandoned houses, telephone poles, trees, and fields.

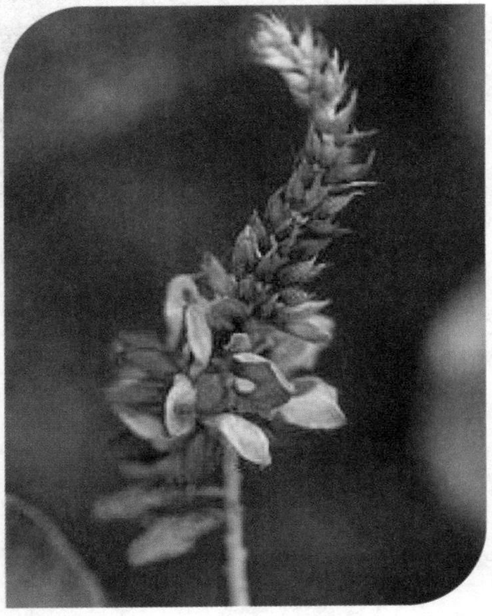

Leaves are grouped into formations of three leaflets at each node. Each leaflet has its own stalk or petiole. The central leaf has 3 lobes and a petiole that is about 3/4 inch (1 cm) long. The leaves on either side have shorter petioles and usually 2 lobes. Leaves may not have any lobes or may have many more. The leaves are medium-green and grow to be about 5 to 6 inches (12.5 cm to 15 cm) long and are covered in very fine hairs. The vines are long and covered in small bristles that help it climb and cling to vertical surfaces. The vines grow rapidly and become thick and woody as they mature. The vines also grow horizontally, putting down roots at each node.

In August or September, purple or reddish-purple flowers appear in clusters. Each cluster is up to 8 inches (20 cm) long and emerges from the central petiole of a leaf trio. Bean-shaped seed pods of approximately 2 inches (5 cm) in length form from each flower cluster. They are greenish-bronze when mature and covered with fine hairs and turn brown when dried.

Edible Use: The leaves, vine tips, flowers, and roots are all edible. The vine stems are not. The roots contain starch and can be roasted and eaten like potatoes, or dried and powdered to make a starch much like cornstarch. The flowers make a delicious jelly.

Medicinal Use: Kudzu root is easily dried and powdered and is the part used for medicine.

Estrogen-like Effects: Kudzu root has estrogen-like effects that are beneficial for pre-menopausal and post-menopausal women.

It alleviates the symptoms of menopause including headaches, hot flashes, and irregular bleeding.

Heart Problems, Cardiovascular System: Kudzu root decoction is useful for increasing blood flow in the body by expanding the arteries and vessels. It increases oxygen supply to the brain and body. It lowers blood pressure and reduces chances of clotting and strokes. It is also a potent weapon against myocardial ischemia.

Relieves Digestive Spasms: Kudzu root soothes digestive spasms and helps treat digestive cramping, Crohn's disease, and Irritable Bowel Syndrome. It works for both acute and chronic conditions.

Measles: Kudzu reduces the infection rate and shortens cases of measles. It also works as a preventative for family members. People who take kudzu root get well faster than those who do not.

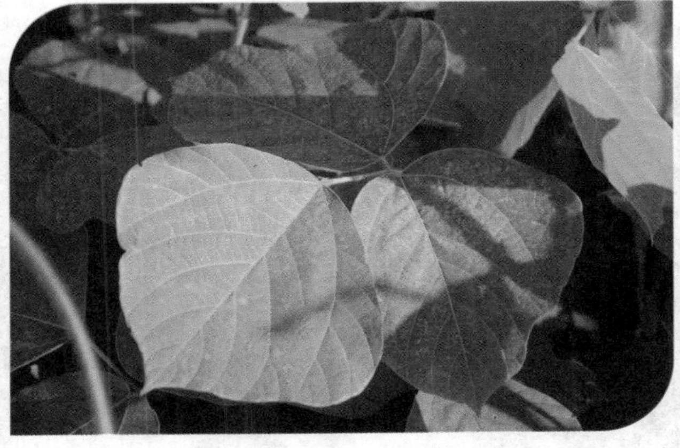

Kudzu leaves, Bubba73 (Jud McCranie) - Own work, CC by SA 3.0

Diabetes: Kudzu root, taken three times daily, helps stabilize blood sugar levels and improves glucose metabolism.

Alcoholism: Kudzu consumption decreases an individual's desire for alcohol. Even a single dose significantly curbs alcohol consumption and may work well for treating people who binge drink or who are alcoholics.

Recipes: Kudzu Decoction: 60 grams dried kudzu root, chopped, 3 cup water. Combine the water and kudzu root and bring to a boil. Lower the heat and simmer for 15 minutes. Turn off the heat and cover tightly. Let the kudzu steep for another 30 minutes. The decoction will be thick. Take 1/3 cup of the decoction, three times a day. Store the remaining decoction in the refrigerator for up to 3 days.

Indian Tobacco, *Lobelia inflata*

Called Indian Tobacco because of its use among Native Americans, this herb is also known as pokeweed, pukeweed, gagroot, vomitwort, asthma weed, and bladderpod. Each seems to refer to one of the properties of the herb, making them easy to remember. It is in the Campanulaceae (Bellflower) Family.

Identification: Indian Tobacco grows to heights of 1 to 2 feet (0.3m to 0.6m), and is erect with a sporadically leaved stem. The stem is angular with white hairs that are less abundant on the upper part, making the stems smooth towards the top, and feathery and rough near the bottom.

The pale green or yellowish leaves of the Indian Tobacco plant grow alternately and become smaller as they ascend the stem. These stems have tiny white dots scattered along the margin and are finely spiked. The upper part of the leaf is almost hairless while the lower part is hairy along the major veins. The delicate flowers of Indian Tobacco are pale bluish to violet in color with a touch of yellow. These flowers are tiny, asymmetrical, and bisexual.

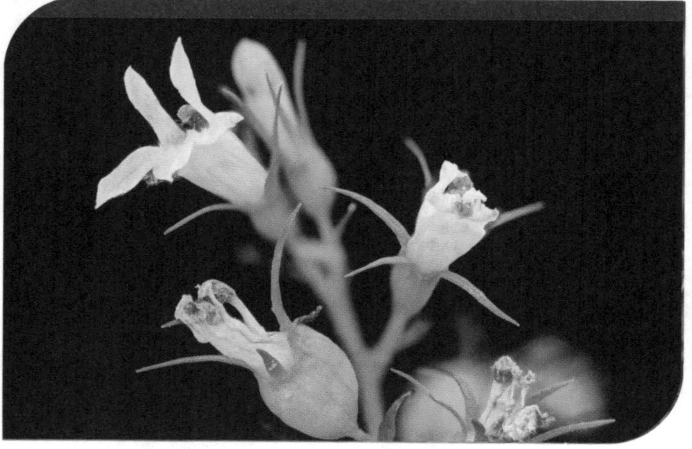

Edible Use: Indian tobacco is not edible, but the leaves are used for flavoring in brewed beverages. They have a mildly bitter taste.

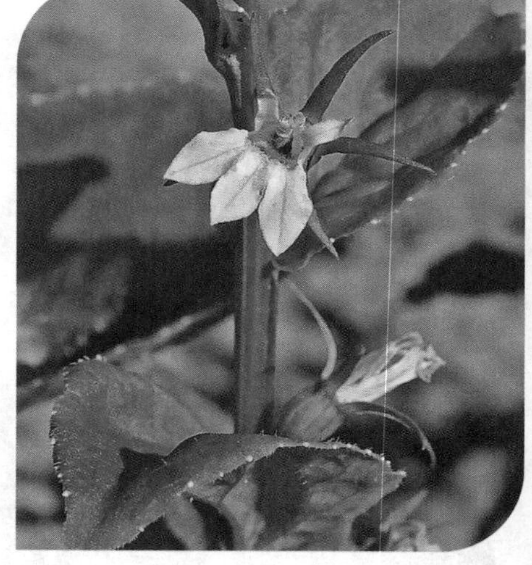

Indian Tobacco, By H. Zell - Own work, CC BY-SA 3.0

Medicinal Use: Many medicinal uses call for Indian Tobacco powder. It can be consumed straight, put into a little water, or packed into a capsule. Traditional use was to smoke the leaves, bur be aware of toxicity and potentially harmful effects. Its aerial parts (leaves, seedpods, flowers, and seeds) are primarily used for medicine. Roots are sometimes used externally.

Respiratory Problems: *Lobelia inflata* treats respiratory disorders such as chronic bronchitis, asthma, pleurisy, and pneumonia. The leaves can be smoked, used as a tea, or swallowed as a powder in a little water to release phlegm from the respiratory system.

Stop Smoking: Some people have found success kicking the nicotine habit using Indian tobacco. Lobeline, found in this plant and similar to nicotine, helps with nicotine withdrawal. It is rarely a successful strategy since this Lobelia also contains addictive substances when used regularly.

Antidepressant: *Lobelia inflata* raises the mood of people with anxiety disorders, dysthymia, eating disorders, OCD, and major depressive disorders.

Body Aches, Muscle and Joint Pain: A decoction or a salve made from the roots of *Lobelia inflata* treats tennis elbow, whiplash injuries, arthritis, and other muscle and joint pain. Apply the salve or decoction directly to the skin over the painful area and rub it in or make a poultice from the roots and rub it into the aching body parts.

Minor Skin Irritations: For minor skin irritations, sores, and boils, make a decoction of boiled crushed roots and use it to wash the affected area, leaving it on to dry in place.

Relaxing the Neuromuscular System: Indian tobacco is nervine and antispasmodic. It relaxes the nerves, calms muscle spasms, and helps with relaxation.

Inducing Vomiting: To release poisons or recently ingested harmful substances from the body, Indian tobacco, also known as vomitwort, is excellent. Use a concentrated tincture form to induce vomiting.

Harvesting: Harvest in the early summer. Wear gloves to avoid the tiny, spiky hairs that prickle your hands. Collect flowers, leaves, seeds, and roots from the plant. Dry before use.

Warning: Due to its lobeline content, *Lobelia inflata* is considered toxic if taken large quantities. Start with small doses and slowly increase the dosage as needed and only if necessary. Side effects are uncommon, but anyone can develop allergies or reactions without warning. Due to its similarities to nicotine, it may be toxic to susceptible individuals, including people with cardiac diseases, children, and pregnant women. Excessive use of this herb will cause vomiting and nausea.

Recipes: Indian Tobacco Decoction: 1-ounce ground root or leaves, 1-quart (1Liter) distilled water. Bring the water to a boil in a non-reactive pot. Add the ground root. Reduce the heat to a very low simmer and cover the pot tightly. Simmer the root mixture for 20 minutes. Remove from the heat. Strain the decoction and discard the root. Keep the decoction in the refrigerator for up to 3 days or freeze it in portions for longer storage. Use topically (roots and/or leaves) or take up 1/4 cup internally (leaves).

Jewelweed, *Impatiens capensis*

Orange jewelweed, also known as garden balsam, jewel balsam weed, and touch-me-not, is a member of the Balsaminaceae (Touch-Me-Not) Family. There are several varieties, including Impatiens capensis, which are medicinally active.

Impatiens are an attractive garden plant popular for their beauty. Their showy flowers attract butterflies and hummingbirds. Jewelweed is often found in moist soil and shady places. Look for it along creek beds, near streams, and at the edge of the woods. It is found throughout most of the United States with the exception of Montana, Wyoming, California, and the southwest.

Identification: Jewelweed is named for its seeds and leaves. Ripe seedpods "pop" when touched, giving it the name Touch-Me-Not. Dew and rain beads up on the leaves, looking like "jewels", hence the name "jewelweed".

Leaves are bluish-green in color, oval or lance shaped, and coarsely toothed. Lower leaves are opposite, while upper leaves are alternate.

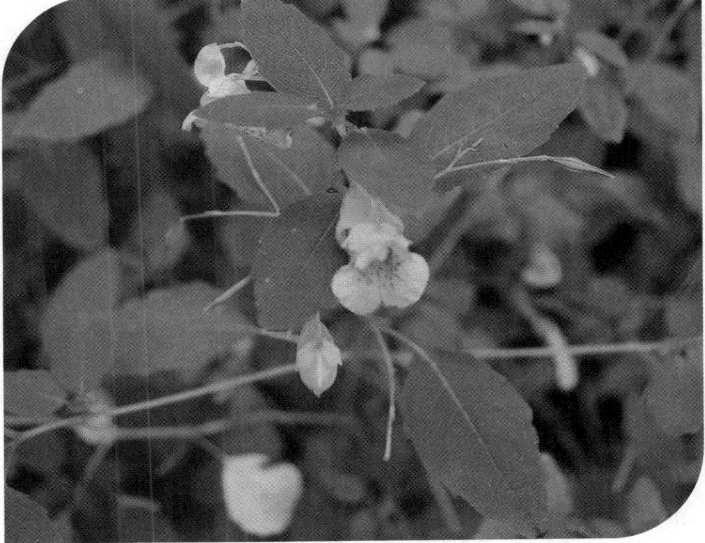

Jewelweed blooms from May through October and produces two kinds of flowers. Showy orange trumpet shaped flowers hang from thin stems. They are about an inch in length and have mottled reddish-brown spots inside the throat of the trumpet. The second flower type is a tiny petal-free flower that stays closed. This small, petal-free flower produces most of the seed pods and has five flaps which, when ripe, open and eject their seeds.

The plant branches extensively, producing smooth, round stems. The entire plant grows to approximately 3 to 5 feet tall (0.9m – 1.5m) and leaves are up to 3.5 inches long (6cm).

Edible Use: Jewelweed is edible, in moderation, but it should be cooked before use. Large portions can have a laxative effect.

The seed pods explode when touched and the small seeds inside can be toasted and eaten. The flavor is similar to walnuts.

The flowers are edible raw in salads or can be cooked in a stir-fry. The stems and leaves should always be boiled for 10 to 20 minutes, changing the water at least twice during cooking. The stems and leaves have high concentrations of oxalates and should be avoided by people prone to kidney stones.

Medicinal Use. Poison Ivy, Poison Oak, Okra Spines, and Stinging Nettle: Jewelweed often grows near poison ivy and stinging nettle, which is fortunate since it is an ideal antidote to the painful sting and rash caused by these plants.

The easiest way to use it is to slice open the stem and rub the juicy inside on all exposed areas. Immediate use is best and stops the irritation and prevents poison ivy rash in most people.

However, I also recommend cutting extra to take home to use again after a thorough shower. The plant can also be made into an infusion, soap, salve, or spray to treat rashes.

The liquid inside the jewelweed stem contains a chemical that neutralizes the urushiol oil contained in poison ivy. Urushiol oil spreads easily and rapidly, transferring the rash to other parts of the body.

Once neutralized with jewelweed, the rash is no longer contagious and will no longer spread. Blisters that have already appeared should heal within a few days.

Jewelweed is a natural herbal remedy for other irritating plants as well. Poison oak, okra spines, and stinging nettles respond well to jewelweed. It is useful to treat acne, eczema, heat rash, ringworm, warts, sores and other skin irritations.

Anti-fungal: Jewelweed's stems and leaves are a good external anti-fungal and treats athlete's foot, ringworm, and other fungal infections.

Bruises, Burns, Eczema, Insect Bites: For skin damaged by bruises, burns and insect bites, try a poultice. Crush the stem of the plant and apply it directly to the affected area or soak a cloth in the juices of the plant and apply it to the area.

Other Medicinal Uses: Traditionally, jewelweed has been used as an aid for kidney, liver, and urinary tract conditions. It has also been used as a diuretic, to promote blood flow after childbirth, and for gastrointestinal upset.

However, most herbalists do not use jewelweed internally and evidence is lacking for many of these traditional uses.

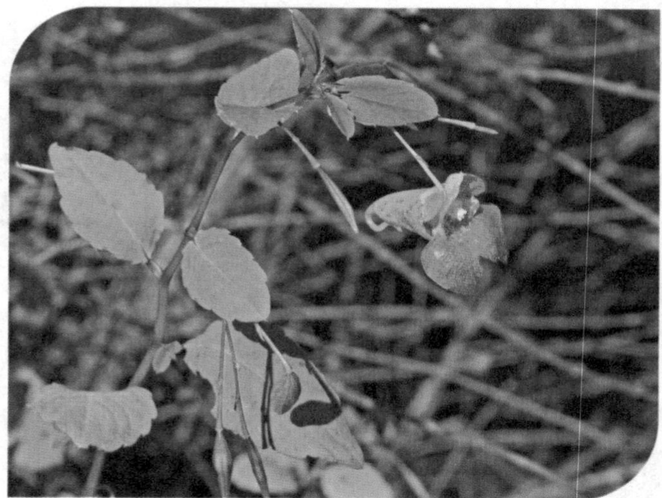

Recipes. Jewelweed Infusion: Chopped jewelweed, boiling water. Chop the stems of orange jewelweed and drop into boiling water. Boil the infusion until the water turns dark orange. Cool the liquid, strain it, and freeze it in ice cubes to use on skin rashes as a cooling and healing rub. Freeze for up to 1 year. The infusion can be stored frozen or it can be canned in a pressure cooker. Jewelweed does not dry well because of its high oil content.

Warning: Both Jewelweed and Potentilla are commonly known as silverweed. Be careful not to confuse the plants. Jewelweed can be used topically or as a water extraction, but do not use it in alcohol tinctures.

Use jewelweed in small amounts and dilute water extracts before using. Concentrated solutions can cause reddening of the skin and irritation.

Maidenhair Fern, *Adiantum capillus-veneris* and *A. pedatum*

Maidenhair fern, also known as rock fern and Venus-hair fern, is native to much of North America and down into Central America and South America. It likes warm damp climates and is most often found in the moist soil of rainforests, woodlands, and along streams.

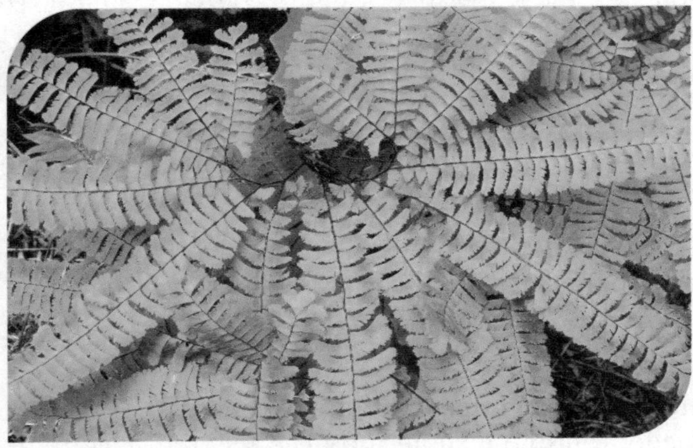

Identification: It grows to 6 to 12 inches (15 cm to 30 cm) tall with clusters of fronds growing from creeping rhizomes. The light green fronds are subdivided into pinnae less than 1/2-inch (1.25 cm) long. The main leaf stalk is thin, black, and polished while its fine stalks are as thin as a hair, giving it a very delicate look.

Medicinal Use: Leaves and rhizomes are used for medicine and are a weak anti-bacterial. The rhizomes have antioxidants.

Respiratory Issues, Bronchitis, Congestion, Sore Throats: Maidenhair fern leaves make a good treatment for coughs and mild respiratory problems like bronchitis, nasal congestion, and sore throats. It is a mild diuretic, and reduces excess mucus. It is also an astringent, anti-tussive, and mild expectorant. Try making a syrup with maidenhair fern leaves. Recipe below.

Urinary Issues, Gallstones, Heartburn, Digestive Disorders: Maidenhair Fern Syrup is useful for the treatment of urinary tract and digestive disorders.

It helps remove toxins from the digestive tract and protects the mucous membranes from irritation. It combines well with red mulberry for the treatment of urinary tract problems.

Circulatory System and Arteriosclerosis: Try an alcohol tincture or a strong decoction of maidenhair fern leaves to treat circulatory problems. It helps open up blocked veins and improves blood circulation to the body.

The infusion is also useful for shrinking varicose veins and hemorrhoids and treating varicose ulcers.

Apply the decoction directly to the affected areas of the body and take the tincture internally as well.

Recipes: Maidenhair Fern Syrup: 1 cup maidenhair fern leaves, dried and crumbled, 1-pint (500ml) water, 1 cup raw honey. Bring the fern leaves and water to a boil and simmer for 5 minutes.

Cover tightly and turn off the heat. Allow the decoction to steep for 3 hours. Strain out the herb and reheat the decoction until hot but not boiling. Add the raw honey and stir until it is fully dissolved. Pour the syrup into a sterile glass jar and store in the refrigerator for up to 2 months.

Standard Dosage: Add 1 to 2 tablespoons to a small amount of water or juice and take 3 times daily.

Male Fern, *Dryopteris filix-mas*

This wood fern grows in shaded, damp soils under the canopy throughout much of Europe, Asia and North and South America. Be careful to correctly identify this fern as it has look-alikes.

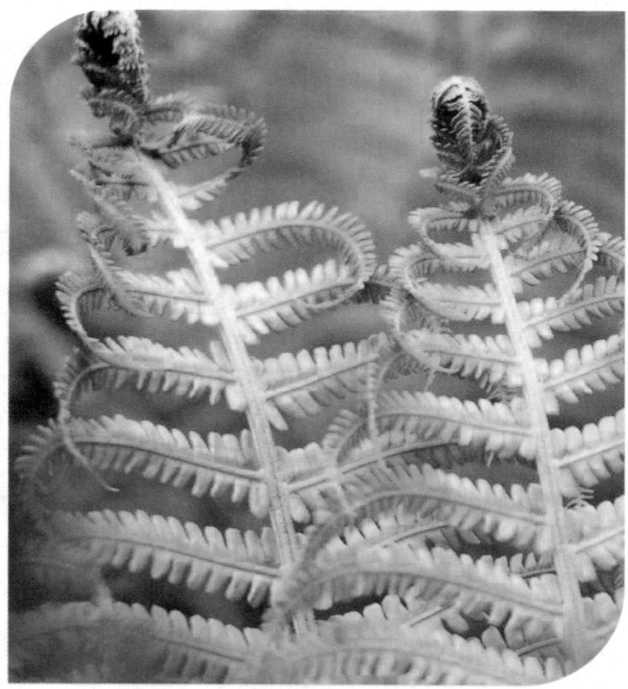

Identification: The Male Fern is a large fern with graceful bands of fronds. It grows to 4 feet (1.2m) in height. The plant does not flower but reproduces by spores and rhizomes. The slowly creeping rootstock forms a crown at the soil surface with a ring of fronds. It grows quite wide and becomes crowded over time, a distinguishing characteristic.

The dull green leaves are usually upright, 8 to 30 inches (10 cm to 75 cm) long, and 4 to 12 inches (10 cm to 30 cm) wide, with its widest section at its middle. They have 20 to 30 pairs of deeply divided tapering leaflets growing on the main stem. The bark on each frond is usually hidden but is dark brown in color. This plant has no smell.

Edible Use: The leaves and roots of the male fern are edible. Cooked young leaves taste like asparagus or artichoke. They should be eaten in moderation, as in large quantities they can be toxic. The rhizomes can be eaten raw or cooked and are sometimes used as a weight-loss strategy. Use with caution.

Medicinal Use: The roots are used internally as a tea or through ingestion. Do not use an alcoholic tincture or oil infusion internally, only externally.

Treating Tapeworms: Treating tapeworms and other parasites is probably the most common way that people use male fern medicinally. Use the rootstalks to paralyze parasites and thus purge them from the body. To use this remedy, eat the root after fasting for at least a few hours. The roots contain oleo-resins, filicin, and filmarone, all of which work to eradicate parasites. It works for pets as well but be careful with dosage for both humans and pets. Do not ingest oils, fats, or alcohols while using this. A light laxative is often used alongside this treatment. Use with great caution.

Colds and Viruses, Fevers, Mumps: The roots of male fern have anti-viral and antibacterial properties. They lower fevers and help heal the body from viral and bacterial diseases.

Hemorrhage: Male fern root is useful for the treatment of internal hemorrhage and uterine bleeding.

Boils, Sores, and Other Skin Conditions: Skin infections and irritations such as boils, carbuncles, sores, and abscesses are treated with a tincture made from the male fern root. Apply the tincture directly onto the affected area. Use this tincture externally only.

Harvesting: Harvest roots in the autumn. Dry for later use.

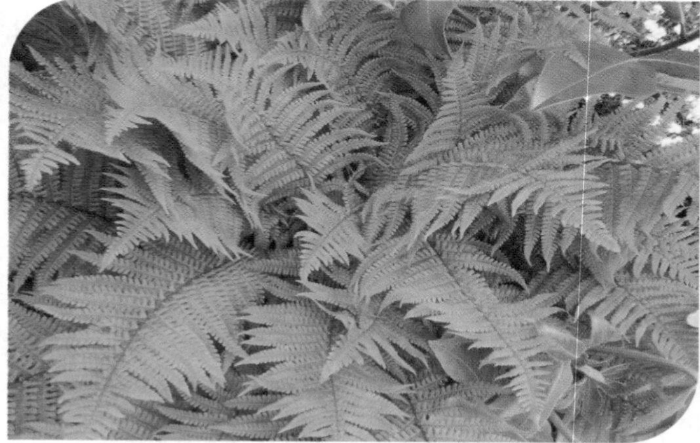

Warning: Caution is advised. Use it in moderation and be very careful with dosage. Best used under medical supervision. Do not use if pregnant or if you have heart issues. Do not take with oil, fats, or alcohol as it increases its toxicity.

Mayapple, Wild Mandrake, *Podophyllum peltatum*

Mayapple should be used internally with great caution if you choose to use it. It is in the Berberidaceae (Barberry) Family. It is widespread in eastern North America. You are most likely to find it in damp meadows and open woods.

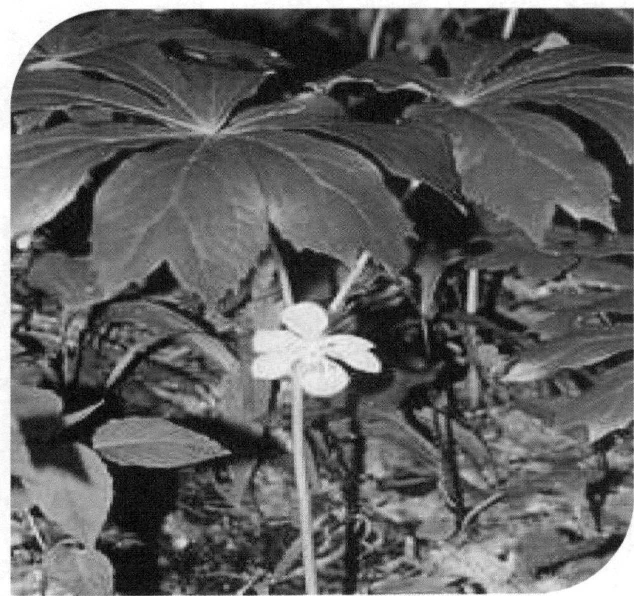

Identification: Mayapple grows 12 to 18 inches (20 cm to 30 cm) tall and has very large leaves. The leaves are smooth, paired, and umbrella-like. Leaves are palmately lobed, 8 to 12 inches (20 cm to 30 cm) in diameter, with 3 to 9 lobes.

Some stems produce a single leaf without any flower or fruit, while others produce two or more leaves and 1 to 8 drooping flowers (often just one) in the axil between the leaves.

The 1-inch (2.5 cm) wide waxy flowers are white, red, or yellow, with 6 to 9 petals and bloom in May. These plants grow in clumps that originate from a single rhizome.

Edible Use: The fruit are edible when ripe, but other parts of the plant are poisonous. Note that the fruits are poisonous until they ripen. They mature into a yellow or red fleshy fruit that is 2 inches (5 cm) long, egg-shaped, and wrinkled.

The fully ripe fruit can be eaten raw or cooked and is often used for jams and pies. The seeds and rind are not edible and must be removed before cooking or eating. The fruit tastes similar to a paw-paw.

Medicinal Use: Warts, Moles, Genital Warts, and Skin Cancer: Mayapple resin from the plant stems is useful for treating warts and moles. Place diluted resin on the wart, mole, or skin cancer, being careful to keep the resin confined to the affected area.

Wear gloves when squeezing the resin from the stems and mix with alcohol at a 20% resin dilution (1 part of resin diluted with 5 parts alcohol). This dilution should be strictly observed. Higher concentrations can do harm to the skin, while lower dilutions may not be effective enough.

Leave the diluted resin on the skin for one to four hours and then wash. Only a single application is needed. The lesions whiten within a few hours and begin to wither away within one to two days. Within three days, the lesions begin to disappear.

Other Cancers: Mayapple has been used in the treatment of other cancers. However, the plant is quite toxic and can be fatal. Only use mayapple under the supervision of a highly qualified medical professional.

Warning: Do not use during pregnancy or on small children. Avoid handling the resin with bare hands, as it is absorbed through the skin and can be toxic or even deadly.

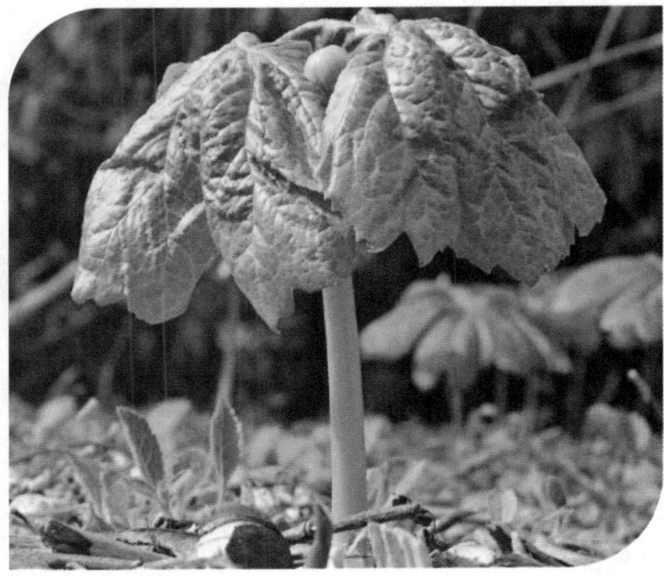

Mugwort, *Artemisia vulgaris* and Western Mugwort, *A. ludoviciana*

Mugwort is the common name for several species of Artemisia. Here we are discussing *Artemisia vulgaris*, Common Mugwort or Felon Herb and *Artemisia ludoviciana*, known as Western Mugwort or White Sagebrush. The two species have similar medicinal properties and can, for the most part, be used interchangeably. Do not confuse these with wormwood, *Artemesia absinthium,* also in this book. They are in the Aster/Daisy Family and are native to Eurasia and naturalized in North America.

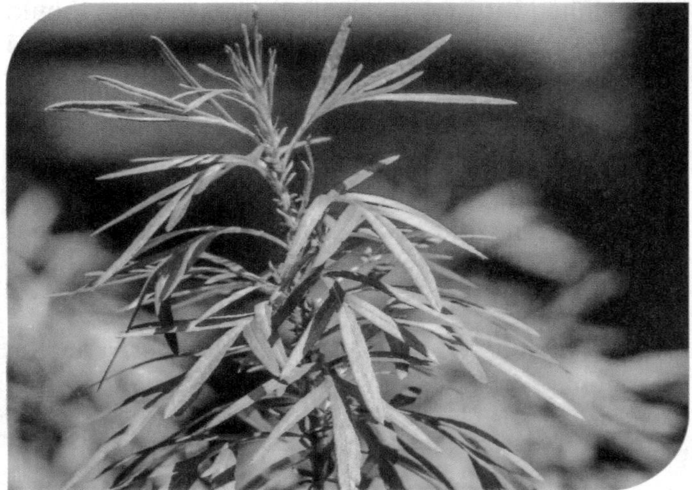

Identification: Common Mugwort grows from 3 to 6 feet (0.9m to 1.8m) tall with an erect upright stem that has a purple or dark reddish-brown tinge that becomes woody with age. It is often found in disturbed areas, along roadsides, and at the edges of woods and sunny meadows. Common Mugwort leaves are deeply lobed, alternate, and grow to about 4 inches (10 cm) in length.

The largest leaves are at the base of the plant, and leaves become smaller and narrower towards the top of the stem. The topside of the leaf is green and is often (but not always) hairless, while the underside is white or silvery with fine hairs (versus wormwood, which has leaves that are silvery on both the top and bottom). The deeply cut lobes are narrow and have smooth edges. The leaves are slightly aromatic. Its flowers are very small, non-showy, reddish-brown or yellow disk flowers that bloom in late summer/early autumn. The flowering stems grow to about 3 feet (0.9m) tall and have hair only on the upper stems. They primarily propagate via rhizomes.

Edible Use: Mugwort leaves are eaten raw or cooked but are usually used as an herb, not as a side dish. They are slightly bitter and best eaten before the plant blooms. Young shoots can be cooked. I make tea from the leaves, flowers, and roots. Mugwort can also be used as a flavoring in beer to replace hops.

Medicinal Use: I use Mugwort as a tea, tincture or, for external use, an oil. You can wrap and burn the leaves as a smudge stick. The smoke is calming and cleansing and is said to promote good dreams and to clear an area of negative energy. Roll and bind the leaves tightly and set fire to the tip. I use the flowers for oil infusions and the leaves and roots for tinctures and teas. You can also smoke it.

Menstrual Issues: Because it helps balance hormones and is an antispasmodic, Mugwort leaf tea is useful for treating menstrual issues. It is slightly toxic, however, and should not be used during pregnancy.

Moderate doses are beneficial in balancing the reproductive system. A tea made from the leaves and flowers works well for the treatment of cramping, excessive bleeding, and bringing on menses. The smoke is also used to move a baby from a breech position.

Digestive Issues: Mugwort leaf tea or tincture is very beneficial for the digestive system and is healing and restorative for the intestine. It treats constipation, diarrhea, gas, bloating, and intestinal worms. It is a natural and gentle laxative that treats the underlying problems by restoring balance.

Liver Health: Mugwort increases bile secretion in the liver and helps detoxify the liver and the body.

Heart Health: Mugwort promotes healthy circulation in the blood stream. It helps increase blood oxygenation and flow throughout the body. It improves blood cell generation, lessens the chance of blood clots, and lowers blood pressure in hypertension.

Respiratory Issues and Asthma: Common Mugwort helps relax bronchial tubes and open airways. It can be made into a leaf tea or the steam can be inhaled to help with bronchial inflammation.

Epilepsy, Convulsions, and Nervine: The sedative effects of mugwort help ease epilepsy and convulsions. It has antispasmodic properties than can control seizures in some epileptics.

It helps decrease the severity of the seizures and increases the time between attacks. Tea or tincture of the leaf seems to work best.

Burns, Itching, Rashes, Poison Ivy/Oak, Fungal Infections: Mugwort is soothing on the skin and helps relieve the pain and itching from poison ivy, skin rashes, burns, and other skin irritations. It reduces scarring and helps the skin heal faster.

Grind the fresh leaves and stems into a fine paste using a mortar and pestle. Apply the paste directly to the affected skin or wound. You may also use a leaf tea or infused flower oil as a topical antifungal and for relief from itching.

Insomnia, Fatigue, and Good Dreams: Mugwort regulates sleep, treating the sources of fatigue and insomnia. The sedative effects help the body to relax, but still allows the user to remain alert when needed. To improve sleep, try taking Mugwort as a tincture or tea, or add it to a long bath soak before bedtime. Hanging Mugwort by the bed is said to promote good vivid dreams.

Antibacterial Properties: Mugwort leaf tincture inhibits the growth of numerous bacteria, including *Staphylococcus aureus*, *Streptococcus*, *Bacillus* spp, *E. coli*, *Pseudomonas*, and others. Acetone extractions seem to work the best.

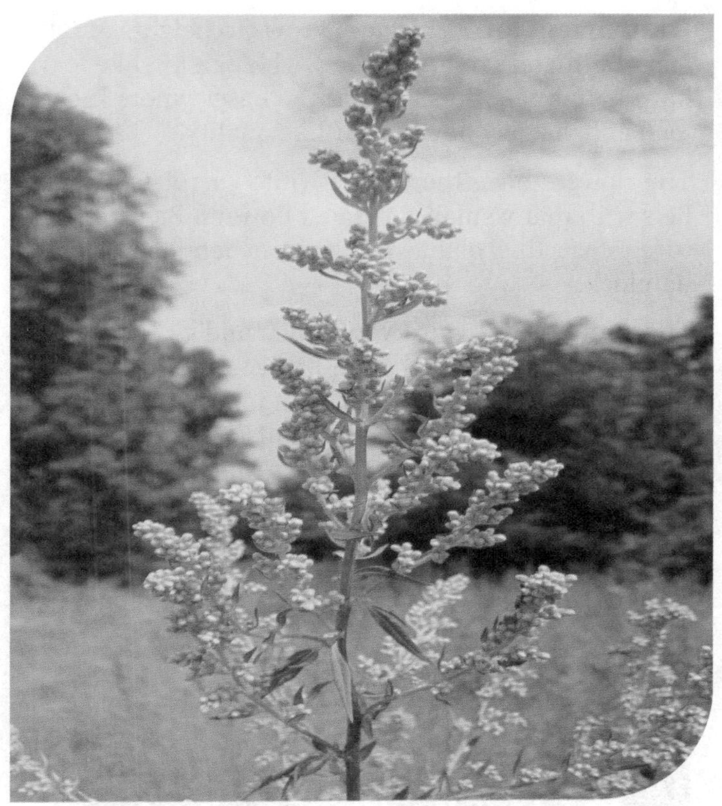

Harvesting: Harvest leaves, stems, and flowers when in flower (end of summer) and dry them for later use. Dig roots in the autumn.

Warning: The plant may be toxic when used in large doses. Do not use if you are pregnant or breast-feeding. Skin dermatitis is sometimes seen. Do not use the plant if you are allergic or if you develop a skin rash.

Osha, *Ligusticum porteri*

This species of osha grows in the Rocky Mountains and the southwestern United States, as well as parts of Mexico.

The Asian variety is also extremely medicinal as is the Western North American species. L. porteri is also called Colorado cough root, bear medicine, bear root, Indian root, Indian parsley lovage, Porter's wild lovage, loveroot, Porter's lovage, Porter's licorice-root, Porter's ligusticum, mountain ginseng, mountain carrot, wild parsley, wild lovage, chuchupate, and empress of the dark forest. It is hard to domesticate. It likes high altitude meadows. Osha is in the Apiaceae/Umbelliferae (Carrot/Parsley) Family and smells strongly like celery.

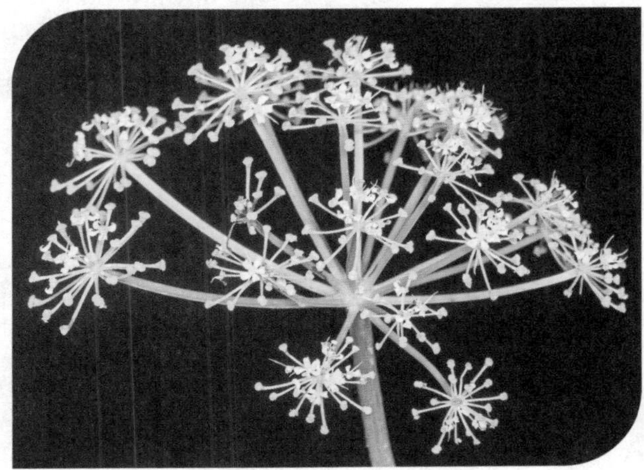

Identification: This herb grows to heights of 6 to 7 feet (1.8 meters to 2.1 meters). The parsley-like leaves have a unique reddish tint at the bases where they attach and visually have a fern-like quality.

The flowers have the classic white carrot-family umbels with many small 5-petaled flowers. Be careful not to confuse this plant with poison hemlock or water hemlock!

The roots of Osha are very hairy and fibrous with a wrinkled, black or chocolate-brown outer skin. When the outer root is peeled off, the inner root tissue is yellowish-white and highly fragrant. Its greenery dies down every winter to its hairy-topped brown root stock.

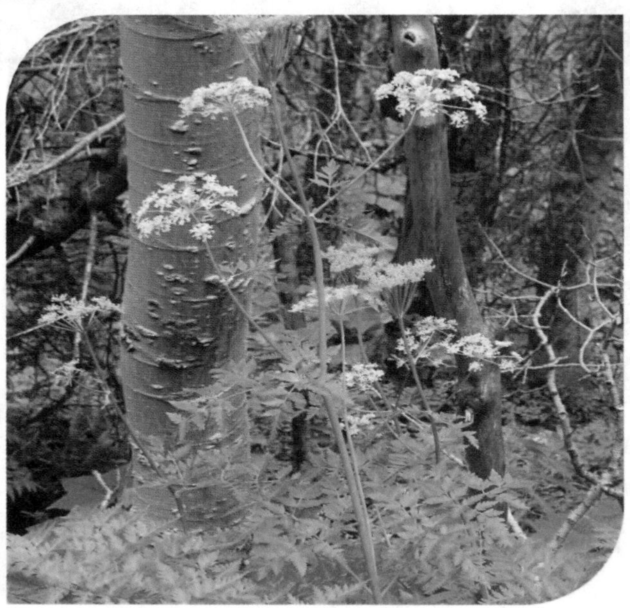

Jerry Friedman - Own work, CC BY-SA 3.0

Edible Use: The leaves and seeds are used as a seasoning and for flavoring various drinks such as mead. The seeds dry well and have a celery-parsley flavor.

Medicinal Use: Osha is one of my favorite medicinal plants. The root is chewed, smoked, powdered, or tinctured. It has anti-bacterial, anti-viral, hemostatic, and anti-inflammatory properties and is best used at the first sign of illness. Osha is my #1 go to for headaches - I light a piece of the dried root and inhale the smoke strongly into each nostril. I always carry it with me in my medicine bag.

Asthma, Colds, Flu, Viral Infections, Sore Throats, and Bronchial Infections: Osha root is a very good anti-bacterial and anti-viral, Osha is also an expectorant. It helps expel mucus that clogs the respiratory tract. It also relieves inflammation in the bronchial tracts making it easier for people with asthma and bronchitis to breathe. It promotes sweating, which gets rid of toxins and helps bring down fevers. To soothe sore throats try sucking on the root, drinking an osha root tea, taking a tincture, or extracting it with raw honey. It is used to manage herpes outbreaks and HIV due to its strong anti-viral properties. Use at the first sign of an outbreak and at the first sign of a cold or flu.

Headaches, Altitude Sickness, and Elevation Changes: Osha helps people breathe better by opening up the bronchial tubes. Chewing the root helps with the symptoms of altitude sickness and assists people performing athletically at higher elevations than they are used to. Osha often gives almost immediate headache relief when the smoke is breathed in deeply. Osha root also has diaphoretic properties, which promote sweating, thus helping to remove toxins from the body.

Skin Wounds, Infections, Boils: Apply Osha Tincture directly on to wounds if it is readily available or dust the area heavily with the powdered root. Osha's antibacterial properties are effective in helping the skin heal.

Arthritis and Carpal Tunnel Syndrome: The anti-inflammatory effects of osha act on the joints to relieve swelling and the pain of arthritis. It also acts on the nerves to relieve the pressure and swelling that causes carpal tunnel syndrome. For these problems, I usually use Osha Tincture, but you can also simply chew on the osha root.

Nicotine Addiction: Smoking is a very addictive habit. Osha helps relieve nicotine cravings. Try chewing on a piece of osha root or adding it to a non-nicotine-based smoking mixture.

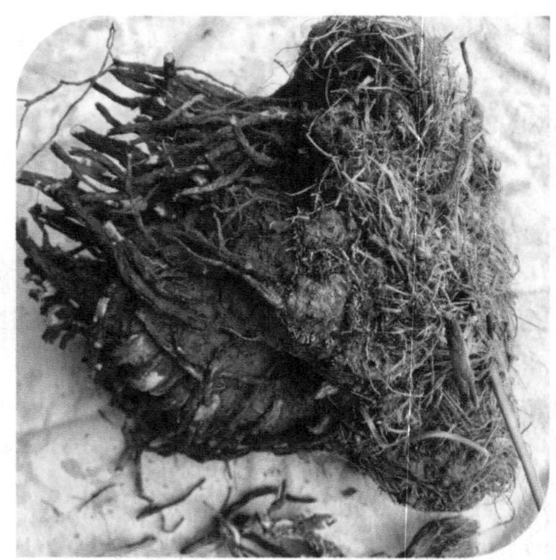

Harvesting: Osha is very hard to cultivate in the garden so please treat this plant with extra care and respect. Harvest the roots late summer to autumn from osha plants that are at least one year old and only take what you need. Dig up the older plants and let the younger plants grow for harvesting another season. Dig deeply. Dry for use. Seeds can be harvested after they have ripened. Spread some seeds around to propagate more osha. As always, tend the wild!

Warning: Safety for pregnant and breastfeeding mothers is unknown. It may trigger menstruation so best to avoid during pregnancy.

Recipes. Osha Decoction: Add 2 ounces (56g) of chopped osha roots and leaves to a pot containing 2 cups of water. Bring the water to a boil and simmer it for approximately 20 minutes. Cool and store the decoction in the refrigerator for up to 3 days. Take 1 to 2 tablespoons of the decoction as needed.

Osha Tincture: 1-pint (500 ml) of 80 proof vodka or other alcohol, chopped roots of the osha plant. Place the chopped dried roots into a glass pint (500ml) jar with a tight-fitting lid, filling the jar 3/4 full. Cover the herbs with alcohol, filling the jar. Store the jar in a cool, dark place such as a cupboard. Shake the jar daily for 6 to 8 weeks. Strain the herbs out of the liquid, cover it tightly and use within seven years.

Parrot's Beak, *Pedicularis racemosa*

Parrot's beak has a unique flower. The petals are shaped like parrot's beaks, giving it its name. The plant is also called leafy lousewort. It is in the Orobanchaceae (Broomrape) Family. It grows in coniferous forests in Western North America at mid-elevations in the mountains. All species of the genus *Pedicularis* have similar medicinal properties.

Identification: Parrot's beak flowers have petals shaped like parrot's beaks. The flowers grow in clusters on a stalk and have a broad three-lobed lower lip and an upper lip that curves over the lower lobes. Flowers are white to cream-colored, yellow, or pink depending on location, and flower in the summer. The alternate leaves are narrow, stalkless (or with short stalks), and have toothed margins. The plant grows from 10 to 20 inches (25 cm to 50 cm) high.

Medicinal Use: The leaves and flower petals are medicinally active. They are relaxing and bring a feeling of peace and contentment. You can use it as a tea, tincture, or a smoking blend. All bring medicinal effects. Smoking it does not produce a "high" feeling, but rather a peaceful feeling of well-being with occasional slight giddiness. My neighbor used to smoke it and nicknamed it "Ridicularis" instead of "Pedicularis", as it worked so ridiculously well.

Emotional Stress and Anxiety: Parrot's beak is relaxing and helps people cope with emotional stress and anxiety.

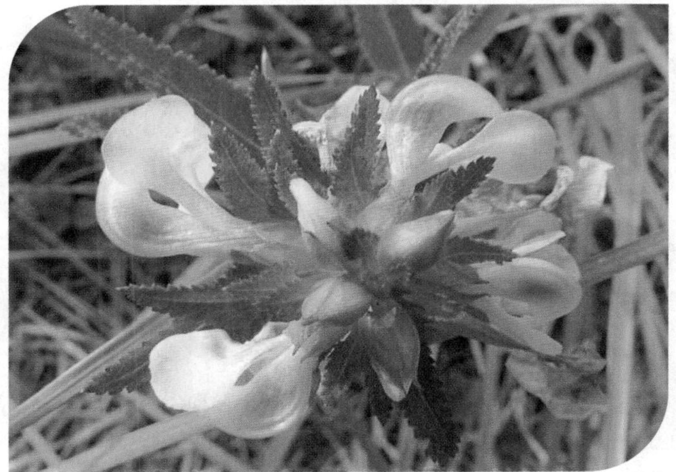

Thayne Tuason, Own Work, Wikipedia Commons cc 4.0

Skeletal Muscle Relaxer: For muscle tension and small muscle tremors, parrot's beak as a tea or tincture works as an excellent muscle relaxer, relieving pain by relaxing the muscles.

Massage therapists often give this to patients before a massage to release muscle tension.

Relaxation and Mild Sedative: This herb acts as a mild sedative, relieving pain, relaxing the body, and bringing a sense of calm.

Tension and Stress Headaches: Parrot's beak is good for treating tension headaches and headaches caused by stress. Low doses are usually quickly effective at relaxing the body and relieving a headache.

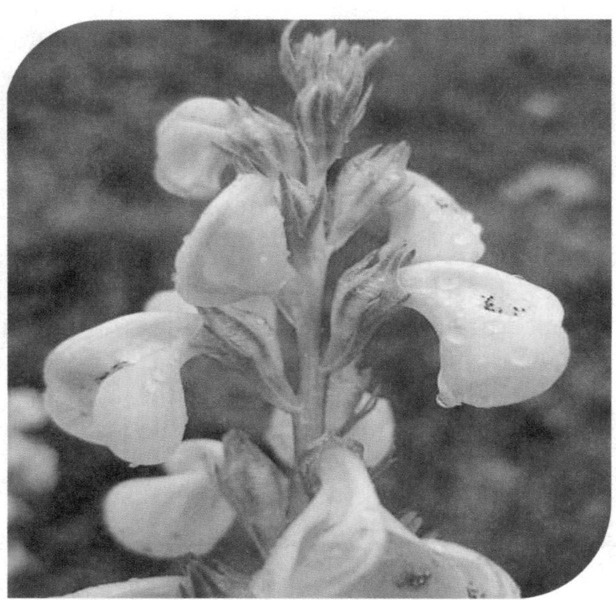

Pedicularis racemosa, Matt Lavin, Wikipedia commons CC 2.0

Smoking and Drug Withdrawal: This herb is calming and relaxing. It helps with some of the withdrawal symptoms from drugs or smoking.

Insomnia: Parrot's beak is a good sleep aid. It helps the body relax and has mild sedative properties.

Harvesting: Harvest the leaves at any time. Flower petals are harvested in the late morning while they are fresh and the dew has dried. Dry the flowers and leaves for future use. Harvest only what you need as it is not a common plant and leave plenty in the area you harvest.

Warning: The plant is relaxing and can give you a "spacey" feeling. Start with a low dose and increase as needed.

Recipes. Parrot's Beak Tea: Ingredients: 1 teaspoon dried and crushed parrot's beak flower petals and leaves and 1 cup boiling water.

Place the herbs in a tea ball. Pour the boiling water over the herbs and allow it to steep for 5 to 10 minutes. Strain out the herbs and drink the tea, as needed.

Partridgeberry, *Mitchella repens*

Partridgeberry is mostly known for its use for menstrual problems and in facilitating childbirth. It is also called Deerberry, Twinberry, and Squaw Vine. It likes sandy soils and is shade-tolerant. It is in the Rubiaceae (Bedstraw/Madder) Family. It grows in Eastern North America.

Identification: Partridgeberry is a creeping broadleaf evergreen that grows as a very low growing ground cover. The plant grows about 2 to 3 inches (5 cm to 7.5 cm) tall and spreads 6 inches (15 cm) to 1 foot across. Opposite leaves are oval to round, dark green, and glossy. Each leaf is up to ¾ inch (1 cm) long with whitish veins growing in pairs along the stems.

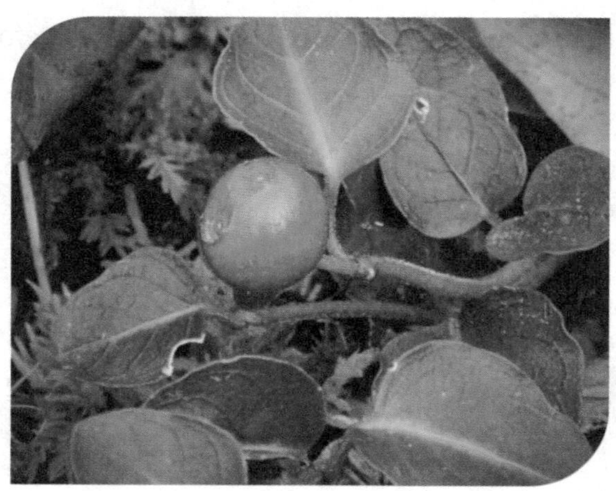

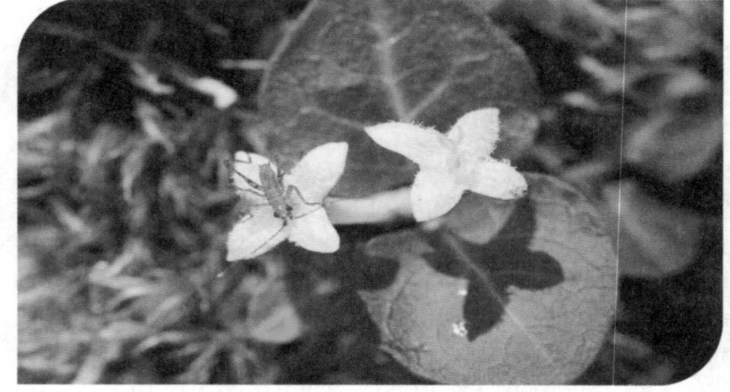

Paired white blossoms appear at the ends of the stems from May to July. Each flower has four lobes and is trumpet-shaped. One pair of flowers forms one bright red berry that ripens in late summer and may stay on the plant until the following spring.

Edible Use: The berries are edible, but rather tasteless, so they are usually only used when food supplies are scarce.

Medicinal Use: Partridgeberry leaves and berries are used to to help with fluid retention, but its main value is to hasten childbirth and treat menstrual problems. It has a tonic effect on the uterus and ovaries, though I prefer other herbs for these uses.

Childbirth and Menstrual Problems: The leaves are used as a tea in the last weeks before childbirth to hasten birth with fewer complications. However, the tea or berries should never be used until the end of the pregnancy; it can cause a miscarriage when used too soon. After delivery, the tea is used externally to wash the breasts and treat sore nipples. Partridgeberry Tea is also used to treat painful or irregular menses and menstrual bloating.

Harvesting: Harvest the leaves during the summer and dry them in the sun or on a dehydrator for later use. Store the dried leaves in a cool, dry place. Harvest berries during the early winter while they are at their peak. Use them fresh or split the berries in half and dry for future use.

Recipes. Partridgeberry Leaf Tea: Use for menstrual problems and childbirth. 1 teaspoon

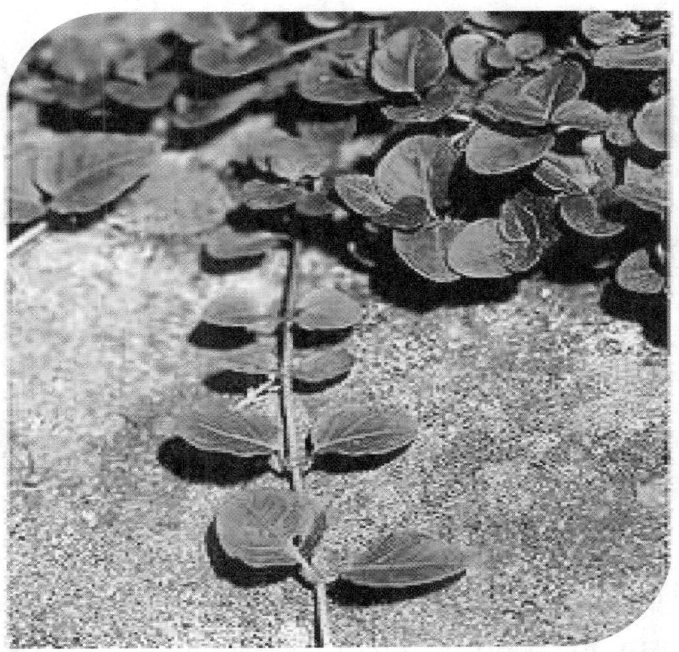

Partridgeberry Leaf, 1 cup boiling water. Pour boiling water over the dried herbs. Allow the tea to steep for 10 minutes Strain and enjoy.

Pipsissewa or Prince's Pine, *Chimaphila umbellata*

Pipsissewa, also known as Prince's Pine, Umbellate Wintergreen, Rheumatism Weed, and Ground Holly, is a member of the Ericaceae (Heath) Family. It is a popular remedy for kidney stones. It is a small perennial found in sandy soils and dry woodlands. It is native throughout the cool and temperate zones of North America.

Identification: Pipsissewa is low growing, 4 to 12 inches (10 cm to 30 cm) tall, and an erect evergreen wildflower. The stems are either simple or branched with whorls of three to seven leaves.

The elongated leaves are leathery, shiny, and sharply toothed with fine hairs on the edges. June brings whitish to pink flowers in loose clusters of four to eight at the end of flower stalks and blooms last through August.

Each stalk produces round seed capsules that remain on the plant until late autumn or even into winter. Each stalk contains four to eight capsules with five-chambers containing numerous tiny seeds. The plant also propagates by underground rhizomes. Prince's pine has a pleasant scent and flavor.

Edible Use: The plant has been used as a flavoring in candy and root beer. It can also be brewed as a tea.

Medicinal Use: All parts of prince's pine are medicinally active. I mostly use the leaves. The plant is an

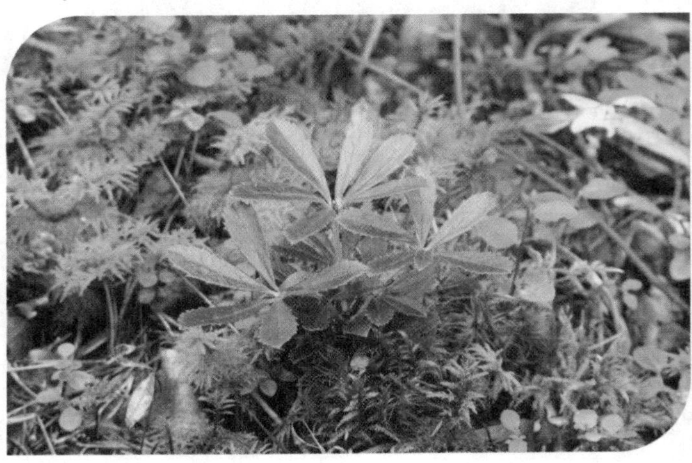

astringent, anti-septic, anti-bacterial, anti-inflammatory, diuretic, and tonic.

Urinary System Problems and Kidney Stones: The name Pipsissewa is a Cree name that means "to break into small pieces" because of its ability to break up and dissolve kidney stones. It contains hydroquinone, which disinfects the urinary system and heals inflammation of the bladder and the urethra. It also treats the presence of blood in the urine. The herb is a diuretic, inducing urination and sweating. Use prince's pine along with cranberry for urinary tract infections in women. It is also useful in the treatment of prostatitis, gonorrhea, and other urinary system infections.

Liver Function: Prince's pine acts as a diuretic to help rid the body of waste products. It helps detoxify the liver and improves its function.

Skin Problems: External application of prince's pine is useful for blisters, skin sores, and other skin problems. Wash the skin with Pipsissewa Tea or apply Pipsissewa Decoction to the affected area. It can also be used to make a wet compress for use on blisters, tumors, ulcers, and to reduce swelling. Caution: for some people it may cause a rash or blistering.

Arthritis, Gout, Muscle Cramps, and Backaches: Prince's pine is an effective treatment for joint and muscle pain, including pain from arthritic joints. Apply a poultice of crushed prince's pine leaves to the joint or rub with Pipsissewa Salve or Pipsissewa Decoction and drink Pipsissewa Tea. It is a mild lymphatic stimulant.

Diabetes: Regular use of prince's pine decoction has the ability to lower blood glucose levels in diabetics. Use at mealtime.

Diuretic Properties: The herb has the same diuretic properties as bearberry, but with a lower tannin content. Used for people with high blood pressure and chronic urinary tract problems. Prince's pine also induces sweating, which helps to reduce fevers, and it helps with edema.

Respiratory Tract Problems: Pipsissewa Tea helps treat respiratory tract infections, colds, whooping cough, and bronchitis.

Harvesting: Prince's pine has been over collected in some areas and is disappearing from the landscape. Always harvest with care and leave behind a healthy plant. Remove leaves as needed year-round for fresh use or harvest and dry leaves for future use when a large supply is available. Take only one whorl at the top of the plant when it is not in flower or in seed.

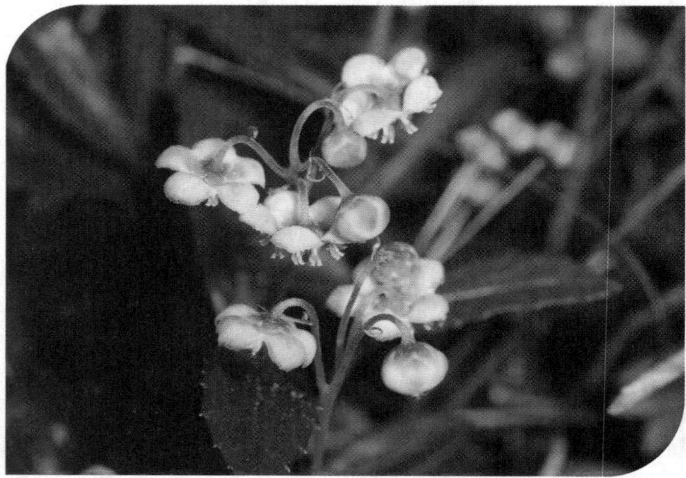

Warning: Occasional side effects include confusion, ringing of the ears, and vomiting. Rarely, seizures can occur. Do not use the herb long-term. In large doses, Pipsissewa can cause diarrhea, nausea and vomiting. Pipsissewa can cause the urine to turn green, but this is not harmful.

Because of its tannin content, it can interfere with the absorption of some medications. Allow several hours between taking the herb and any medications. People with poor nutrient absorption should avoid using Pipsissewa, as it can reduce the absorption of minerals from the gut. Do not use while pregnant or nursing. Some people are allergic to Pipsissewa and can develop a contact rash or blistering.

Recipes. Pipsissewa Tea. Ingredients: 1 teaspoon dried crushed leaves and 1 cup boiling water. Pour the boiling water over the dried, crushed leaves and allow it to steep until the water is cold. Strain the tea and take one to two cups of the cold tea daily.

Pipsissewa Decoction. Ingredients: 2 teaspoons dried crushed leaves and 1 cup boiling water. This is a stronger version of the tea. The effects are the same, but less is needed for people who don't like the taste.

Pour the boiling water over the dried, crushed leaves and allow it to steep until the water is cold. Strain the tea and take from 2 to four 4 (60 ml to 120 ml), three times a day. Store the decoction in the refrigerator for up to three days.

Red Raspberry, *Rubus idaeus*

Red raspberry grows wild in forests, but is most often found in cultivated gardens. It is grown mainly for the sweet-tart fruit, but also for the leaves and roots. It is in the Rosaceae (Rose) Family.

Identification: The red raspberry grows from a central cane. Side shoots produce compound leaves with three, five, or seven leaflets. In the wild, it forms open stands when shaded under the tree canopy, but in the open it forms very dense groupings. The plants grow to approximately five to eight feet (2.4 meters) in height and have thorns.

Flowers appear in the late spring, growing on short racemes forming on the side shoots. Flowers are less than 1/2 inch (1.25 cm) in diameter with five white petals. Fruit develops in the summer and early autumn. Each fruit is actually an aggregate fruit made up of drupelets around a central core. The drupelets separate from the core when picked leaving a hollow center.

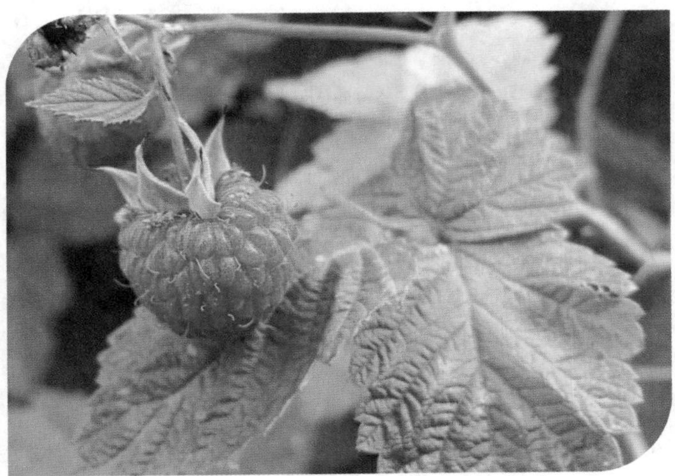

Edible Use: The berries are delicious raw or cooked. Raspberry leaves are used to make an herbal tea.

Medicinal Use: Red raspberry is full of healthy compounds, vitamins, and minerals. It gives the immune system a boost, is an astringent, and increases health and uterine tone during pregnancy.

Late Pregnancy and Labor: Raspberry Leaf Tea is widely used by expectant mothers, especially in the last few months of pregnancy. It helps with morning

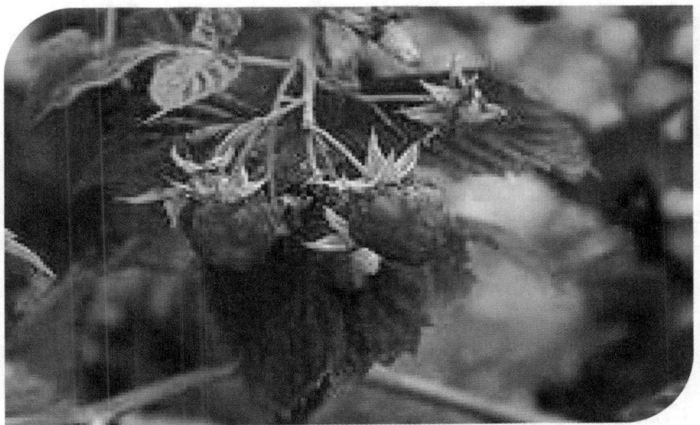

sickness and tones the uterine muscles to help ease labor pain. Mothers who take Raspberry Leaf Tea in the last few months of pregnancy have fewer miscarriages and easier births. Most mothers continue using it after birthing to reduce cramping, reduce bleeding, and tone the uterus and pelvic muscles. Only start use after the 3rd month of pregnancy.

Diarrhea: For diarrhea, use a decoction of the leaves or raspberry vinegar.

High Blood Pressure: Compounds in raspberries are very heart healthy. They improve the tone of the circulatory system and help lower blood pressure.

Wounds, Skin Lesions, Ulcers and Minor Skin Infections. Raspberry Leaf Tea works as a wash for skin wounds, lesions, bites, and itchy skin.

Recipes. Raspberry Leaf Decoction: 1/2 ounce of dried raspberry leaves or 1 ounce of fresh leaves, chopped, 1-pint (500 ml) of water. Bring the water and raspberry leaves to a boil, reduce the heat and cover the pot. Simmer the decoction for 20 minutes. Remove from the heat and allow to cool. Strain out the leaves and store in the refrigerator for up to 3 days. General dosage is 1/4 cup to 1 cup.

Raspberry Vinegar. 2 cups apple cider vinegar, 8 ounces (230g) red raspberries, 8 ounces (230g) brown sugar or raw honey. Crush the raspberries and add the vinegar. Allow the mixture to steep for 10 days.

Strain out the raspberries and bring the vinegar mixture to a low simmer. Add the sugar and simmer until dissolved. Cool. Store Raspberry Vinegar in a tightly closed jar in a dark place. Use the vinegar straight or diluted. General dosage is 3 tablespoons, 3 times daily.

Red Root, New Jersey Tea, *Ceanothus americanus* and other *Ceanothus* spp.

Red root, also known as New Jersey Tea, is found on dry, gravelly banks and open woods. Many species of *Ceanothus* species have the same medicinal properties. It is in the Rhamnaceae (Buckthorn) Family.

Identification: You can recognize Red Root by its lacy white flowers and the wintergreen scent of its leaves. It grows to a height of 4 feet (1.2 meters), although many plants are shorter. It tends to grow very wide. The slender branches are herbaceous in the upper part and woody at the base. The root system is substantial and deep with fiber-like root hairs near the surface.

Deeper roots are plump and woody with small lumps. The large and deep root system increases the plant's ability to survive wildfires. The plant produces lacy white flowers in clustered inflorescences on long peduncles. These small white flowers appear in oval clusters at the tip of the branches. The fruits produced are dry and burst open naturally to release the seeds.

Edible Use: The leaves have a refreshing flavor and wintergreen scent. They make a good tea without the caffeine.

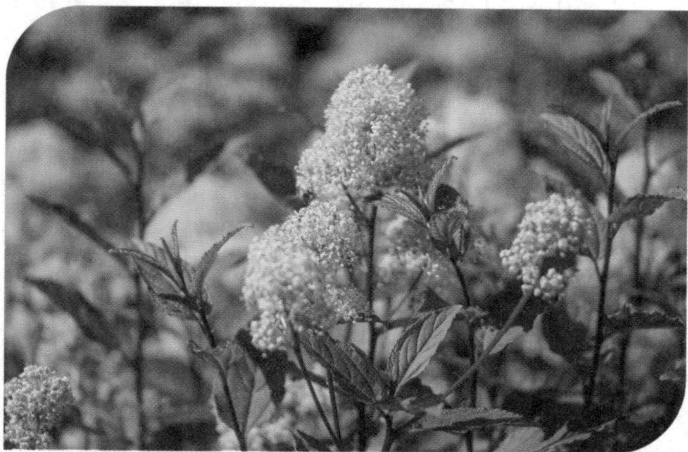

Medicinal Use: The root and root bark are used medicinally. The flowers can be used as a soap.

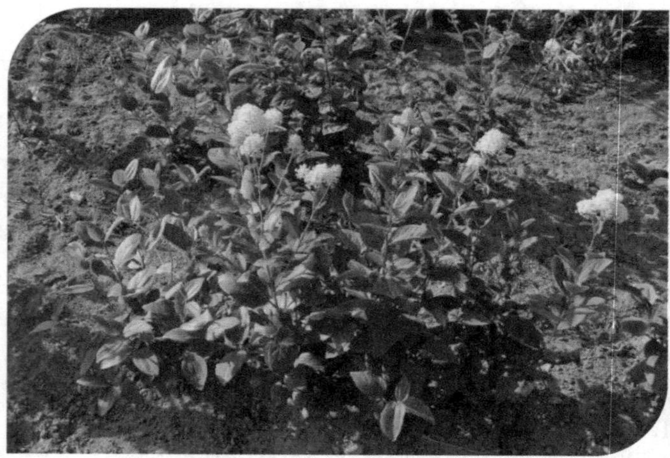

Fevers, Coughs, Bronchitis, Sore Throats, Whooping Cough, and Tonsillitis: The root and bark of Red Root are both used for treating fevers, sore throats, and mucous problems. It also works to treat infections of the upper respiratory tract. The roots are astringent and anti-spasmodic with expectorant properties. It has a high tannin content. Try Red Root Tea or a Red Root Bark Decoction and use as a gargle.

Stimulates the Lymphatic System, Mononucleosis: A tea from the roots and root bark stimulate the lymphatic system and the immune system. It works to support healing from mononucleosis.

High Blood Pressure: The roots and root bark contain gentle hypotensive properties that reduce the blood pressure.

Hemorrhoids: The combination of tannins and the anti-inflammatory properties of Ret Root help reduce the swelling and relieve the pain of hemorrhoids. Use topically.

Skin Wounds, Dermatitis, Herpes, and Skin Tumors: A decoction made from the root bark of Red Root treats skin wounds and diseases. The high tannin content reduces fluid in the lesions and the astringent properties reduce the symptoms. The dried and powdered bark can also be dusted onto skin wounds.

Body Wash: The flowers have high levels of saponins and lather well for use in cleaning the body or clothing.

To use them for cleaning, mash the flowers and soak in water. Use the lather as a mild soap. Alternately, rub the flowers all over the body to produce a lather. Using the flowers in this way has the added benefit of leaving your body and clothes nicely scented.

Toothache: Take one mouthful of Red Root Bark Decoction and swish it gently in the mouth to relieve pain and reduce swelling. Hold it in the mouth for a few minutes, then spit it out.

Harvesting: Harvest the roots during spring or autumn, when their color is the deepest red, and dry them for future use. Make sure to cut the roots prior to drying them as they are difficult to cut once they have dried.

Warning: Do not use if on an anti-coagulant medication.

Recipes. Red Root Tea. 1 teaspoon of dried, ground Red Root, 1 cup of water. Combine the water and root and bring to a simmer. Simmer the tea for 5 minutes, then allow to cool to drinking temperature and strain.

Red Root Bark Decoction. 1-ounce New Jersey Tea plant root bark, ground or chopped fine, 1-pint (500 ml) water. Bring the root bark and water to a boil and reduce the heat to a low simmer. Simmer the root bark for 30 minutes for ground bark or 45 minutes for finely chopped root bark. Strain the decoction.

Rhodiola rosea, Golden Root

Rhodiola rosea, also called Golden Root, Rose Root, or Arctic Root, can sometimes be difficult to find. It likes sea cliffs and high elevations in sandy areas in Northeastern America, Europe, and Asia. It is a perennial flowering plant that is sometimes planted as a groundcover. It is in the Crassulaceae (Stonecrop) Family. Golden root likes cold weather, and is most often found it on sunny river and stream banks, in snow beds, and rocky shelves.

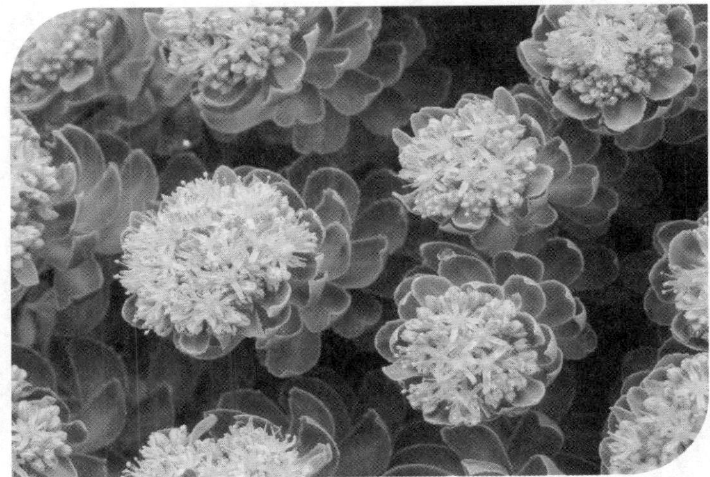

Golden Root Plant, Dolina Tomanowa, CC by SA 2.5

Identification: This plant grows from 4 to 15 inches (10 cm to 37.5 cm) tall, with several stems growing from thick rootstock. The stems are erect with succulent leaves and a waxy coating that helps the plant conserve water. The leaves are flat and smooth, alternate and stalkless, with a slightly blue tint. The lowest leaves are scale-like, and stem leaves are ovate with a sharp tip and saw-like teeth. Rhodiola flowers from July to August, forming greenish yellow to yellow flowers with four sepals and four petals. The staminate flowers have 8 stamens and are taller than the pistillate flowers. The flowers are massed together into a semispherical flower head. Fruits are four united follicles with many seeds.

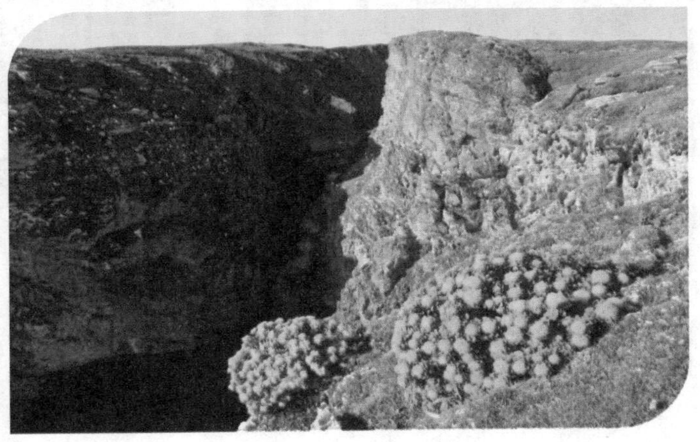

Edible Use: The leaves, stems, flowers, and roots are edible. Young leaves and shoots are good eaten raw or cooked like a vegetable. Older plants are slightly bitter. The stems can be steamed like asparagus. The roots are good raw, cooked, or fermented like sauerkraut.

Medicinal Use: Rhodiola root is a powerful adaptogen. It is good for lifting the mood, increasing mental concentration, and it regulates the body's reaction to stress and normalizes hormones. Rhodiola's effects are often best at lower doses, so it is important to start with a lower dose and increase it only if needed.

Physical Endurance and Sexual Potency: Athletes take Rhodiola root to enhance their physical strength and endurance. It increases energy levels and decreases the effects of strenuous exercise on the body. It allows the athlete to push harder without feeling the physical stress. It also promotes sexual health, libido, and stamina. It may increase fertility.

Fatigue and Adrenal Fatigue: Fatigue can be caused by a number of factors, everything from anemia to generally poor health or even stress. The adaptogenic properties of Rhodiola root helps increase energy and reduce fatigue in almost all of these cases.

Healthy Thyroid Function: Rhodiola root promotes healthy immune system function and regulates many of the hormones that allow the body to function normally, including the thyroid. It promotes healthy function of the thyroid and helps to balance the hormones. This is part of the reason that it increases energy, but it also does far more to help the thyroid function properly.

Memory and Brain Function: Rhodiola increases the mental capacity of the brain and helps with mental clarity. It improves memory retention, boosts the mood, reduces fatigue, and calms anxiety. This calm and improved function helps people relax.

Relieves Anxiety and Depression: For people suffering from anxiety and depression, Rhodiola can be a lifesaver. It calms anxiety, helps the person think clearly, and lifts the mood. It is not suitable for use with people who have manic episodes, but for others it is often considered a cure. Warning: Do not take golden root with prescription anti-depressants or SSRIs as they can interact.

Post-Traumatic Stress Disorder (PTSD): Rhodiola regulates the brain hormones that cause anxiety, flashbacks, and other symptoms of PTSD. Start at a low dose.

Treatment of Tuberculosis: A combination of Rhodiola flowers and Astragalus root is used as a treatment for tuberculosis. Eat the raw flowers from the golden root plant and take Astragalus root powder daily.

Harvesting: Harvest golden root in the autumn after the first frost when the plant is dying back. Look for older plants with large roots, as older roots have more medicinal value. Slice them into thin slices before drying. The roots will turn a light brown; this is ok. Store them wrapped in a paper bag for up to three years.

Warning: Do not use if you have an autoimmune disorder as it may cause a flare up. Do not use if on SSRIs or if you have bipolar. Do not use if you are on thyroid medications. Consult with a doctor if you are on anti-coagulants or ACE inhibitors.

It may have stimulating effects so best taken in the morning so as not to interfere with sleep.

Solomon's Seal, *Polygonatum* spp.

Solomon's seal grows in the temperate zones of the United States, Europe, and Asia. It is a member of the Asparagus family and the young shoots can be eaten like asparagus. It is a different plant than False Solomon's Seal, also in this book. You can tell easily them apart when in flower or seed as Solomon's Seal carries their bell-shaped flowers and dark blue berries on the underside of their stem while False Solomon's Seal has terminal feathery flower clusters with red berries.

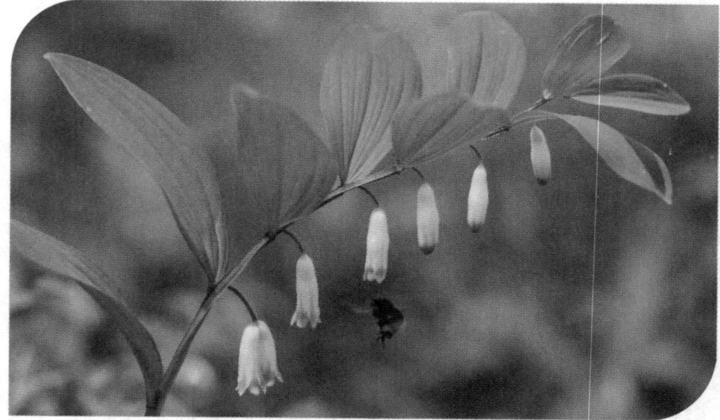

Identification: Solomon's Seal grows to 3 feet (0.9 meters) in height and up to 10 inches (25 cm) across. The stems arch gracefully and the light green smooth leaves are large and oval shaped, growing alternately on the stem. The leaf base clasps the stem and the leaves have parallel veins. Its white or yellow-green flowers are tubular, growing in small clusters of two to 10 flowers that grow from the underside of the stem at the leaf axils. The small drooping bell-shaped flowers bloom from April to June and produce a blackish-blue berry that is the size of a small pea. Solomon's seal

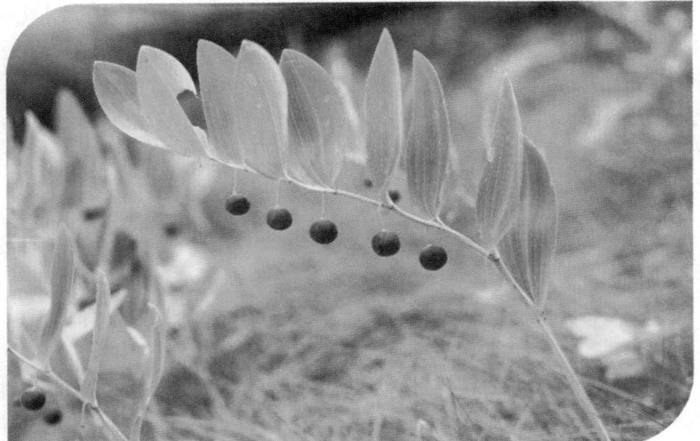

grows from a thick, multi-scarred rhizome that spreads underground.

Edible Use: The young shoots are eaten cooked as a vegetable and the rhizomes can also be eaten cooked, after soaking in water to remove the bitterness. The rhizomes can be dried, powdered and used as a flour to make bread. The berries should not be eaten and large amounts can be toxic.

Medical Use: I primarily use Solomon's seal as a poultice or salve for external use. It can also be used internally as a tea or tincture. Most people use the rhizome for medicine. It is a lubricating herb.

Prevents Bruising, Heals Blemishes, and Repairs Tissue: For bruised skin, inflammations and swellings, infections, hemorrhoids, and boils, try a poultice made with the powdered roots mixed with a little water or oil. A salve from the bruised leaves and oil can be used to treat a black eye. An application of tea directly on the skin is used for acne and blemishes. People with recurring acne can use the tea as a wash.

Stomach Inflammations, Dysentery: Solomon's seal root has mucilaginous properties that are anti-inflammatory and soothe irritation in the digestive tract. Try Solomon's Seal Cold Infusion Tea for helping heal gastrointestinal problems including indigestion, heartburn, inflammations of the digestive tract, diarrhea, and ulcers.

Respiratory Issues, Tuberculosis: The anti-inflammatory properties of Solomon's Seal help soothe irritated airways in the pulmonary system while its expectorant properties loosen mucus in the lungs and help the body expel it. Solomon's Seal Cold Infusion Tea treats both a dry cough and a productive couth, respiratory infections, and sore throats. It has been used as an effective treatment for tuberculosis and bleeding in the lungs. Settlers and Native Americans used the dried and powdered roots and flowers as a snuff to clear the nasal and bronchial passages.

Muscular Trauma, Weaknesses, Torn Muscles and Ligaments: Torn, bruised, or over stretched muscles, tendons, ligaments, and joints are helped by taking fresh Solomon's Seal Root Tincture or Solomon's Seal Tea. Rub the tincture or tea into the inflamed tissue 2 or 3 times a day until the tissue heals. It is also useful for treating sprains, broken bones, herniated discs, painful joints, arthritis, and tendonitis. It soothes irritation and inflammation in the connective tissues and cartilage.

Reproductive Problems: Solomon's seal is used as a treatment for reproductive problems in both men and women. It helps with vaginal dryness, heals inflamed tissue, and helps with conception. It is also effective for treating menstrual cramps and problems during or after menopause. Try Solomon's Seal Tea or Solomon's Seal Tincture for use in fertility problems or problems with premature ejaculation.

Cardiovascular System, Diuretic, and Detoxification: Solomon's seal acts as a heart tonic to regulate the heart and lower high blood pressure. It also works as a mild diuretic to rid the body of excess fluids and detoxify the body. Use Solomon's Seal Tea for this purpose. Consult your doctor if you are using any prescription medications or have a known heart problem.

Mild Sedative: Solomon's Seal Tea and Tincture soothes the nervous system and calms the body. It also relieves pain and discomfort, while having a tonic effect that strengthens the body.

Strengthens the Immune System: The tincture and tea are helpful in regulating stresses on the immune system. It strengthens the immune response, works as an anti-inflammatory, and allows tissue to heal.

Harvesting: Allow several years for the plant to grow into a large clump in need of division. Harvest in the autumn after the flowers begin to fade. Dig up the rhizomes, leaving several buds on each plant for a future crop. Dry for future use.

Warning: Do not use Solomon's Seal if you are pregnant or breast feeding. Solomon's seal can cause problems for diabetics, reducing blood sugar levels and interfering with blood sugar control. Do not use Solomon's seal just before surgery. It can interfere with blood sugar control during and after the surgery. Do not eat large quantities of the fruit; they are poisonous.

Recipes: A little goes a long way with this herb and too much can be irritating.

Solomon's Seal Cold Infused Tea: The cold infusion retains more of the mucilaginous properties and is more beneficial for treating bronchial problems and digestive problems. For other issues a hot tea works well. Ingredients: 1 1/2 teaspoon Solomon's Seal root, chopped fine, 3 cups cold water. In the evening, place 1 ½ teaspoons of Solomon's seal root into a 24-ounce bottle or a quart (liter) jar. Add 3 cups of cold water to the jar or bottle and cap tightly. Allow the tea to steep overnight at room temperature. The next day, sip the tea throughout the day, drinking the entire bottle by early evening. You can drink the tea cold or warm it gently as desired.

Spanish Moss, *Tillandsia usneoides*

Spanish moss is in the Bromeliaceae (Bromeliad) Family. It is not actually a moss. It is a tropical and subtropical epiphyte. It is found in humid savannas, swamps, and lowlands. It likes sun and partial-shade.

Identification: Spanish moss is the beard-like silvery-grey string-like that hangs from trees all over the south-eastern United States. Do not confuse it with the Usnea lichen. The stems are 20 to 25 feet (7.6m) long and thread-like with 1 to 3 inch (2.5 cm to 7.5 cm) long leaves. Plants are covered by small scales, which absorb water from the air. It has no roots and absorbs its nutrients from the air, rain, and sun. The plant does flower, but rarely. Their flowers have three yellow petals and three sepals.

Medicinal Use: It is mostly used as a leaf tea. It also works as a good makeshift menstrual pad or diaper.

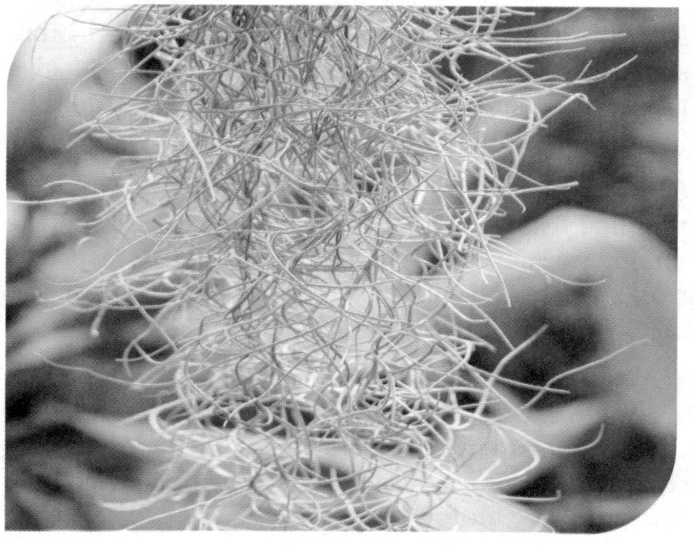

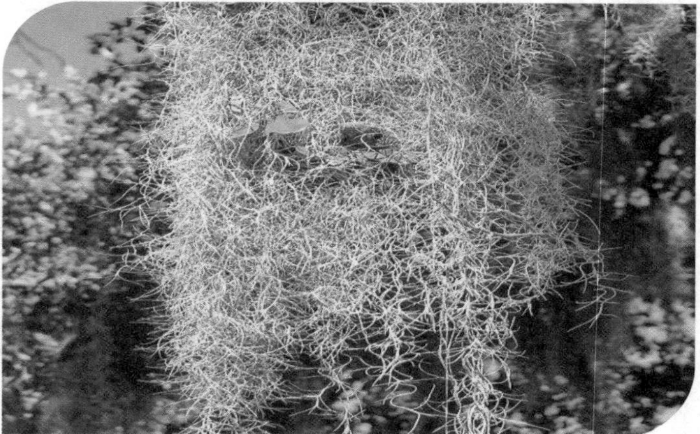

Lowering Cholesterol: Spanish moss contains substances (like HMG/3-hydroxy-3-methylglutaric acid) that lower blood cholesterol.

Balances Female Hormones, Labor: Spanish moss helps ease labor and promotes the production of breast milk. It is known to act as an estrogen supplement.

Diabetes: Spanish Moss is useful for diabetes treatment by lowering blood glucose levels. It is beneficial, but not always strong enough to treat diabetes alone. It is used in combination with other herbs such as bottle gourd, prickly pear, red mulberry, and American ginseng. Spanish moss alone helps lower the blood sugar, while these other herbs also help increase the production of insulin. Spanish Moss Tea is especially helpful for diabetics who have problems with acidosis and ketosis.

Arthritis and Hemorrhoids: Spanish Moss Tea is beneficial in the treatment of arthritis (rheumatism). It has anti-inflammatory benefits that help relieve joint inflammation and pain and is commonly used externally to treat hemorrhoids.

Stone Root, Richweed, *Collinsonia canadensis*

Stone root, also known as richweed, horse balm, and ox balm is an herb with a lemon-like scent. It is a member of the Lamiaceae (Mint) Family. It likes damp places and shady woodland areas across eastern North America.

Identification: The plant grows to 4 feet (1.2 meters) tall when mature and grows from a single, straight stem. Oval-shaped jagged-edges leaves are oppositely arranged on a square stem. At the top of the stem is a cone-shaped group of pale-yellow flowers that bloom from July to September. The roots justify their name as they are as hard as a rock.

Medicinal Use: The leaves and root are brewed to make medicinal teas and washes.

Bladder Infections, Kidney Stones, and Fluid Retention: The root tea has antibiotic effects as well as being a powerful diuretic. It expels toxins and bacteria from the body and is good for bladder and kidney problems.

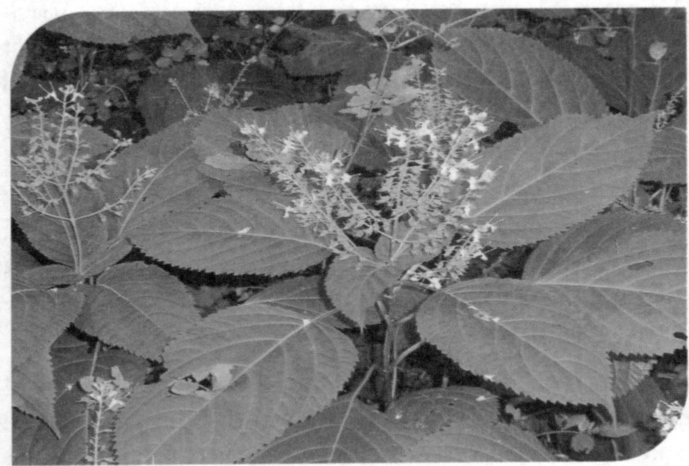

Stone root flowers, R. A. Nonenmacher, CC by SA 4.0

Healing Wounds: Try a Stone Root Tea wash for wounds and minor skin infections. It has antibiotic and antiseptic effects for healing.

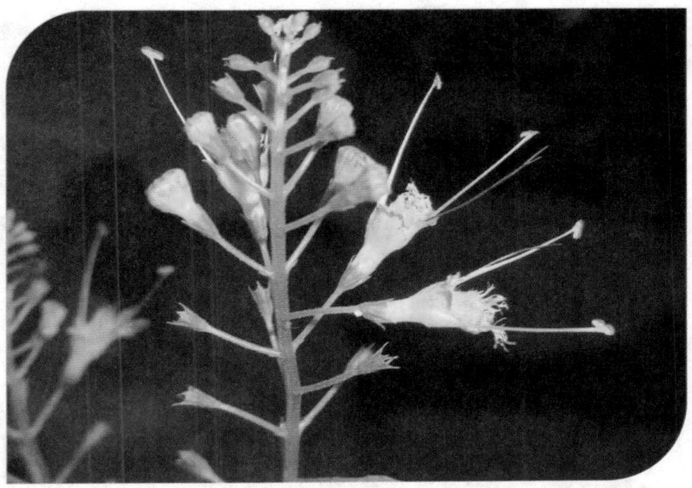

Collinsonia canadensis, by R. A. Nonenmacher, Own work, CC-BY-SA-4.0

Hemorrhoids, Varicose Veins, Circulation, and Inflammation: Stone root is excellent at reducing inflammations, especially those caused by hemorrhoids and varicose veins. Taken internally the root tea improves circulation and strengthens the veins and reduces blood pooling.

Use as a tea internally and also as an external wash or compress on the affected areas.

Sore Throats: Stone root tea, used as a gargle, gives immediate relief for a strained larynx and for sore throats.

Digestive Problems: Stone root tea relieves a wide variety of digestive problems including indigestion, heartburn, constipation, diarrhea, and excessive flatulence. It soothes muscle spasms and improves circulation to the digestive organs.

Reducing Stress and Anxiety: Stone root tea elevates the mood and increases feelings of well-being while decreasing stress, panic, nervousness, and feelings of anxiety. Some people report that it increases energy levels and the libido.

Recipes. Stone Root Tea. 2 teaspoons grated stone root, 3 cups water. Bring the water and stone root to a boil and reduce the heat to a simmer and cover tightly. Simmer the root for 30 to 45 minutes.

Unicorn Root, *Aletris farinosa*

Unicorn root is a member of the Nartheciaceae Family and is found in eastern North America in sunny locations. It goes by many names including ague root, colic root, starwort, stargrass, white-tube stargrass, Ague grass, crow corn, blazing star, Devil's bit, mealy starwort, and husk-wort. Do not confuse it with false unicorn root, *Chamaelirium luteum*.

Identification: True unicorn root has yellow-green, radial, grass-like leaves 2 to 6 inches (5 cm to 15 cm) long. The leaves are smooth and firm. Its parallel veins are quite prominent with 6 to 10 veins per leaf. The radial leaves grow directly from the upper part of the growing end of the crawling rhizome. It spreads using underground rhizomes.

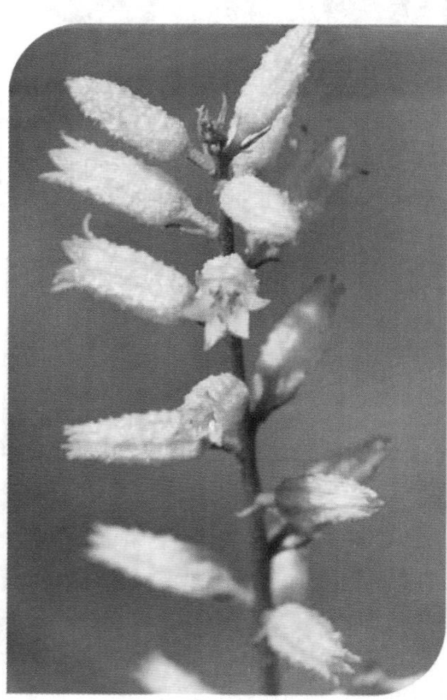

By John Flannery CC BY-SA 2.0

The erect stem of the Unicorn root is round near the base, but it is angular above, and grows 1 to 3 feet (0.3m to 0.9 meters) tall. When unicorn root is in bloom it is easily identified, so if you are not sure, wait for the flowers. Its round stem has a spike-like cluster of white, small, urn-shaped flowers. The flowers have an unusual appearance because of their warty-textured outer surface. Flowers are cylindrical, with a yellowish tinge at its rough and wrinkled apex and six divisions at the top.

Edible Use: The root is edible. Cook before eating. It has a bitter-sweet soapy flavor. The leaves are used to make tea.

Medicinal Use: Unicorn Root is used as a laxative, anti-flatulent, estrogen-replacer, sedative, treatment for diarrhea, arthritis, and as an antispasmodic. It is a pain killer and has narcotic effects. The root can be taken orally as a dried root, powdered root, tea, or tincture. You can also use the leaf as a tea. The infused oil of unicorn root makes a nice salve.

Habitual Miscarriage: The estrogenic properties of unicorn root make it valuable in treating a wide assortment of female related issues. It is a tonic for the female reproductive organs and of great use in treating cases of habitual miscarriages when taken throughout pregnancy.

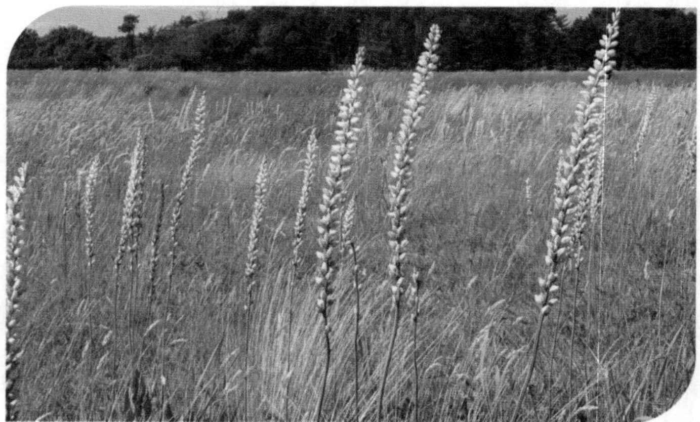

Menstrual Disorders, Menopause, PCOS, Vaginal Dryness, and Skin Aging: The estrogenic activity of unicorn root makes it a good treatment for many menstrual disorders and for the symptoms of menopause including vaginal dryness and hot flashes. Use the root tincture.

It is also used to treat other gynecological disorders such as amenorrhea, dysmenorrhea, PCOS, prolapsed vagina, and other female gynecological complications. It can be used on the skin in an oil or salve as an anti-aging cream.

Arthritis, Muscle and Joint Pain: The roots of unicorn root act as a pain killer and sedative. Use the root to make a salve, which you can rub on aching muscles and joints. The salve relieves the pain and calms the muscles.

Colic and Flatulence: The root of this herb causes gastric pain when fresh. However, the dried leaves are a treatment for colic and flatulence. Use the leaves only to make a tea and give in small doses. The amount of tea needed depends on the size and age of the child, start with a few drops, increasing the dose slowly. You can also use small amounts of powdered root.

Inducing Vomiting to Remove Toxins and Poison: When taken in large doses or used fresh, unicorn root acts as an emetic and induces vomiting. In smaller doses of the dried plant, it relieves stomach contractions and calms inflammation. It is important to note that the herb itself can be toxic, so it is best to follow a medical professional's advice.

Promotes Appetite: Unicorn Root is well known for its ability to encourage appetite.

Harvesting: Wear gloves when harvesting the roots and leaves to avoid being injured by the spike-like leaves of the plant. Dig up the roots in the late summer and dry them for later use. Do not use fresh unless you are trying to induce vomiting.

Warning: Because unicorn root has narcotic and sedative properties, it is easy to take too much. Use with care and always start with small doses. It can be toxic in large doses. Dry the roots and leaves before using.

Recipes: Unicorn Root Tea: For medicinal purposes only, not to be consumed as a routine beverage.

A few sprigs of shredded dried unicorn root, 1 cup water. Place the unicorn root into the water and heat to boiling. Remove from the heat and allow the tea to steep for 10 to 15 minutes. Strain out the root and use the tea as desired for medicinal purposes.

Unicorn Root Leaf Tea: 1/2 teaspoon dried unicorn root leaves, 1 cup boiling water. Pour boiling water over the unicorn root leaves and allow the tea to steep for 8 to 10 minutes. Strain out the leaves and enjoy.

Unicorn Root Salve: Making Unicorn Root Salve is a two-step process. First, you must infuse the oil, then make the salve.

Infusing the Oil: 1 cup Organic Olive Oil or another carrier oil, 1/4 cup dried unicorn root. Shred or grind the unicorn root into small pieces; grinding is best. Place the root into a glass jar and cover it with a suitable carrier oil such as olive oil. Allow the oil to steep for 4 to 6 weeks to release the beneficial oils from the root. If you need to speed up the process, you can heat the oil gently for 10 to 12 hours. Strain the oil through a coffee filter or cheesecloth to remove the root. Store the oil in a cool, dark place. Follow our Salve-Making Recipe on page 38.

Wild Comfrey, Hound's Tongue, *Cynoglossum virginianum*

Wild Comfrey is also known as blue houndstongue, as its leaves are said to look like a dog's tongue. It is native to eastern North America and much of Europe. It primarily grows in deciduous forests and open upland areas.

Note that this is not the same plant as Comfrey (Knitbone), *Symphytum officinale,* which is also in this book, though they are both in the Borage Family.

Identification: Wild comfrey grows on an erect simple stem with fine hairs on both the leaves and stem. The alternate leaves are simple, 4 to 8 inches (10 cm to 20 cm long and 1 to 3 inches (2.5 cm to 7.5 cm) wide with smooth edges.

The leaves are larger and stalked at the lower end of the stem and grow in a rosette. As you move up the stem the leaves are smaller, clasp the stem, and are unstalked. It is biennial. The blue-purple to white flowers appear in late spring/early summer. Each flower has five deep lobes connected to an ovary, which is connected to the style. Flowers are approximately 1/3 inch (0.8 cm) across and have ragged edges. Fruits are produced in mid-late summer. There are one to four prickly nutlets per flower, each having one seed that is covered with bristles that cling to clothing. The plant grows from a taproot.

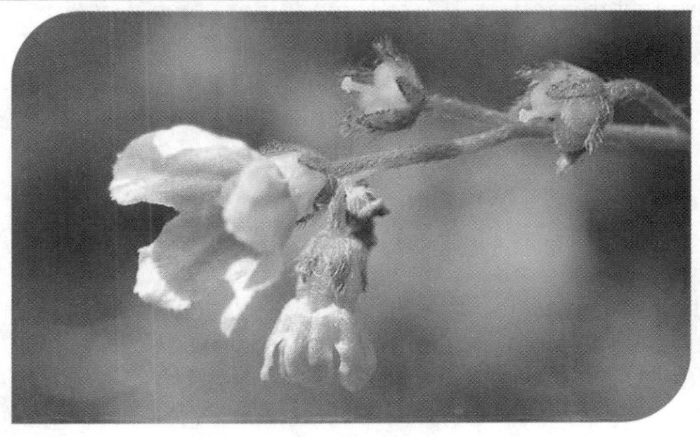

Cynoglossum virginianum by AlbertHerring

Medicinal Use: While both the root and the leaves can be used medicinally, the root is more powerful and best used fresh.

Note that this is a different plant than the medicinal comfrey, also in this book. I do not use this particular wild comfrey species as reports of medicinal uses are not backed up by as much research. I do use comfrey, *Symphytum officinale*, quite often.

Itchy Skin: Wild Comfrey Root Decoction is said to treat itchy skin.

Burns, Bruises, and Contusions: Wild comfrey leaves have been used as a poultice for burns, and bruises. Again, I prefer *Symphytum officinale* and don't use Wild Comfrey.

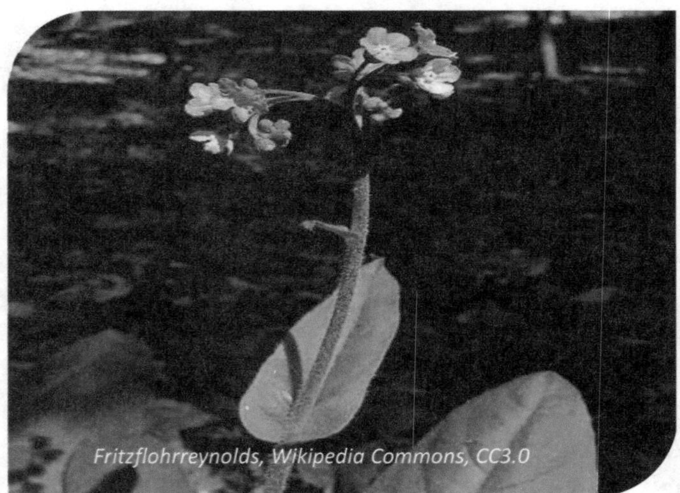

Fritzflohrreynolds, Wikipedia Commons, CC3.0

Warning: Avoid large doses and long-term use, which can result in liver problems.

Wild Ginger, *Asarum caudatum*

Also known as Canadian snakeroot, wild ginger is a member of the Birthwort family. It is not a true ginger, but tastes and smells like the popular spice. I like it as a flavoring and have never experienced any side effects, but many consider it potentially dangerous because of its aristolochic acid content. Use with caution. It is in the Aristolochiaceae (Birthwort) Family.

Identification: Wild ginger is a low growing ground cover that loves the shade. The plant grows from a rhizome, producing two opposite slightly hairy heart-shaped leaves about 3 to 5 inches (7.5 cm to 12.5 cm) in size. In the spring, it produces single reddish- brown flowers 1 to 1 1/2 inches (2.5 cm to 3.75 cm) in diameter. The flowers are easy to miss, growing below the leaf cover.

Edible Use: The root should not be eaten in large quantities, but used as a flavoring. It has a strong aromatic smell that is a combination of ginger and pepper. The leaves and roots make an excellent tea. Do not infuse in vinegar or alcohol. Aristolochic acid is not very soluble in water thus a tea is the preferred method of ingestion.

Medicinal Use: Wild ginger root is best known for its effect on the digestive system. It is soothing, laxative, and tonic.

Colds and Flu: The root tea promotes sweating and is useful in the treatment of colds and flu. It is an anti-inflammatory, antioxidant, and antimicrobial, helping to fight the underlying illness.

Fights Infections: Compounds in the wild ginger root inhibit the growth of many bacterial strains, lowering the risk of infections and helping to rid the body of existing infections. It does not kill existing germs, but prevents them from reproducing.

Gingivitis and Periodontitis: Oral bacteria that cause gingivitis and periodontitis respond to treatment with wild ginger. Try using the unsweetened Wild Ginger Root Tea as a mouthwash at least twice daily, after brushing. Rinse and spit.

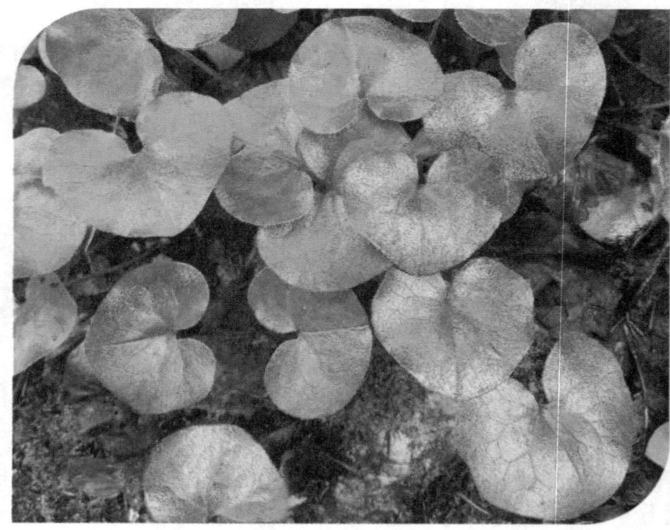

Nausea, Indigestion, and Food Poisoning: Wild ginger is effective in settling the stomach and calming nausea. Wild ginger tea helps empty the stomach, preventing or reducing indigestion. It helps alleviate the pain and discomfort caused by indigestion and bloating. Do not use if pregnant as it stimulates the uterus.

Diabetes, High Blood Sugar and Cholesterol: Wild ginger tea can help regulate blood sugar levels in diabetics and lower cholesterol and triglyceride levels, especially the "bad" LDL cholesterols.

Menstrual Cramping: Wild ginger reduces muscle cramping, relaxing the muscles and relieving inflammation and pain. It also helps to bring on menses.

Wounds and Skin Infections: Wild ginger root helps prevent external infections.

Chop or grate the root and apply as a poultice directly on the affected skin or make a strong tea to use as a wash or compress.

Harvesting: Wild ginger leaves can cause an allergic reaction or skin irritation in some people, so use gloves when harvesting the plant. I prefer to gather roots in the spring, but they can be dug at any time. Use them fresh or dry them for future use.

Leaves for tea can be harvested throughout the spring and summer.

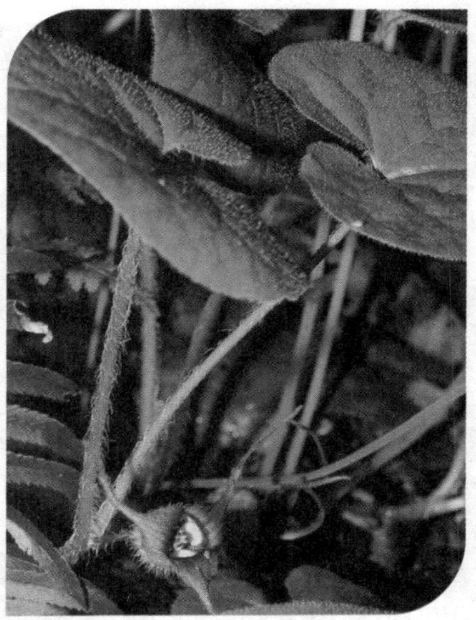

Wild Ginger with flower, Walter Siegmund [CC BY-SA 3.0]

Warning: Wild ginger is considered safe in small doses, but it does contain aristolochic acid, a toxin that can cause kidney problems or even be fatal in extremely high doses. Use wild ginger in medicinal doses as a tea and avoid eating large amounts. Wild ginger stimulates the menstrual cycle and can cause miscarriages in high doses. It has been used as a contraceptive and should be used with caution.

Recipes. Wild Ginger Root Tea: You'll need: 1 teaspoon chopped or grated ginger root,1 cup boiling water, and raw honey, if desired for sweetness. Pour boiling water directly over the grated ginger root and allow it to steep for 5 to 10 minutes. Strain the tea and enjoy. To use the tea as a compress or wash, use 1 tablespoon of grated or chopped ginger root and allow it to steep until cold

---

Wild Strawberries, *Fragaria vesca*

Wild strawberries, also called alpine strawberry, mountain strawberry, pineapple strawberry, and woodland strawberry, are mostly known for their delicious fruit. They are in the Rose Family.

Identification: Wild strawberries have light green leaves arranged in groups of three. The leaves are oblong and toothed. The plant spreads by runners that take root and produce a new plant. Wild strawberries bloom in April and May.

The small white flowers have five white petals and a yellow center. The berries usually mature in June to July.

Edible Use: I usually eat wild strawberries raw, however they can also be made into jams, fermented into wine or liqueur, or dried.

Medicinal Use: The berries, leaves, and roots are all used medicinally. The leaves are astringent.

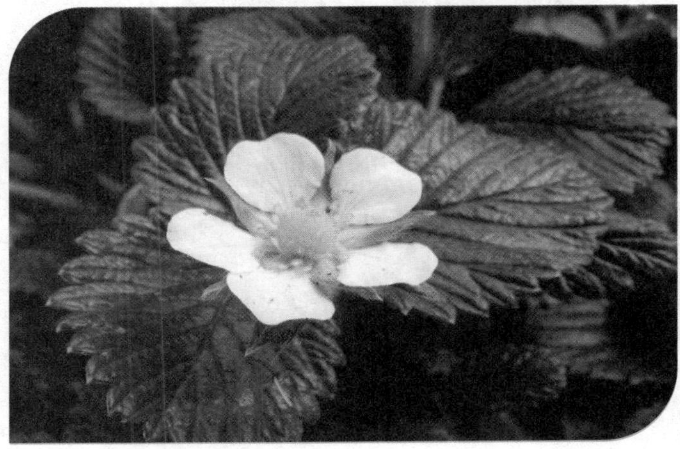

Stomach Problems, Diarrhea, Dysentery: Strawberry Leaf and Root Tea is beneficial in treating dysentery, diarrhea, and other stomach disorders. The berries and juice of the plant treat gastritis.

Sore Throat: Try using strawberry tea as a gargle to cure a sore throat. One teaspoon of dried strawberry leaves brewed with one cup of boiling water and strained works well to calm irritation and inflammation in the throat.

Diuretic and Increased Urine Flow: The leaves and roots of the wild strawberry have diuretic and astringent properties that flush excess water and toxins from the body.

Burns, Cuts, and Wounds: The antiseptic and mildly anti-bacterial properties of wild strawberry leaves work to heal skin wounds such as burns, cuts, and minor infections. Use the infusion as a wash to clean and sanitize the wound then use fresh chopped leaves as a poultice to reduce inflammation and help it heal. For sunburns, apply the crushed fruit on to the skin.

Toothpaste: Fresh strawberries can be rubbed on teeth as a regular tooth cleaner and stain remover. Leave for 5 to 10 minutes and then brush off.

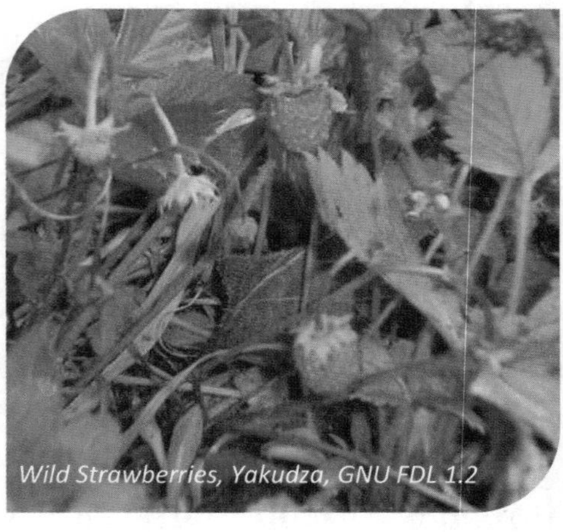
Wild Strawberries, Yakudza, GNU FDL 1.2

Joint Pain, Arthritis, and Gout: Wild strawberry leaves help treat arthritic and other joint pain. Try combining them with St. John's wort to drink as a tea for this purpose. Strawberry fruit is anti-inflammatory and helps prevent the formation of uric acid crystals in the body. Eating a serving of strawberries daily is protective.

Recipes. Wild Strawberry and St. John's Wort Infusion:1 teaspoon dried wild strawberry leaves, crushed, 1 teaspoon fresh or dried St. John's Wort flowers, 1 cup boiling water, lemon, and raw honey, as desired. Pour the boiling water over the wild strawberry leaves and St. John's Wort. Steep them for 10 minutes. Strain out the herbs and sweeten if desired. This tea is bitter. Honey and lemon help the flavor.

Wild Yam, *Dioscorea villosa*

Wild yam is in the Dioscoreaceae (Yam) Family. It is found in wet, wooded areas in eastern and mid North America. The plant has been overused and is becoming harder to find, so be careful when harvesting to replant tubers for future growth or find alternative herbs to use.

Identification: Wild yam grows on a variable twining vine with smooth stems. Its alternate, heart-shaped leaves have prominent veins radiating out from the stem. They occur in whorls of three and are hairy on the underside.

The vine produces separate male and female flowers from May to August. Prominent three-winged fruit appears in the fall. Roots are tubers.

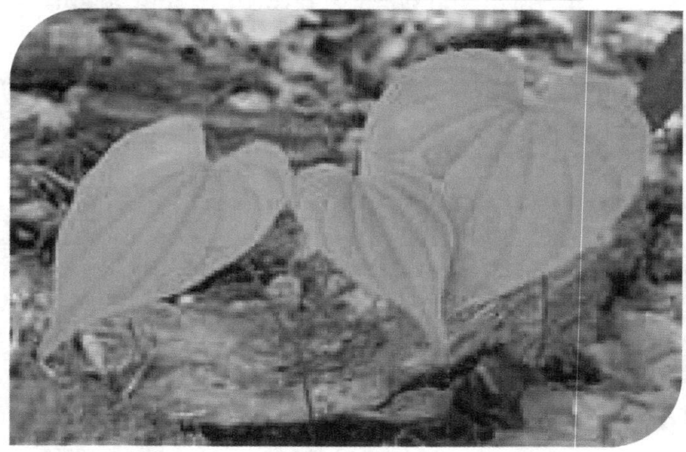
Wild Yam, Phyzome, CC by SA 3.0

Medicinal Use: Wild yam root is an anti-inflammatory and pain-reliever and is good for digestive issues. Use wild yam either as a dried powdered root or as a tincture made from the root. Not for long term use.

Colic, Crohn's Disease, Ulcerative Colitis and Other Digestive Issues: Wild yam is also known as colic root, indicating its value in treating colic and other digestive illnesses. It is known to treat digestive problems involving cramping, muscle spasms, inflammation, and bloating. It also works well for irritable bowel syndrome, Crohn's, Ulcerative Colitis, and diverticulitis.

Arthritis: Wild yam root contains anti-inflammatories and pain-relieving substances that make it effective in the relief of arthritis symptoms.

Wild Yam Tincture: 4 ounces (113g) powdered wild yam root, 1-pint (500 ml) 80 proof or better vodka. Place the powdered wild yam root in a glass jar and cover with vodka. Seal the jar tightly and place it in a cool dark place to brew. Allow to steep for 4 to 6 weeks, shaking the jar daily. Strain the tincture through a coffee filter. Store it in a cool, dark place for up to 3 years.

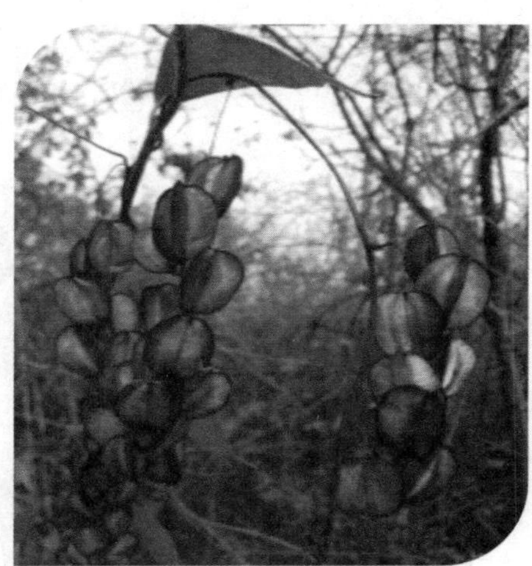

Wintergreen, *Gaultheria procumbens*

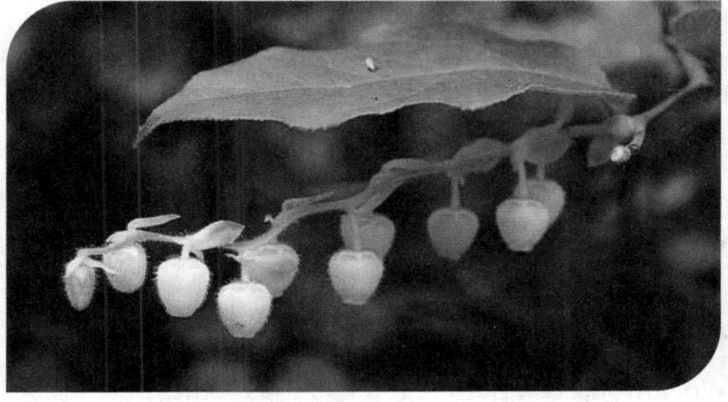

Wintergreen Flowers, Wing-Chi Poon, CC by SA 2.5

This member of the Heath Family (Ericaceae) is often identified by its scent. Although most wintergreen oil is now synthetically made, most people can readily identify the distinctive smell. It is also known as Eastern teaberry, checkerberry, mountain tea, deerberry, boxberry, ground berry, or spice berry. It grows in eastern and mid North America.

Identification: This semi-woody plant forms low growing leafy mats. The plants are approximately 6 inches (15 cm) tall with evergreen leaves, making them a popular choice for a groundcover. They like woodlands with moist, acidic soil and filtered sunlight or partial shade.

Bright green ovals or spoon-shaped leaves have a glossy appearance and a waxy or leathery feel. The leaves are attached in groups near the tip of a small reddish stalk. Waxy flowers with a droopy, bell-like appearance appear in June or July but are often hidden beneath the ground cover.

The brilliant scarlet-red berries ripen in late autumn through winter.

Edible Use: Wintergreen berries can be eaten raw or cooked and the leaves make a nice tea.

Medicinal Use: Distilled wintergreen oil contains a high concentration of methyl salicylate, a chemical compound used in the production of aspirin. It is used in creams and ointments for pain relief of sore muscles and joints. Because of its toxicity, wintergreen essential oil should never be taken internally. Wintergreen essential oil is metabolized into salicylic acid, which is a Non-steroidal Anti-Inflammatory Drug (NSAID).

Thirty milliliters of the oil, approximately 1 ounce, contains the equivalent of 171 adult aspirin tablets, a highly toxic amount. This illustrates how concentrated the oil is and why it should never be taken internally, even in small amounts. Because the oil is so potent, even small doses taken internally can be toxic. Wintergreen Essential Oil is obtained from the leaves by steam distillation.

Wintergreen berries and leaves are effective against pain and help reduce swelling and inflammation. Use it topically as a poultice, and in creams and ointments.

Sore Throat: Wintergreen tea is an excellent remedy to relieve pain and inflammation in a sore throat.

Gargle with one mouthful of the tea at a time, using the entire cup of tea over the course of a day, as needed. Do not swallow.

Headaches, Aches, and Pains: Wintergreen leaf tea provides quick relief of headaches and other aches and pains associated with arthritis, sciatica, and lumbago.

It acts quickly to relieve pain and long-term to reduce inflammation and swelling that causes the pain. Not for long term use.

Colic: Care must be taken when using any herbal remedy with children, so consult a qualified medical professional before using wintergreen or any herb on a child.

Wintergreen infusion is useful in relieving colic. Use only a few drops of a weak infusion to relieve gas pains and ease digestion, even less for young children. Best to consult a medical professional or to simply use a different, safer herb.

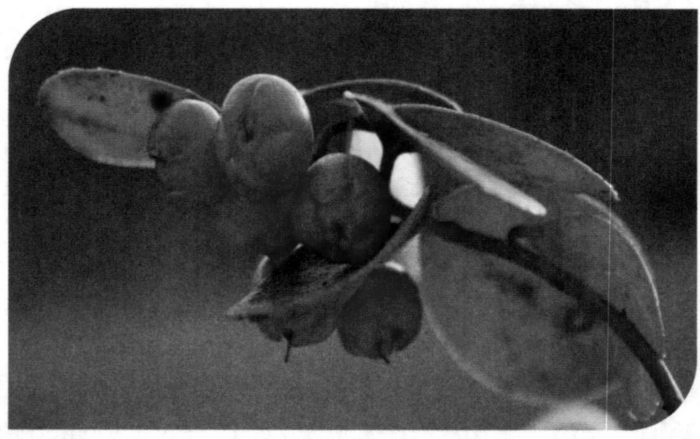

Poultice for Skin Inflammation: Either dried or fresh leaves can be used as a poultice for boils, swellings, skin ulcers, wounds, and sores.

Warning: Wintergreen essential oil is a concentrated form of methyl salicylate and should not be used internally. Undiluted use can also trigger contact dermatitis in some people. Always dilute the oil with a carrier oil or use it in a cream or ointment.

Wormwood, *Artemisia absinthium*

Wormwood is a powerful medicinal plant. It is a relative of mugwort, also in this book. This plant has a strong odor and a bitter taste. It is the primary ingredient in absinthe liqueur and is the responsible part for its hallucinogenic effects. It is in the Aster/Daisy Family. It grows wild in meadows and along roadsides in full sun throughout much of Europe and North America.

Identification: Wormwood is a shrubby plant with multiple stems that grows from a woody base to 1 to 5 feet (0.3m to 1.5m) tall. The stems are white or grey-green and covered by fine hairs. Its hairy alternate leaves are silvery or greyish-green on both the top and bottom (unlike mugwort, which are green on top and white on the bottom). The leaves produce resinous particles that act as a natural insecticide. The plant has three different types of leaves. At the bottom of the stem, the leaves are bipinnate or tripinnate with long petioles. In the middle of the stem, the leaves become smaller and less divided with shorter petioles. At the top of the plant, the leaves are simple with no petioles. This plant has small yellow flower clusters at the branch tops from mid-summer through autumn.

Medicinal Use: Wormwood is used fresh and dried. The leaves, stems, and flowers are all medicinally active. I use the dried leaves and flowers to make tinctures, tea, decoctions, and infused oils.

The wormwood plant contains thujone, toxic at a dosage higher than 35mg/kg. Alcohol distillation, like people use in making absinthe, increases the thujone concentration. The plant contains Vitamin C, carotenoids, flavonoids, phenolic acids, tannins, and many other healthy compounds. It is excellent for treating parasites, Crohn's, and intestinal and stomach ailments.

Malaria and Artemisinin for Lyme Protocol: Anti-parasitic compounds in wormwood have a powerful action against the malaria parasite. It quickly reduces the parasite population in the blood and helps treat the disease. Artemisinin, the effective compound against malaria, is one of the most effective herbal treatments for malaria. Wormwood is my first-choice herb in the treatment and prevention of malaria. Artemisinin is also often used as part of a Lyme Protocol, though it is often extracted from *Artemisia annua* (sweet wormwood).

Kills Parasites: In addition to the malaria parasite, wormwood is effective in eliminating intestinal worms, pinworms, and roundworms. I make a tincture with wormwood, garlic, cloves, turmeric, cayenne, oregano oil, and Oregon grape root to kill intestinal worms and parasites. Black walnut hulls are also effective.

Fights Breast Cancer: The artemisinin in wormwood has been found to be effective in killing breast cancer cells and from stopping the cancer from metastasizing.

Crohn's Disease, IBS, Stomach Issues, Acid Reflux: Wormwood has been found to accelerate healing for those with Crohn's Disease, even leading to complete remission in many people. It also spared the need for steroid treatment in Crohn's patients. It is an excellent anti-inflammatory. It is helpful for people with inflammatory bowel syndrome and treats indigestion, flatulence, acid reflux, and heartburn. It also stimulates the appetite.

Antimicrobial and Antifungal Properties: Try the infused oil or tea for use against microbes, including *Salmonella* and *E. coli*. The external oil is good to treat fungal infections and internally can be used to treat *Candida*.

Balances the Intestinal Flora: Overgrowth of bacteria in the intestinal tract is a common cause of

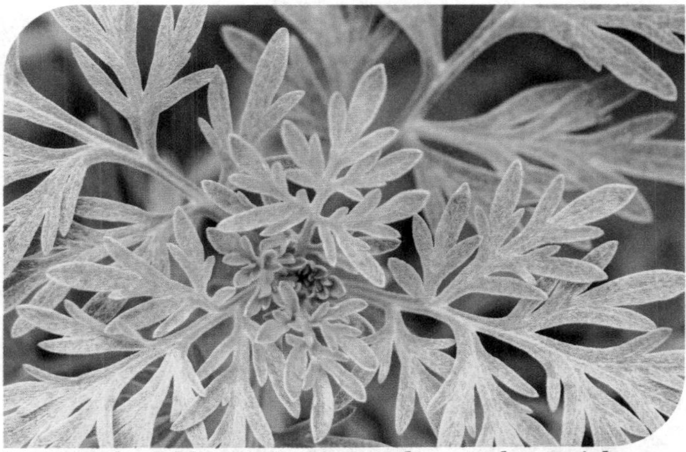

intestinal problems. Wormwood treats bacterial overgrowth, restoring and rebalancing the intestinal tract.

Harvesting: Allow the plants to grow for at least two years before harvesting. The medicinal properties are stronger as the plant matures. Harvest when the plant is in bloom on a dry day.

Warning: Take wormwood under the supervision of a medical professional. Use small doses and take it for no longer than 4 weeks at a time, then give the body a rest before repeating treatment if needed. Do not take wormwood if you are pregnant or breastfeeding. It can cause miscarriages. Do not use wormwood if you are allergic to it or other members of the daisy family.

Wormwood Tea: You'll need 1 teaspoon of dried wormwood leaves, 1 cup boiling water and dried peppermint or fennel, as desired for taste. Add the wormwood leaves to the boiling water and allow it to simmer for five to 15 minutes. Note that the longer it steeps, the more bitter it tastes. Use dried peppermint or fennel to flavor the tea and to help with intestinal upset.

Yellow Jessamine, *Gelsemium sempervirens*

Yellow Jessamine is a beautiful plant, but it can be deadly. It looks similar to honeysuckle and children sometimes confuse the plants and ingest the poisonous plant. Use with caution.

Yellow Jessamine is a twining, slender vine found throughout the southern United States. It is also called Poor Man's Rope, Evening Trumpetflower, Woodbine,

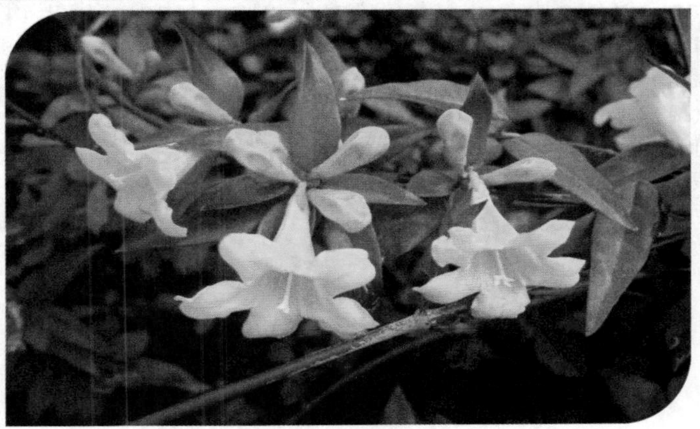

By KENPEI - KENPEI's photo, CC BY-SA 3.0,

and the Carolina Jessamine, because of its prevalence throughout the Carolinas. It is in the Gelsemiaceae Family.

Identification: Yellow Jessamine is often found climbing over fences, sign posts, trees, trellises, and up the sides of buildings. Yellow Jessamine vines like to climb, reaching up to the very tops of trees.

However, they are narrow enough that they do not starve the plants beneath them for sunlight. Without a tall, supporting structure to climb, it will simply grow into a tangled mound.

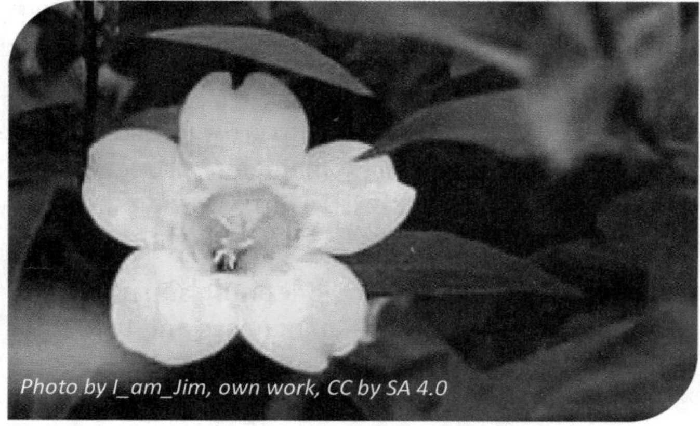

Photo by I_am_Jim, own work, CC by SA 4.0

Its leaves are simple and blade shaped with a shiny, waxy texture. Each leaf is 2 to 4 inches (5 cm to 10 cm) long and less than half an inch (1.25 cm) wide.

The leaves develop a yellow or purple shade in the winter months, but otherwise, the plants have deep green foliage. It is a semi-evergreen vine, keeping its leaves through most of the winter. Yellow Jessamine flowers begin to bloom as early as December and last through the spring.

Clusters of the fragrant yellow flowers bloom into tunnel-shaped, five-pointed stars. Toward the end of their bloom, little capsule-shaped fruits develop. The fruit is typically flattened and pod-like, growing about 1 inch (2.5 cm) in length. The flowers give off a scent like honey.

Medicinal Use: Caution should always be used when working with Yellow Jessamine. The entire plant is poisonous, and even small amounts of the extract can be deadly. I don't personally use this plant since safer preparations are almost always available.

Skin Care: A salve made from yellow Jessamine is used to treat boils and acne.

Muscle Pain and Arthritis: Yellow Jessamine can be helpful in treating muscle pain and arthritis using a diluted tincture or salve. If too strong a dose is used these preparations sometimes relax the muscles to the point of paralysis.

Sedative, Fevers, and Headaches: Yellow Jessamine depresses the nervous system and acts as a sedative.

This is the source of its powers and also the source of its poison. A tiny amount can relieve pain and reduce fevers, while too much has deadly effects. A small amount of dilute salve applied to the forehead works to reduce headache pain.

Warning: It is important to remember that all parts of yellow Jessamine are considered highly toxic and ingestion can be fatal.

Under no circumstances should any portion of the plant be eaten in any form. In the Southern States, it is not uncommon for young children to confuse yellow Jessamine for Honeysuckle and require immediate medical attention. The plant is so toxic it can even kill the bees that pollinate it, resulting in colony collapse. Consumption of fewer than 4 milliliters of Yellow Jessamine extract can prove fatal.

Symptoms include sweating, nausea, muscle paralysis, convulsions and muscular spasms, and dilated pupils. If consumed, or if you experience any of these symptoms, immediate medical treatment is required.

Yerba Santa, *Eriodictyon californicum*

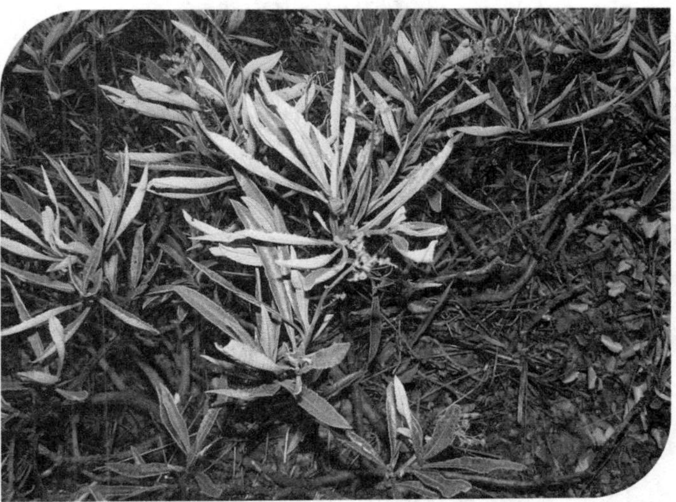

Yerba Santa is my number one plant to dry up mucous.

Yerba Santa, also known as Mountain Balm, Consumptive Weed, or Bear Weed, is an evergreen shrub native to the coastal chaparral and Redwood forests of the Pacific Northwest. It is in the Hydrophyllaceae (Waterleaf) Family.

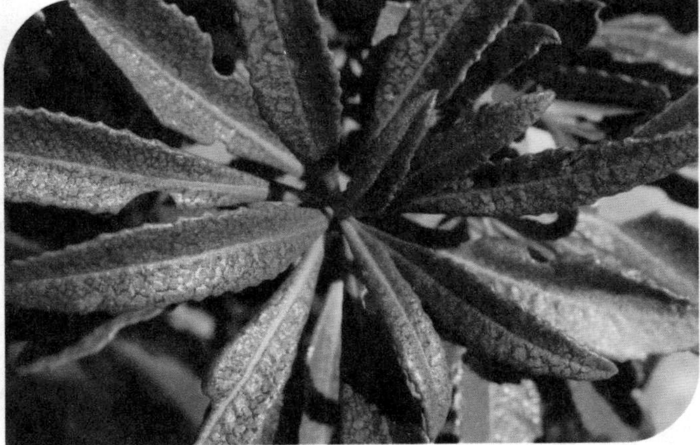

Yerba Santa, Wikipedia Commons

Identification: Yerba Santa grows in small colonies along dry, rocky slopes, ridges, and hillsides. It is especially common on eastern and southern facing surfaces. It grows from 3 to 8 feet (0.9m to 2.4m) in height, with many straight, protruding branches. Its long, lance-shaped leaves are dark green, growing from a short stem. The more mature leaves often feel sticky to the touch and may even appear sooty or black. This is the result of a common fungal growth that forms on mature Yerba Santa shrubs.

The pink and purple flowers of Yerba Santa bloom in the spring. The gray fruit surrounds a small seed capsule containing small hard black seeds. The shrub itself is an occasional source of nutrition for some animals, especially deer in the winter, but the leaves have a pungent and unpleasant odor and a bitter taste.

Edible Use: Surprisingly, because of the bitter leaves, Yerba Santa extract can be used as a taste enhancer, especially effective in masking unpleasant flavors. To make the extract, take about an ounce of the leaves and place them in a mason jar. Pour boiling water to the top and let steep overnight. Strain and store the extract. Use the extract to mask objectionable flavors in teas or extracts.

Medicinal Use: The leaves are used for medicine.

Mucous, Asthma, Fevers, Allergies, Sinus, and Respiratory Infections: Yerba Santa contains chemical components that alleviate and loosen mucus in the chest and sinus due to infection, colds, allergies, etc. I use a very effective leaf tincture to dry up mucous but you can also apply the plant as a poultice by crushing the steeped leaves and rubbing it on the chest.

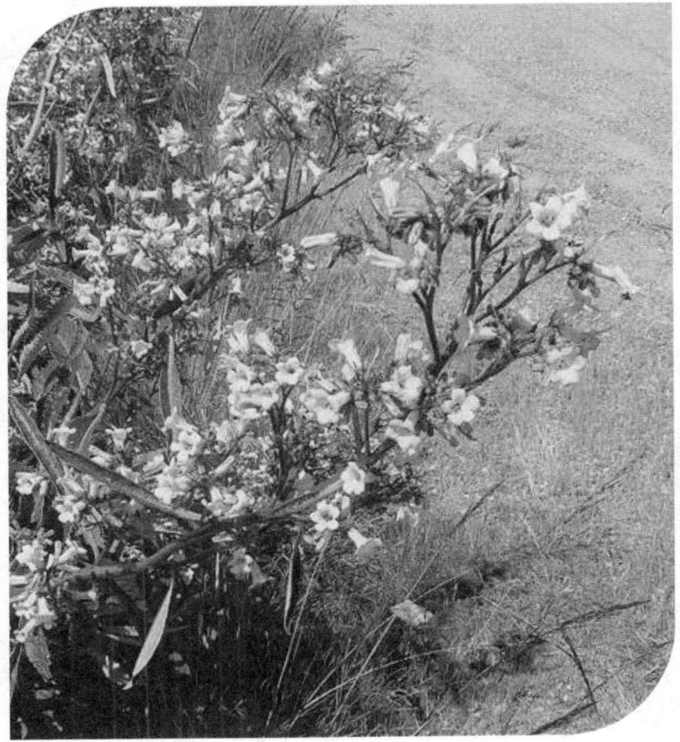

Topical Skin and Pain Relief: Yerba Santa leaves can relieve arthritis and muscle spasms by applying the leaves directly on the afflicted area. Mature leaves should stick naturally to the skin thanks to their sticky residue.

Fever Relief: Yerba Santa tea can be used to relieve fevers.

Mouthwash: A natural mouth freshener is made by balling up washed leaves and letting them dry in the sun. Once dried, chew these balls. The initial taste is bitter, but after chewing briefly, spit out the leaf ball and drink some water. The taste gives way to a pleasant, natural sweetness.

Warning: Yerba Santa can negatively affect the body's ability to take in iron and other important minerals, so it is not advised for women who are nursing or pregnant.

Trees and Shrubs

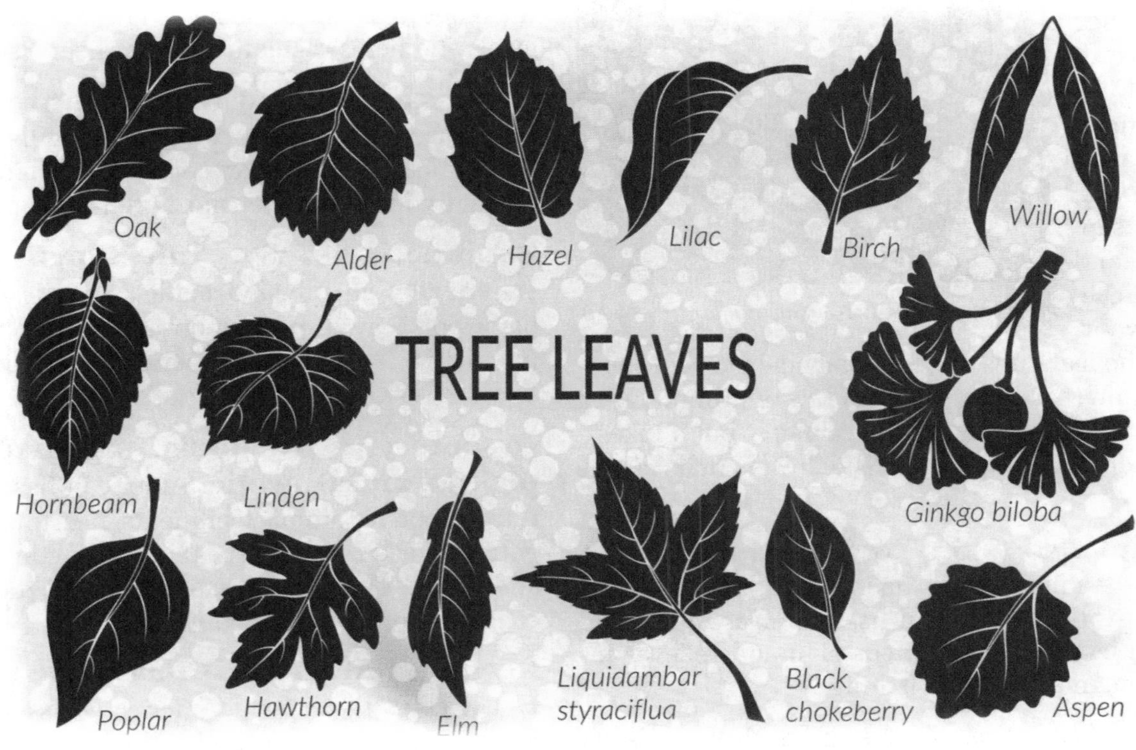

American Basswood or American Linden, *Tilia americana*

Tilia americana belongs to the Malvaceae (Mallow/Hibiscus) Family. It is most commonly known as American Basswood, American Linden, and American Lime Tree. The common name of this plant is from "bastwood," referring to use of the inner bark, the "bast," for weaving rope and baskets. The tree is a native to eastern and mid North America.

Identification: American Basswood is a large deciduous tree that reaches a height of 60 to 100 feet (18m to 30m). It has a trunk diameter of 3 to 6 feet (0.9m to 1.8m) at maturity. It has gray furrowed bark with flat ridges.

Leaves of American Basswood are deciduous, alternate, and unevenly heart-shaped. Leaves are 4 to 6 inches (10 cm) long, about 3 inches (7.5 cm) wide, thick and slightly leathery, with sharply serrated margins. They are usually smooth and hairless on both sides but occasionally have soft downy hairs on the lower surface.

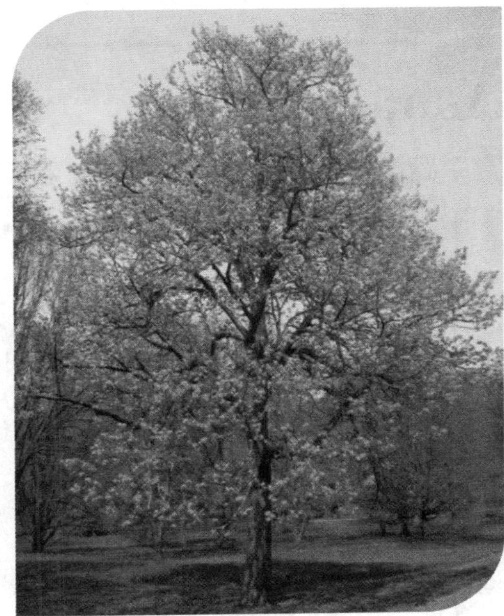

Yellowish-white fragrant flowers grow in drooping clusters of 5 to 20 and are about ½ inch (1.25 cm) wide. It flowers May thru June for about 2 weeks. Fruits are small dry round nutlets that ripen in autumn, with each fruit bearing one seed.

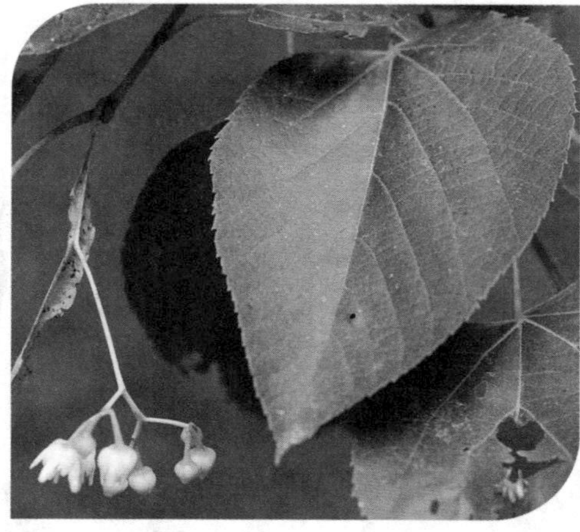

Plant Image Library - Tilia americana, CC by SA 2.0

Edible Use: Edible parts of this plant include its flowers, leaves, seeds, bark, and sap. Leaves and flowers can be eaten raw or cooked. The leaf buds are especially delicious. The inner cambium (bark) can be eaten raw or ground into a flour. The tree can be tapped like a maple but it takes a lot more sap to make a syrup. The flowers make a nice tea.

Medicinal Use: Skin Treatments Burns. A poultice or tea made from the inner bark of American basswood works well for burns, sunburns, boils, and other skin irritations. It softens skin and relieves inflammation, infection, and itching.

Sedative, Anticonvulsant, and Nerve Pain: American Basswood is a sedative, an antispasmodic, and an analgesic. It helps with nerve pain, anxiety, insomnia, and seizures. A tincture made from the leaves and flowers effectively treats seizures and other problems related to the nervous system.

Hypertension, High Cholesterol, and Heart Tonic: An American Basswood flower and leaf tincture helps lower high blood pressure. Its calming effects extend to the cardiovascular system as they relax the blood vessels. It also helps lower blood cholesterol levels and helps regulate irregular heartbeats.

Coughs and Throat Irritation: The flowers and leaves are used to treat coughs, laryngitis, and throat irritations, though *Tilia cordata*, the European littleleaf linden, is the tree most often used for this.

Conjunctivitis, Eye Infections, and Eyewash: Try an infusion made from fresh American basswood leaves to clear up eye infections and conjunctivitis. A recipe for American Basswood Infusion Eyewash is below.

Dysentery, Heartburn, Stomach Complaints, and Diuretic: American Basswood Tincture is good for stomach ailments, heartburn, and dysentery. For stomach issues, use a tincture of flowers and leaves. The inner bark infusion has diuretic properties and promotes urination.

Recipes. American Basswood Infusion Eyewash: 1 teaspoon American basswood leaves, crushed but not ground and 1 cup distilled water. Bring the water and fresh leaves to a full boil, then reduce the heat and simmer for 10 minutes. Strain the infusion to remove all of the plant material. Allow the mixture to cool completely before using. Use fresh.

Ash, *Fraxinus americana* or *Fraxinus excelsior*

The ash tree, also known as the American Ash (*F. americana*), Common Ash, Weeping Ash, White Ash, and European Ash (F. excelsior), is a tall, fast-growing tree that can reach up to 100 feet (30m) in height. The tree grows tall and thin when young, and it spreads and becomes more rounded as it ages. It is in the Oleaceae (Olive) Family.

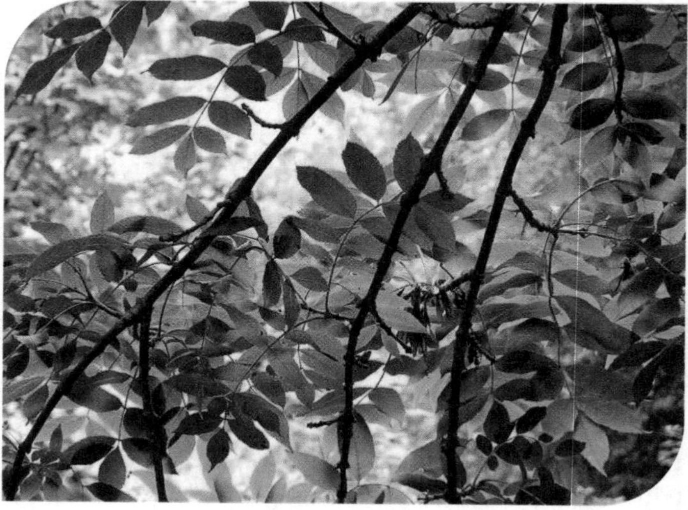

Copyright Andrew Curtis and licensed for reuse under this Creative Commons Licence

Identification: In the early spring, before the leaves have fully formed, the branches display clusters of flowers, with male and female flowers on separate plants. It has large 8 to 12 inch (20 cm to 30 cm) dark green opposite pinnately compound leaves that each have 5 to 11 oval-shaped leaflets. The leaflets are 2 to 5 inches (5 cm to 12.5 cm) long, stalked, and shiny green on top and pale green below. Margins may be slightly toothed. The fruit is a tan winged achene, called a samara, one to two inches (5 cm) long. Each fruit contains a single seed.

Medicinal Use: Leaves, seeds, inner bark, and sap are used for medicine.

Childbirth, PCOS, Uterine Fibroids: Ash Leaf Extract is used as a tonic after childbirth. It is used homeopathically for PCOS and uterine fibroids.

Fevers, Stomach Cramps, Laxative: Ash tree inner bark has tonic and astringent properties. It can be taken as a tea to treat fevers and stomach cramps. Ash Leaf Tea is a diuretic and useful for flushing excess water and toxins from the body. The inner bark is a laxative.

Harvesting: Gather the leaves during the summer when the leaves are fully open, but before they begin to change color. Gather the bark in the spring.

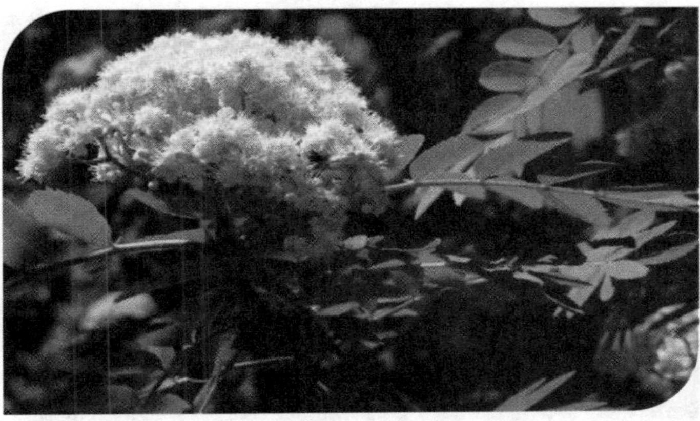

Warning: Ash can cause vomiting when taken internally. Use caution. Ash is very potent and should not be combined with other medicines without the advice of a doctor or qualified health professional. Do not give ash to pregnant women, nursing mothers, or young children. Do not use ash for people with kidney or liver problems.

Ash Tree Bark Tonic: 1 teaspoon dried inner bark of the ash tree, 1 cup boiling water. Add the inner bark to the boiling water and turn off the heat. Allow the tonic to brew for 15 minutes. Strain out the bark.

Balsam Fir, *Abies balsamea*

The balsam fir is popular as a Christmas tree. It is also known as the Canada balsam, fir pine, silver fir, or silver pine. It is easily recognized by its cone-shape, short needle-like leaves, and its fir fragrance. It is in the Pinaceae.

Identification: Most balsam firs grow 45 to 65 feet (13.7m to 19.8m) tall when mature. The Christmas trees sold for indoor use are only a few years old and still immature. The tree grows in the classic Christmas tree shape, although trees grown for sale are shaped. In nature, the tree forms a narrow crown that is more rounded than the single point that most commercial trees have.

Leaves are short dark green, flat needles, each approximately an inch (2.5 cm) long and silver-blue on the underside. The bark is smooth and grey with resin-filled blisters that form a rough, scaly appearance on older trees.

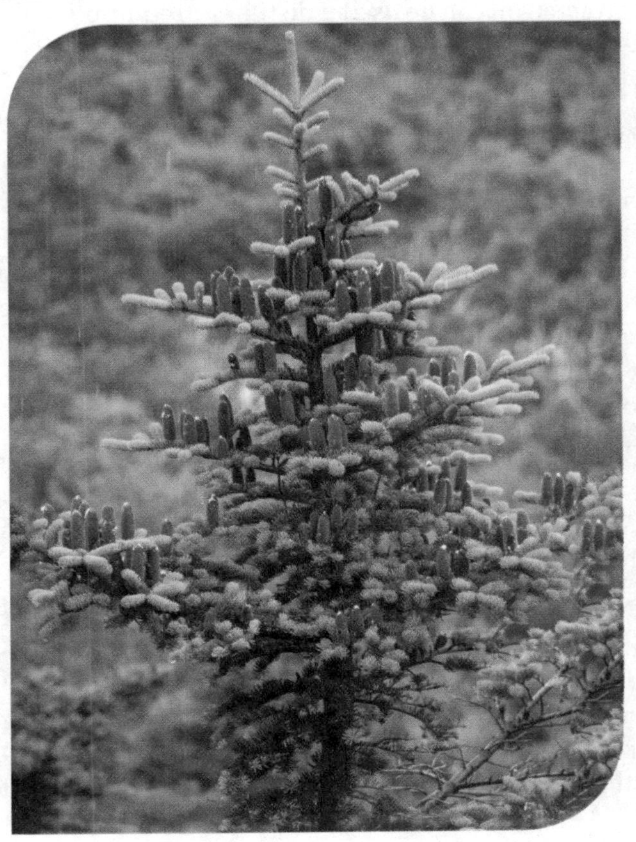

Seed cones are about 1 1/2 inch- to 3 inches-long (3.75 cm to 7.5 cm) and dark purple, turning brown and opening to release the seeds when mature. The seeds are winged and release in September.

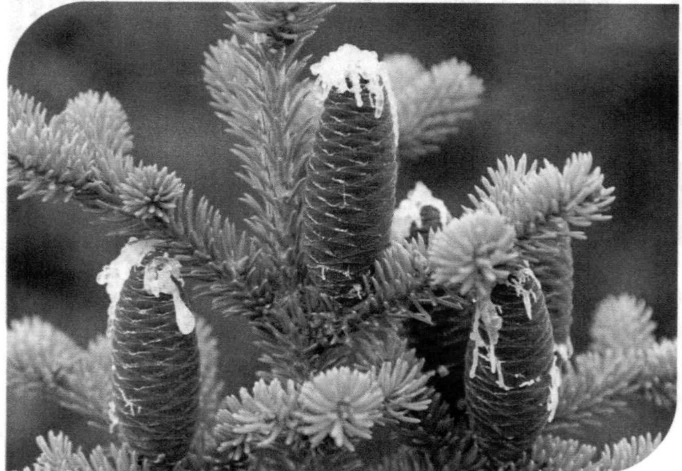

Balsam Fir Seed Cones with Resin, Cephas - Own work, CC by SA 3.0

Medicinal Use: The leaves and twigs can be used to make medicinal teas, tinctures, and extracts, and the pitch is used as it is or to make a medicinal tea. It has antibiotic, analgesic, and anti-cancer properties. The distilled essential oil and extracted oil are also valuable medicines. The distilled essential oil is strongest, but extracted oil can be used if distillation equipment is not available.

Healing and Infections: Cuts, Sores, Wounds, and Abrasions. Balsam fir pitch or resin is easy to use as is as on cuts, sores, and wounds of all kinds. Cover the affected area with the pitch. It forms a protective cover, helps prevent and heal infection, and helps wounds heal quickly. It has antiseptic and healing properties. For large cuts, use the stickiness to "glue" the edges of the wound together to help it heal once it is clean. Infused oil can also be applied for infection.

Chapped Lips and Cold Sores: In winter, smear a little balsam fir pitch on your lips to prevent chapping. If your lips are chapped, or if you have a cold sore, the pitch helps the area to heal quickly.

Bronchitis, Coughs, and Sore Throats: For bronchial and chest congestion, coughs, tuberculosis, and sore throats, use either Balsam Fir Tincture or Balsam Fir Pitch Tea. If using tea, sip as needed to calm sore throat pain, coughs, and bronchial spasms. Another treatment for bronchial congestion is to add balsam needles to water and use it in a sweat bath or sauna. The essential oils in the needles will sweeten the air and loosen phlegm from the lungs, easing breathing.

Gonorrhea: Balsam Fir Pitch Tea is useful for curing the sexually transmitted disease Gonorrhea.

Anti-Cancer Agent: Balsam fir essential oil has many anti-cancer and anti-tumor properties. The oil stops the growth of cancer cells, prevents cancer from spreading, and kills existing tumor cells. The oil also has anti-inflammatory properties, which calm the inflammation in the nearby skin. Common dosage is to take one to two drops of distilled balsam fir essential oil in a tablespoon of organic olive oil or add one to two drops to a cup of balsam fir tea. Take two to three times daily. Start with one drop, then increase it to two when you are sure you are not allergic. Balsam fir essential oil can be used along with conventional cancer treatments.

Painful Muscles and Body Aches: Balsam fir essential oil is an excellent pain killer for muscle and body aches. Put a small amount of the diluted essential oil (always dilute essential oils in a carrier oil) onto the achy area and massage it into the skin.

Harvesting. To Harvest Balsam Fir Pitch: The pitch is found in blisters on the tree bark. Simply open the blisters with a knife, cutting gently into the blister. If the blister is forcefully popped, the pitch can spray out. The pitch is clear, runny, and sticky. In cold weather, it is thick and almost gel-like in texture. I collect the pitch into a small glass jar with a tight lid.

To Harvest Balsam Fir Leaves: The young leaves and shoots are best for making teas and

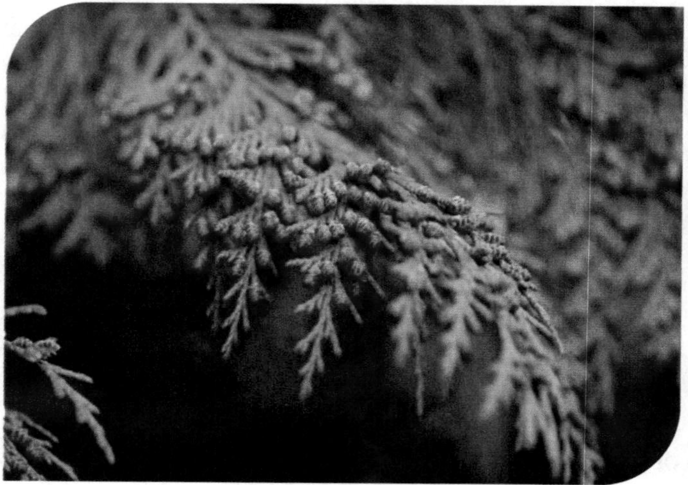

tinctures. It is best to harvest leaves and young shoots in the spring. Use them fresh to make tinctures and dry some leaves for use throughout the year.

Recipes. Balsam Fir Pitch Tea: Dissolve a small amount of balsam fir pitch, approximately 1/8 to 1/4 teaspoon, into a cup of warm water or an herbal tea. Drink pitch tea as needed to calm throat pain and bronchial spasms.

Extracted Balsam Fir Oil (Cold or Warm Extraction). Cold Extraction: Balsam fir leaves, twigs, and/or bark, dried, organic olive oil, or another suitable carrier oil. Fill a glass jar 2/3rds full of dried balsam fir needles and small pieces of twig or bark. Cover the fir needles and twigs with organic olive oil, filling the jar to within ½ inch (1.25 cm) of the top. Stir the oil and herbs to make sure no air pockets remain. Place the jar in a sunny window for 6 to 8 weeks. Strain the oil through a fine sieve to remove the leaves, twigs, and bark. Store in a cool, dark place, and use the oil within one year.

Warm Extraction: Place the herbs and oil in the top of a double boiler. Fill the bottom of the double boiler with water and heat to a low simmer. Heat the oil and herbs slowly for 2 hours, checking frequently. Simmer. Do not boil. Strain the oil through a fine sieve or cheesecloth. Discard the herbs. Store in a cool, dark place, and use the oil within one year.

Balsam Poplar, *Populus balsamifera*

Balsam poplar is a member of the Salicaceae (Willow) Family. It is also commonly known as bamtree or eastern balsam poplar. It has similar uses as Cottonwood Trees (also in this book). It is most commonly found in Northern North America. It likes moist sites along rivers and in floodplains.

Identification: If you live in an area where balsam grows, you probably already know this tree. *Populus balsamifera* is a deciduous tree growing up to 100 feet (30m) tall. It has brown bark on the branches in the first year that turns grey as it ages. This fast-growing tree can grow several feet in height each year. The simple, toothed, alternate leaves are narrow to broadly oval-shaped and pointed. They are 3 to 5 inches long and 1.5 to 3 inches (4.5 cm to 7.5 cm) wide. Their bases taper in a heart shape and are usually rounded at the base. The underside is whitish or pale green and the tops are a shiny green. Its flowers are borne in catkins. The male catkins are 1 to 2 inches (2.5 cm to 5 cm) long. The female catkins are nearly 3 inches (7.5 cm) long.

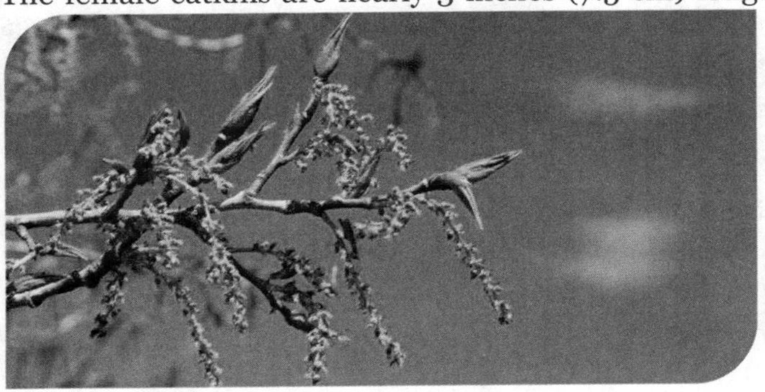

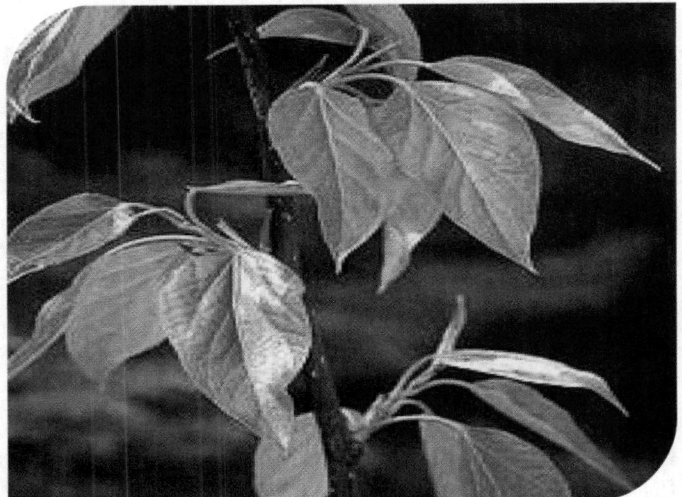

Their blooms form in mid-spring. Their fruits are egg-shaped capsules with two to three carpels each. They are usually hairy.

Edible Use: You can dry the inner bark of balsam poplar and grind it into a flour to use as a thickener or add it to flour for making bread. Catkins can be eaten raw or cooked.

Medicinal Use: The inner bark, leaf buds, and resin are most often used.

Coughs, Colds, Bronchitis, and Respiratory Diseases: The inner bark and buds of balsam poplar have proven to be a highly effective treatment for respiratory illness. The anti-inflammatory effects soothe swollen airways, while the herb expels mucus and relieves pain and fever. It also has anti-microbial effects that combat the causes of the disease. When treating severe congestion, try a steam treatment. Put poplar balsam buds into boiling water and breathe in the cooled steam. This releases the phlegm and gives quick relief.

Arthritis: Balsam poplar reduces the pain and inflammation of arthritic joints. For joint pain, try drinking inner bark tea daily and using the buds as an external infused oil or salve.

Skin Conditions: For skin diseases, inflamed skin, cuts, wounds, burns, bruises, acne, rashes, and other related skin conditions, balsam poplar is a good herbal treatment. The resin from the buds soothes and moisturizes irritated skin and burns, and the tea makes a good wash for general skin irritations. It relieves pain and itching while calming the inflammation. The resin can be used fresh or extracted with alcohol.

Harvesting and Warning: See Cottonwood

Bayberry and Wax Myrtle, *Myrica carolinensis* and *M. cerifera*

Southern Bayberry/Wax Myrtle fruit is a favorite among the local bird populations. It grows in wet bogs, marshes, and thickets near sandy coasts They also grow along the banks of the great lakes. The wax is used for candle-making and provides the "bayberry scent". It is in the Myricaceae (Wax Myrtle) Family.

Identification: The plant is an evergreen shrub, sometimes deciduous, growing 6 to 12 feet (1.8m to 3.65m) tall. It has long elongated leathery dark green leaves with jagged edges, hanging from thin, small trunks. The shrubs produce either all male or all female flowers.

Male flowers have 3 to 5 stamens, while female flowers produce globular fruit that is coated with wax. Flowers appear in the spring to early summer, and fruit follows in the late summer and fall. Another bayberry, *Myrica pensylvanica*, grows further north, but the range overlaps.

You can easily tell the shrubs apart by examining the leaves. The *Myrica pensylvanica* leaves are greener and lack hairs on the fruit wall and papillae.

They are also rounder at the tips, while the Southern Bayberry come to a point. *Myrica pensylvanica* does not have all of the healing properties of *Myrica carolinensis*. Below Bayberry and Wax Myrtle are used interchangeably and taxinomically they are often lumped together under *M. cerifera*.

Edible Use: The berries can be eaten raw or cooked and the leaves can be used for flavoring like bay leaves.

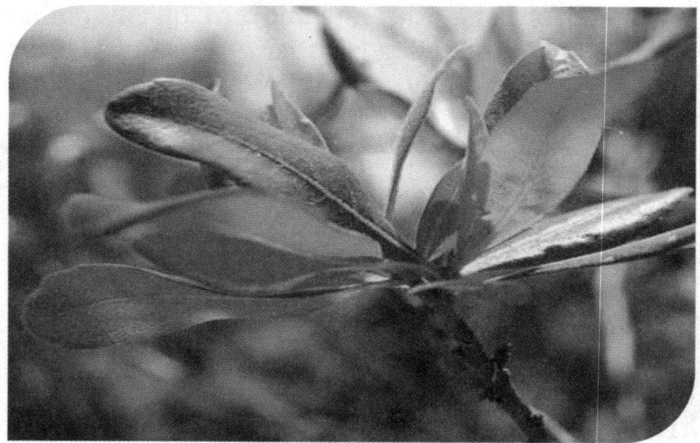

4 Northern Bayberry, Myrica Pensylvanica, Photo by Derek Ramsey - Own work, CC BY-SA 2.5

Medicinal Use. Bayberry root bark, leaves, and berries are used.

Diarrhea, Colitis and Digestive Issues: Try bayberry root mixed in a glass or water for bowel and digestive issues. It is effective in the treatment of diarrhea and colitis. When bayberry root is not available, you may use the leaves.

Dysentery and Ulcers: A concentrated extract made from the bayberry fruit is used (see recipe below).

Common Cold and Sore Throats: Powdered bayberry root in a glass of cold water makes a soothing gargle for sore throats and colds. Cold bayberry leaf tea can also be used.

The root bark is an astringent that brings blood to the area to speed healing.

Reduce Fevers: Those same qualities that bring blood to the surface and speed healing also dilate the capillaries in the skin and induce sweating, cooling the body.

Muscle Aches and Arthritic Joints: The wax of the bayberries contains pain-relieving agents. Combined with the healing benefits of the powdered root, it makes an excellent salve for aching joints and muscles.

Harvesting: Collect the root bark in the late autumn or early winter and dry it for future use. Store the pieces in sections, then chop it or powder it when needed to keep it fresh. Store the bark in a tightly sealed container in a cool, dark place. Harvest the bayberries when they are at the peak of ripeness and extract the wax as soon as possible. Retain both the wax and the water for medicinal use.

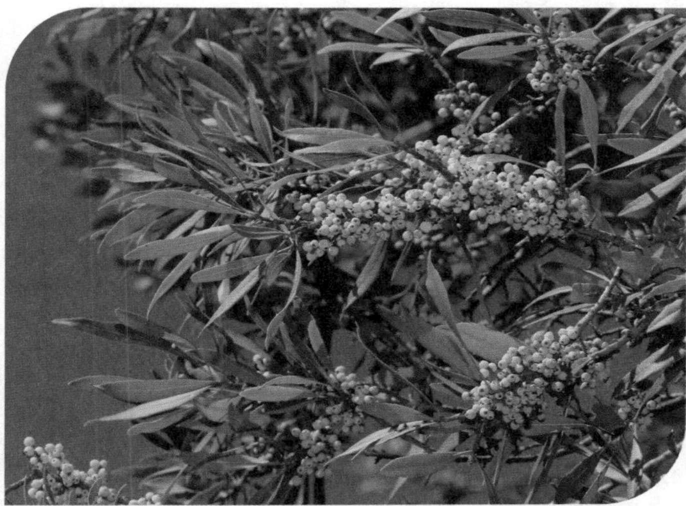

Recipes. Bayberry Tea: 1 tablespoon dried bayberry leaves or crushed root, 1 cup water. Bring the water to a boil and pour it over the leaves or root. Allow leaves to steep for 10 to 15 minutes and root bark to steep for 20 to 30 minutes. Strain the tea. Use hot or cold.

Bayberry Fruit Extract and Wax Extraction: Around five pounds of berries are needed to yield about one pound of wax. Gather bayberries in the mid-fall when the fruit is fully ripe. Wash the berries in cold water and place them in an old pot, preferably one reserved for wax making, and cover them with at least 2 inches (5 cm) of water. Bring the pot to a simmer, but do not boil. Simmer for at least one hour.

Turn off the heat and cool overnight. In the morning, remove the solid wax from the water and keep it for other uses. Put the water back over low heat and simmer it again to reduce the volume greatly, leaving a few cups of water only. This concentrates the medicinal qualities so that only a few drops are needed per dose. Store the extract for up to 3 days in the refrigerator or divide it into smaller containers and freeze it for future use. The dosage depends on how concentrated the extract is made. Try using a few drops of a concentrated solution in tea. Use the saved wax below to make salve.

Bayberry Salve – for external use only. 1/4 to 1/2 cup extracted bayberry wax (see above recipe), 1 cup organic olive oil or another carrier oil, more if needed, 1 tablespoon powdered bayberry root. Add the powdered bayberry root to the organic olive oil and place over low heat. Warm the oil and powdered root together for 30 minutes. Add the bayberry wax, stirring, until it is melted and the wax and oil are thoroughly combined. Cool the mixture and test the consistency. Add more wax if the salve is too runny or more oil if it is too hard. The consistency will depend on your extracted wax and may vary between batches.

Bilberry, *Vaccinium myrtillus*

Bilberry is sometimes called whortleberry, dyeberry, and European blueberry. It is often confused with true blueberries. This plant is a powerhouse of nutrition and medicine. There is no better reason to eat jam and jelly every morning than the medicinal benefits found in this little berry. Watch closely for them to ripen, as the birds also love them. It is in the Ericaceae (Heath) Family. The bilberry plant is found in meadows and moist northern coniferous forests, and is a common arctic and subarctic shrub. It likes acidic soil. It is a European plant but is commonly found in North America

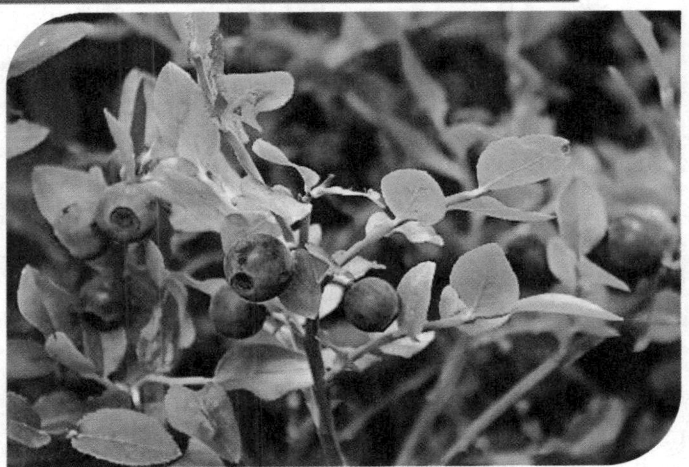

5 Anneli Salo [CC BY-SA 3.0]

today. The plant is a close relative to blueberries, huckleberries, and cranberries.

Identification: This deciduous shrub grows low to the ground, usually less than 2 feet (0.6 meters) tall. Flowers are pink and urn-shaped. The fruit are small, blue-black in color, and contain many seeds. The flesh is dark red or blue, versus the pale-green inner fruit of blueberries. Bright green leaves are alternate with finely-toothed margins.

Edible Use: Bilberry is a relative of blueberry, but has a slightly tart bitter flavor, so it is mostly used cooked with sugar, though I quite like them raw. They are often used for pies and jams. The leaves are used for tea.

Medical Use: Bilberry is a strong anti-oxidant, anti-inflammatory, anti-bacterial, and anti-fungal that has many beneficial properties. It is also a natural antihistamine.

The berries are very high in anthocyanins, which give it its blue-black color, and are a strong anti-oxidant and heavy metal chelator. Berries and leaves are used for medicine. Medicinally, you can eat the berries raw, in jams or jellies, or eat them dried and powdered in capsule form.

Powerful Anti-Inflammatory: Bilberries are rich in antioxidants and help reduce free radical damage. They also fight inflammation in the body. By reducing inflammation, they protect against many the many chronic diseases that are caused or aggravated by inflammation, including many autoimmune diseases.

Diabetes: Compounds in both bilberry berries and leaves help reduce blood glucose levels and insulin resistance. Reducing blood sugar levels helps protect the kidneys, eyes, nerves, and blood vessels. Bilberries may also help combat obesity by decreasing fat absorption and have been shown to both treat and prevent Type 2 diabetes.

Improves Vision: Bilberries are remarkable for their ability to improve the health and function of the eyes. It can help treat night blindness, cataracts, macular degeneration, poor vision, and chronic eye strain.

Bilberry protects the cells of the eye, reduces inflammation, and helps prevent damage to the ocular nerves in diabetics. Use it internally; it is not used topically in the eyes.

Anti-Cancer: The anti-inflammatory and antioxidant properties of bilberries help lower the risk of cancer. Bilberries help reduce inflammation and reduce free radical damage in the body. They also inhibit the growth of cancerous cells as well as help kill off cancerous cells.

Liver and Kidneys and Detox Heavy Metals: Bilberry berry compounds help the body remove toxins and help improve function of the liver and kidneys. It helps balance chemicals in the kidneys and the anthocyanins help organs chelate heavy metals like arsenic, lead, cadmium, and iron from the blood.

Heart Health: Bilberries have many benefits for the heart and circulatory system. It supports the blood vessels, lowers blood pressure, and helps regulate cholesterol levels and the plaque that causes atherosclerosis. It also contributes to the formation of healthy blood platelets and reduces the chances of a heart attack or stroke. Bilberry compounds help strengthen blood vessel walls, improving varicose veins and hemorrhoids.

Gastrointestinal Problems, Irritable Bowel Syndrome, and Ulcers: Bilberries help soothe the gastro-intestinal system. Tannins and anti-inflammatory compounds reduce inflammation and irritation in the intestinal tract. It helps relieve symptoms such as nausea, indigestion, diarrhea, and IBS. Internally, the leaves are both preventative and curative of ulcers. A leaf extraction can be applied topically to ulcers in the mouth.

Alzheimer's Disease and Dementia: Antioxidants in bilberries help slow cognitive decline and reduce the effects of existing symptoms. It may also improve overall mental focus and clarity.

Promotes Healthy Gums: Bilberries are anti-inflammatory and help reduce inflammation and swelling in the mouth and gums. The anti-inflammatory, astringent, and antibacterial compounds help fight gingivitis.

Harvesting: Harvest green bilberry leaves at any time before winter. Pick the berries when they are fully mature and blue-black in color. Cut or prick each berry and dry them on a dehydrator for future use.

Warning: Bilberries are safe, with no known side effects, and are often eaten as a fruit. However, they can interfere with some medications. Consult your health care professional before eating bilberries if you have problems related to blood clotting or if you take blood-thinning medications or aspirin.

Consult your doctor if you are pregnant or breastfeeding. Diabetics should also discuss bilberry prior to use. Leaves should only be utilized short-term.

Birch, *Betula* spp.

Birch trees are members of the Betulaceae (Birch) Family and are related to alders and hazelnuts. They are found throughout most of the Northern Hemisphere. There are over 60 species worldwide.

Identification: Birch trees are deciduous and grow quickly, but they don't reach the towering heights of many trees. Most grow to about 30 feet (9.1 meters) tall or less, though yellow birch and paper birches reach about 80 feet (24 meters). They often grow in stands (groupings).

Birch trees often have several main stems or trunks, giving the tree an irregular shape. Some look bushy, others have a rounded crown. Birch bark can be quite varied. The paper birch has a thin, white bark that peels into paper-like strips. Yellow birch bark curls into small strips of bronze-colored bark. Mature river birch trees have a scaly blackish-gray bark. Birch leaves are alternate, toothed, and pinnately veined.

Leaves are oval or triangular, broad at the top and pointed at the end. Birch trees have male and female flowers on the same tree. The male flowers appear in late summer and remain on the tree. The female flowers are smaller green catkins that form on the end of the branch. Once pollinated, they become cone-like, open, and fall apart.

Edible and Other Use: The sap of the birch tree can be tapped and made into a syrup. The sap can also be consumed as is. It is nutritious, containing vitamins, minerals, and amino acids. The inner bark of birch contains xylitol, a sweetener that also kills unwanted bacteria in the mouth when used orally (like in gum). The bark is used for making baskets and containers and birch bark is an excellent firestarter.

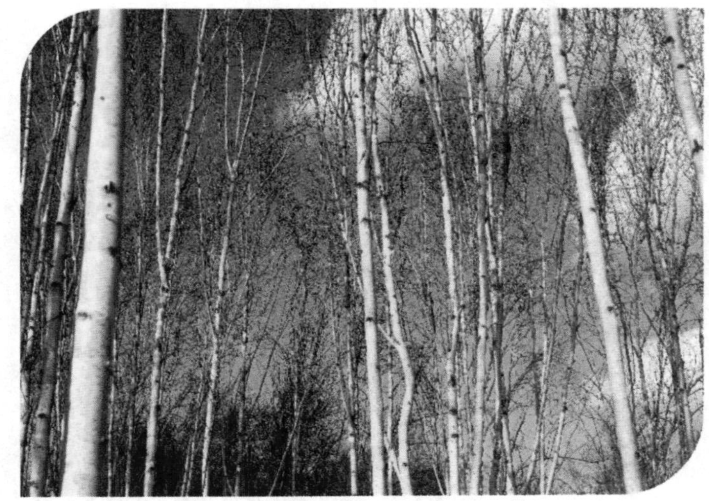

Medicinal Use: The leaves, twigs, catkins, bark, buds, and sap are all used medicinally. They have anti-inflammatory, astringent, and diuretic properties. Birch contains salicin, which helps with pain and is an anti-coagulant. Inner birch bark also contains betulin, which is a triterpene and is best extracted in oil, vinegar, or alcohol as it does not extract well in water. We best utilize it as betulinic acid. Chaga mushroom, which grows on birch trees, is a good source of betulinic acid, which is antiviral, anticancer, and antibacterial.

Anti-Inflammatory, Arthritis, Eczema, and Sore Muscles: Birch leaves, buds, bark, and twigs have anti-inflammatory properties that are easily accessed by boiling the twigs, buds, and leaves. A medicinal tea or decoction can be used internally or as a wash on the skin. It is used to treat arthritis, painful joints, eczema, and sore muscles. You can make a salve using infused birch oil made from the buds.

Diuretic, Edema, Heart and Kidney Problems: The diuretic properties of birch trees help the body release excess fluids, which helps lower blood pressure and helps the kidneys. Birch also helps lower cholesterol and break up kidney stones.

Urinary Tract and Kidney Infections: Birch Bark is useful in treating urinary tract infections and cystitis. It helps first by removing excess water from the body, increasing the urine and flushing out infections. It has anti-inflammatory and anti-bacterial properties that help treat the underlying disease.

Stimulates the Digestive System: Birch tree extracts stimulate the digestive system and aid digestion. Its anti-inflammatory properties are beneficial in calming the digestive system and relieving cramping, abdominal pain, bloating, and diarrhea. Try the recipe below for Birch Leaf Vinegar Extract.

Coughs and Congestion: Birch Leaf Vinegar Extract, recipe below, is effective in treating coughs. Add leaves to a water steam and inhale to help relieve congestion.

Burns and Frostbite: The inner bark of the birch tree is useful in treating frostbite and burns. It soothes the damaged skin, reduces pain and inflammation, and helps the skin heal. Remove the bark from the tree and mash it to a pulp adding sap from the tree if necessary, to form a wet pulp. Apply the pulp to the damaged skin and cover with a clean cloth. If the area is infected, use a poultice of leaves and leaf buds in the same way.

Supports the Immune System: Birch Leaf Tea is excellent at supporting the immune system. It is anti-inflammatory, anti-bacterial and contains many vitamins, minerals, saponins, flavonoids, tannins, and other compounds that are excellent for the immune system. It helps cleanse and heal the body.

Cancer: Betulinic acid from birch is being actively researched as an anti-cancer drug. Note that the Chaga mushroom, which grows on birch trees, effectively converts the betulin found in birch into betulinic acid. See page 268 for Chaga.

Harvesting: Harvest sap in early spring, and buds and branches in late spring, before the buds open. Harvest inner bark in spring or autumn. Collect birch leaves in the summer when the leaves are fresh and bright green, and harvest in the morning before the heat dissipates their oil. Use them fresh (best) or dry for future use. Strip the bark in shallow thin strips using a sharp knife.

Warning: Birch leaf is considered safe for external and internal use. However, pregnant or nursing mothers should not use it.

Some people are allergic to birch and should not use it. Birch leaves can increase salt retention in the body and may increase blood pressure in sensitive individuals. Avoid birch if you have high blood pressure. Do not use if you are taking diuretics or water pills. Drink plenty of water when using birch.

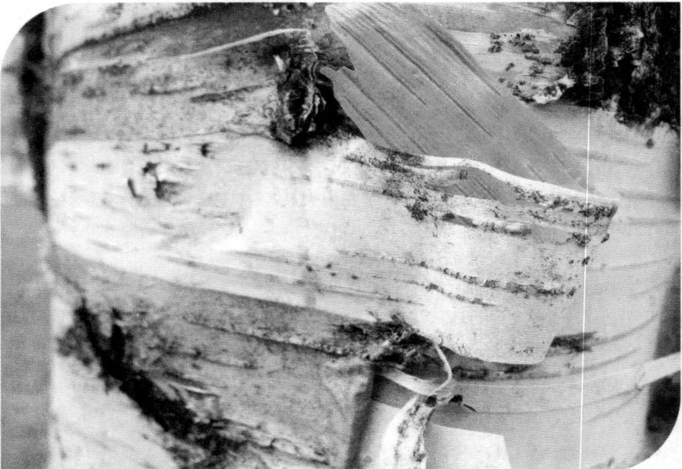

Recipes: Birch Leaf Vinegar Extract. Birch tree leaves, crushed, Apple cider vinegar. Crush birch leaves and stuff into a jar, about 3-quarters full. Cover the leaves with apple cider vinegar and stir to release air bubbles. Add more vinegar until the jar is full. Cap tightly. Let the leaves soak for 4 to 6 weeks, shaking the jar every day or two. Strain out the leaves and label the vinegar. Use the vinegar with meals, in salad dressings, or drink in water with meals. Good for 1 year.

Birch Leaf Oil or Inner Bark Extract: Pack a jar about 3-quarters full with fresh birch leaves and/or inner bark. Cover the leaves with organic olive oil or almond oil and fill to the top. Cover the jar and place it in a sunny spot on a windowsill and allow it to steep for 6 to 8 weeks, shaking the jar every day or two. Strain the oil into a glass jar with a tight-fitting lid and label it. Store in a cool, dark place.

Black Crowberry, *Empetrum nigrum*

Black crowberry, crowberry, or mossberry, is a low evergreen shrub that is usually 4 to 10 inches (10 cm to 25 cm) high and forms a dense mat on the ground. It is in the Ericaceae (Heath) Family and is found throughout North America, Europe, and Asia.

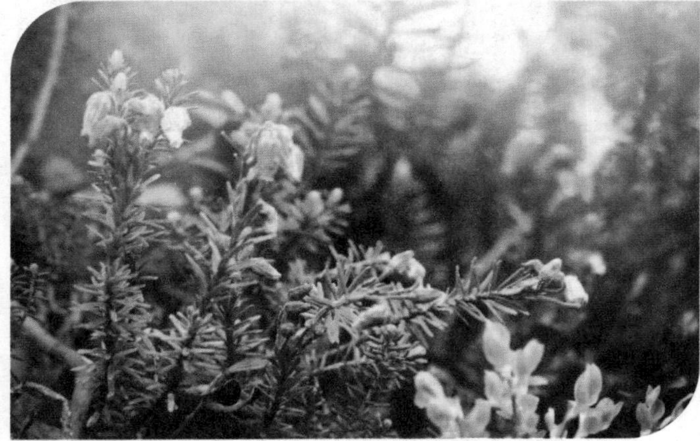

Identification: The light green needle-like leaves are simple and narrow, with side margins that are strongly curled under. It likes to grow in rocky areas. The leaves have glands that produce toxic substances and leaves are shed every 2 to 4 years.

Black crowberry produces small, individual pink-purple flowers during the summer and a sour blue-black fruit.

Edible Use: The berries are the only edible part of the plant, but the twigs can be used for tea. Crowberries have an acrid bitter taste, which is why they are rarely eaten fresh. They are usually used for pies, jams, juice, and wine.

Berries ripen in autumn and remain throughout much of the winter, making them a good Vitamin C source in wintertime. The berries are very high in anthocyanins and are an excellent antioxidant.

Medicinal Use: The fruit, branches/twigs/stems, and roots are used for medicine.

Diarrhea, Dysentery, and Gastroenteritis: Diarrhea and other stomach illnesses respond well to a Crowberry Leaf Infusion made from the leaves and stems. The infusion stimulates mucous, calms the digestive tract, and reduces inflammation. The cooked berries are used for gastroenteritis.

Antibacterial and Antifungal: Crowberry branches are both antibacterial and antifungal.

Eye Wash: A tea made from the roots of crowberry can be used as an eye wash for sore eyes.

Antihistamine, Anti-inflammatory, and Pain Relief: The berries contain the antihistamine and anti-inflammatory quercetin. This anti-inflammatory also helps with pain relief and can be used for any disease resulting from inflammation.

Harvesting: The fruits of black crowberries are ripe and ready to harvest between August and September. They can be harvested until the onset of winter or they can be allowed to winter on the plant for harvesting in the spring.

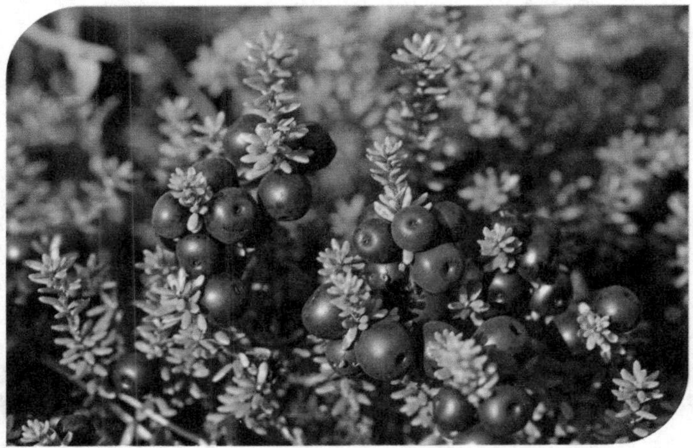

Recipes. Crowberry Leaf Infusion: 1 ounce of the leaves and stems of the crowberry plant, 1 cup boiling water. Chop the leaves and stems into fine pieces and cover them with boiling water.

Cover the container tightly. Let the herbs steep until the liquid has cooled to room temperature. Strain out the herbs.

Black Walnut, Eastern, *Juglans nigra*

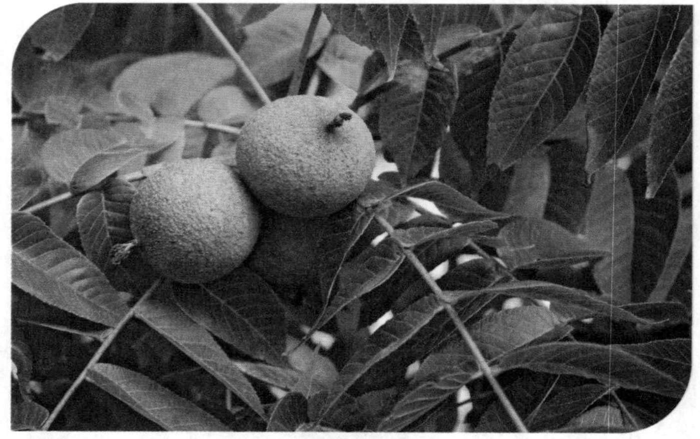

The eastern black walnut is a deciduous tree in the Juglandaceae (Walnut) Family. It is widespread in Eastern North America.

Identification: Black walnut trees grow to 100 feet (30 meters) tall and have a tall, straight trunk with an oval crown. The bark is grey-black with deep, thin ridges that appear to give the bark a diamond-shaped pattern. It usually doesn't have lower branching – just the top crown. Buds are pale colored and covered in hairs.

Terminal buds are 1/4 inch (0.75 cm) long and oval shaped. Lateral buds are smaller. Its large (1 to 2 foot) pinnately compound leaves are alternately arranged with 13 to 23 leaflets, each 3 to 4 inches (7.5 cm to 10 cm) long. Leaflets have a rounded base, pointed tip, and a serrated margin. Leaves are dark green, smooth on top and hairy on the bottom.

The black walnut has both male and female flowers. Male flowers appear first on drooping catkins, approximately 3 to 4 inches (7.5 cm to 10 cm) long, on the previous year's growth. Female flowers appear on new growth in clusters of two to five flowers.

The fruit (nuts) ripen in the fall. A brownish-green husk covers the brown nut. The nut, including the husk, falls to the ground in October or November and is harvested from the ground. The seed is small and hard. While the nut lacks odor, most parts of the tree have a characteristic pungent or spicy odor.

Edible Use and Other Use: The seed is edible, either raw or cooked. The flavor is rich and sweet. The sap of the tree can be tapped and drunk or concentrated into syrup or sugar. Black walnut hulls work well as a dye.

Medicinal Use: Black walnut is an anti-inflammatory, anti-fungal, antiviral, astringent, emetic, laxative, painkiller, and vermifuge. The green hulls are more potent than the mature black hulls, and are what I use for medicine.

To Treat and Prevent Parasites: Black walnut hull, used along with garlic, cloves, Oregon grape root, and wormwood, is an excellent remedy for parasite and worm infections. I have used this herbal blend for many types of parasitic infections. This remedy will kill the eggs, larva, and adult worms and parasites.

Skin Care: For preventing and treating blemishes, acne, psoriasis, eczema, warts, poison ivy, and other skin conditions, use a poultice from ground black walnut husks and water. For sensitive skin, try mixing a little of the powdered husk with a carrier oil.

Antifungal: Black walnut hull is an excellent choice for treating fungal infections. Black walnut contains juglone and tannins that are very effective for treating yeast infections, including *Candida*, in the gut and on the skin. Externally, black walnut is effective against athlete's foot, ringworm, jock itch, and other common fungal infections. Use the juice from the fruit husk externally as a treatment for ringworm or make a poultice or salve from powdered husks when fresh hulls aren't available. Apply the absorbent powdered hulls into the folds of the skin for surface yeast infections and heat rashes.

Digestion and Laxative: The anti-inflammatory activity of black walnut is useful in treating upset stomach, inflamed colon or gut, and normalizing the digestive process. Black walnut hull also treats constipation, diarrhea, and is a laxative.

Heart Health: Black walnuts contain beneficial omega-3 fatty acids and other heart healthy compounds.

Anti-Viral, HPV, HIV: People have long been using black walnut to prevent and treat viral infections. Black walnuts and black walnut hulls inhibit the reproduction of viruses, including herpes. A study published in Phytotherapy Research found that juglone in black walnut hulls inhibits replication of the HIV virus. While there are no therapeutic recommendations yet, it would be advisable for those exposed or infected by HIV to take Black Walnut Hull Tincture. In addition to the hulls, the roots and buds also contain juglone. Juglone is not soluble in water so best to use an alcohol extract/tincture.

Harvesting: Wear gloves when collecting black walnuts since the husk will stain your hands. Collect nuts that have fallen to the ground, nuts that remain on the tree are not yet mature. Remove the green to yellowish hull from the nut. Eat the nuts and dry and save the husk for use in poultices, tinctures, and to powder when needed.

To store black walnuts inside their shell, lay them out and allow them to dry for a few days after harvesting. Store them in a dry, squirrel-proof area. To crack nuts, use a hammer, nut cracker, or a vise to crack the shell. Remove the meat inside. Black walnut leaves can be picked for use throughout the season.

Warning: Side effects associated with black walnut use are not common. However, it is important to note that nut allergies are very common. Black walnuts or any of their products should not be given to anyone allergic to tree nuts. Risk during pregnancy is deemed low, but it is best to avoid black walnut internally if you are pregnant or nursing.

Recipes. Black Walnut Hull Tincture: Ground walnut hulls, vodka or another 80 proof or higher alcohol. Place the ground hulls in a clean, dry jar with a tight-fitting lid. Fill the jar 1/3rd full. Pour 80 proof or higher vodka or other alcohol over the hulls to within ½ inch (1.25 cm) of the top. Cover tightly and place the jar in a cool, dark place. Shake the jar every few days. Watch the alcohol level and add more if needed. Soak the hulls for 6 to 8 weeks. Strain the mixture through a fine sieve or cheesecloth. Squeeze out all liquid.

Discard the hulls. Place the alcohol extract in a cool place, undisturbed overnight. Strain again through a coffee filter or decant to remove any remaining hull residue. Store the tincture in a tightly capped glass bottle in a cool, dark place.

Blue & Black Elderberry, *Sambucus nigra ssp. caerulea* (blue) and *Sambucus nigra ssp. canadensis* (black)

Sambucus nigra tincture is with me 24/7 as an antiviral. I dose with it when traveling or at the first sign of illness. It is in the Adoxacaeae (Moschatel) Family and is one of my family's most important herbal medicines.

Identification: Elderberry grows as a wide woody shrub to about 12 feet (3.1 meters) tall. The segmented stems have a soft white pith. The bark is smooth and green when young. As the wood ages, the bark becomes smooth and brown, and you will notice round lumps on the bark. As the shrub continues to age, the bark develops vertical furrows.

Opposite compound leaves have 5 to 11 toothed lance-like leaflets per stem. Veins in the leaves may disappear after leaving the midrib, or they may continue to the tip of the teeth. The elderberry blossom is a dense head of white to cream-colored flowers. Flowers are radially symmetrical with five flat white petals and five protruding stamens. The flower head is 6 to 12 inches (15 cm to 30 cm) across. Elderberries are black or purplish-blue when ripe and occur in clusters.

Important Differentiation: Some people confuse elderberry with the deadly poisonous water hemlock. Water hemlock is an herbaceous plant, not woody, and it does not have bark. The main stem of water hemlock is hollow, while elderberry is filled with a soft pith. Water hemlock stems often have purple streaks/splotches and purple nodes. Older plants may be entirely purple.

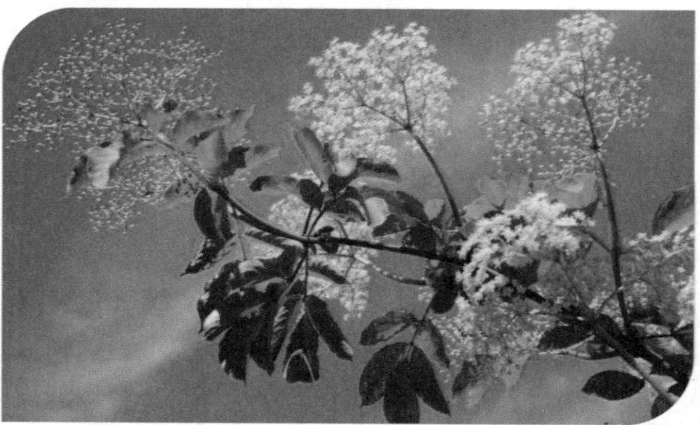

Edible Use: The *Sambucus nigra* variety of elderberry is considered non-toxic when used fresh, but I always cook all varieties, and some people become ill from fresh berries. Other varieties of elderberry's fruit pulp and skin are edible when picked fully ripe and then cooked. However, uncooked berries and other parts of the plant are poisonous. The flowers are edible when they are completely dried; do not use them fresh. I use cooked fresh berries to make elderberry syrup, elderberry wine, and cordials.

Medicinal Use: The flowers, leaves, and cooked berries are all useful. I use elderberry berry tincture once a day as a preventative during flu season or during travel, and 3x per day if feeling a cold or flu coming on. I extract the berries in glycerin or alcohol.

Colds and Flu, Anti-Viral: Taken early blue elderberry reduces the chance of catching the flu. Taken after a flu infection, it reduces the spread of the disease throughout the body and lessens the severity and duration of the virus. Blue elderberry is one of the best anti-virals out there and there has been much research supporting its effectiveness. It is deemed safe for children and my kids take it in the form of a tincture or syrup. The flowers also reduce inflammation, help drain mucous, and promote perspiration. They have anti-viral, anti-inflammatory, and anti-cancer properties. Elderberry is most effective in combination with yarrow to bring down fever.

Bruises, Sprains, and Hemorrhoids: For bruised tissue, muscle sprains, and hemorrhoids, use chopped elderberry leaves applied as a poultice to the affected area or infuse the leaves in oil to apply (my preference). Leaves are only for external use.

Eye Irritation and Conjunctivitis: Elderberry Flower Tea makes a gentle eyewash for eye irritations and conjunctivitis.

Strengthens the Immune System: Elderberries have long been recognized as a therapy for a variety of illnesses. It is thought that their beneficial effects are due to their ability to strengthen the immune system.

Harvesting: Harvest the berries during the early autumn when they are fully ripe. I like to harvest and then put the berries in the freezer. Once frozen it is easy to remove the berries from their stems. Remove all stems before using!

Warning: All parts of the fresh plant are mildly toxic. Dry or boil berries before use and dry the flowers. Do not use the fresh plant without cooking or drying. The bark and root are emetic, causing vomiting, and should not be used internally. The leaves and unripe berries are toxic.

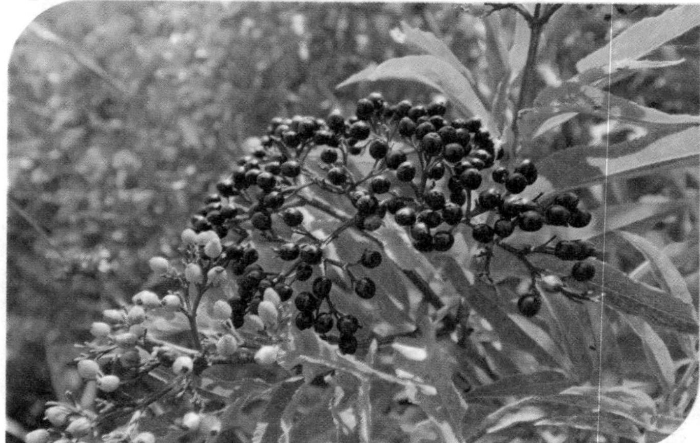

Recipes: Elderberry Syrup. Use 1 to 2 teaspoons for adults and ½ to 1 teaspoon for kids. Take once a day as a flu preventative and 3 to 4 times daily if infected. 1 cup of elderberries, water, 1 cup of raw honey, and ½ tsp of ground cinnamon. Place fresh elderberries, with all stems removed, in a pot and add a small amount of water to cover. Heat the berries over low heat for 2 hours. Mash the berries to release the juice or puree the berries in a blender. When all the juice is released, strain the juice through several layers of cheesecloth. Squeeze the cloth to extract all the juice.

Measure the juice and mix in an equal amount of raw honey. Add cinnamon if desired. Put the syrup in clean pint canning jars and seal.

Place the jars in a boiling water bath, completely covered with water and boil for 15 minutes at sea level to 1000 feet (300 meters) in elevation, 20 minutes at higher elevations. Remove the jars from the water and place on a towel to cool. Allow the jars to cool undisturbed. When cool, check the jar seals. Re-process any jar that did not seal or refrigerate it for immediate use. Label.

Burning Bush, Western, *Euonymus occidentalis*

Western burning bush grows in Western North America. It is also called spindle tree, western wahoo and strawberry bush. It is found in shaded streambanks, moist woods, canyons, and high in the mountains. It is in the Celastraceae (Bittersweet) Family. *E. alatus* is used in Asia.

Identification: Western burning bush is a deciduous straggly shrub, growing to 6 to 15 feet (1.8 m to 4.5 meters) when mature. It has slender branches, often climbing, and twigs are usually 4-angled. It has opposite finely-toothed leaves that are 2 to 4 inches 5 cm to 10 cm) long, sometimes with rolled edges, with pointed tips and rounded or tapered bases. The flowers form on the end of a long peduncle with one to five flowers. Each flower has five rounded brownish purple petals, sometimes dotted. Flowers bloom April to June. The fruit is a rounded capsule with three lobes. Each of the three lobes opens to reveal a brown seed surrounded by red pulp.

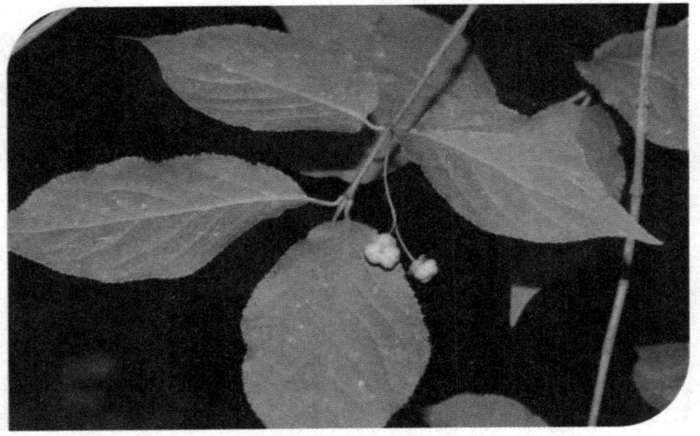

Western Burning Bush, Dean Wm. Taylor, Ph.D. University of California, Berkeley, CC by SA 3.0

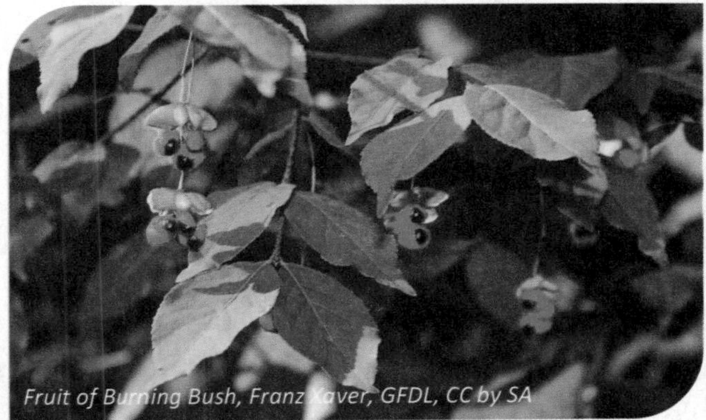

Fruit of Burning Bush, Franz Xaver, GFDL, CC by SA

Medicinal Use: The root bark and the leaves are used for medicine.

Stomach Tonic and Liver: Root bark infusions, syrup, and tinctures are all useful as a stomach tonic for indigestion and constipation. It also stimulates the flow of bile and improves the appetite.

Irregular Menstruation: For suppressed or irregular menstruation, the leaves of burning bush were traditionally used. Do not use if pregnant as it may induce miscarriage.

Warning. Do not use during pregnancy. Do not ingest the fruits of burning bush.

Cascara Sagrada, *Rhamnus* or *Frangula purshiana*

Also called sacred bark and chittam stick, cascara sagrada is well known for its use as a laxative. It is very effective, but carries risks when used long-term, especially if a person's health is already compromised. Cascara is native to the Pacific Northwest, but it is cultivated in other parts of North America. It prefers moist, acidic soils and is usually found on the edges of clearings and forests. It is in the Rhamnaceae (Buckthorn) Family.

Identification: Cascara grows up to 30 feet (9.1 meters) tall. It has finely toothed ovate leaves, each 3 to 5 inches (7.5 cm to 12.5 cm) long, with prominent parallel veins leading off the central vein. Leaves are shiny green on top and a lighter, dull green on the bottom. The smooth bark is reddish-brown to silver-grey. In early to mid-spring, the tree produces tiny flowers with five greenish-yellow petals that grow in umbel-shaped clusters. Red berries appear and ripen to dark purple or black. The berries have yellow pulp and two to three seeds each.

Edible Use: The fruit is sometimes eaten raw or cooked, but is reported to be slightly toxic and also has a laxative effect. Tea is made from the bark after drying or aging. It has a bitter taste. Do not use fresh bark.

Medicinal Use: Cascara is usually prescribed as tea, however many people cannot tolerate the intense bitterness. The bark can be powdered and taken in a capsule as a more palatable alternative. Its medicinal effects are usually felt within 6 to 8 hours. Cascara is recommended only for short-term use, no more than 2 weeks. Always use the smallest effective dose. Only used aged cascara bark (see harvesting).

Natural Laxative: Cascara bark is a natural laxative for the treatment of constipation. The herb acts as a stimulant on the large intestine, stimulating contractions and moving food through the digestive system.

Gallbladder, Liver, Stomach, and Pancreas Stimulation: Cascara stimulates the gallbladder to produce more bile. This action aids digestion and prevents and breaks up gallstones. It improves secretions from the stomach, liver, and pancreas, treating issues such as enlarged liver and poor digestion.

Lowers Cholesterol: Cascara is said to have a beneficial effect on cholesterol levels. However, it is not recommended for this purpose because of its long-term side effects and potential risks.

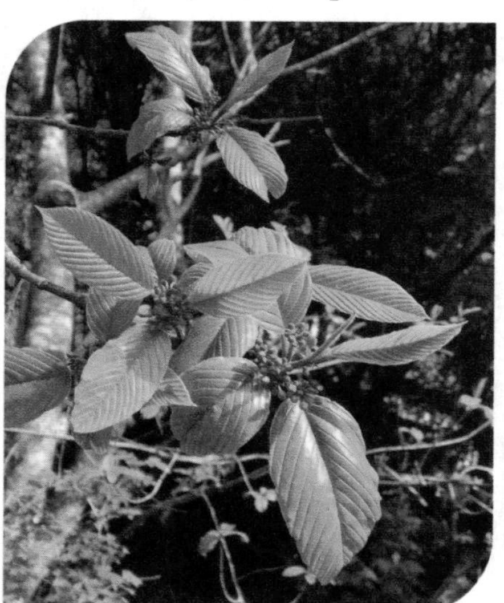

Hemorrhoids: Because of cascara's laxative properties, it is helpful, temporarily, in the treatment of hemorrhoids. It reduces the need to bear down, which eases the condition.

Antimicrobial Properties: Cascara has antibacterial and anti-fungal properties. It is effective against *Helicobacter pylori*,

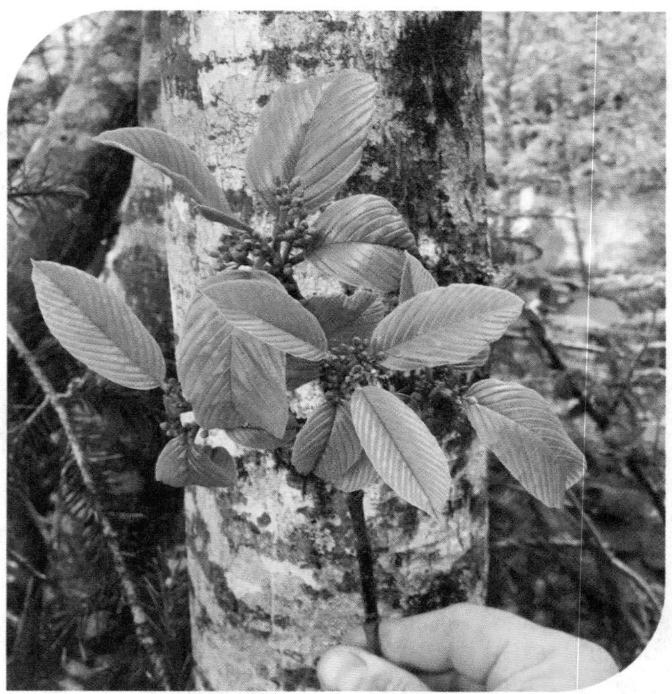

which causes ulcers, *E. coli*, *Staphylococcus aureus*, and others. It is also effective against *Candida* yeast.

Central Nervous System: Cascara sagrada improves anxiety, emotional well-being, and other central nervous system problems in some people

Anti-Inflammatory Effects: The herb is an anti-inflammatory, however, there are more effective anti-inflammatories with fewer risks available.

Cancer: Cascara has been used to inhibit the growth and spread of cancer. It can be used in addition to traditional cancer treatments with medical supervision.

Harvesting: Harvest cascara in the spring, at least a year before using it medicinally. Aging is necessary to reduce gastrointestinal irritation. Fresh cascara causes nausea, vomiting, diarrhea, and intense intestinal spasms. Dry the bark or bake at low heat until completely dry.

Warning: Cascara sagrada is a stimulant and should be used for the short-term only, less than 2 weeks. Cascara should never be used during pregnancy or lactation. It can stimulate menstruation and miscarriage. Cascara should not be given to children. Long term use can result in chronic diarrhea, electrolyte imbalances, dehydration, and severe intestinal pain. It can also cause toxic hepatitis. Cascara can interact with some prescription medications and should not be combined with other medications except under the advice of a medical professional.

Recipes. Cascara Tea: For this tea, you need bark that has been aged for at least 1 year. Do not use fresh bark. Ingredients: 1 teaspoon aged cascara sagrada bark, 1 cup spring water or distilled water. Bring the water and bark to a boil and reduce the heat to a simmer. Simmer for 30 minutes, then strain and allow to cool. Sweeten the tea with raw honey or fennel to mask the bitterness.

Chaparral or Creosote Bush, *Larrea tridentata*

Larrea tridentata belongs to the Zygophyllaceae (Caltrops) Family. It is also known as creosote bush and greasewood. It has a strong creosote smell. This plant is a prominent species in southwestern North America.

Identification: Chaparral bush is an evergreen shrub that grows from 3 to 10 feet (0.9 meters to 3 meters) tall. The stems of this plant bear resinous, small, dark green, compound, opposite leaves. Each leaf has 2 leaflets, which join at the base. The flowers have five yellow petals. The fruit is covered in dense white hairs.

Edible Use: Not generally considered edible. I do add some leaves to my water bottle when this plant is around. It helps keep my water bottle clean and microbe-free.

Medicinal Use: The leaves are used for medicine. They are antimicrobial, antibacterial, antioxidant, and active against protozoa.

Treating Toothaches: For sensitive teeth and toothaches due to cavities, heat the young shoot tips of the plant to produce sap, then drip the sap resin into the tooth cavity. This seals the tooth temporarily and stops the pain.

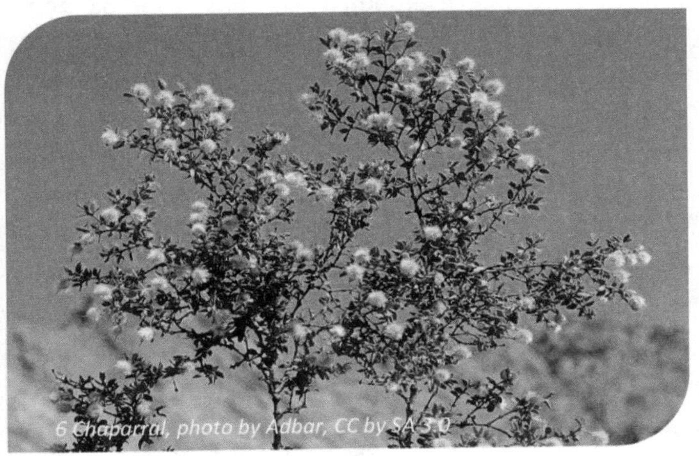

6 Chaparral, photo by Adbar, CC by SA 3.0

Wounds, Burns, Bruises, Rashes: Antibacterial and Antimicrobial: A salve made from chaparral leaves is a good choice for wounds, burns, bruises, and rashes. An external tincture is also a good choice if the skin is not broken. Chaparral has antimicrobial and antibacterial benefits on the skin's surface. I primarily extract it in oil for external use but you can also make a poultice from the ground leaves, apply it to the skin, and cover it with a clean cloth.

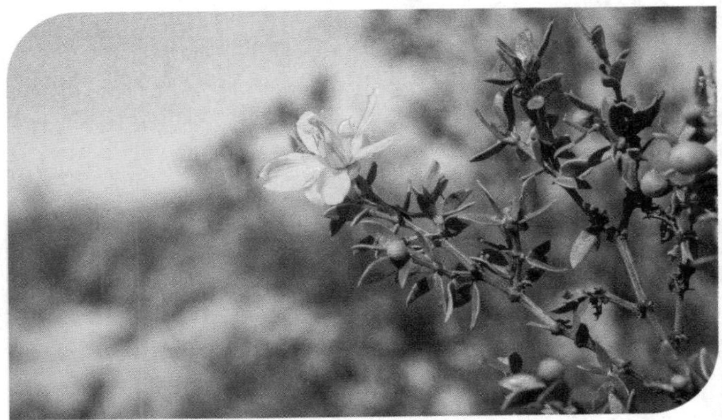

Acne, Psoriasis, Eczema, Dandruff: Anti-Fungal: Chaparral Tincture or Oil can be used externally on acne, eczema, psoriasis, and dandruff. The antibiotic and anti-inflammatory properties are beneficial as well as its tannins. It is a very good external antifungal.

Arthritis: Chaparral Tincture made with alcohol or oil works as a rub to relieve the pain of arthritis.

Pulmonary and Respiratory Problems, Venereal Diseases, and Urinary Tract Infections: In the past, Chaparral Tea and Chaparral Tincture were used as an expectorant for respiratory problems and as a pulmonary antiseptic, as well as a treatment for VD, rheumatism, and UTIs. In recent years (since the 1960s), there has been some concern over possible toxic effects on the liver, so I strongly suggest limiting its internal use.

Harvesting: I prefer to harvest chaparral in dry-weather before the plant has flowered so that the highest concentration of the active ingredients is in the leaves. Collection is best undertaken at midday when the chemical activity of the plant is the highest. It can be dried in a warm, shady place, or in the artificial heat at temperatures less than 130 degrees Fahrenheit. One of the simplest methods of drying the herb is to collect the leaves, put them into a large paper sack and then put the sack in a warm, dry place for a few days. Store in an airtight glass jar in a cool, dark place.

Recipes. Chaparral Salve: Carrier oil such as organic olive oil or liquid coconut oil, dried chaparral leaves, beeswax. Fill the jar half-full with dried chaparral. Cover the herbs with organic olive oil, filling the jar to near the top. Cover the jar with a tight-fitting lid and label. Place the jar in a sunny location for 6 to 8 weeks, shaking every few days. Strain out the herbs. Measure the oil and add 1/4 the amount of beeswax (if you have 1 cup of oil, add ¼ cup of beeswax). Heat the two together gently until the wax melts using a double boiler. Mix the wax and oil, and pour into your containers to harden. Use within two years.

Chokecherry, *Prunus virginiana*

Chokecherry is edible but rarely eaten these days because of its acidity and astringency. It is a North American native that grows across the northern US and Canada and as far south as North Carolina. It is in the Rosaceae (Rose) Family.

Identification: *Prunus virginiana* is a small tree or a deciduous shrub that grows as tall as 30 feet (9.1 meters). It has simple large elliptical leaves that are 4 inches (10 cm) long by 2.5 inches (6.4 cm) wide. They are dark green, have a glossy upper side and paler underside, and have toothed margins. They turn yellow in the autumn.

Between the clusters of leaves are white showy flowers that are approximately 3 to 6 inches (7.5 cm to 15 cm) long. The flowers bloom in May and June, and the fruit appears in August.

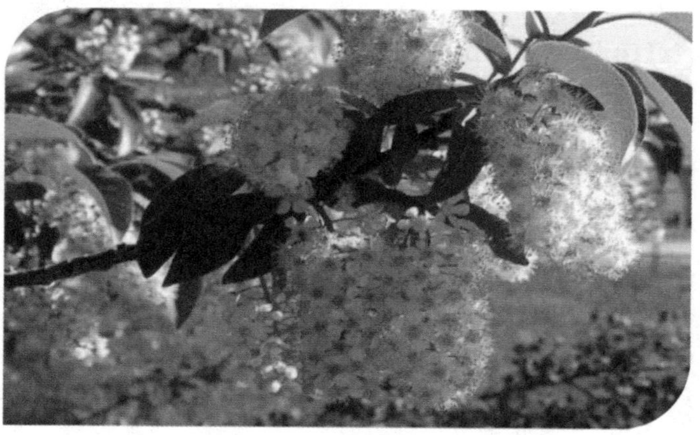

Chokecherry bark ranges in color from brown or gray, to purple and red, and the texture of the bark is smooth

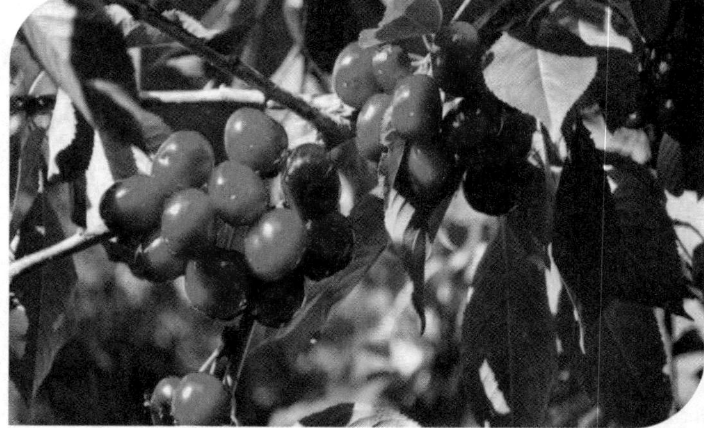

and thin in appearance when young. Bark becomes more uneven and creased with age.

Edible Use: The edible parts of chokecherry are the fruits and seeds. The raw berry is edible and has a good flavor, but is highly astringent. In cooking they are used in pies and jellies where sugar counters their sour flavor.

The berries contain high amounts of pectin, so they are often combined with lower pectin fruits when making syrups, jams, and jellies. The fruit is also used to make wine and syrups. Dried berries are used to make pemmican, and the twigs and bark make a good tea. Do not eat the seeds if they are bitter-tasting.

Medicinal Use: In addition to the uses below the inner bark is used as a flavoring agent for cough syrups and other bitter medicines. It is not used often used in other ways these days.

Stomach Illness: Dried chokecherry fruits and bark are used for diarrhea, bloating, heartburn, and stomach ulcers.

Wet Coughs and Bronchitis: Chokecherry bark is used as a base for cough medicine and also directly treats wet coughs and bronchitis. Best paired with other, more potent, herbs.

Warning: The seeds are said to have a high concentration of hydrogen cyanide, which is a poison that gives almonds their characteristic flavor. This toxin can be easily detected by the bitter taste. It is usually present in small quantity. In large amounts, it can be deadly; however, in small quantities, hydrogen cyanide has been shown to stimulate respiration, improve digestion, and suppress cancer growth. Use it carefully.

Cottonwood, *Populus trichocarpa* and *P. deltoides*

Some consider the cottonwood a sacred tree; at the least it is an important plant for medicinal purposes. Its roots run deep and are said to find water while the tree absorbs the energy of experiences happening nearby. "Balm of Gilead" is made from cottonwood buds and smells wonderful!

Cottonwoods grow along streams, rivers, and flood plains. It loves water, but also grows in dry sites. Black cottonwood grows in the Northwest from Alaska to the Rocky Mountains. Other species are found throughout the United States and Canada. All varieties can be used for medicinal purposes. It is in the Salicaceae (Willow) Family.

Identification: The cottonwood is a large tree, growing 150 to 200 feet (45 meters to 60 meters) tall when mature. It has deeply furrowed grey bark and shiny, dark green, triangular leaves with course teeth along the margin. The leaves turn yellow in the fall before falling. In winter and early spring, the tree produces large buds that are long and pointed. The buds are filled with fragrant resin, yellow-orange to red in color, and are greatly revered for medicine.

Each tree is either male or female. Male flowers are reddish, drooping into a catkin shape. Female flowers form 4-inch (10 cm) catkins followed by light green seed capsules. Ripe capsules open into three parts, releasing white, fluffy down covered seeds that float on the wind. When the seeds are released the tree is covered in cottony fluff. Many people think they are allergic to cottonwood but usually it is the grasses releasing pollen at the same time that are the culprit.

Edible Use: Cottonwood leaves are edible and very nutritious and are rich in protein – they have a higher amino acid content that of barley, wheat or rice. However, the taste is very bitter. Boiling the leaves and discarding the water relieves some of the bitterness as well as adding seasoning. It can be used in soups or eaten as a green. The inner bark is harvested in the spring. Dried and powdered it is used as a thickener for soups. The catkins, which are high in Vitamin C, can be eaten raw like Alder catkins (they have a nutty flavor) or added to a soup, steamed, or sautéed.

Medicinal Use: Cottonwood buds and bark are rich in salicylic acids, known for pain relief and treating fevers. The resinous leaf buds are used to create oils and salves for topical treatment of muscles, joints, tendons,

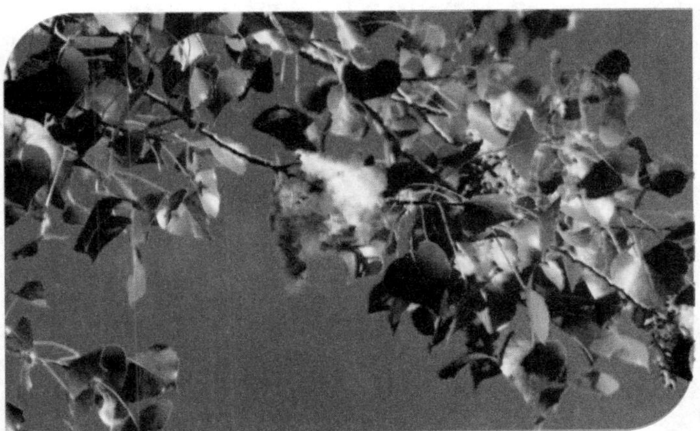

and inflammation or pain. The recipe below is a very cooling and soothing ointment for inflamed tissues. Extracts also can be made with oil or alcohol to make pain relievers similar to aspirin. The inner bark is also used as a tea to being down a fever and as an expectorant.

Joint Pain, Sore Muscles and Arthritis: Cottonwood bud oil is very effective for relieving pain and inflammation in swollen joints, carpal tunnel, arthritis, and muscles. Massage the oil or salve into the affected area 3x/day. A poultice made from crushed fresh leaves is also effective in the treatment of arthritis and other joint issues. Cottonwood bark decoction can be used to relieve menstrual cramping.

Skin Injuries: The anti-bacterial, anti-microbial, anti-fungal, and antioxidant properties of cottonwood bud oil or salve make it useful in treating skin injuries including rashes, irritations, chapped lips, cracked skin, sunburn, and other burns. It helps the skin heal and prevents infection. For boils, sores, and infected skin, make a poultice from crushed leaves. Washing the skin with cottonwood decoction is also effective. Cottonwood buds also helps regenerate cells for healing and I use it along with Calendula Oil as an anti-aging face and neck cream.

Pneumonia, Flu, and Other Respiratory Ailments: Cottonwood Bark Infusion or Tincture is useful in the treatment of whooping cough, tuberculosis, colds, flu and Pneumonia. It kills and inhibits both bacteria and the influenza virus when used early in the disease and helps alleviate pain, reduce fever, and works as an expectorant.

Sore Throats: An infusion of cottonwood inner bark is used as a gargle for sore throats and mouth sores.

Intestinal Worms: Cottonwood Bark Decoction is effective in ridding the body of intestinal worms.

Harvesting: Harvest cottonwood leaf buds in late winter to early spring. The buds are ready to harvest when you can pinch the bud and see resin inside. The largest buds are at the top of the tree and difficult to harvest but after a windstorm you can easily find newly downed branches on the ground. Like willow they root easily, so I plant back small limbs when I gather so that new trees can grow. It's always a good idea to tend the wild when you harvest! Snap the buds off the branches (I leave the terminal buds on the tree) and place them in a container. Sticky resin will adhere to your hands and the container. You can wear gloves for this, coat your hands with salve or oil before harvesting, or remove the resin with rubbing alcohol.

Warning: Some people may be allergic to cottonwood sap. Cottonwood should not be used by people allergic to aspirin or bees.

Recipes. Cottonwood Bud Oil and Salve: Use this salve externally to treat skin ailments and to relieve inflammation and pain in arthritic joints. Ingredients: 1 cup cottonwood buds, 3 cups carrier oil: organic olive oil, coconut oil, or other skin friendly oil, beeswax. Infuse the oil with cottonwood buds. Place the oil in an old double-boiler over very low heat. Add the cottonwood buds and allow the oil to infuse. You should be able to smell the resinous odor and the oil should change color. I like to do this step in a small crockpot or double boiler that I use for this purpose or in a mason jar placed in water. Note that the resin will stick to the pot or jar and will be forever resinous (you can actually clean it with alcohol). I often kick-start my buds with heat and then cold-infuse them in a cupboard for another 6 to 8 weeks. You can also keep it on low for a few days.

When the oil is infused, let it cool and strain out the

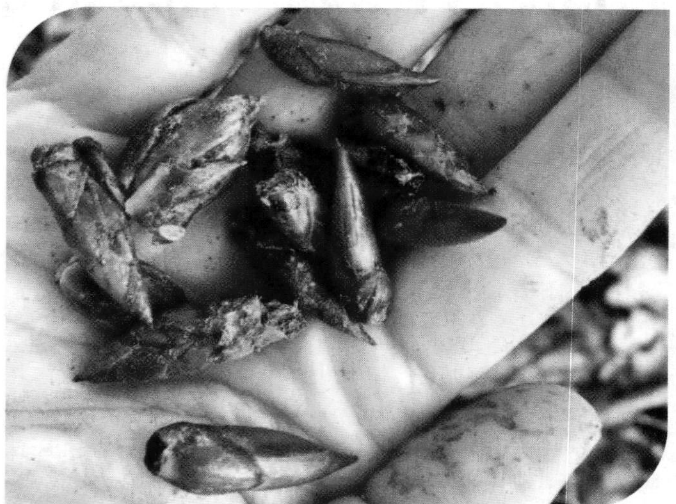

buds. Heat the oil again and add your beeswax. It will take approximately one-half to one cup of beeswax to reach the desired stiffness (ratio of 4:1 oil to beeswax). Once the beeswax is melted, test the salve by placing a spoonful in the freezer for a minute. It will thicken and indicate the consistency of the salve. If you want it thicker, add more beeswax. If you want it thinner, add more oil. How thick or thin you make it is up to you and how you plan to use it. A good rule-of thumb is 4 parts oil to1 part beeswax for a salve. Place the salve in a shallow glass jar or a tin with a wide mouth. Tighten the lid and leave it to cool and harden.

Cottonwood Decoction. Ingredients: ¾ ounce of cottonwood leaf buds and/or bark, 2 cups water. Bring the leaf buds and water to a boil and turn the heat down to a simmer. Simmer the decoction for 10 to 15 minutes. Strain out the herbs and allow the decoction to cool. Make a compress by soaking a washcloth in the decoction, wring it out and place on the affected skin. Allow it to sit for 20 minutes, repeating as necessary to relieve the pain and inflammation. You can also use the decoction directly on the skin.

Cranberry, *Vaccinium macrocarpon*

The cranberry shrub is a member of the Ericaceae (Heath) family. It grows in acidic bogs, swamps, wetlands, and poorly drained meadows throughout the colder climates of Northern North America.

Identification: These low growing, creeping shrubs rarely top 8 inches (20 cm) in height. They have long wiry stems, or vines, that stretch to 7 feet (2.1 meters) long. The plant has small, oblong, evergreen leaves that are speckled with tiny dots on the underside. The leathery leaves are 1/4 to 1/2-inch (0.75 cm to 1.25 cm) long. Dark pink flowers with distinct reflexed petals appear June through August. The style and stamens are exposed and point forward. The cranberry fruit is a small berry that is larger than the leaves. The berry is white when immature, usually turning dark red when ripe.

Edible Use: The berries are edible, but they are very acidic. The addition of sugar makes them more palatable, as does drying them.

Medicinal Use: Cranberries are an effective preventative and remedy for early stage urinary tract infections. They work by preventing the adhesion of bacteria to the lining of the bladder and gut, thereby preventing infection. If the infection is too well entrenched, other remedies may be required, such as Usnea, Bearberry/Uva Ursi, and Oregon Grape Root. Cranberries have high levels of antioxidants, vitamin C, and salicylic acid, which help relieve pain and heal.

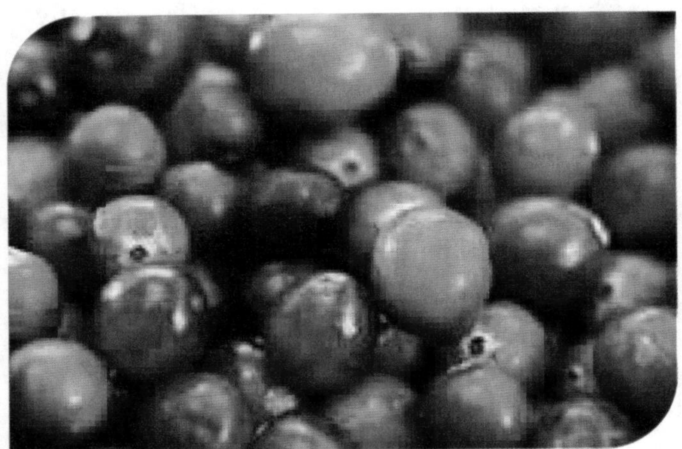

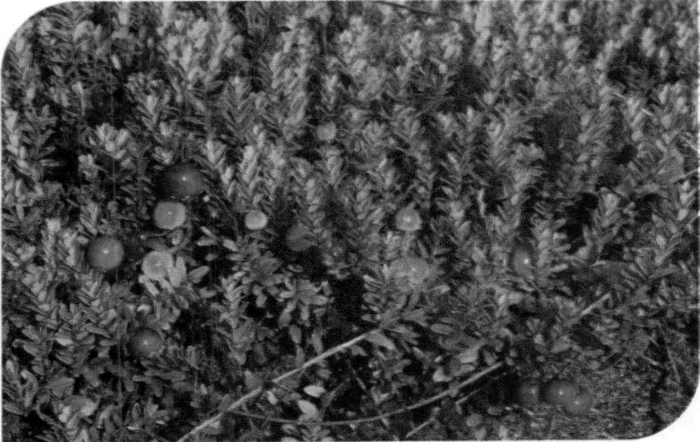

Cjboffoli, CC by 3.0

To get all of the benefits of cranberries for medicinal purposes, simply consume the fruit or its unsweetened juice daily for as long as needed. Cranberry juice is sour, but more palatable when diluted in water.

Urinary Tract Infections: Consumption of cranberries, their juice, or a concentrated cranberry pill prevents the bacteria in the urinary tract from multiplying and clinging to the walls of the bladder, allowing them to be easily flushed out of the system. Regular consumption of unsweetened cranberry juice prevents urinary tract diseases and can keep you from needing antibiotics. Cranberries are not as effective in treating established UTIs. The juice does not kill the bacteria, and reinfection can occur if cranberry is discontinued while bacteria are still in the system. You may need to add in an herbal antibiotic blend (see above).

Cardiovascular Health: The flavonoids in cranberries are high in antioxidant and anti-inflammatory properties and decrease the risk of atherosclerosis. They also boost HDL ("good") cholesterol levels.

Respiratory Bacterial Infections: Cranberry juice inhibits *Haemophilus influenza*, which is a common cause of childhood respiratory and ear infections. The juice prevents these bacteria from adhering to the skin's surface.

Treats and Prevents Peptic Ulcers: Cranberries help reduce the risk of peptic ulcers caused by *Helicobacter pylori*. Along with preventing the adhesion of bacteria to the stomach lining, the high flavonoid content of cranberries suppresses infection and helps the body heal.

Antitumor and Anticancer Effects: Cranberry is a powerful anti-tumor agent and is also a cancer preventative. Medicinal compounds within the fruit inhibit the growth and spread of many types of cancers.

Warning: Patients who take Coumadin (Warfarin) need to be careful when taking cranberry. The additional anti-clotting effects of cranberry compound the Coumadin. Cranberries contain salicylic acid, a component of aspirin. People who are allergic to aspirin should not consume cranberries.

Recipes. Fresh Cranberry Juice. 4 cups cranberries, 4 cups water, 1/4 cup lemon juice, 1/4 cup orange juice, sugar to taste. Bring the cranberries and water to a boil, turn down the heat and simmer the berries for 25 minutes or until all the berries have popped and the berries are cooked. Pass the cranberry mixture through a food mill on the smallest setting. Pass the mixture through a fine-mesh sieve. Mash the pulp slightly to increase draining, but not hard enough to push the pulp through. Mix in the orange juice and lemon juice. Add sugar to sweeten the juice, if desired.

Devil's Club, *Oplopanax horridus, (Echinopanax horridus, Fatsia horrida)*

Devil's Club is a relative of American ginseng and is beginning to be marketed as "Alaskan ginseng". While the plants are similar, Devil's Club is not a true ginseng (*Panax*). Until recently, its covering of thorns has protected it, but as it becomes more well known for medicinal use, it may become over-harvested. It is in the Araliaceae (Ginseng) Family.

Identification: Also known as devil's walking stick and devil's root, this plant thrives in the damp woodlands of the North America's Pacific Northwest. The plant is a large understory shrub with large leaves and woody stems covered completely in irritating spines. It usually grows slowly to a mature height of up to 5 feet (1.5m) tall, but can grow up to 15 feet (4.5m) in height.

Leaves are simple, palmate and spirally arranged. Each has 5 to 13 lobes and is 8 to 16 inches (20 cm to 40 cm) across. Spines are found on the upper and lower veins in the leaves and on the stems. Flowers appear in dense umbels, from 4 to 8 inches (10 cm to 20 cm) in diameter, with small green-white petals. The ripe fruit is a small red drupe about 1/4 inch (0.75 cm) in diameter.

Edible Use: The very young shoots are delicious and edible cooked, but are only available for a few days each spring. The shoots are edible when the leaf buds break through their sheath and are between 1 to 2 inches (2.5 cm to 5 cm) long. The leaf spines are soft and edible at this point, but quickly harden and the shoots become inedible. The berries are poisonous.

Medicinal Use and Adaptogenic Herb: The inner bark and stems of the root are used medicinally. This adaptogen is a pain reliever, anti-inflammatory, blood purifier, regulates blood sugar levels, helps with adrenal fatigue, and treats infections. Devil's Club is known as a panacea ("cure-all") plant.

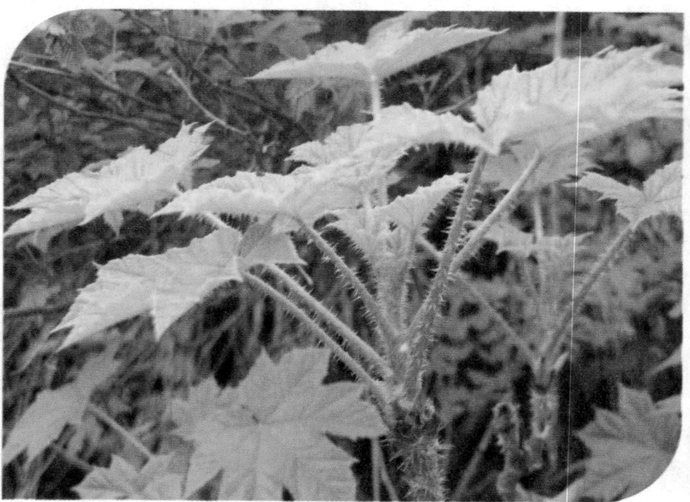

Skin Infections, Swollen Glands, Boils, Sores, and Burns: Apply Devil's Club directly to the skin as a poultice or as a wash to treat skin infections, boils, sores, and swollen glands. It treats the underlying infections, reduces inflammation and helps the area heal. For burns, dust root bark ashes directly onto the burn. Ashes can also be mixed with oil and used as a salve for skin problems. The root bark can also be baked and powdered to use this way.

Lowers Blood Sugar Levels: Root bark extract and infusion balance blood sugar levels in diabetics and can be used to treat the disease. The infusion also has a tonic effect.

Coughs, Colds, Bronchitis, and Tuberculosis: Respiratory problems respond to an infusion made with the inner root bark and stems. Try Devil's Club Tea, as needed, for respiratory symptoms. It helps treat excess mucous and eliminates toxins. A decoction of the inner root bark is used to treat tuberculosis and other respiratory diseases.

Arthritis: Treat arthritis internally and externally with Devil's Club. Use a strong decoction as a wash on painful joints. It can also be applied to joints as a poultice of crushed bark. Use it carefully as it has a laxative effect.

Head Lice: To get rid of head lice, mash the berries into a pulp and massage the pulp into the scalp. It will get rid of lice, dandruff, and leave the hair shiny and healthy.

Fever: A decoction of stems is useful for treating fevers. If the underlying cause is infectious, it will help get rid of the infection and heal the body.

Tooth Pain: Dried inner bark can be chewed or laid into the tooth cavity to relieve the pain.

Cancer and Hormone Regulation: Devil's Club has been shown to kill cancer cells and regulate hormone levels. There are many new research studies focusing on this.

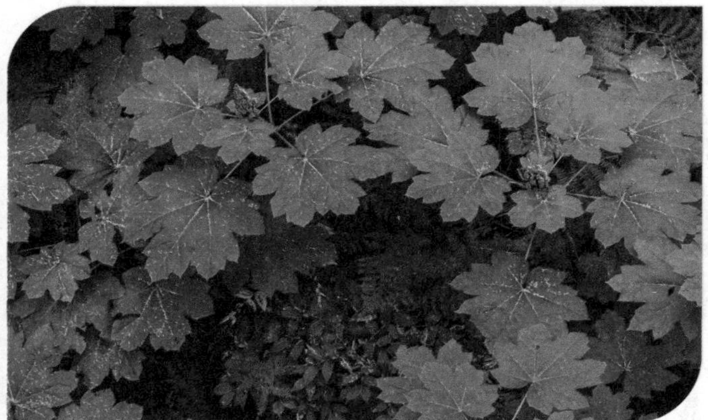

Harvesting: Wear heavy leather gloves and protective clothing to harvest Devil's Club as the spines are irritating. I harvest mid-autumn through early spring.

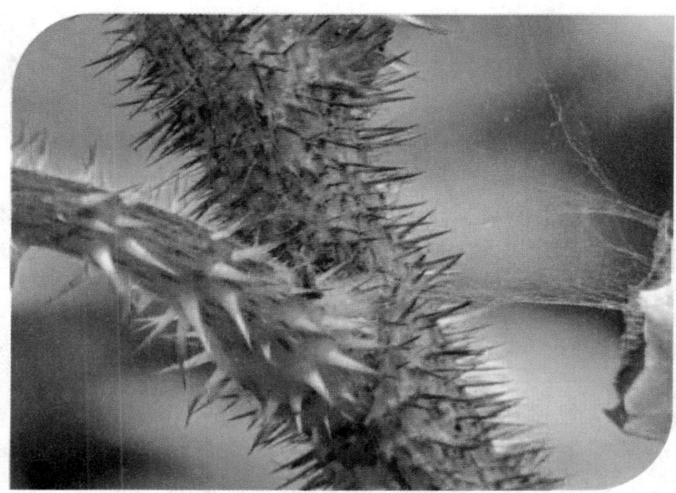

Devil's club covered in spines

For medicinal purposes, harvest the inner bark of the root and the stems that lie along the ground that have lost their spines. The stems are also valuable, but the spines must be stripped first. Dig around the roots and expose them, removing spiny branches. Cut any small roots holding it in place on both ends.

Pull up the root. Tend the wild! Re-plant the cut end of any stalks that you have cut back into the soil. They will grow roots and survive for the next year's harvest. The berries are poisonous to people, leave them to propagate the plant.

Warning: The main hazard is the presence of spikes, which are an irritant. Women should avoid this in their first trimester of pregnancy.

Devil's Club Decoction: You'll need 4 tablespoons Devil's Club root bark, 2 cups spring water. Chop or grind the root bark into very small pieces. Mix with the spring water and bring to a boil. Reduce the heat to a simmer and simmer for 20 to 40 minutes. Cool. This is a strong decoction for external use or take internally in small doses as needed.

Devil's Club Tea or Infusion: Ingredients: 1 teaspoon Devil's Club root bark, 1 cup boiling water. Pour the boiling water over the root bark and allow the tea to infuse for 10 to 15 minutes or until cool. Drink as needed.

Dogwood, *Cornus florida*

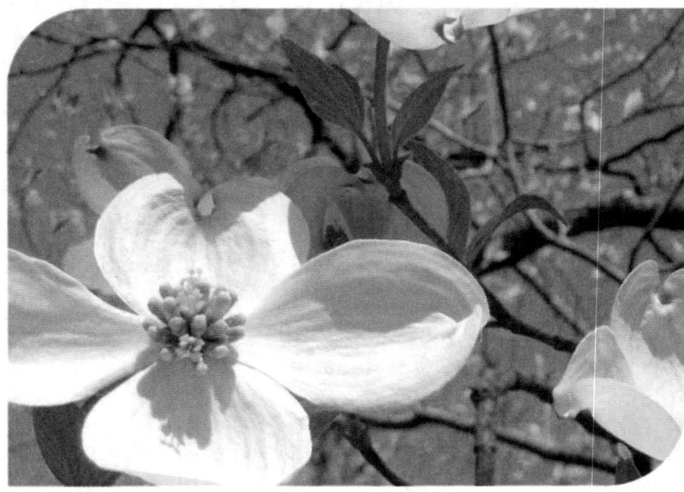

Flowering or American dogwoods are in the Cornaceae (Dogwood) Family.

Identification: Dogwood grows as a shrub or as a small deciduous tree. The opposite smooth leaves are oval-shaped and have prominent parallel veins with a pointed end. Leaves are deep green on the upper surface and a velvety white on the underside and are 2 to 5 inches (5 to 12.5 cm) long. Their veins curve under as they approach the leaf margins. White or pink flowers appear in April or May. The flowers appear before the leaves. The small blooms are at the center of four showy, creamy white bracts that appear as petals. Small red drupes form containing one or two seeds each.

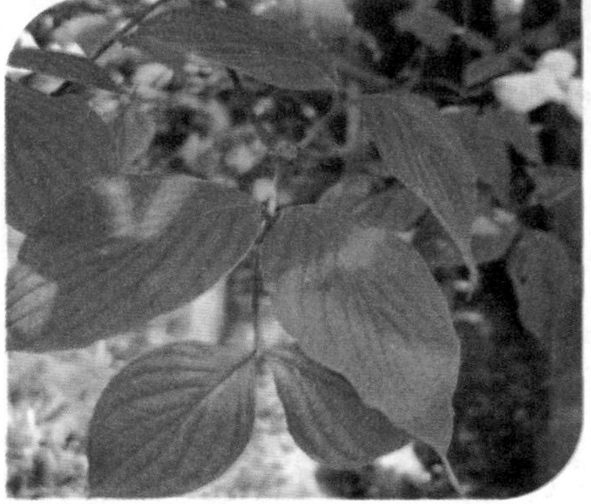

Dogwood Leaves, KENPEI, CC by SA 3.0

Edible and Other Use: The fruits can be eaten if cooked. Peeled and chewed dogwood twigs make a good toothbrush and help whiten teeth.

Medicinal Use: The fruit, leaves, bark, and root bark are used medicinally.

Malaria and Fever Reduction: The bark of dogwood trees contains quinine, useful in treating malaria. The tea also induces sweating, which cools the body.

Wound Care and Sore Muscles: For cuts, burns, and other skin wounds, try a poultice made from dogwood leaves. It is an anti-inflammatory and an analgesic.

Dogwood Bark Decoction is useful for easing the pain of sore muscles. Rub the decoction into sore muscles or use it on sore joints.

Hardy Kiwi, *Actinidia arguta*

The hardy kiwi is a perennial fruiting vine that is known for its vigorous growth and ability to withstand the cold. It is also known as baby kiwi, arctic kiwi, cocktail kiwi, or kiwi berry. It is a popular cultivated fruit. It is in the Actinidiaceae (Chinese Gooseberry) Family.

Identification: The plant is a deciduous twinning vine with a woody stem. It easily climbs to heights of 25 to 30 feet (7.6m to 9.1m), but can reach much higher if sufficient support is available.

The oval leaves are 3 to 5 inches (7.5 cm to 12.5 cm) long. The leaves are bright green with reddish stems and the fruits can be brown, green, or reddish. The fruits are similar in size to a large grape with a smooth skin and sweet flavor. The plants are either male or female. The small white flowers appear in May.

Edible Use: The hardy kiwi fruit has a flavor like the true kiwi fruit, only sweeter. It can be eaten whole, with no need to remove the peel.

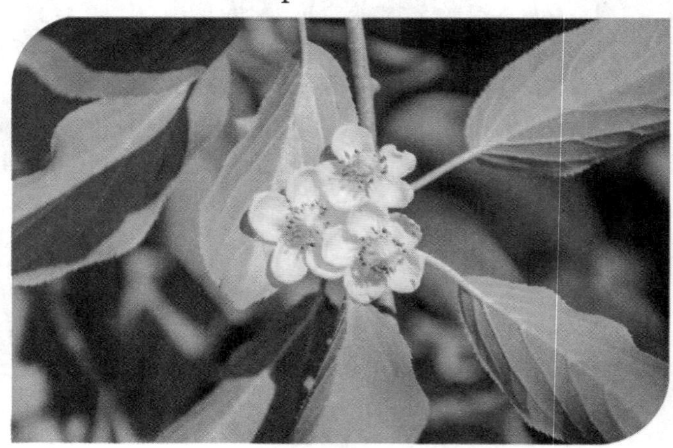

It is usually consumed raw, but is also used for jams and chutneys.

Medicinal Use: Hardy kiwi fruit contains many beneficial vitamins and antioxidants that protect the body from disease. Unless otherwise noted, eating the fruit provides the beneficial effects.

Cancer: These kiwi fruits provide protection against and treatment for cancer. They are particularly effective for treating cancers of the stomach, intestines, colon, and breast. Eat a serving of kiwi fruit daily. Eating too many may cause a laxative effect.

Constipation: Kiwi has a laxative effect when eaten in excess and makes a good treatment for constipation. Eat a large serving of the fruit to relieve constipation.

Irritable Bowel Syndrome (IBS): The protective nature of kiwi on the digestive tract is a great help for people who suffer with IBS. It helps restore normal bowel movements and calms inflammation of the intestinal tract.

Insomnia and Sleep Disorders: The hardy kiwi is rich in serotonin and other compounds that are beneficial to an uninterrupted sleep. It helps with insomnia and increases beneficial REM sleep. Insomniacs can simply include a serving of hardy kiwi in their daily diet.

Anemia: The hardy kiwi is a rich source of both iron and vitamin C, making it a good dietary source for people with iron deficiency anemia. The vitamin C increases the absorption of iron.

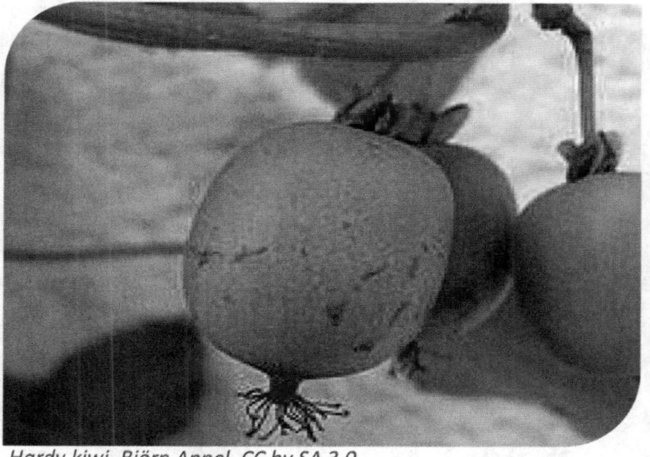

Hardy kiwi, Björn Appel, CC by SA 3.0

Boosts the Immune System: Hardy kiwis boost the function of the immune system and help prevent the common cold and other related illnesses, especially in children. This effect is probably due to the high concentrations of vitamin C; however, other protective compounds may also be involved.

High Blood Pressure, Cholesterol, and Triglycerides: The protective nature of hardy kiwi extends to the cardiovascular system where kiwis prevent or lower high blood pressure, prevent blood clot formation, and help cholesterol and triglyceride levels. It protects the cardiovascular system and reduces the threat of heart attacks and cardiovascular disease.

Hawthorn, *Crataegus monogyna*

Like its family members in the rose and apple family, hawthorn is both nutritious and medicinal. They also share the long woody thorns that can be quite painful if not avoided. The hawthorn bush, also called the May-tree or thorn-apple, is a deciduous member of the Rosaceae (Rose) Family.

Identification: Hawthorn can grow as a thorny bush or a tree. I often find it along sunny paths in the woods and it is often planted on parking strips in towns. White, red, or pink flowers bloom in May. Its numerous flowers are usually white and less than 1 inch (2.5 cm) in diameter. The calyx has 5 lobes and five petals. Small berries ripen to a bright deep red color or sometimes even black. The berries are edible and have a sweet-sour flavor that is often cooked with sugar.

The leaves are alternate, serrated and ovate, 2 to 3 inches (5 cm to 7.5 cm) in length, and can be lobed or sharply cut with teeth. They are dark green with bluish-green bases and vary in size and shape. The entire tree rarely reaches 30 feet (9.1 meters) and may be much smaller. It is covered with sharp thorns that grow up to 2 inches (5 cm) in length.

Edible Use: The fruit are edible raw or cooked, but are more pleasant when cooked

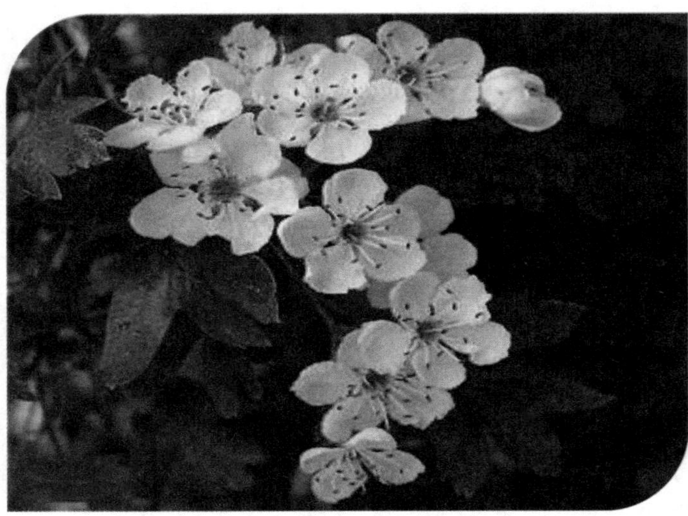

EugeneZelenko, CC by SA 3.0

as a jam or jelly. They can be dried and ground for adding to breads. Young shoots are good eaten raw. The dried leaves make a pleasant tea and the seeds can be roasted and used as a coffee substitute. Use the flowers as flavoring for syrups and puddings.

Medicinal Use: Hawthorn has many medicinal uses, but its value for heart patients is its most significant. For heart patients, it is usually taken daily as a tea or tincture and is considered a very safe herb. Long term, consistent use is necessary to get the benefits. People who do not like the tea or tincture can use hawthorn powder in a capsule. The berries, flowers, and leaves are all used medicinally.

Hawthorn for Your Heart. Heart Failure: Hawthorn is a common herbal go to for heart ailments. People who follow a daily regimen of hawthorn along with moderate exercise and a good diet do very well. Editor's Note: Heart failure is a serious condition and should not be self-treated. Please see your doctor and follow his or her advice.

Heart Disease: Hawthorn has many beneficial effects for the heart and treats multiple causes and symptoms, including: lowering blood pressure, improving heart rate, cardiac output, and tolerance for moderate exercise.

Angina Pectoris: Angina is caused by decreased blood flow to the heart and can be a symptom of heart disease. Treatment with hawthorn is effective in preventing and treating the underlying causes and the symptoms. It dilates the blood vessels, improving blood flow to the heart and the rest of the body. Hawthorn works best for people who do mild aerobic exercise (always talk to a doctor first.)

Irregular Heart Rhythms: People who take hawthorn for heart related problems report a significant decline in heart palpitations.

Atherosclerosis: Hawthorn helps open up the blood vessels and increase blood flow, which relieves or reduces the symptoms of atherosclerosis.

High Blood Pressure: Hawthorn berries, flowers, and leaves are all effective at reducing diastolic blood pressure. Hawthorn must be used regularly over a number of weeks to see results.

High Cholesterol: People who take hawthorn berries have a reduction of LDL (bad) cholesterol and overall cholesterol levels. It also has a beneficial effect on triglycerides, liver cholesterol, and loss of body fat.

Overall Health Tonic: Hawthorn berries are anti-inflammatory and contain powerful antioxidants that remove free radicals that cause damage in the body. These two properties are extremely beneficial in maintaining health and preventing chronic disease in the body. Hawthorn berry protects the body from oxidative stress, kills off many strains of bacteria, and protects the organs.

Immune System: The antioxidants in hawthorn help boost the immune system and eliminate toxins from the body. Additionally, hawthorn contains high amounts of vitamin C, which improves the ability of your white blood cells to fight infections.

Improved Digestion, Intestinal Infections: Hawthorn tea improves the digestive process. It helps reduce constipation, bloating, and cramping along with treating intestinal infections and parasites such as tapeworms.

Skin Conditions: Hawthorn berries can be used topically to relieve skin conditions like eczema and psoriasis. The anti-inflammatory properties help relieve swelling, rashes, itching, and help wounds heal.

Malaria and Other Fevers: The bark of the hawthorn tree is an astringent and provokes sweating. This property makes it useful in treating fevers from malaria and other causes.

Harvesting: Collect flowers and leaves when available and dry in a dehydrator on low or hang to dry. Collect fruit when ripe for drying. Fruit needs to be pierced or halved for drying and will take longer to dry. Dry the fruit on a dehydrator on low or in the oven at the lowest setting. Store dried fruit, flowers, and leaves in sealed containers in a cool, dark, and dry place.

Warning: Hawthorn is usually well tolerated, but it does have side effects in some people. These include stomach upset, sweating, fatigue, nausea, dizziness or agitation. Serious side effects include shortness of breath, allergic reactions, heart irregularities, and mood swings. Consult with a medical professional before taking hawthorn, especially if you are taking any medications.

Recipes. Hawthorn Berry Tincture: You'll need: 1-pint (500ml) fresh hawthorn berries, 80 proof or higher vodka, brandy or other alcohol*and a sterile glass jar and tight-fitting lid. Place the berries in a sterile glass jar up to 1/2 inch (1.25 cm) below the rim.

Cover the berries with 80 proof vodka and cover with a tight-fitting lid. Allow the berries and alcohol to steep for 6 to 8 weeks in a cool, dark place. Shake the jar daily. Filter the berries out and place the alcohol in a clean glass jar. Label and date the tincture.

*Apple cider vinegar can also be used, but the tincture will not be as potent, nor last as long.

Honey Locust, *Gleditsia triacanthos*

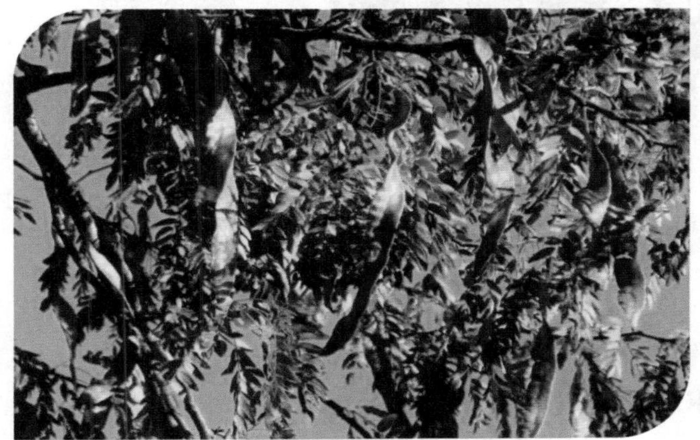

Honey Locust is a deciduous tree that is in the Fabaceae family. It is also known as the Thorny Locust. It is a native to eastern and central North America. The leaves turn a brilliant yellow in autumn. Honey locust is most commonly found on moist, fertile soils in upland woodlands, rocky hillsides, old fields, river floodplains and rich, moist bottomlands.

Identification: Honey locusts can reach a height of nearly 100 feet (30 meters) and grow quickly. Honey locust trees are prone to losing large branches in windstorms. They are armed with thick-branched thorns up to 3 inches (7.5 cm) long. The bark is blackish or grayish-brown in color, with smooth, long, plate-like patches of bark separated by furrows.

Its sharp thorns grow on the main trunk and at the bases of the branches. One-year-old twigs have single spines, but older branches have spines arranged in clusters of three. The spines grow from the wood and decrease in number as the tree ages. Young spines are green, but they mature to red, brown, or gray.

Its leaves are deciduous, alternate, pinnately or bipinnately compound and are 4 to 8 inches (10 cm to 20 cm) long. They often have 3 to 6 pairs of side branches; with pairs of shiny, dark green leaflets. The small numerous flowers are greenish yellow and hang in clusters. They are 2 to 5 inches (5 cm to 12.5 cm) long, either staminate (male) or pistillate (female) borne on separate trees. However, each tree will have a few perfect flowers (male and female). The flowers have a pleasant fragrance. Fruits of Honey locust are flattened and strap-like pods 6 to 16 inches long (15 to 40 cm) and 1 to 1 1/2 (2.5 cm to 3.75 cm) inches wide.

They are dark brown at maturity, pendulous and usually twisted or spiraled, with a sticky, sweet, and flavorful pulp. The seeds inside the pod are beanlike and about 1/3 to 1/2-inch (0.8 cm to 0.75 cm) long. The trees flower in May to June and bear fruit in September to October. The pods sometimes remain on the tree through February.

Edible Use: The seeds and seedpods are edible. The young seeds taste like raw peas. You can roast the seeds as a coffee substitute. The pulp of the young seedpods is sweet and can be eaten raw or made into a sweet drink. As the seedpods mature the pulp turns bitter.

Medicinal Use: The prominent medicinal properties of Honey Locust are as an anesthetic, antiseptic, anti-cancer, and as a digestive.

Cough, Colds, and Sore Throats: An infusion made from honey locust bark and roots treats colds and coughs. The inner bark is useful for treating sore throats.

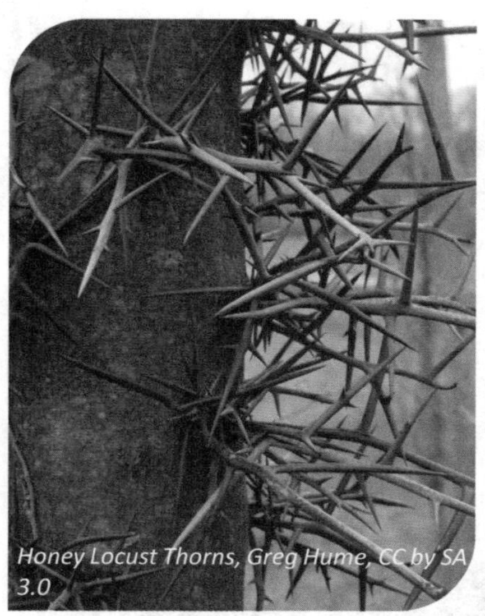
Honey Locust Thorns, Greg Hume, CC by SA 3.0

Anti-Cancer Treatment: The leaves, inner bark, and spines of the honey locust tree are all effective against the growth of cancer cells. Use the leaves and inner bark to make an anti-cancer decoction that inhibits the growth of cancer cells.

Smallpox and Measles: The seedpods are valuable in the treatment of smallpox and measles. Add enough water to 1/2 teaspoon of Honey Locust Seedpod Powder (see recipe below) to make a thick syrup or use the seedpod pulp fresh.

Indigestion and Whooping Cough: Honey Locust Bark Infusion is used to treat both indigestion and whooping cough.

Recipes. Honey Locust Extract: 1 1/2 pints (750ml) honey locust leaves and spines, crushed, 1-quart (1 Liter) of 80-100 proof vodka. Place the honey locust leaves and spines in a quart (1 Liter) jar, filling it 3/4 full. Fill the jar with the vodka or other suitable drinking alcohol. Seal the jar tightly. Place the jar in a warm, sunny spot, like a windowsill, and let the herbs marinate for 4 to 6 weeks, shaking every day or two. Strain the alcohol through a fine sieve or a coffee filter to remove the leaves and spines. Store the extract in a cool, dark place for up to 7 years.

Honey Locust Seedpod Powder. To prepare seedpod powder, the pods must be boiled, soaked, and the seeds removed. Then dry and grind the pods.

Bring a pot of water to a boil and add the pods. Turn off the heat and soak the pods for at least 4 hours, or overnight. Split the pods lengthwise and remove the seeds. Discard the seeds. Chop the pods into small pieces. Dehydrate the pod pieces at low heat (135 degrees F). Grind the dried pods in a coffee grinder or mortar and pestle until you have a fine powder.

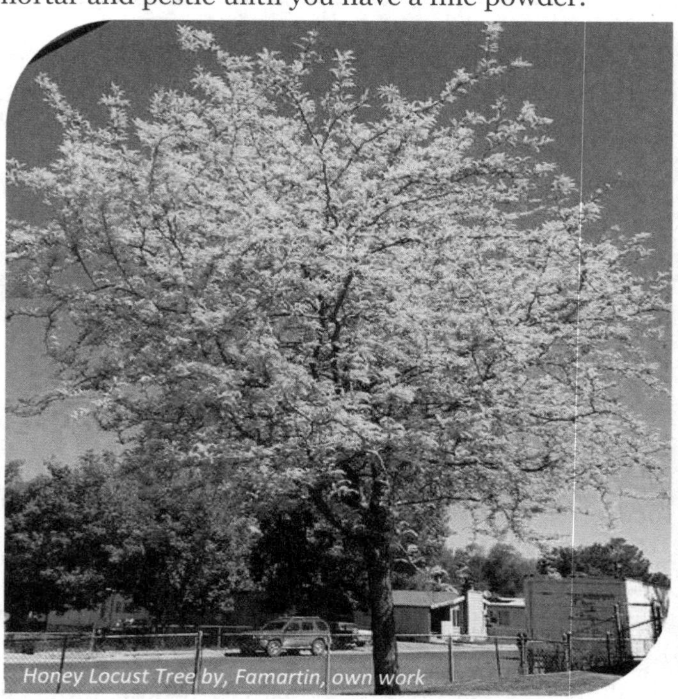
Honey Locust Tree by, Famartin, own work

Horse Chestnut, *Aesculus hippocastanum*

Horse chestnut is also known as a conker tree, Horse chestnut is a large deciduous tree and is a member of the Sapindaceae (Soapberry) Family. It is often used as an ornamental tree in parks and landscaping.

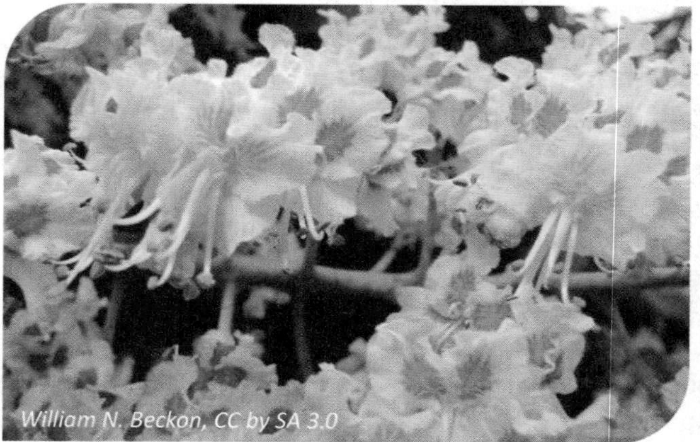
William N. Beckon, CC by SA 3.0

Identification: Horse Chestnut is a large tree reaching 50 to 75 feet (15 meters to 22.8 meters) when mature, and is often as wide as it is tall. Beautiful clusters of white flowers with a yellow splotch of color in their center cover the tree in early to mid-May. The yellow color slowly changes pink-red as the bloom matures. Flower clusters are 5 to 12 inches (12.5 cm to 20 cm) across with 20 to 50 flowers in each cluster. Leaves are palmately compound with 5 to 7 oval leaflets. Leaflets are doubly serrated and 4 to 10 inches (10 cm to 25 cm) long, and the entire leaf is 12 to 24 inches (30 cm to 60 cm) long. The trunk and branches develop exfoliating bark as the tree matures, with outer bark peeling away to show the orange bark below.

Each flower cluster produces one to five fruits. The fruits are about 2 inches (5 cm) in diameter and are covered with a light green spiny shell that turns brown as the nuts mature. The spiny shell contains one or two nut-like seeds. Each glossy brown seed is 1 to 2 inches (2.5 cm to 5 cm) in diameter with a light-colored scar at the base.

Edible Use: Horse chestnuts are not edible. The seeds are slightly poisonous and cause illness when eaten.

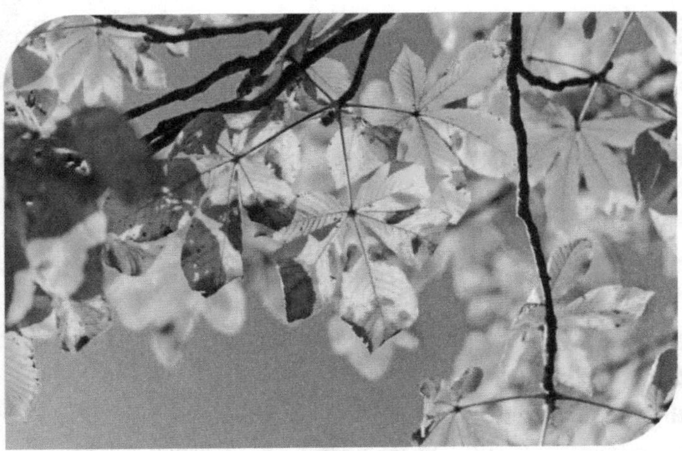

Medicinal Use: Horse chestnut is a tonic that is used specifically to treat vascular system problems. It helps control varicose veins and hemorrhoids, and it improves the general tone of veins. Used both topically and internally.

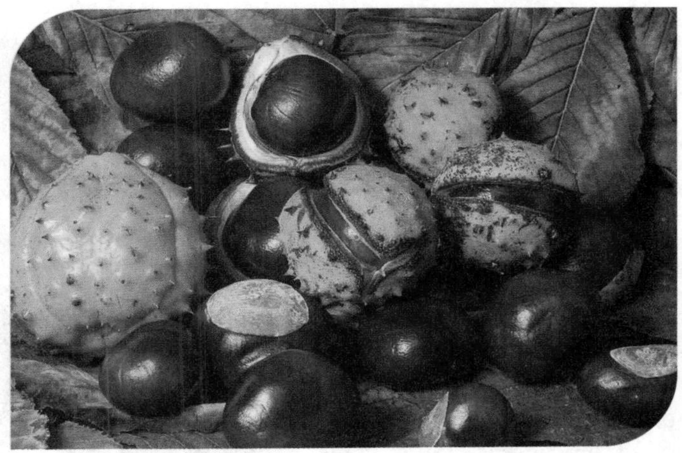

Solipsist, CC by SA 2.0

Chronic Venous Insufficiency: Horse chestnut is used as a treatment for venous insufficiency; use carefully dosed seed tinctures. Medicinal preparations can be made at home but should be used with care, starting at low doses and increasing slowly as implicated.

Lowers Blood Sugar: Horse chestnut lowers blood sugar and can be beneficial for people with diabetes when used carefully and blood sugar is closely monitored. Monitoring is necessary for anyone taking horse chestnut because hypoglycemia can result from overdosing. There are better choices.

Varicose Veins: Horse chestnut seed is a treatment for varicose veins. It reduces pain and swelling in the legs and strengthens the veins.

Harvesting: Only harvest nuts that have dropped to the ground and released their seed. Nuts that are still on the tree are not mature.

Warning: The horse chestnut is known to be mildly toxic, but carefully prepared seed extracts are safe when used properly. Do not use on children, during pregnancy, or while nursing.

Use cautiously with people taking blood-thinning medications. Monitor blood sugar levels closely, especially when beginning treatment or when increasing dose.

Juniper, *Juniperus* spp.

Juniper is usually a small shrub, growing between 2 to 20 feet (6 meters) high, and found throughout the Northern Hemisphere. It is a member of the Cupressaceae (Cypress) Family.

MPF, CC by 2.5

Identification: The shrub has reddish-brown bark that peels off in papery pieces. The leaves are needles, tapering to a spiny point, in whorls of 3, with white bands down the center. Cones appear on short stalks. The berries are small, round to oval and up to ½ inch (1.25 cm) in diameter. Berries are green when young and purple-black when mature. They take up to 3 years to ripen, so both green and ripe berries are often on the same shrub. Each berry usually has three seeds.

Edible Use: Use crushed berries in cooking to flavor meats and sauces. Juniper berries are used as a flavoring for gin. The berries can be used either dried or fresh, and crushing them releases their bitter flavor. The astringency is strongest in fresh berries and declines with drying and storage.

Medicinal Use: Juniper berries for medicinal use can be incorporated as a flavoring in cooking or taken as an infusion. The needles are also medicinal and, unlike the fruits, can be gathered year-round.

Heartburn, Indigestion, and Flatulence: Juniper berries are a bitter astringent that improves digestion. The bitters cause saliva, digestive enzymes, and stomach acids to increase, which aids in the digestion of food and helps with flatulence and gas. Use Juniper Infusion, Juniper Oil, or eat dried, crushed ripe juniper berries.

Diuretic: Eating juniper berries relieves bloating. It increases urine output and relieves water retention caused by injury, inflammation, or excess sodium in the diet.

Bladder and Urinary Tract Infections: Because of its diuretic action, juniper helps flush out toxins and bacteria in the urinary tract, which helps prevent urinary tract infections. It also clears uric acid, helping gout, and helps clear the bladder and prostate.

Anti-Bacterial and Anti-Fungal Properties: Juniper berry is an effective treatment against many bacterial strains, both gram-positive and gram-negative. These include common bacteria such as *E. coli*, *Staphylococcus aureus*, pneumonia, gonorrhea, and antibiotic-resistant bacteria. It is also a strong internal and external anti-fungal.

Skin Infections, Irritations, and Wounds: A mixture of Juniper Essential Oil in lard or a carrier oil is used to treat skin infections and wounds.

Edema (Dropsy). Juniper Infusion treats edema.

Anti-Inflammatory, Antioxidant, and Anti-Aging: Juniper berries are high in antioxidant and anti-inflammatory properties. Antioxidants neutralize free radicals, which are responsible for cell damage and aging that leads to the development of diseases like cancer, arthritis, and heart disease. They also help keep the skin healthy and fight the fine lines and wrinkles that result from aging.

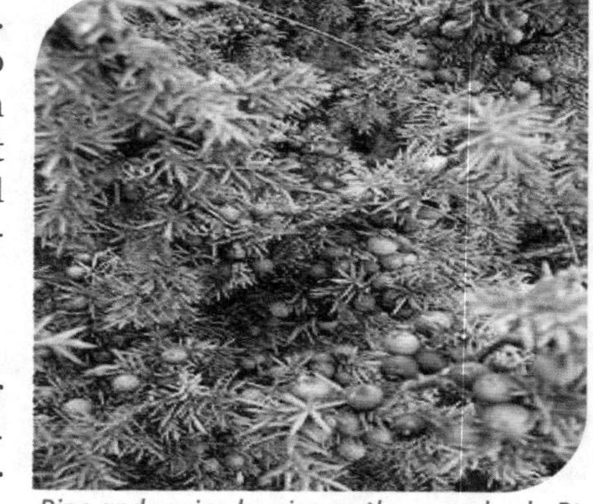
Ripe and unripe berries on the same bush, Pt, CC by SA 3.0

Respiratory Issues: Juniper needles can be infused in water and the steam inhaled to relieve respiratory issues and to clear mucous.

Harvesting: Pick only the ripe, dark-blue berries and lay them out to dry. As they dry, they lose some of their blue color and turn blackish. The berries contain the most oil just as they begin to ripen, so use them fresh whenever possible.

Warning: Excessive consumption may cause kidney irritation. Use Plantain leaf or Mallow root to help minimize kidney irritation. Juniper berries should not be used by pregnant or nursing women. Diabetics and people with bleeding disorders should avoid Juniper. It should also be avoided after surgery.

Meadowsweet, *Filipendula ulmaria*

Meadowsweet is a perennial shrub known for its sweet smell and medicinal uses. It is also known as queen of the meadow because of its ability to take over a low-lying meadow and as meadwort due to its use in flavoring alcoholic beverages. It is in the Rose Family, and is native throughout Europe and Western Asia, and naturalized in Eastern North America. It likes damp soil.

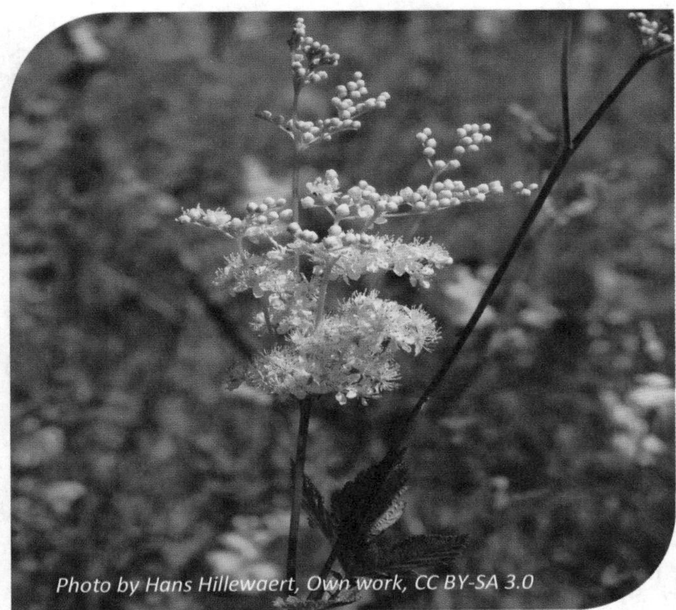

Photo by Hans Hillewaert, Own work, CC BY-SA 3.0

Identification: Meadowsweet grows up to 4 feet (1.2m) in height. The flowers are a creamy pastel yellow or white and have an almond-like scent. It blooms from June to August. Its pinnate leaves are alternate and have 5 to 7 serrated leaflet blade pairs with a terminal leaflet.

Edible Use: Meadowsweet buds and flowers are used as a flavoring for stewed fruit, jams, vinegar, wine, and beer. It has a mild almond flavor. The leaves can also be used as a stewing herb. The entire plant is often dried for use as a potpourri.

Medicinal Use: The buds and blooms are most often used medicinally, but the leaves are also valuable for medicinal use and the fresh root is sometimes ground and used. This plant contains chemicals that are similar to salicylic acid and are used to create acetylsalicylic acid, a synthetic chemical known as aspirin. These chemicals give the plant additional medicinal properties, including pain relief, fever reduction, and use as an anti-inflammatory.

Colds and Flu: The anti-inflammatory, analgesic, and antipyretic (fever-reducing) actions of meadowsweet make it an effective supportive treatment for colds and the aches and pains of the flu.

Use the buds and flowers to treat most symptoms, but the roots are best for treating respiratory symptoms such as coughing, wheezing, and hoarseness.

Indigestion and Peptic Ulcers: Meadowsweet is a digestive treatment for acid indigestion and for peptic ulcers. It protects the lining of the stomach, discourages inflammation, and promotes healing when used properly.

For stomach upsets, indigestion, nausea, and peptic ulcers use the ground root. It can be taken in capsules, as a tea, or as a tincture.

Meadowsweet also has antibacterial properties known to be active against the bacteria Helicobacter pylori. Overuse can irritate the stomach lining and allow ulceration to begin, so it must be used wisely.

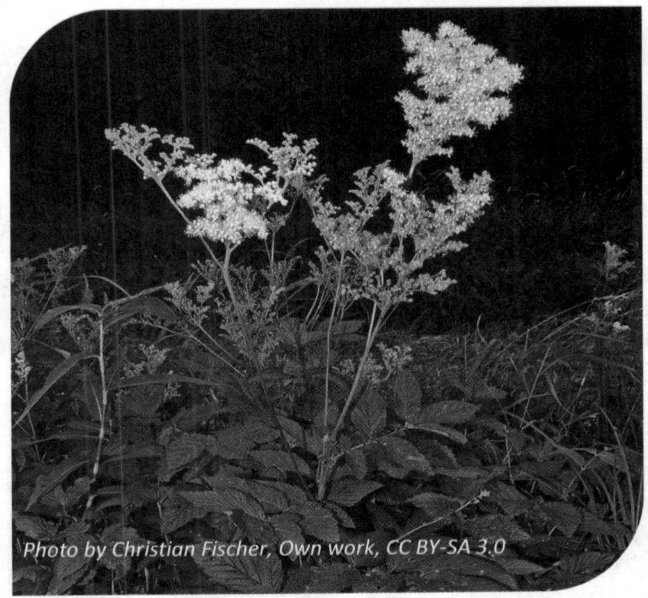

Photo by Christian Fischer, Own work, CC BY-SA 3.0

Joint Pain and Arthritis: Meadowsweet has been used as a treatment for joint pain for hundreds of years. It gives temporary relief from the swelling and pain, while also healing the connective joint tissue.

Bacterial Infections, UTIS, Skin Infections: Meadowsweet works against *E. coli, Staphylococcus aureus, Staphylococcus epidermidis, Proteus* *vulgaris,* and *Pseudomonas aeruginosa.* It also inhibits the growth of *Helicobacter pylori.*

Warning: Patients with Aspirin or sulfite sensitivity should not use meadowsweet. Patients with asthma should use with caution. Do not use meadowsweet if you are pregnant or breast-feeding. Do not use meadowsweet if you are taking anticoagulant drugs, NSAIDS, or any herbal remedies with blood-thinning properties. Overuse can cause GI bleeding. The plant can be used as a disinfectant for wounds and skin diseases and infections.

Anti-coagulant – Blood Clots: Meadowsweet has heparin, which is an anti-coagulant. Its highest levels are in the seeds, and flowers may also be used.

Meadowsweet Tea: 1.5 to 2 grams of dried meadowsweet herb, 1 cup boiling water. Pour the boiling water over the dried herbs and allow it to steep for 5 to 7 minutes. Strain the tea and drink 1 cup, 3 times daily. Sweeten with honey if desired.

Moringa oleifera, Drumstick Tree

Moringa oleifera is commonly known as drumstick tree, horseradish tree, benzoil tree, or ben oil tree. It is an extremely useful tree because of its healing properties, nutrition, and for the oil produced from the seed pods. This deciduous tree is very fast growing, going from a seedling to maturity in a single year. The roots taste like horseradish and the leaves are eaten as a green vegetable. It is also useful for water purification. The plant is now widely cultivated in the tropical and subtropical areas of the United States and is often grown in greenhouses in cooler areas. It is the only genus in its own family, the Moringaceae. It is native to India.

Identification: Mature trees reach a height of up to 40 feet (12.1 meters) if not pruned and have a trunk diameter of 1 1/2 feet (0.45m). Most growers trim the trees back to a maximum of 6 feet (1.8 meters), so that the leaves and seed pods are easily harvested. The tree

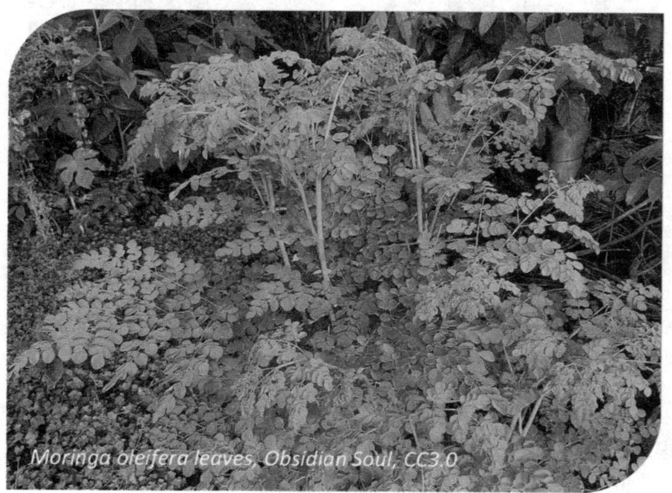

Moringa oleifera leaves, Obsidian Soul, CC3.0

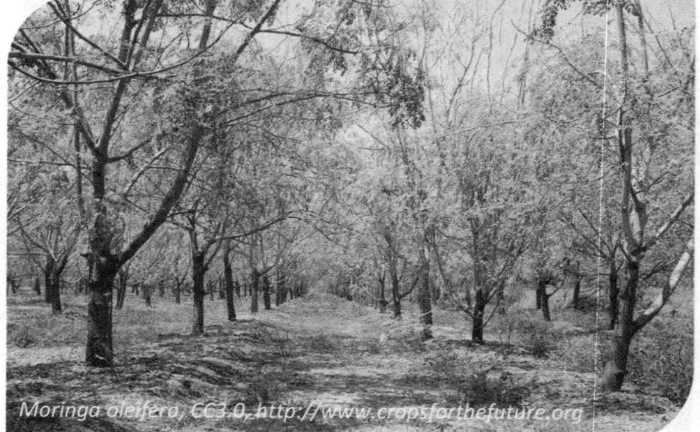

Moringa oleifera, CC3.0, http://www.cropsforthefuture.org

bark is whitish-grey in color and surrounded by thick cork. Young shoots have a purplish or green-white hairy bark. Branches are drooping and fragile, while leaves are feathery and tri-pinnate. Asexual flowers appear within the first 6 months of planting. They grow in thin, hairy stalks in drooping clusters. Each flower is approximately 1/2-inch (1.25 cm) long and 3/4-inch (1 cm) across. Five yellowish-white petals of varying sizes surround the fragrant center. In cool regions, flowers appear between April and June, but in warm regions flowering happens twice a year or year-round when the weather is hot without significant cool temperatures. Fruit pod production usually occurs in the second year and increases in the third year. The seed pods hang from the former flower clusters, forming a three-sided brown pod of 10 to 20 inches (25 cm to 50 cm) in length. Each seed is approximately 1/3 to 1/2 inch (0.8 cm to 1.25 cm) in diameter with papery wings that aid dispersion. Moringa propagates easily from seed or cuttings and the germination rate is high when planted in well-drained soil.

Edible Use: Moringa leaves are cooked and eaten as a green. In areas where nutrition is poor, moringa is often used as a seasoning for rice or other foods. The dried leaves are sprinkled on top of the food at every meal to add vitamins.

Medicinal Use: Moringa is reported to reverse or cure many different health problems, especially those caused by environmental pollution and toxins. It is also highly effective for diseases caused by poor nutrition, as it is high in vitamin and mineral content. Nearly every part of the plant can be used medicinally.

Anti-Inflammatory, Anti-aging, and Antioxidant: Moringa has earned the nickname "the miracle plant" due to its ability to fight inflammation and the effects of aging, including age-related eye problems.

Diabetes: Moringa consumption has a positive effect on insulin when eaten with a high-carbohydrate, low fat meal. It helps control blood sugar levels.

Detoxing the Body and Improving Digestion: Moringa is helpful for a wide variety of medical conditions due to its anti-inflammatory properties and purifying effects. Moringa is useful for the treatment of cancer, stomach ulcers, liver disease, urinary tract infections, edema, and kidney disease. It is also helpful in the treatment of problems with the digestive tract, including diarrhea, constipation, and fungal infections like *Candida*.

Moringa oil is especially beneficial to liver function and helps the body rid itself of heavy metals and other toxins.

Joint Problems and Arthritis: Arthritis and other joint problems are improved with daily use of moringa. It is highly effective at reducing inflammation, and its readily available vitamins and minerals help rebuild joints and stop further damage. People report that pain is reduced within 2 to 4 weeks with daily use.

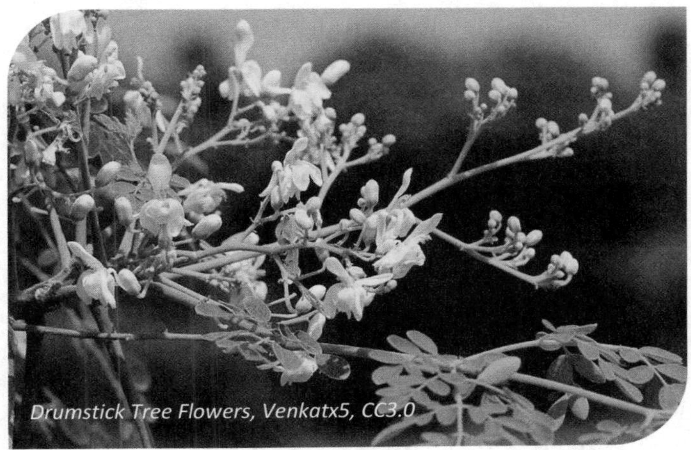
Drumstick Tree Flowers, Venkatx5, CC3.0

Treats Skin Problems: Moringa contains natural antibacterial, antifungal and antiviral compounds that protect the skin from infections. Moringa oil works well for these purposes and is effective at reducing inflammation and treating acne, skin infections, gum disease, dandruff, abscesses, and eliminating viral warts, athlete's feet and jock itch. It also helps soothe and heal wounds, bites, and burns. Applied regularly, the oil hydrates the skin and eliminates dry, itchy patches.

Stabilizes the Nervous System and Improves Brain Health: Moringa's high levels of tryptophan help stabilize nerve and brain function and increase the production of serotonin. It is used for mood swings, insomnia, fatigue, and depression.

Water Purification: Moringa seeds can be used to purify water. Heavy metals, toxins, and salts in water bind to the moringa seeds and remove them from the water. The seeds also have antibacterial, antiviral, and antifungal effects. Reportedly, only 1/2 gram of ground moringa seed is needed to purify 1/2 gallon (2 Liters) of contaminated water

Oregon Grape, *Mahonia (Berberis) aquifolium* and *M. nervosa*

Tall or Shiny Oregon grape (*M. aquifolium*), also called mountain grape or Oregon grape holly, is an upright shrub that grows 6 feet (1.8 meters) high. It is in the Berberidaceae (Barberry) Family. *M. nervosa* (Dwarf/Dull Oregon grape or Cascade barberry) has the same medicinal properties. It is found in forests in the Pacific NW of North America.

Identification: Their leaflets look a lot like holly: dark green, spiky, leathery and shiny. They have compound pinnate leaves; each pinnate leaf is about 12 inches (30 cm) long with 7 to 9 leaflets. The small yellow flowers are grouped in a raceme at the tips of branches and produce dark bluish-purple berries when mature. The fruit grows in small clusters like grapes.

Edible Use: The small purplish berries are edible, although they are very tart and contain large seeds. They are sometimes used to make jelly and wine. Its flowers are edible.

Medicinal Use: The root of the Oregon Grape is used for medicinal purposes. It contains berberine, an alkaloid that is antifungal, antibacterial and antiviral. It is yellow in color and helps regulate blood sugar and metabolism, lower cholesterol, is a neuroprotective, anti-parasite, anti-cancer, is an ACE inhibitor, and is used for Type 2 Diabetes. I use Oregon Grape root often as it grows in my backyard and is such a versatile plant.

Cleans and Stimulates the Liver, Gallbladder, Spleen, and Blood: Oregon Grape stimulates the liver and the secretion of bile, and helps with non-alcohol induced fatty liver. It cleans the blood, gallbladder, and spleen. It alleviates symptoms caused by weakness in these organs, including headaches, digestive problems, and accumulated toxins.

Anti-bacterial, UTIs, Staph, Strep: Oregon Grape Root is an antibacterial and helps urinary tract infections, bladder infections, lung infections, staph, strep, MRSA, and more.

Anti-viral: The berberine in Oregon Grape acts as an neuraminidase inhibitor and inhibits viral replication. It also inhibits the inflammatory response due to viral infection, and decreases the production of inflammatory cytokines. It has been shown to act against the herpes virus, Zika, HIV, and Influenza A (including H1N1/Swine Flu).

Digestive Disorders: Oregon Grape Root tea is used for issues such as dysentery, diarrhea, and gastritis. It also helps balance intestinal flora.

Skin Conditions, Wound Care, Anti-Fungal: Oregon Grape works externally and internally to treat skin conditions like acne, wounds, psoriasis, eczema, herpes, and fungal conditions.

Lowering Blood Glucose Levels: The berberine in Oregon Grape Root has similar effects as the drug Metformin, which is used for Type 2 Diabetes.

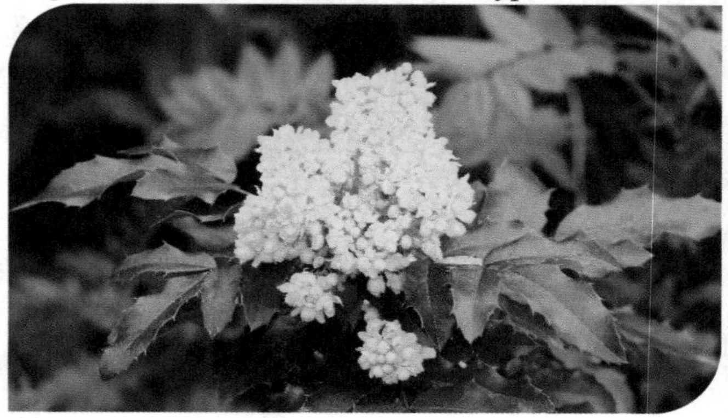

Cardiovascular Disease: The berberine in Oregon Grape Root is an ACE inhibitor. ACE inhibitors widen blood vessels increasing blood flow.

Anti-Cancer: Oregon Grape helps with cancer via inhibition of tumor growth. It can be used in conjunction with modern therapies, and has a similar effect as Metformin (it activates AMPK-AMP activated protein kinase).

Parasites: Oregon grape root is a good internal anti-microbial. It works well for giardia, and targets protozoans as well as worms.

Harvesting: I prefer to use roots from mature plants that are at least a year old. I look for older plants that have attained their full height and have produced fruit. Harvest the roots in the late fall, digging up the entire root system and then replanting the crown roots and any other unused pieces to grow again.

Warning: Not for use during pregnancy or nursing due to berberine. Limit usage of the berries to reasonable servings and be careful not to over-consume.

Recipes. Oregon Grape Root Tea. 1/2-ounce Oregon grape root, dried and crushed, 1-quart (1 Liter) water. Combine the root and water in a pot with a tight-fitting lid. Bring to a boil and turn the heat down to a slow simmer. Simmer the tea for 10 to 15 minutes. Strain out the root.

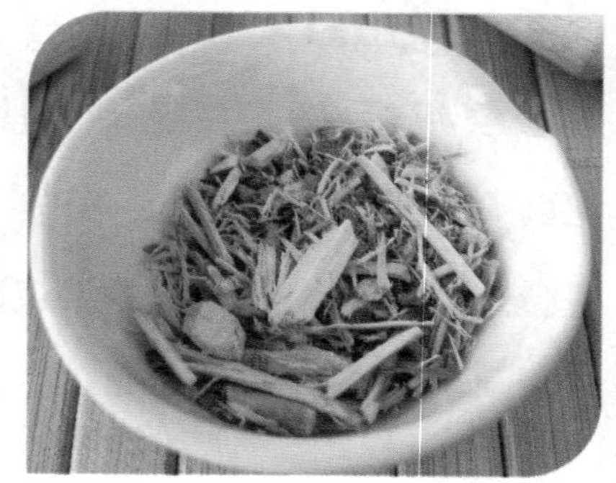

Quaking Aspen, *Populus tremuloides*

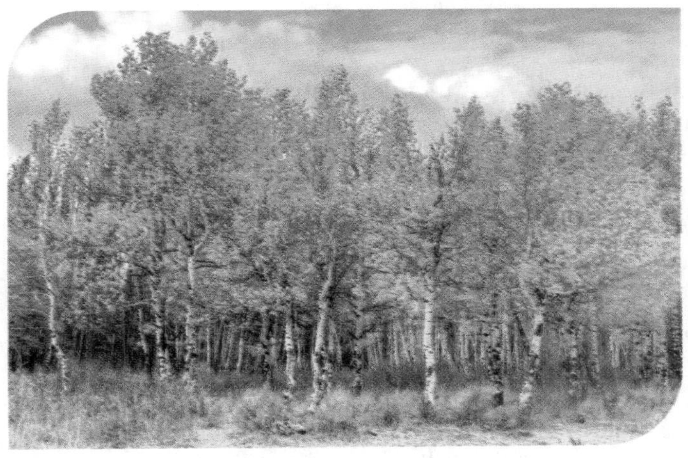

Quaking aspen belongs to the Salicaceae (Willow) Family. It is a deciduous tree native to cooler regions of North America. It is also known as trembling aspen and American aspen, It's one of several species referred to as aspen. The tree is named quaking because of its flexible flattened petioles, causing its leaves to shake in the wind. The leaves turn bright yellow in autumn.

Identification: Quaking aspen is a native tree that usually grows 20 to 50 feet (15 meters) high with a rounded crown.

Its lateral roots may extend out over 100 feet (30 meters), and an aspen grove may all be clones of the original. The bark is usually whiteish in color and is often peeling and thin, becoming thicker and furrowed with age, especially toward the base of this tree. Its leaves are simple, deciduous and are broadly ovate to nearly round. They are usually 1 1/2 to 3 inches (7.75 cm to 7.5 cm) long with small rounded teeth on the margins. Leaves are dark green and shiny on top and pale green on the underside. The male flower (staminate) and female flowers (pistillate) are on separate trees. Flowers of each type are borne in hanging catkins. The small fruits are narrowly ovoid to flask shaped capsules that are nearly 2/10 to 3/10 inches (0.5 cm to 0.75 cm) long. They split to release the seeds. Each seed has a tuft of long, white, silky hairs that are easily blown by the wind.

Edible Use: Like many inner barks, quaking aspen can be dried and ground into a powder that is added to flour. It can be eaten raw or cooked in moderate amounts and makes a good thickener for soups and stews. The sap can be tapped and used for drinking or as a flavoring. The catkins can be eaten raw and cooked.

Medicinal Use: It is used to treat wounds, skin problems, and respiratory problems and is valued for its antiseptic and analgesic properties.

Rheumatoid Arthritis: Quaking aspen bark contains anti-inflammatory and pain-relieving properties. This is a powerful combination for treating rheumatoid arthritis. It can be used externally on a painful joint, as well as internally.

Chilblains, Wounds, and Hemorrhoids: Quaking Aspen Bark Infusion is a good external treatment for chilblains, wounds, and hemorrhoids. Application to the skin reduces swelling, increases blood flow, and disinfects the wound. For an infected wound, apply a poultice made of crushed roots to the wound and hold in place with a clean cloth.

Respiratory Problems, Coughs, and Fevers: For coughs, colds, congestion, and other respiratory problems, try an infusion of quaking aspen bark. It treats coughs and congestion because of its anti-inflammatory properties. It also effectively reduces fevers.

Menstrual Problems and Menopause: For menstrual problems and menopause, try a combination of quaking aspen and black cohosh. The two together act to relieve pain and cramping, hot flashes, moodiness, night sweats, headaches, heart palpitations, vaginal dryness, and mental fog. They balance the hormones and normalize menstrual cycles. Do not use Black Cohosh for treatment of women with endometriosis.

Harvesting: Always be careful when harvesting bark from trees. Bark taken too liberally kills the branch or, if taken from the trunk, it can kill the tree. Only remove a side branch from the tree, then remove the bark and dry it for later use.

Red Alder, *Alnus rubra*

Red Alder is a distinctive tree native to the northwest coast of North America. It is a deciduous broadleaf member of the Betulaceae (Birch) Family and gets its name from the distinctive rusty-red coloring that develops on the bruised or scraped bark.

Identification: Red Alder grows quickly and usually grows 25 to 50 feet (7.6 meters to 15 meters) high. Trees that grow in the forest develop a tapered trunk that extends up to a narrow and round shaped crown, while trees growing in the open have a broad cone-shaped crown and can be scrubby.

Its broad alternate leaves are greyish underneath and bright green on the top. They have an oval-shape and pointed tips. The coarsely toothed edges curl downward and are a distinguishing trait. Its veins form a ladder-like pattern.

Flowers develop as female or male clusters. Female flowers are on woody brown cones, while male flowers are long, drooping reddish catkins. The oval-shaped female cones are just under an inch (2.5 cm) long and produce 50 to 100 seeds that look like a narrow, winged nut.

Edible Use: The catkins of red alder trees can be eaten raw or fresh. They are rich in protein and nutrients, and although they are bitter I have gotten used to the taste. The inner bark is sometimes dried and powdered, and used as a flour to thicken soups and sauces. The sap of the red alder has a sweet flavor. Collect in late winter and consume raw.

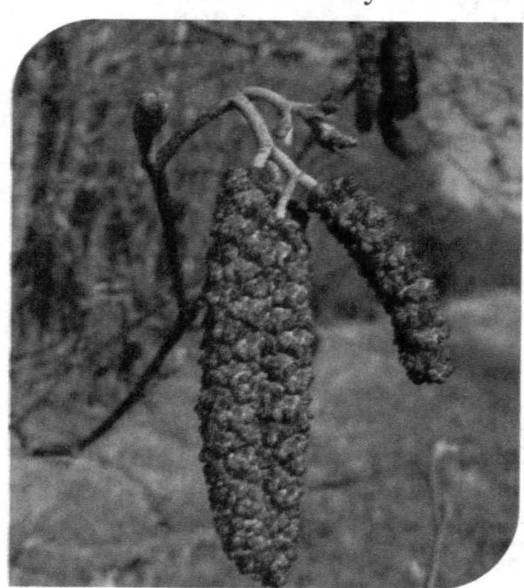

Walter Siegmund - Own work, CC by 2.5

Medicinal Use: An extract or decoction of the dried bark is used in most cases. The bark contains salicin.

Diarrhea and Indigestion: A Red Alder Bark Decoction relieves indigestion, calms the stomach muscles, and treats diarrhea.

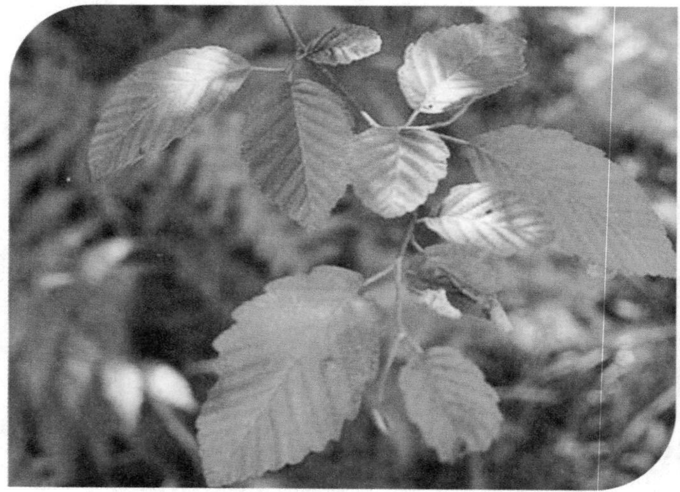

Fevers, Headaches, Arthritis Pain: Red Alder bark contains a painkiller that works like aspirin to reduce fevers and relieve pain.

Insect Bites, Poison Oak, Rashes, Eczema, and Other Skin Irritations: For skin irritations, bites, swellings, eczema, and rashes, use a Red Alder Bark Infusion or poultice directly on the skin. The red alder soothes the skin, relieves the pain, and reduces swelling and inflammation.

Lice, Scabies, and Mites: To get rid of lice, scabies, and mites, boil the inner bark and leaves of the red alder in vinegar and allow it to cool. Massage into the affected areas. It kills them and eliminates the problem.

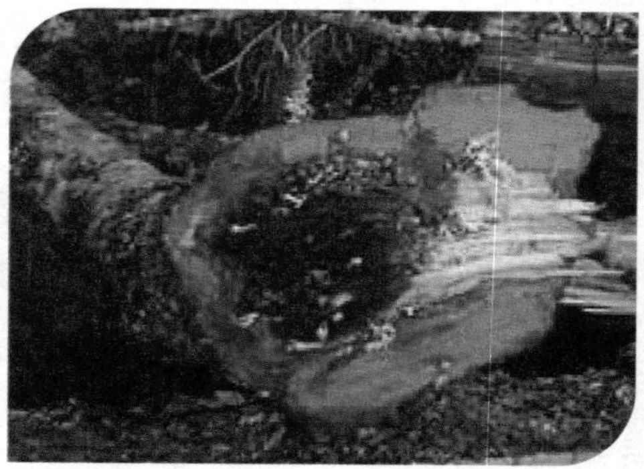

Red Coloration on bark, Walter Siegmund, CC by 2.5

Tuberculosis: Red alder decoction has been traditionally used to treat tuberculosis, lymphatic problems, and syphilis.

Harvesting: Collect red alder leaves during the summer and use fresh. Collect the bark in the spring when new growth is occurring. Choose a young branch, about 2 to 3 years old. Remove the branch from the tree and remove the outer and inner bark. Dry the bark for future use. Fresh bark can cause vomiting and stomach upset; only use dried bark.

Recipes. Red Alder Decoction: 1 ounce of Red Alder Dried Bark, 1-pint (500 ml) (2 cups) of Water. Crush or grind the dried bark into small pieces. Place it in a non-reactive pot with the water over medium heat. Bring the mixture to a simmer. Simmer the herbs until the water has reduced by 1/4 to 1/3, leaving 1 1/3 to 1 1/2 cups of liquid. Cool the decoction and strain out the bark. Store in the refrigerator for up to 3 days.

Red Elderberry, *Sambucus racemosa*

Red Elderberry is also known as a scarlet elder, stinking elderberry, and bunchberry elder. It is native throughout North America, Europe, and temperate Asia. It is in the Adoxaceae (Moschatel) Family and grows very quickly.

Identification: Red elderberry is a deciduous shrub that grows in milder climates along rivers and in forests. It appears treelike when mature, growing up to nearly twenty feet (6 meters) in height. The branches of the red elderberry are often broad and tend to arch outwards from the center of the plant. The branches are soft to the touch and pliable, with a pithy center and a bumpy jointed surface. The oval shaped compound green leaves cluster along the branches, growing outwards from the base in groups with 3 to 7 leaflets per cluster. Leaflets are toothed and lance-shaped.

The growing season of the Red Elderberry begins in the early months of spring and, once blooming, generates numerous tiny off-white flowers in pyramid-like clusters during the spring and summer months. Clusters of fleshy, drupe fruit grow bright red and occasionally purple during these months. The foliage has a potent odor, which is the source of one of the Red Elderberry's nicknames, the stinking elderberry.

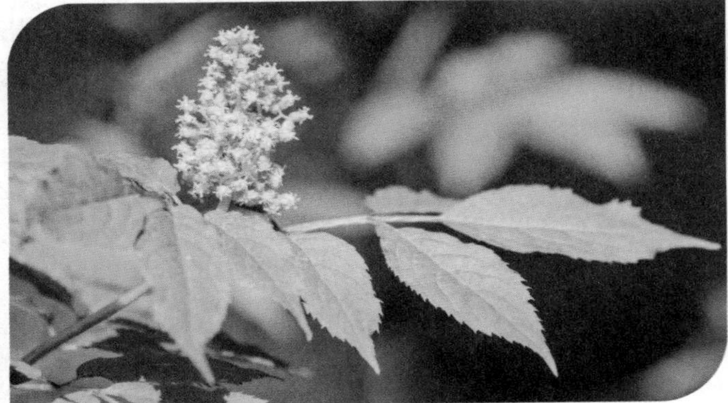

Edible and Other Use: The berries are edible when cooked and are used in jellies, syrups, and pies.

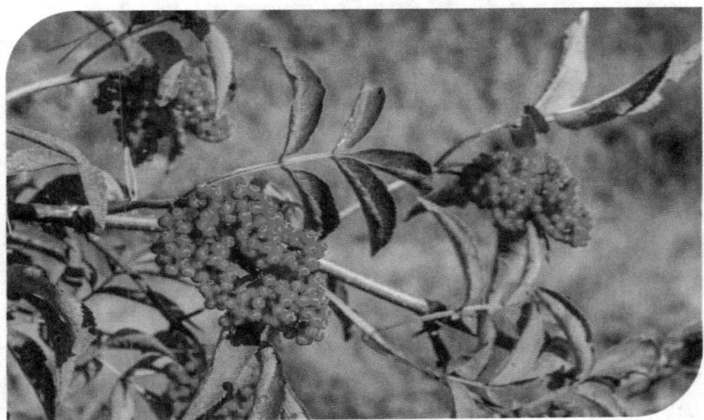

Spit the seeds out for safety. Cooked red elderberries have a bitter taste and pungent odor, so it is best to mix the berries with other fruits or sweeten them with honey while cooking. The flowers are dried and used to make wine and can be cooked and eaten in moderation. Dry the flowers before cooking. Do not eat any other parts of this plant as they have cyanide-producing toxins.

I use the stems to make fireblowers as it is easy to clean out their pithy center. They are also used for making instruments, like flutes.

Medicinal Use. Fever Reduction, Cold Remedy, and Laxative: Tea or thin syrup made by boiling red elderberries and consuming the liquid works as a tonic for colds, fevers, and also as a laxative. Strain out the seeds and drink the liquid fresh after cooking. The tea causes the body to sweat, which cools the body. Healing compounds in the berries ease the symptoms and help the body heal faster.

Boils, Abscesses, and Skin Infections: The leaves of the red elderberry draw out fluid and pus from boils and abscesses, helping to reduce swelling and relieve pain while encouraging healing. Apply bruised fresh leaves as a poultice. External use only.

Warning: Red elderberry berries are toxic when raw and can cause upset stomach and indigestion; however, they are safe and edible when cooked and deseeded. The leaves, shoots, and roots are considered toxic and should not be eaten, even after cooking.

Red Mulberry, *Morus rubus*

The deciduous thornless red mulberry tree grows to 50 feet (15 meters) high. I had one near my house where I grew up in New England and have cultivated one where I now live in the PNW. They are native to Eastern North America. They are in the Moraceae (Mulberry) Family.

Identification: The heart-shaped leaves are alternate and approximately 3 to 6 inches (7.5 cm to 15 cm) long and 2 to 5 inches (5 cm to 12.5 cm) wide. They are broadly cordate with a notch at the base and a pointed tip. Most leaves on mature trees are unlobed but leaves on young trees often have 2 to 3 lobes with a serrated margin. The leaves have a rough upper surface while the underside is covered with soft hairs. The leaf petiole secretes a milky sap when cut or injured. The flowers are small, yellow-green or red-green, with male and female flowers usually on separate trees. The flowers open in the early spring as the leaves emerge. The trunk is covered with dark brown bark that is scaly or sometimes smooth.

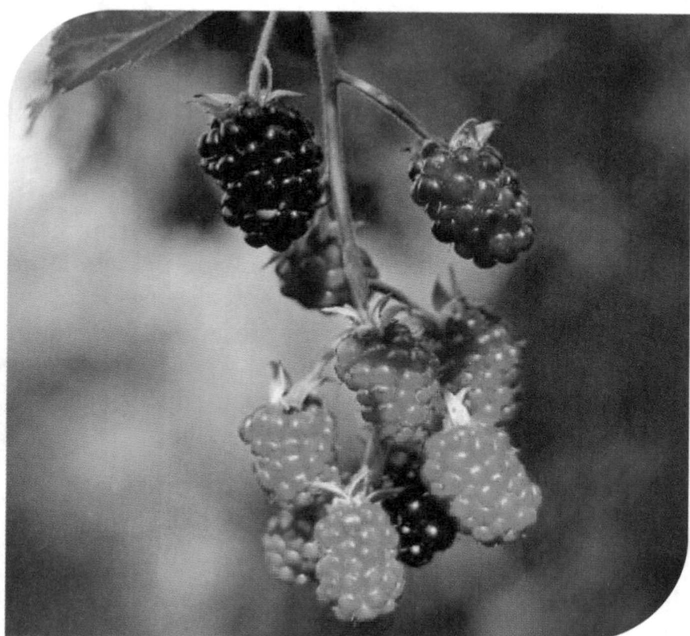

Edible Use: You can eat mulberries both raw and cooked. They are most often used to make pies, pastries, and jellies, but I like them raw. They also make a very nice sweet fruit wine. The dried wood is useful for barbecue and smoking meats. It adds a smoky flavor that is sweet and mild.

Medicinal Use: The leaves, fruit, and bark all have medicinal value. Use the fruit and leaves during the summer months when they are readily available and switch to bark tea during the winter when the trees are bare.

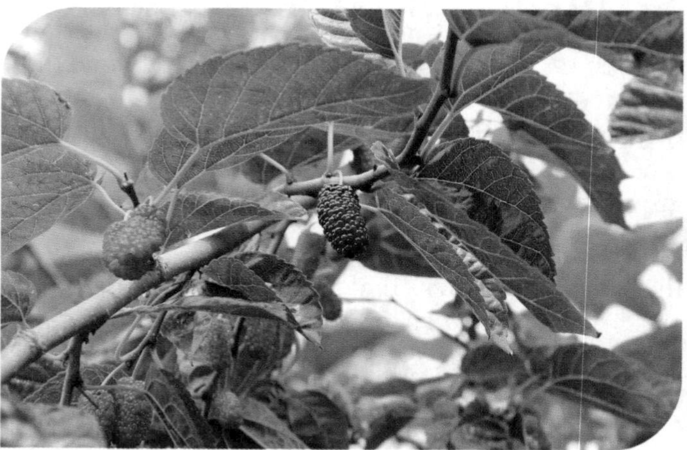

Heart Disease: Mulberries are beneficial for the heart. They reduce inflammation in the arteries and veins, lower cholesterol, and lower the risk of heart disease. Eating the berries or drinking the wine, in moderation, confers all the benefits.

Alzheimer's Disease and Parkinson's: Eating mulberries regularly protects the brain from inflammation and its effects. They reduce chronic inflammation and slow down the disease process.

Urinary Tract Problems: Mulberry Leaf Tea is a potent weapon against urinary tract infections and other problems. The leaves are anti-inflammatory and anti-microbial. Combined with their healing properties and superior nutrition, the leaf tea resolves the problem quickly.

Ringworm: Ringworm responds well to the application of mulberry sap taken from the cut leaf petiole. Apply the sap directly to the affected area as needed.

Diabetes: The leaves and bark of the red mulberry tree help reduce blood sugar levels in diabetics and increase the production of insulin. They also protect the heart, liver, and kidneys from damage by the disease. Use leaf or bark tea.

Salal, *Gaultheria shallon*

Salal is also known as Oregon wintergreen, and is in the Ericaceae (Heath) Family. Commonly found in the Pacific Northwest of North America, it likes a warm, moist climate. It holds great medicinal value, but is known mostly for its use in floral arrangements. I love snacking on the berries as I wander through the woods.

Identification: Salal grows between 2 to 10 feet (0.6m to 3 m) tall and has dark green leathery leaves that are thick, shiny, and waxy on top.

This evergreen shrub produces white, rose, or pink clusters of small flowers that look like urn-shaped bells. The flowers are slightly sticky and hairy. They give way to berries that are red, purple, or dark blue in color and covered in tiny hairs. The plant grows in lush thickets, preferring sunny areas with moisture and good drainage.

Edible Use: The berries are sweetest in the fall, after the first frost, but are edible throughout the summer and fall. They are quite tart, similar to cranberries or blueberries but with a mild flavor. Berries are eaten fresh but can also be cooked. The flavor can vary from plant to plant, so if you don't like them, try the next plant over. Lemon juice seems to brighten the flavor greatly. The berries can be dried for future use.

Medicinal Use: Both the berry and the leaf are useful for medicine. The leaves are astringent in nature.

Strengthens the Immune System: Salal has an astringent effect that helps treat infections of all kinds. It is also a strong anti-inflammatory and contains tannic acid and many vitamins and anti-oxidants. It can strengthen the immune function and speed healing.

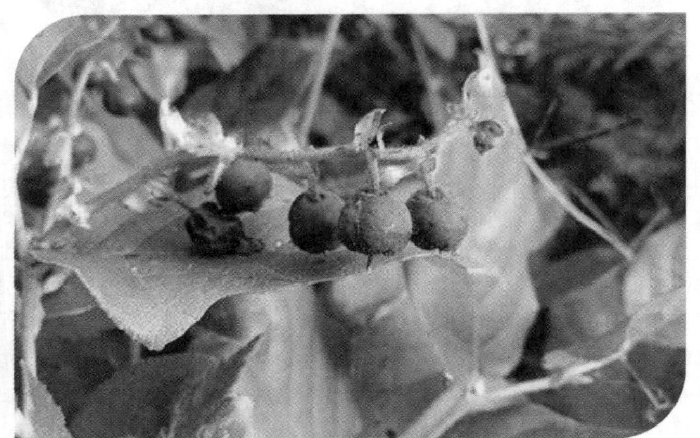

Salal Berries, by Darren Giles [CC BY-SA 3.0]

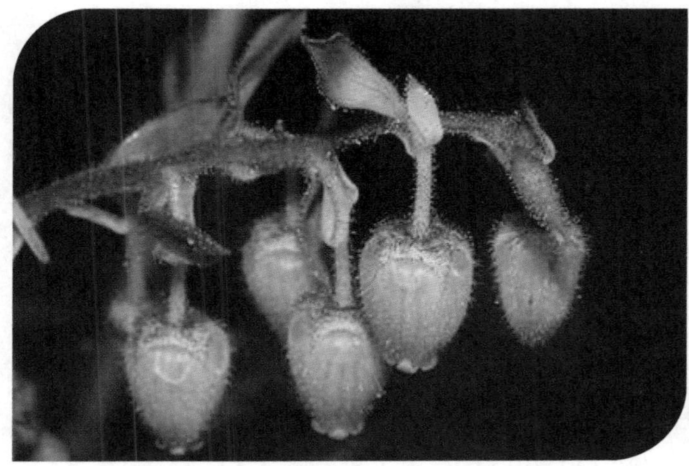

Salal Flowers, by Walter Siegmund, CC by SA 3.0

Skin Treatments, Abrasions, Burns, and Wounds: For skin treatment, make a poultice with powdered leaves or wash the skin with an infusion made from crushed leaves. Allow the infusion to dry on the skin or leave the poultice in place for 20 minutes or more, as needed.

Chronic Skin Problems: Eating a handful of Salal berries daily is helpful for chronic skin problems. The berries increase blood circulation to the skin and help the skin to heal.

Anti-diarrhea, Gas Pain, Colic, Digestive Ailments: For digestive ailments, try Salal Leaf Tea. The tea is safe for children and can be given as needed or 2 to 3 hours after a meal for gastric distress. Give the tea frequently to treat diarrhea, until symptoms are gone.

Dry Cough: An infusion of Salal Leaf Tea treats a raspy, dry cough in children and adults.

Respiratory Problems: Salal Leaf Tea is a good choice for respiratory problems, including tuberculosis and colic

Heartburn: Heartburn can be relieved by chewing the leaves or by taking Salal Leaf Tea as need to relieve symptoms.

Obesity and Appetite Suppressant: Chewing the young leaves acts as an appetite suppressant and helps aid weight loss.

Bladder Inflammation: Salal leaves help reduce inflammation and relieve infections in the urinary tract, particularly the bladder. In most cases, Salal Leaf Tea taken several times a day will solve the problem.

Reduces Inflammation and Promotes Health: The flavonoids and anti-oxidants in salal berries are anti-inflammatory and help boost the immune system. They promote health and help prevent disease. Eat the berries and drink Salal Leaf Tea for optimal health.

Relieves Insect Stings and Bites: For reducing the pain and inflammation of insect bites make the powdered leaves into a paste and apply it directly to the affected area. This is a good remedy when Plantain (*Plantago* spp.) isn't available.

Reduces the Effects of Aging: Salal berries are filled with vitamins and antioxidants that reduce free radical damage and the effects of aging.

Harvesting: Berries are best gathered in the fall when they turn deep blue. They are sweetest after the first frost, but can be eaten throughout the fall. Pick the entire stem of berries and place in a basket. Remove the berries by pinching them off the stem instead of pulling. The berries can be crushed and dried for future use. Gather healthy green leaves from spring to summer. Cut the stems and bundle them together with a rubber band or string and hang to dry in a cool, dark place. When the leaves are dry and crumbly, remove them from the stems and store them in a sealed glass jar for future use. They will remain medicinally active for several years if stored properly.

Warning: The leaves are considered safe, but should not be consumed in excess.

Recipes. Salal Leaf Tea. Ingredients: 5 to 6 dry leaves or 1 Tablespoon crushed leaves, 1 cup boiling water. Pour the boiling water over the dry leaves and steep for 20 minutes. Strain out the leaves and drink as needed.

Sassafras, *Sassafras albidum*

Some believe sassafras to be a cure-all, others value the tree for its flavor and calming aroma. Sassafras is a deciduous tree native to North America. It is famous for its aroma and brilliant displays of color in autumn, when the leaves turn yellow, orange, deep red, and even purple before they fall. Sassafras has many uses including traditional root beer. The wood is used to repel insects much like cedar is used. It is in the Lauraceae (Laurel) Family.

Identification: Most parts of the sassafras tree will give off a faint citrus smell when crushed. However, if you pull a sassafras shrub up by the root, you will get a whiff of old-fashioned root beer. Sassafras can be identified by its unique leaf characteristics. Each leaf can have anywhere from a single lobe up to five lobes, all occurring on the same tree. The most recognized shape of a sassafras leaf is the two or three-lobed leaves that look like a mitten. Sassafras blooms in early spring, with groups of little yellow flowers that grow 1-2 inches (5 cm) long. In the fall, sassafras yields small berry-sized blue drupe fruit, with a fleshy outside and a small seed inside. The fruit is a favorite snack of deer and other wildlife.

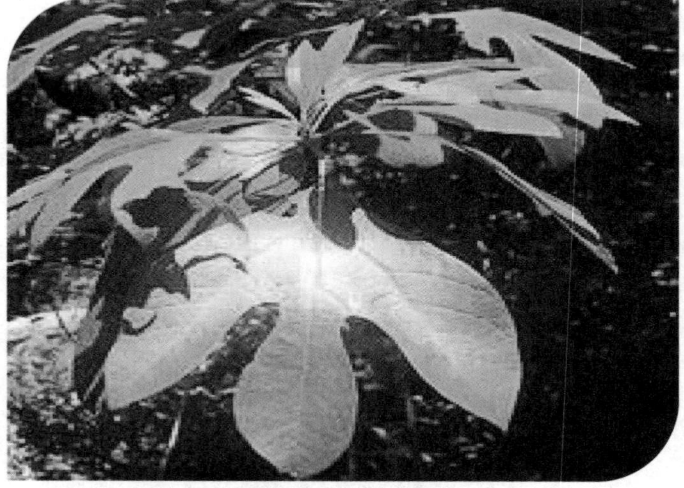

7Sassafras, by Wowbobwow12, CC by SA 3.0

Edible Use: Nearly every part of the tree is useful for food or medicine. The powdered leaves of the tree are used as a thickener and flavoring. The flavor is both earthy and spicy, and is similar to coriander seed. The most famous use of sassafras root is in traditional root beer recipes. However, the use of sassafras root was banned in 1960 by the Food and Drug Administration after studies found safrole, the chemical component of sassafras root, to be a possible carcinogen and linked safrole use to higher rates of cancer and liver damage with extended use. It is considered safe for short-term use only with proper dosage.

Medicinal Use: The leaves, root bark, and mucilaginous pith from the tree are used medicinally.

Skin Inflammations and Irritations: Make a thick mucilage from the pith of the sassafras tree for the treatment of skin irritations and inflammations and apply it directly to the wound. Alternately, a poultice made from bruised fresh leaves can be applied to large areas or the leaves can be rubbed onto itchy bug bites and small irritations.

Heals Wounds: For wound healing, apply a poultice made from the fresh, crushed leaves and cover it with a clean cloth to keep it in place. The sassafras leaves stimulate the flow of blood to the area and speeds healing. The poultice also relieves the pain.

Headaches and Menstrual Pain: The pain-relieving properties of Sassafras Leaf and Root Bark Tea are helpful for headaches and many menstrual symptoms including cramping, bloating, and heavy bleeding.

Kidney Problems, Swelling, and Fluid Retention: Sassafras Leaf and Root Bark Tea is an excellent diuretic, and helps flush toxins from the body.

Dental Care: A sassafras twig makes a great toothbrush. The twig not only leaves behind a pleasant flavor and clean teeth, but it also has anti-microbial and anti-inflammatory benefits.

Lice Treatment: Sassafras Oil (see below for recipe), diluted with a carrier oil, is used to get rid of head lice. To use this treatment, add 1/4 teaspoon of sassafras oil to ½ cup of warm coconut oil. Mix and apply to the scalp. Cover the head and wait 30 minutes to 1 hour. Shampoo the hair thoroughly to remove the oil, then use a nit comb to remove the dead lice and nits.

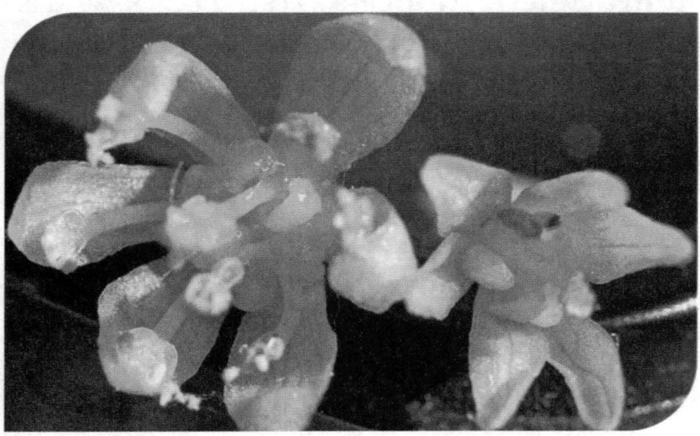

Sassafras male and female flowers, by Ittiz, CC by SA 3.0

Arthritis and Anti-inflammatory: Sassafras root bark works well to reduce joint pain and inflammation throughout the body.

Harvesting: If you can find a downed Sassafras tree after a storm, harvest the roots then. Roots peel more easily in the winter and early spring. Or harvest one in the shade where it won't likely thrive. Harvest the bark in spring and leaves when they are green.

Warning: Safrole can cause liver damage, is a carcinogen, can cause stomach upset, vomiting, increased blood pressure, hallucinations, and death. It should not be used by pregnant or nursing women. There are safrole-free sassafras products that are safer to use. Some people are allergic.

Recipes. Extracting Sassafras Oil for External Use. A large piece of sassafrass root, water. Dig up a large piece of sassafras root, at least two inches (5 cm) thick and as long as possible. Clean the root, then peel off the bark. Keep the root bark. Allow the bark shavings to dry. Place the dried bark in a pot of simmering water and allow it to simmer for 4 to 6 hours. The oil will be released from the bark. Allow the water and oil to cool undisturbed in the refrigerator overnight. Skim off the oily layer on the top of the water. This oil is very potent, dilute it before use and do not take internally.

Sassafras Root Tea: Sassafras root tea is prepared differently than most teas. Sassafras roots, small pinch of salt, optional and water. Pot with a lid. Clean the roots with a brush under running water to remove all dirt. Place the sassafras roots in the pot and cover with cold water, filling the pot about 3/4 full. Add a small pinch of salt. Use more roots for a stronger tea or more water for a weaker tea. Make a weak tea if you have not had it previously. Put the water and roots on high heat until it comes to a boil, then turn down the heat. Keep the roots at a high simmer until the water turns a deep red color. This may take a few hours. Turn off the heat and cover the pot with a lid. Allow the tea to steep for 5 to 10 minutes while it slowly cools a little. Strain the tea and drink hot, as it takes on a more bitter flavor when cool. The tea can be refrigerated and reheated for later use. Sweeten the tea with raw honey, if desired. Use with care (see warning section).

Saw Palmetto, *Serenoa repens*

Saw Palmetto, a fan palm, grows in the Southern Atlantic and Gulf Coast areas of the USA. It grows in dense thickets of low-growing plants from 2 to 10 feet (0.6 to 3m) tall. It is in the Arecaceae (Palm) Family.

Identification: The light green or silvery-white saw palmetto leaves form a rounded fan containing approximately 20 leaflets. The petiole (leaf stalk) is covered with sharp teeth or spines, hence its name. The petioles can grow 2 to 3 feet (0.6m to 0.9m) long. Leaves are 2 to 3 feet (0.6m to 0.9m) across and are divided into leaflets that are 2 to 4 feet(0.6m to 1.2m) long. Small flowers are yellow-white on densely covered compound panicles up to 2 feet (0.6m) long. Saw palmetto fruit is a large reddish-black drupe when ripe. Berries about 1 inch (2.5 cm) in size appear at the end of the summer as green to brown berries, ripening to a purple-black color.

Edible and Other Use: The heart is edible raw or cooked as is the ripe fruit, which is described as having a blue cheese-like or soapy flavor. To access the delicious heart cut the trunk and peel away the outer husk. The new shoots are also edible. The palm stems/stalks are used for cordage (rope) and basketmaking.

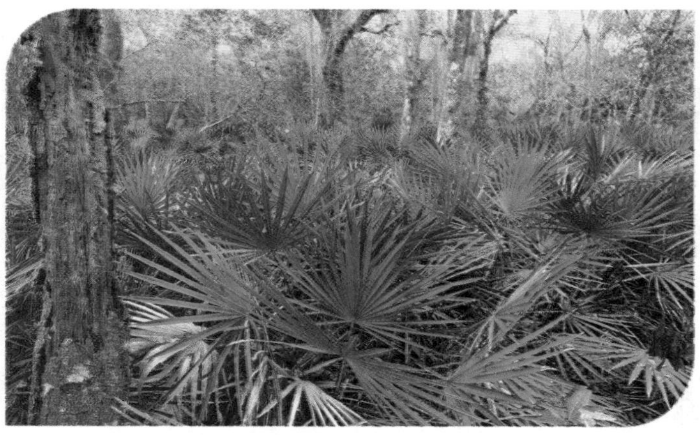

Medicinal Use: Saw palmetto berries are used for medicine.

General Tonic, Coughs, and Indigestion: Try the juice of crushed berries as a general tonic for health. It also relieves even the most troublesome coughs and is an expectorant. It is also used for

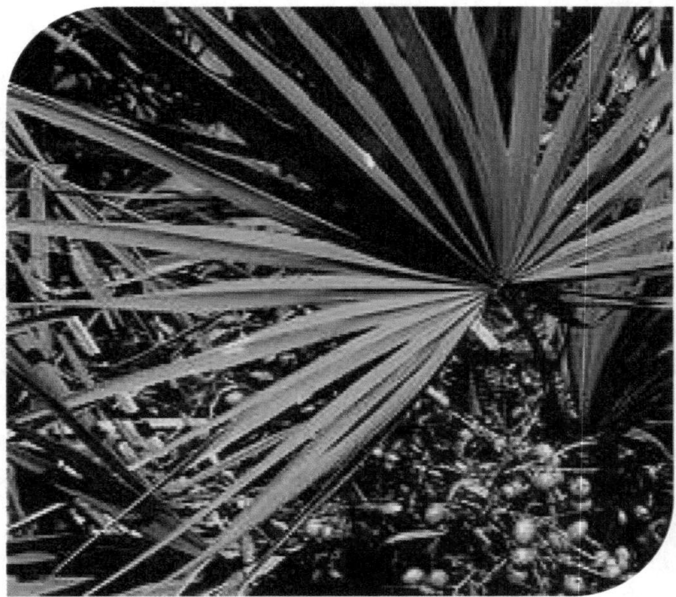

Ted Bodner, CC by 3.0

stomachaches, indigestion, and dysentery. It has both sedative and diuretic properties.

Prostate Problems: Saw Palmetto is used for prostate swelling, prostate cancer, and other prostate problems. It is a safe treatment for men with mild to moderate Benign Prostatic Hyperplasia. It improves the need for frequent urination.

Increased Libido and Delayed Menopause: Saw palmetto has long been believed to increase the libido in both men and women. It is said to increase fertility in women and delay the onset of menopause.

Androgenetic Alopecia (Hair Loss): Saw Palmetto berries treat Androgenetic Alopecia in some people. This is a type of hair loss and baldness caused by hormone imbalance.

Weight Gain and Failure to Thrive: Saw palmetto berries are anabolic, and help increase muscle mass and aid in weight gain.

Harvesting: Pick the ripe purplish-black berries by hand in August and September spreading them out to dry. Store them in a cool, dry, and dark place.

Warning: Avoid use of saw palmetto if you have a blood clotting disorder, liver disease, or pancreas disorder. Do not use saw palmetto if pregnant or breastfeeding. Saw palmetto increases fertility and makes birth control pills less effective. Do not give saw palmetto to children.

Slippery Elm, *Ulmus rubra*

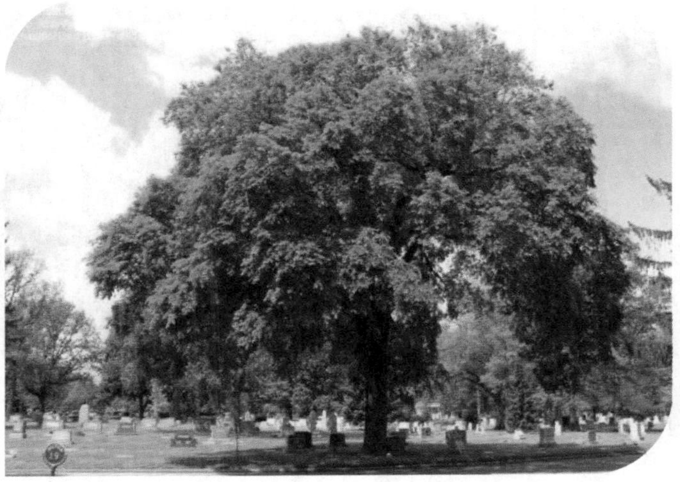

Many people with Crohn's Disease and other digestive upsets feel that Slippery Elm is a miracle herb. After one cup of tea, it is easy to understand the origin of the name; the inner bark makes a thick, slippery mucilage of a tea that you can almost eat with a spoon. Native to Eastern North America, slippery elm prefers moist forests. It is also called Indian Elm, Moose Elm, and Sweet Elm. It is in the Ulmaceae (Elm) Family.

Identification: This deciduous tree grows to between 40 to 60 feet (12.1 meters to 18 meters). The alternate leaves are oval and approximately 4 to 7 inches (10 cm to 17.5 cm) long. The leaves have a rough, sandpaper-like texture on top and are soft and hairy on the underside. The edges are sharply double-toothed and distinctly uneven at the base. The leaves are often reddish when emerging from the bud, turning dark green as they mature, and then a dull yellow in the autumn. Flowers are drooping clusters and fruits appear in March to May and are papery, winged, circular, flat, and yellowish-green. Each fruit has one seed about 1/2 inch (1.25 cm) wide and hairless.

Medicinal Use: The medicinally valuable inner bark is white and mucilaginous. I use slippery elm most often as bark tea, by chewing on a piece of bark, or as a tincture.

Coughs and Sore Throats, Bronchitis, Pleurisy, and Tuberculosis: When the fresh bark is available, chew on a small piece to relieve a cough or a sore throat. Slippery elm is even used in modern-day throat lozenges. Slippery Elm Inner Bark Tea will relieve throat irritation and helps treat respiratory diseases. It produces mucilage that coats the throat.

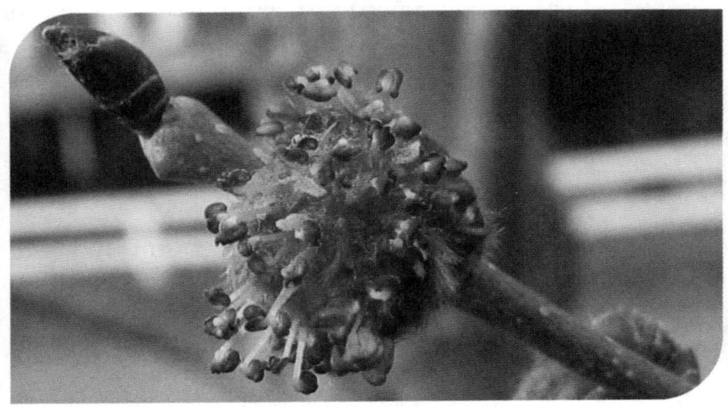

Crohn's Disease, Digestive Disorders, Leaky Gut, and Diverticulitis: Here is where slippery elm really shines. People with Crohn's and irritable bowel disease achieve great relief from Slippery Elm Bark Tea or Tincture, often describing it as a miracle cure. It also works for other forms of digestive problems and stomach pain. It has a calming effect on the digestive tract and helps with leaky gut repair as well.

Colic: Slippery elm is safe for use with children and is nourishing. It comforts the digestive tract and soothes the distress of colic.

Heartburn and GERD: Slippery elm bark coats the esophagus, helping with irritation from acid reflux.

Urinary Tract Infections: Slippery elm has medicinal compounds that release the UTI from the body and help it heal. It isn't antibacterial but helps coat the urinary tract for healing and to stop bacteria from attaching.

Boils, Cold Sores, and Cuts: Mix a small portion of powdered slippery elm bark with a small amount of boiling water. Allow it to sit for a few minutes to cool and thicken. Place the thickened paste on boils, cold sores, cuts, and other skin irritations.

Joint Pain, Gout, Arthritis, and Bruises: The Slippery Elm Paste described above can be used on the skin to relieve joint pain and bruises. Slippery Elm Tea taken internally hastens healing and provides relief from gout and arthritis pain.

Harvesting: For best results, collect the inner bark from older trees.

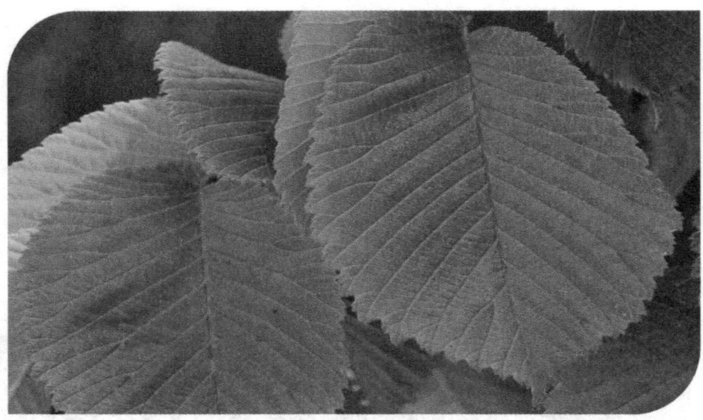

Remove the inner bark from larger branches as they are harvested from the tree or cut a rectangle of bark from the tree without cutting around the tree. If the bark is removed all the way around the tree, it will die. Once the bark is free, remove the outer bark, keeping the inner bark that is closest to the wood. Cut the harvested bark into small pieces and dry it for future use.

Slippery Elm Bark Tea/Pudding: Combine 1 teaspoon to several tablespoons of ground inner bark from slippery elm, 1 cup of warm water or milk (almond, coconut, hemp, etc.)

Mix the water or milk with the ground bark and simmer the mixture gently for 10 to 15 minutes. Add less bark for a thinner drink or more to thicken it to pudding consistency. Flavor it as desired with cinnamon, ginger, or raw honey.

Sugar Maple, *Acer saccharum*

The sugar maple is a surprisingly healthy tree. Many people think of sugar when they think of sugar maple and assume that the sweet syrup is unhealthy. Instead, the opposite is true and I have used maple syrup as a remedy when the sap is not available. Maples are in the Sapindaceae (Soapberry) Family.

Identification: Yellowish-green flower clusters appear in April or May, growing on umbels. The flowers produce a dry fruit called a samara that contains two seeds and paper-like wings (like a helicopter) that help dispersal. The trunk, branches and leaves produce a sweet sap, which is tapped, boiled, and concentrated to produce maple syrup.

Edible Use: Maple syrup made from the sap serves as a popular sweetener, but the sap can also be used as a drink in its raw form. The seeds are edible raw or cooked – just remove the "wings". Pieces of the inner bark can be cooked, dried, and ground into flour for thickening or mixed with grains for baking. I love the blossoms and young buds of the Big Leaf Maple (*Acer macrophyllum*) both raw and cooked. They are one of my favorite sweet spring greens where I live.

Medicinal Use: The inner bark and sap are the parts used for medicine.

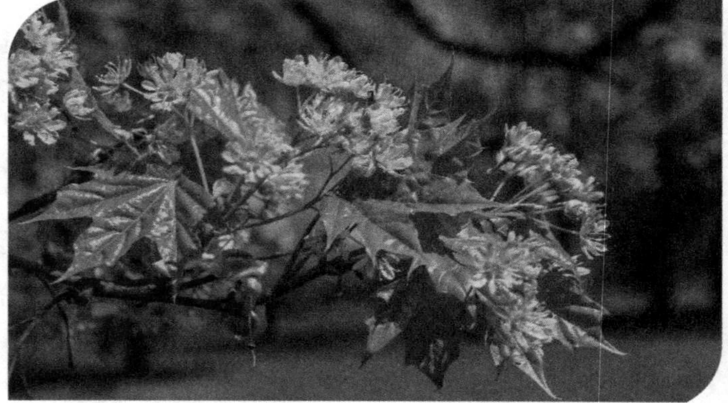

Sugar Maple Leaves, photo by Superior National Forest [CC BY 2.0]

Blood Tonic and Diuretic: A tea made from the inner bark is used as a blood tonic. It helps remove toxins from the body and cleans the blood. It also has diuretic effects so it should be taken early in the day and in moderation.

Coughs, Bronchial Congestion: Maple Bark Tea, made from the inner bark of the sugar maple, has expectorant properties. It loosens phlegm in the lungs and helps the body get rid of it. It makes the cough more productive and relieves the need for excessive coughing. In addition to the tea, maple syrup is soothing on the throat and for coughs. I use it as a base in cough syrups.

Eye Remedy: Traditionally, a compound infusion of the bark was used as an eye drop to treat blindness, though a reference for what type of blindness is not known. The sap is useful to treat sore eyes.

Osteoporosis: The sap from the sugar maple tree is rich in minerals that are necessary for bone health, including calcium, potassium, and magnesium.

Gastric Ulcers and Gastric Cancer: Gastric ulcers caused by injury to the stomach lining and infection by *Helicobacter pylori* bacteria sometimes progress to gastric cancer. Both the ulcer and cancer can be prevented by regular consumption of sugar maple sap and the sap can heal existing gastric ulcers.

Blood Pressure: The high mineral content in maple sap is beneficial for keeping blood pressure levels regulated.

Protects the Heart: Zinc, potassium, magnesium, and other minerals that are necessary for healthy heart function are present in the sap. In addition, maple sap helps control high blood pressure.

Helps Prevent Diabetes and Regulate Blood Sugar: Maple syrup and maple sap are healthy for blood sugar control. They do not raise the blood sugar as much as other sweeteners and they actually prevent type 2 diabetes when used in moderate amounts. Ascorbic acid present in the sap helps increase insulin sensitivity and stimulates the pancreas to produce more insulin.

Immune System Support: Regular use of maple sap stimulates the immune system and helps the body eliminate harmful microbes. It can also be used when fighting an infection or when exposed to infectious agents.

Acne and Skin Blemishes: Maple sap and maple syrup contain antioxidants and anti-inflammatory properties that help heal acne blemishes and prevent new ones from forming. Apply maple syrup directly to the infected blemish and leave it in place for 10 to 20 minutes. Rinse it away with lukewarm water.

Reducing Stress and Depression: Maple sap and maple syrup contain minerals and antioxidants that help the body deal with the effects of stress and calm the nervous system to reduce depression.

Fights Chronic Inflammatory and Degenerative Diseases: Inflammatory diseases such as arthritis, inflammatory bowel disease, heart disease, and many autoimmune diseases are calmed by the anti-inflammatory and antioxidant contents of maple sap. It protects the brain and body from oxidative stress, chronic inflammation, and the effects of aging.

Increases the Effects of Antibiotics: When taken with antibiotics, maple sap enhances the effects and seemingly makes the antibiotics more potent. The combination of antibiotics and maple sap works better and faster than antibiotics alone.

Harvesting Maple: The maple tree makes sugar during the summer and stores it in the tree roots in the form of starch. During the winter, the tree uses the stored sap to provide energy for the tree. We can "tap" the tree to gather that energy for ourselves. In the

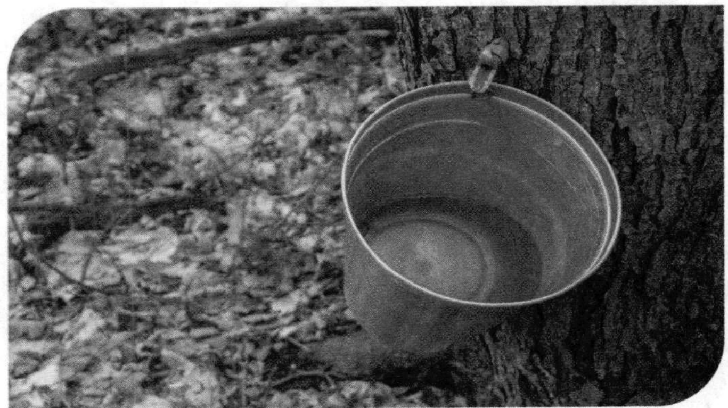

spring, drill a tap hole and insert a spout with a bucket below for catching the sap. As the weather becomes warmer the sap will flow from the tap hole into the bucket via the spout. The best time to collect the sap is from March through April. The sap can be used fresh as it is or boiled down to make syrup. It takes about 10 gallons (37 Liters) of sap to make a quart (liter) of maple syrup.

Western Red Cedar, *Thuja plicata*

Western Red Cedar is an incredibly useful and spiritual tree with a rich history as a building material. Many people value the tree for its beautiful and useful wood, and its bark for basketry, clothing, and rope. At 200 feet (60 meters) tall, there is a lot to admire in the Western Red Cedar.

I always take note when I see one. It is in the Cupressaceae (Cypress) Family. It prefers moist soil and cooler climates.

Identification: At up to 200 feet (60 meters) tall and up to 20 feet (6 meters) in diameter, this tree stands out. You probably already know if there is one in your area. It is a distinctive evergreen with a wide base, fluted trunk and gray to cinnamon-red bark. The leaves are greenish-yellow with flat, opposite scales. Branches are often J-shaped curving toward the sky. In late autumn, the tree fills with round flowers that give the tree a golden appearance, especially when the pollen is released in a thick yellow cloud. The flowers become small seed cones with 8 to 12 scales. Each cone is about 1 1/2 inches (3.75 cm) long.

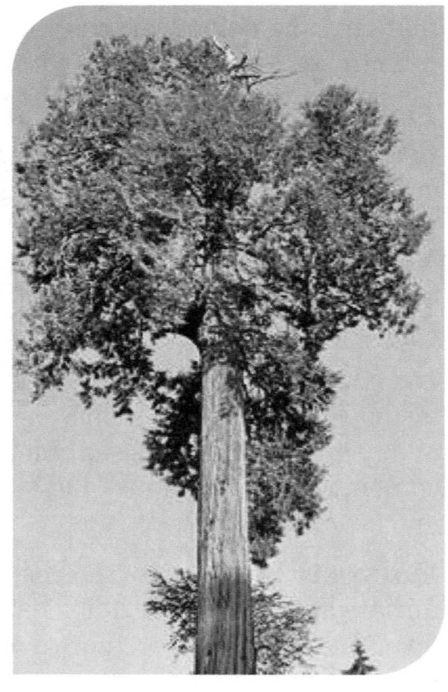
Abdallahh from Montréal, Canada

Medicinal Use: Western red cedar is an antifungal, antiviral, antibacterial, and antioxidant. It has been used for centuries by Native Americans and continues to be used today.

Treating Skin Problems: Red cedar bark is useful to treat boils, ringworm, fungal skin infections, sores, and swellings. Make the powdered bark into a paste for application directly onto an infection. You can also use dry bark powder to cauterize sores and stop bleeding. An infusion of the inner bark works as a wash to soothe irritated skin. A poultice of ground inner bark is useful for carbuncles and boils.

Healthy Tonic: Red Cedar Tea is a good medicine to support the health of the heart and body. I make tea from the bark and twigs for a good overall body tonic. Do not use if you have weak kidneys and if it causes stomach upset try a tincture instead.

Reduces Inflammation, Pain, and Swelling: A strong decoction of red cedar leaves applied directly to the skin helps relieve sore muscles and joints. For arthritis, a weak tea is prescribed several times a day until the joint pain is relieved.

Treat Dandruff: For dandruff relief, use a decoction of the twigs and leaves. It improves the scalp and stops the itching and flaking of dandruff.

Warts, Fungal & Yeast Infections, and Viral Infections of the Skin: Red cedar has strong antiviral properties that kill the virus that causes warts. Apply a leaf tincture or oil infusion 3 times a day until the wart falls off. It also treats fungal infections of the skin and nails and other viral infections of the skin. Apply Western Red Cedar Oil directly to the affected area several times a day and continue to apply it for at least a week after all symptoms are gone. Couple this with internal use as a tincture. A brew of the leaves can also be used as a douche for vaginal infections.

Foot Fungus: For foot fungus, use a salve or soak your feet in cedar tea. Make your external tea with one cup of red cedar leaves in 10 cups of boiling water. Let the tea cool until it is the right temperature for a warm soak. Place it in a basin and soak your feet for 10 to 15 minutes.

Stimulates the Immune System: Red cedar improves immune function by stimulating white blood cells to fight infection, clean up debris, and attack cancer cells.

Respiratory Infections: Respiratory infections readily respond to steam infused with red cedar bark or oil. Cedar improves the blood flow to the lungs and allows the body to take in more oxygen. Place chopped cedar leaf in your steam vaporizer and breathe the steam deeply for at least 5 minutes per sitting. Use the steam up to 5 times daily to clear the respiratory tracts.

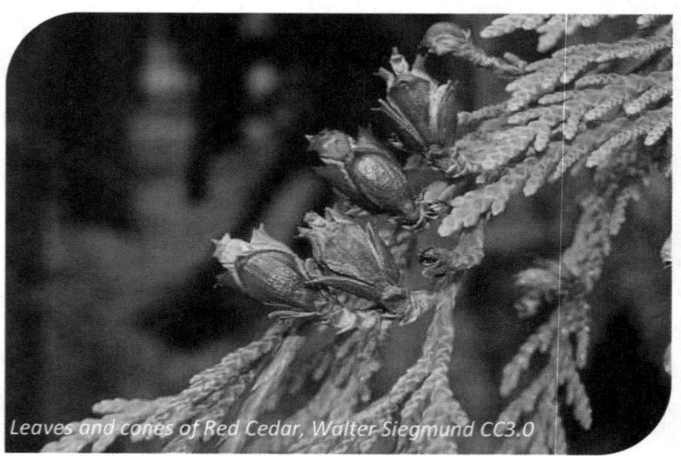
Leaves and cones of Red Cedar, Walter Siegmund CC3.0

For sinus congestion or chronic coughs, you may need to steam more often.

Harvesting: All parts of the tree are useful, including the wood, bark, roots, and leaves. The easiest parts to use medicinally are the leaves and the bark, so I concentrate on those. Gather leaves in the late summer or early fall when the oil content is highest, or as needed throughout the year. Prune off small branches until you have the desired amount. Use them fresh or dry them for future use. Crush just before use to release the oils.

Warning: Red cedar is strong medicine and should be used in moderation and carefully. Do not use red cedar in any form if you may be pregnant. It stimulates uterine contractions and could cause miscarriage. Some people are allergic to red cedar. Skin irritations can be severe. Test the oil on a very small patch of skin and check it for a few days before using it on a larger area. Use red cedar in low doses and for short periods of time. Do not use red cedar if you have weak kidneys.

Recipes. Western Red Cedar Oil: Ingredients: fresh cedar leaves, finely chopped, carrier oil such as organic olive oil or coconut oil. Finely chop fresh cedar leaves and place them in the top of a double boiler. Fill the lower pot with water so that the water doesn't touch the bottom of the top pot. Cover the leaves with olive oil or other carrier oil. Gently heat the oil so that it gets warm, but do not boil. Turn the pot on and off throughout the day to keep the oil warm without excess heat.

Check and refill the water level in the bottom pot throughout the day. Heat the oil gently, turning it on and off for a week or until the oil is dark green and has a strong cedar odor. Strain the cedar oil through cheesecloth and squeeze the cloth to remove as much oil as possible. Label and date the oil and store it in a cool, dark place.

Western Red Cedar Tea: Ingredients: 1 tablespoon fresh or dried cedar tea leaves, chopped, 1 cup cold water. Put the chopped cedar leaves into the cold water and cover. Allow it to steep several hours or overnight. Drink ¼ to ½ cup, twice a day. Store the remaining tea in the refrigerator.

White Pine, *Pinus strobus*

Pinus strobus belongs to the Pinaceae (Pine) Family. It is also known as the eastern white pine, northern white pine, white pine, and soft pine. The Native American Haudenosaunee tribe called it the Tree of Peace. It is a large pine native to Eastern North America.

Identification: The white pine is a very large conifer and reaches over 150 feet (45.7 meters) in height and nearly up to 40 inches (100 cm) in diameter. The trees have tall, cylindrical stems with pyramidal-shaped crowns, characterized by distinctive, plate-like branching that is especially noticeable as the trees become older. On young growth, the bark of white pine remains rather thin, smooth, and greenish-brown in color. On older trees, the bark becomes dark grayish-brown in color and deeply fissured. The evergreen leaves or needles of white pine are in bundles of 5, soft and flexible, 2.5 to 5 inches (6.25 cm to 12.5 cm) long, and are usually bluish-green in appearance. The cones of this plant are nearly 4 to 8 inches (10 cm to 20 cm) long and about 1 inch (2.5 cm) thick. They can remain attached for several months after ripening in the autumn of the second season. The small seeds are dispersed by the wind when the cones open.

Edible Use: The flowers, inner bark, and seeds are all edible. It is used as a condiment and tea. The dried inner bark can be ground to make a flour. The flour can be used in baking and as a thickener.

Medicinal Use: The inner bark, needles, and sap/pitch are used for medicine. The inner bark is the most valuable because of its high tannin content and other medicinal qualities.

Wounds, Skin Infections, and Swelling: Externally white pine is a very useful treatment for various skin issues like wounds, sores, burns, boils, etc. It is used as a poultice, herbal steam bath, and by putting the sap/pitch directly on a wound. A poultice or plaster

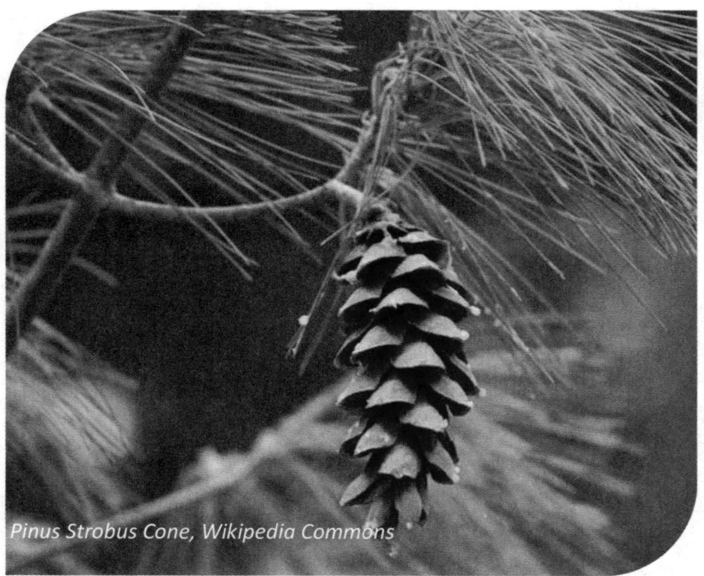
Pinus Strobus Cone, Wikipedia Commons

is easily made by soaking a piece of inner bark in water and applying it to the wound, or an inner bark decoction can be used as a wash to clean and treat wounds. For infected wounds, use both. The tannins are astringent, drawing out the infection and helping the wound heal. A poultice of the sap/pitch has proven to be effective in drawing out toxins and reducing pain.

Respiratory Tract Issues, Mucous, Wet Coughs, Expectorant: The inner bark contains mucilage and other compounds that relax the mucous membranes and the openings of the respiratory tract. It also helps reduce phlegm so that the body can expel it. If you are seriously congested, add white pine bark to a steam bath and breathe in the steam. It helps relieve congestion allowing you to breathe easier. Often used in combination with other herbs. Do not use for dry coughs.

Arthritis and Joint Pain: White pine pitch/sap is an effective remedy for arthritis and sore joints. Boil the resin in water to make an internal dose and mix the resin with oil or fat to use externally. This mixture is also good for treating and preventing infections.

Worms: Tapeworms, flatworms, and roundworms are supposedly killed and expelled from the body with a mixture of pine tar and beer. I have never used this (I use more common parasite remedies) but it sure sounds like a fun cure!

Colds and Flu: White pine needle and bark tea is used as a preventative and remedy for the cold and flu. Best to combine with blue elderberry. It also gives a good dose of Vitamins A and C.

Sore Throats: Treat sore throats with a tea made from the young needles.

Harvesting the Seeds and Inner Bark: Eastern white pine has a fruit that is a large elongated cone. Harvest the fruit in the autumn as the scales in the cone begin to open, but before the small winged seeds have been shed. If you allow the cones to dry, the scales will open and shed the seeds. For a small quantity of white pine seeds, the cone scales can be pulled apart to retrieve the seeds. Store in a dry place in an airtight container in the refrigerator.

Collect the inner bark in the spring when new growth is occurring. Choose a young branch, about 2 to 3 years old. Remove the branch from the tree and peel off the bark. Peel off the outer bark and dry the inner bark for future use.

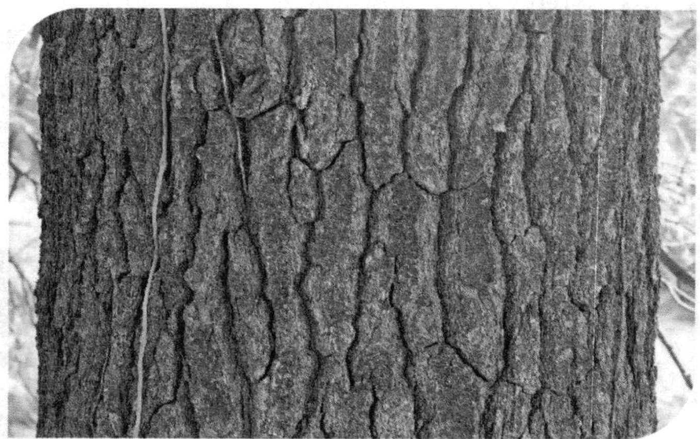
White Pine Bark, Derek Ramsey, CC by SA 4.0

To Extract Pine Resin: The resin extracted from pine can be used as water-proofing and building fires, as well as for medicinal use. The resin is a powerful antibiotic. Look for where the tree has been injured or simply collect some that has dripped down, making sure you leave plenty for the tree. If you are in an area you go to often you may "wound" the tree and return to collect the pitch later. Ask first.

White Sage, *Salvia apiana*

White sage, also known as sacred sage or bee sage, is an evergreen perennial shrub found in the southwestern United States. It is in the *Lamiaceae* (Mint) Family.

Identification: This shrub grows to between 4 and 5 feet tall and about 4 feet (1.2 meters) wide. The whitish leaves release oils and resins when rubbed, giving them a strong scent. White to pale lavender flowers appear in the spring and bloom through the summer. They grow on many 3 to 4-foot flower stalks that are sometimes pinkish in color. The flower petals pucker back and the stamens dangle on the sides.

Edible Use: The pounded seeds of white sage are used to supplement flour. The leaves and stems are also edible.

Medicinal Use: White Sage Infusion is good for coughs and colds. The seeds are used medicinally to cleanse the eyes.

Childbirth: The root tea of white sage is said to give strength and healing during childbirth. The herb is avoided during pregnancy, then consumed when the time for delivery is at hand.

Coughs and Colds: White Sage Infusion made from the leaves of the plant is good for treating cold and coughs. It has antibacterial qualities that speed healing. Use the leaves in a steam bath to release mucus and open up congested airways.

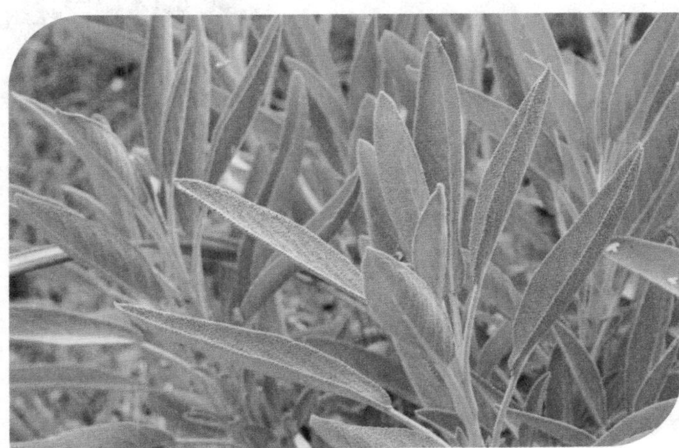

Cleaning the Body and Home: White sage leaves are used as a form of hair shampoo and for cleansing. The leaves are crushed in water and then rubbed into the hair and body. To clean a house or space of negative energy, purify the area by burning a white sage leaf smudge in the space.

White Willow, *Salix alba*

White willow is a deciduous tree that grows to 90 feet (27 meters) tall. It grows in moist areas like riverbanks and low-lying areas. It is native to Europe and Asia. Most willows can be used interchangeably for medicine. It is in the Salicaceae (Willow) Family.

Identification: The branches are pliable and lean downward, and the trunk often leans as well. The pliable and leaning branches give this tree a graceful appearance with flashes of green and white. Willow is often used for basketry. The leaves are lance-shaped and pale green. They are covered in white hairs on the top and bottom of the leaf. The undersides of the leaves are white, giving the tree its name. Leaves are 2 to 4 inches (5 cm to 10 cm) long and approximately 1/2 inch (1.25 cm) wide.

Flowers grow on catkins in the early spring, producing male and female catkins on separate trees. Male catkins are 1 ½ to 2 inches (3.75 cm to 5 cm) long and

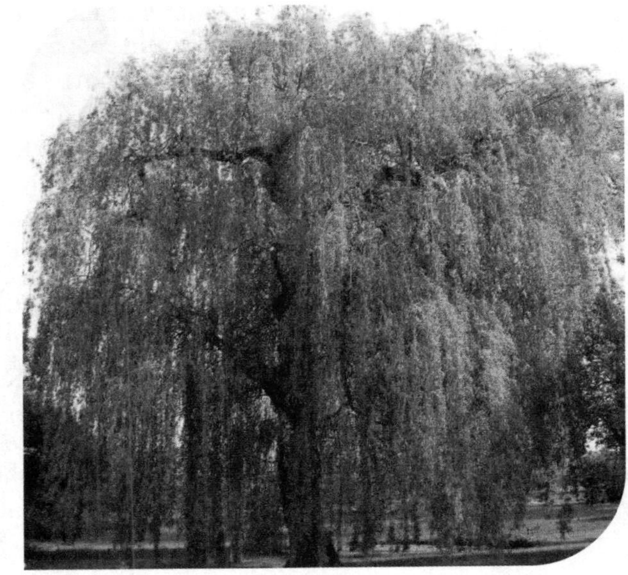

White Willow, MPF, CC by SA 3.0

female catkins are a little shorter. In mid-summer, the female catkins produce small capsules containing minute seeds covered in white down. The tree bark is green-brown to grey-brown.

Medicinal Use: The bark and dried leaves are used for medicinal purposes.

Headaches, Fevers, Joint Pain, and Arthritis: White willow bark has aspirin-like compounds that relieve pain and reduce fevers.

White Willow Bark Tea works well for pain and fever relief, as does chewing on the tip of a willow branch. Unlike aspirin, it doesn't cause gastric damage.

Menopause and Menstrual Symptoms: White Willow Bark Tea helps symptoms of menopause and menstruation, including night sweats, hot flashes, cramping, and headaches.

Digestive Problems: White Willow Bark Tea is taken after meals to relieve indigestion. The tea enhances the digestive process.

Warning: Do not use white willow in children suffering from low-grade fevers. Do not take white willow if you are allergic to aspirin. Do not use long-term.

Recipes. White Willow Bark Tea: 1 to 2 grams white willow tree bark, 1 cup water. Simmer the tree bark and water together for about 10 minutes. Cool, strain, and drink warm or cold.

Wild Rose, *Rosa* spp.

There are many varieties of wild rose. All have similar healing properties. Garden varieties of roses have some of the medicinal benefits of wild varieties but have lost some from hybridization. Wild varieties have strongly fragrant petals and high medicinal content. If necessary, use whatever rose varieties you have available, but the most fragrant have the highest medicinal activity. They are in the Rosaceae (Rose) Family.

Identification: Unlike most garden roses, wild roses have only 5 petals, but many stamens. The flowers are a beautiful pink and its compound leaves are alternate with 5 to 9 toothed leaflets. It has thorns that are wide at the base. The fruit, called hips, are orange to red with attached sepal lobes and have a pear-like shape. It grows in open, dry or moist locations, including woodlands, in low to middle elevations and may form dense thickets.

Edible Use: Roses are well appreciated for their edible use. Rose syrups, jams, and flavoring agents are very popular. Rose hips are nutritious with a tangy, fruity flavor similar to cranberry. Crushed rose hips make an excellent Rose Hip Tea. Note that the seed hairs can be irritating both on the way in and on the way out. The petals are beautiful and tasty in fresh salads.

Medicinal Use: Roses are antiseptic, anti-inflammatory, anti-oxidant, antiviral, digestive, nervine,

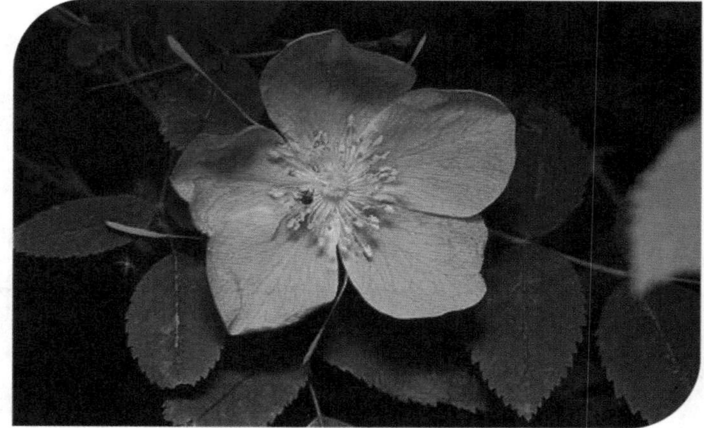

Wild Rose, Rosa acicularis, by Walter Siegmund [CC BY-SA 3.0

sedative, vulnerary (wound-healing), and a rich source of vitamins, especially vitamin C.

Cold and Flu Remedy: Roses support the immune system to help people recover quickly from cold and flu symptoms.

Use Rose Petal Tea with 1 or 2 teaspoons of added raw honey and a squeeze of lemon for coughs, colds, and the flu. Infusing rosehips along with elderberries in brandy makes a great cold tonic, and is one I use at home.

Asthma and Bronchial Infections: Rose petals and hips act as a fever reducer and anti-spasmodic, relieving the bronchial spasms of coughs and asthma and the muscle cramping and aches that often result. The antibacterial and antiviral properties help cure the underlying causes of colds and flu. Rose Petal Tea or Rose Hip Tea help treat bronchial infections and congestion.

Relieves Menstrual Problems: Rose petals, hips, and leaves relieve menstrual congestion and pain while supporting reproductive health.

Use rose petals to help regulate menstruation and bring on delayed menstrual cycles. They are also a good uterine tonic for healing infections, bleeding, and cysts. They soothe and calm the nervous system, easing the tension and pain of PMS and uterine cramping.

Tonic: Rose petals and rose hips are high in vitamin C and also contain vitamins A, B-3, D, and E, along with various minerals, anti-oxidants, and pectin. They are a natural mild diuretic and laxative. These properties and nutrients help the body remove toxins, excess fluids, and drain the lymph nodes.

Lifts the Mood: Roses have a very soothing effect on the nerves and lift depression. Use rose water, rose oil, or rose tincture, along with infusions from the petals and hips.

Promotes Circulation: Rose Petal Tea promotes blood circulation and reduces swelling in the capillaries just beneath the skin. Drink the tea and apply rose water to the skin as needed.

Supports the Liver and Gall Bladder: Rose petals increase the production of bile, which helps the body eliminate toxins. It supports the liver and gall bladder and helps in detoxification. Drink Rose Petal Tea as needed.

Treatment for the Skin: Rose petals are antiseptic, anti-inflammatory, and antiviral. They are an excellent treatment for wounds, bruises, incisions, and skin rashes. Wash the area with rose water or Rose Petal Tea and make a poultice of bruised rose petals to apply directly to the affected area.

Eye Wash: Rose water is soothing and cooling to the eyes and can be used to treat eye infections and irritations. Make sterile rose water from chlorine-free water for use as an eye wash.

Ulcers, Bacterial Infections of the Stomach, Colon, or Urinary Tract: Rose Oil made with a suitable carrier oil is used to treat bacterial infections of the internal organs. Its anti-inflammatory

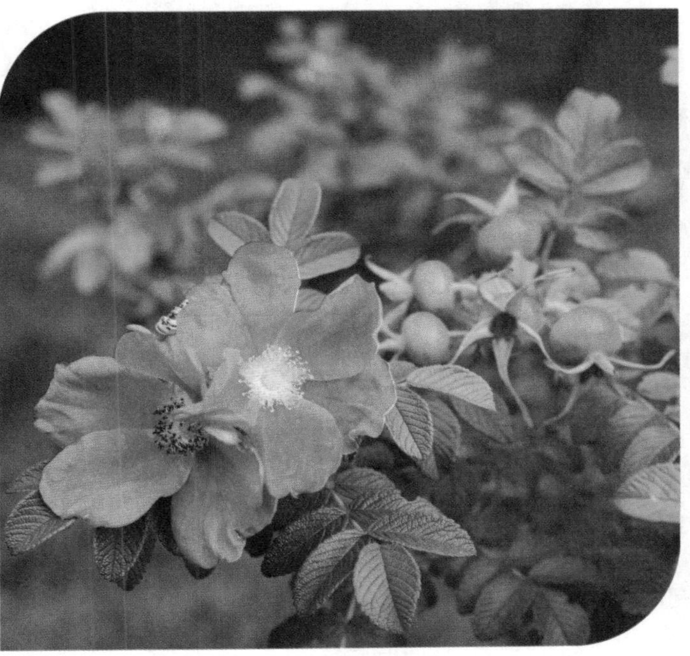

and antiseptic properties make it valuable for these purposes. Rose hips are a good treatment for diarrhea.

Harvesting: The best time to harvest wild rose petals is in the morning while the dew is still on the roses. During the spring and early summer, when they have just opened, pick up to 1/3 the petals from each plant. Leave the stamen and hips on the plant. This way the bees will pollinate the flowers and the rose hips will mature for harvesting later. Harvest the rose hips in the autumn when they are fully mature and ripe. Rose leaves can be gathered in spring through early fall. Do not harvest rose petals, hips, or leaves from plants that are near the road or that have been sprayed.

Recipes. Rose Petal Tea. Ingredients: 2 to 4 teaspoons dried, crushed rose petals or 3 to 4 tablespoons fresh and 1 cup boiling water. Cover the rose petals with boiling water and infuse for 10 to 15 minutes. Take as needed.

Rose Oil: There are several ways to make rose oil, but I like this one for its simplicity. You will need freshly picked rose petals, organic olive or almond oil, ¼ teaspoon vitamin E, and a wide mouth glass jar with a tight-fitting lid. Fill a sterile wide-mouth jar with rose petals. Pack them in to completely fill the jar.

Cover the petals with a good quality oil. Run a spatula around the inside edge and stir slightly to remove any trapped air. Cover the jar with the lid and allow the oil to steep for 2 weeks, shaking daily. Strain the oil though cheesecloth to remove the petals. Pack the jar again with fresh rose petals and return the oil to the jar to repeat the process. After the second steeping, strain the oil and add a 1/4 teaspoon of natural vitamin E as a preservative. The oil should have a mild rose fragrance. Store the oil in a cool, dark place and use it alone or to make ointments, balms, and salves.

Rose Water: You'll need fresh rose petals, spring water to cover, and a glass jar with a tight-fitting lid. Fill a saucepan with rose petals and cover with water. Bring the water to a simmer over low heat. Simmer for 5 minutes. Allow the rose water to cool naturally, then strain out the petals, squeezing to remove all moisture. Pour the rosewater into a glass jar and store in the refrigerator.

Witch Hazel, *Hamamelis virginiana*

Witch hazel is such a welcome sight in the winter, as its bright yellow flowers appear in the late fall, and often until early spring. *Hamamelis virginiana* is a tall shrub or a small tree, which is usually 20 to 30 feet (6 meters) high and spread as wide. It is native to Eastern North America and is in the Hamamelidaceae (Witch Hazel) Family.

Identification: It is quite easy to identify witch hazel because of its unique canopy-like shape and its elongated, 3 to 6-inch-long (7.5 cm to 15 cm) alternate leaf with a dark green upper layer and a pale-green lower surface. Leaves have coarsely toothed margins. My favorite way is to look for the plant is to hunt in the dead of winter. It is usually the only tree blooming. Mark the location and come back whenever you like.

The plant grows with multiple trunks and forms a disorganized cluster. It has bright yellow flower with strap-like petals and becomes leggy when it does not

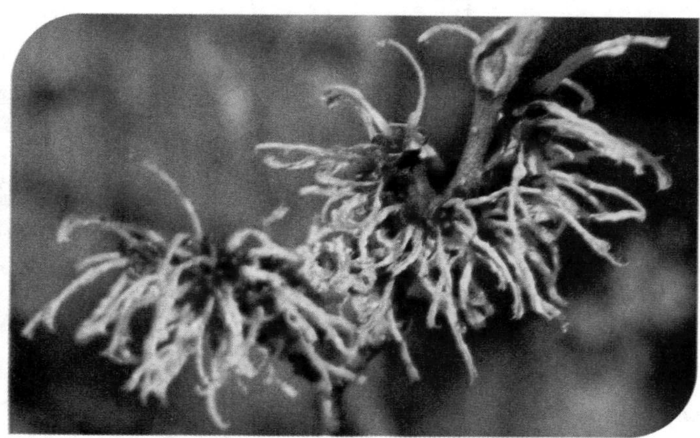

Witch Hazel Flowers, Wikipedia Commons

get enough sunshine. The bark and twigs are usually light brown and gray, depending on the habitat. The

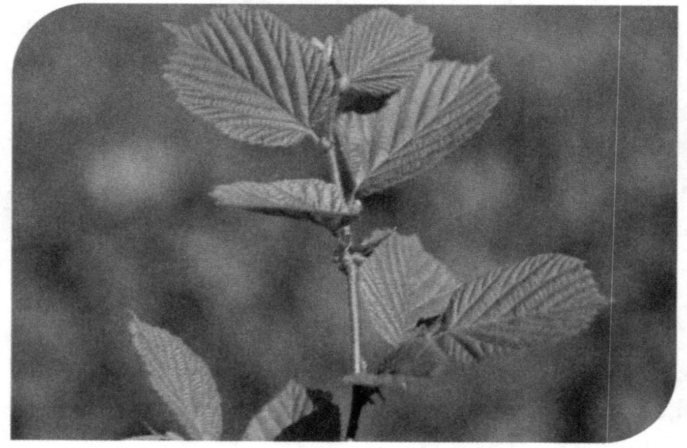

bark develops rough patches and becomes scaly as the tree ages.

Edible Use: The capsule-like fruit of the witch hazel tree can be opened to expose the edible nutty seed.

Medicinal Use: Skin Care: For cosmetics and skin/personal care products, Witch Hazel Astringent, made from the bark of the tree, works as a skin conditioning agent that is used as a toner on dry and damaged skin to restore the suppleness of the skin. It reduces inflammation and irritation and soothes the skin.

Sore Muscles: Applying witch hazel to sore muscles relieves pain and inflammation. You can also boil the bark in water use it in a sauna or steam bath. Add pieces of bark or small twigs onto hot rocks for a relaxing and soothing steam bath.

Colds and Coughs: Witch hazel bark is a tannin-containing astringent. It tightens the tissues and reduces mucous and inflammation from a cold or flu. It soothes inflamed airways and reduces swelling. Warm (not hot) witch hazel tea can be applied as a compress for respiratory illnesses, including coughs, colds, and even asthma. Place the compress on the chest and throat and breathe in the vapors.

Stop Bleeding from Wounds: Apply witch hazel astringent to bleeding wounds to tighten the tissues and stop the bleeding. For large wounds, soak a cloth in Witch Hazel Astringent or Witch Hazel Tea and cover the wound.

Hemorrhoids and Other Itching: Witch Hazel Astringent reduces the swelling of hemorrhoids and soothes the itching caused by hemorrhoids and other skin irritations. To use Witch Hazel Astringent for hemorrhoids, soak a soft cloth or cotton pad in the astringent and use it as a poultice. Replace as needed.

Other Uses: Some people are able to use a forked witch hazel branch as a divining rod to find water underground. The diviner holds each end of the Y-shaped branch, using the tail to point to water. When the ends are held gently, the divining end points downward to indicate when water is below

Harvesting: Removing the bark from a witch hazel tree will kill the tree, so it is important only to collect branches that have fallen or to prune a branch carefully, using sanitized tools. Do not remove bark from the trunks or main branches.

Recipes. Witch Hazel Astringent: This witch hazel astringent is much stronger than the store-bought variety. It contains concentrated tannins and is for external use only. Best used without alcohol but it can be added for preservation. Collect 1 pound of fresh twigs as soon as the tree has flowered. The tonic properties are strongest immediately after flowering. Remove leaves and flowers. Chop the twigs into small pieces. Place the chopped twigs into an extra-large stainless steel or enamel pot. Cover the twigs with one gallon (4 Liters) of distilled water and bring to a boil. Reduce the heat, cover the pot, and simmer the water for at least 6 hours, adding water as needed to keep the twigs covered. You can use a crockpot on medium or high for this step if you have one. Allow the mixture to cool, then strain the mixture to remove the twigs. Keep the witch hazel refrigerated and use within a few weeks. Yields one gallon (4 Liters). For longer-term storage, add 8 ounces (250ml) of vodka or grain alcohol to 16 (500ml) ounces of tonic.

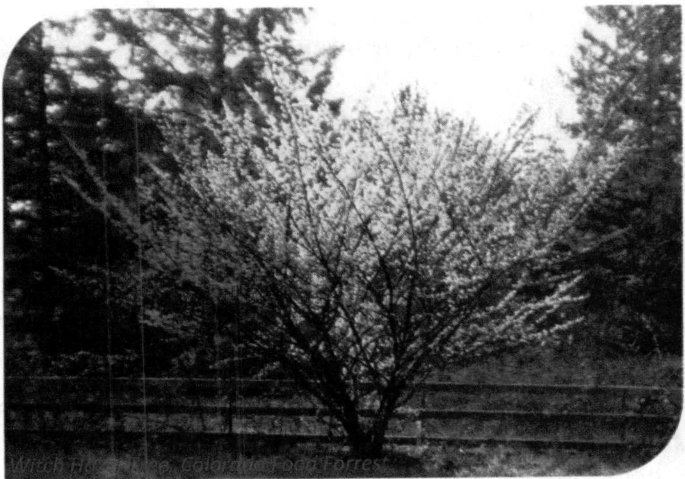

Mushrooms and Lichens

A note on extracting mushrooms and lichens:
Many lichens and mushrooms need to be double/dual-extracted both in water and in alcohol in order to access all of the necessary medicinal compounds. For example, in Reishi (*Ganoderma lucidum*), the main components with pharmacological activity are polysaccharides and triterpenoids. The polysaccharides (including beta-glucans) extract in water while the triterpenoids, like ganoderic acid, extract in alcohol. Below is a recipe for a double-extraction.

Double/Dual Extraction Method:
Feel free to scale down this recipe for at-home use. You'll need: 8 ounces (225g) or more of dried mushroom or lichen, 24 ounces (650g) of 80 to 100 proof alcohol (40 to 50 % alcohol), and 16 ounces (500ml) of distilled water.

1. Fill a quart-sized (32 oz – 900g) canning jar half-full with diced dried mushrooms, then fill it to ½ inch (1.25cm) of the top with alcohol. Stir and cap it, shaking it every few days for 2 months. Then strain out the alcohol and set it aside to keep.
2. Make the decoction. Put 16 ounces (0.5L) of water into a ceramic or glass pot with a lid and put the mushrooms into it. Cover and simmer the mixture on low until half of the water has simmered off. This will take a few hours. If the water level drops too quickly, add more so that you can continue simmering your mushrooms. The end result should be 8 ounces (250ml) of your decoction. Do not boil.
3. Allow the water to cool, and then strain out the mushrooms, pressing them to remove all of the liquid. Mix this water (8 oz –250 ml) and the alcoholic tincture you have set aside (you should have about 24 oz – 0.75L of alcohol tincture) together to create the finished double-extraction. It has a high enough alcohol content (30%) that it should be shelf-stable for many years, as long as it is stored in a sealed container. The ratio of the alcoholic tincture to the decoction is 3:1.

Chaga Mushroom, *Inonotus obliquus*

Chaga mushroom, also known as cancer polypore and tinder conk, grows on live birch trees in temperate zones throughout the Northern Hemisphere. It looks like charcoal bursting from the tree. It grows in the form of a woody conk.

The fungus grows slowly; only harvest from large growths and leave plenty on the tree.

It is a valuable mushroom for use in treating cancer and for immune system problems. It is also an excellent firestarter.

Identification: Chaga grows almost exclusively on live birch trees. Tree burls are often mistaken for chaga mushrooms. The burl is an outgrowth of the tree, while the chaga mushroom grows inside the tree then bursts forth from it.

There is a distinct difference between the mushroom and the tree. The outside surface of the fungus is black, brittle, and has a cracked appearance. The interior is gold-orange, and woody. The gold-orange interior is sometimes visible where the mushroom attaches to the tree. It feels like cork when freshly cut.

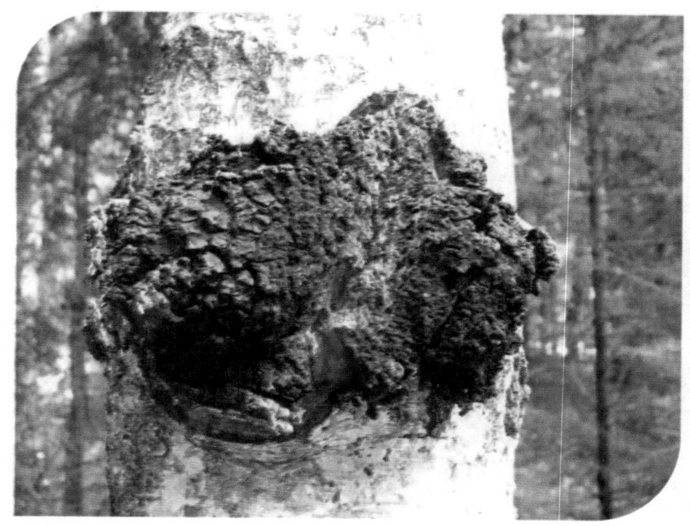

Medicinal Use: Chaga must be collected from birch trees, as the relationship between the birch and the parasitic chaga helps form some of the medicinal compounds found in chaga, like the terpenes betulin and betulinic acid. Chaga is best taken as a double-extracted tincture to access all of its medicinal compounds (see page 39 or page 268 for the recipe).

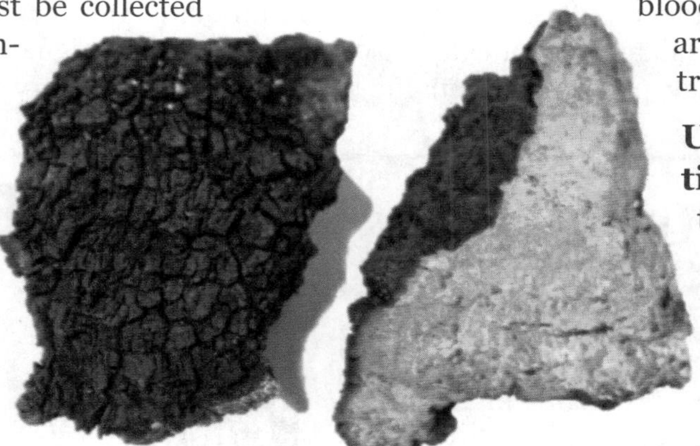

Cancer Treatment: Chaga mushrooms treat cancers of all types, including Hodgkin's Disease. Chaga helps prevent and treat cancer through increased antioxidant activity, by slowing or stopping the growth of the cancerous tissue and metastasis to other parts of the body, by killing off existing cancerous cells and reducing tumors, through boosting the immune system, and by helping eliminate cancer cells from the body.

Powerful Adaptogen: Adaptogens help the body adapt to changing conditions, increased work, and stress in general. Chaga is a powerful adaptogen that helps reduce the effects of these stressors on the body and improves overall body health. Chaga also has antioxidant, anti-inflammatory, and anti-viral properties.

Boosts the Immune System and Anti-inflammatory: Chaga mushroom stimulates the immune system and helps the body heal itself. It has anti-inflammatory and antioxidant properties that reduce chronic inflammation in the body and help prevent further damage. It is valuable for patients with immune system dysfunction and weak immune systems, but it is still unclear if people with autoimmune disorders should use it due to the way it boosts the immune system. Until more research is done, best to use the adaptogenic Reishi mushroom instead.

Anti-Viral, HIV, Herpes, and Flu: Chaga is an excellent anti-viral. It has demonstrated efficacy against Influenza A and B, HSV (Herpes Simplex Virus), and inhibits HIV protease.

Reduces the Blood Sugar: Chaga helps lower blood sugar levels significantly and quickly. This can be helpful for people with diabetes, but it can also cause problems. Monitor blood sugars carefully when taking chaga, especially if you have had problems with blood sugars in the past or if you are taking medications to control blood sugar levels.

Ulcers, Ulcerative Colitis, and the Gastrointestinal Tract: Chaga protects the gastrointestinal tract and stops the formation of ulcers. Its anti-inflammatory effects work well for people with ulcerative colitis.

Protects the Liver and Hepatitis C: Because of its anti-inflammatory and anti-oxidant properties, chaga is beneficial for most body organs, however it is especially protective of the liver. It helps the body get rid of toxins, prevents hardening and scarring in the liver, and inhibits the production of chemicals that cause inflammation in the liver.

It is also effective against Hepatitis C. One of the ways chaga boosts the immune system is by protecting the liver and activating the white blood cells to destroy foreign substances in the body.

Reduces Fatigue and Increases Physical Endurance: Chaga helps reduce fatigue in people who have low energy levels. It may also boost endurance by lowering lactic acid levels and boosting glycogen stores.

Harvesting: The chaga mushroom takes a long time to grow to maturity, so only harvest large mushrooms (it grows up to 16 inches (40 cm) in size). Do not harvest any mushroom that is less than 6 inches (15 cm) across and always leave enough of the mushroom on the tree to cover the opening on the tree where the chaga is growing.

Take care not to damage the birch tree when collecting chaga and only harvest from living trees in a very environmentally clean area. It may be collected year-round, but it is more potent in the autumn. Using a saw or hatchet, remove the mushroom from the tree and break it into small pieces to dry.

Make sure that there are no tree parts still attached to the mushroom. If you find tree bark or wood, cut it away before drying. Use a dehydrator on its lowest setting, or dry them in a warm, dry place in your house. Store in a sealed container placed in a cool, dry place.

Chaga mushrooms must be taken with care for long term use. They are high in oxalates, which can cause kidney stones or other kidney problems when they accumulate. They can also inhibit absorption of some nutrients. Very high doses may be toxic but it is generally considered a very safe herb.

Lion's Mane Mushroom, *Hericium erinaceus*

Lion's Mane is a popular food and medicine throughout Asia. It is also called bearded tooth mushroom, bearded hedgehog mushroom, bearded tooth fungus, and pom pom mushroom. Its strengths lie in healing the brain and nervous system, but it has many other useful benefits. It is a powerful antioxidant and anti-inflammatory.

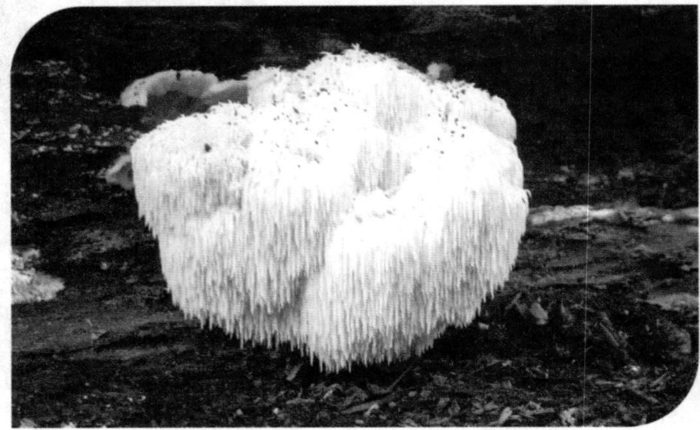

Identification: Look for lion's mane mushrooms around the middle of August through the autumn. They grow on dead and wounded hardwood trees of all kinds, but they prefer beech, oak, and maple trees. These fungi look like a clump of white icicles flowing downward to a point. Each spine is about ½ inch to 2 inches (1.25 cm to 5 cm) long and is soft and pliable. The spines and spores are white, with the spines turning yellowish to light pink as they mature. There are a few mushrooms that are similar to lion's mane in looks. They are all related and considered edible. One identifying characteristic of the lion's mane mushroom is the downward growing spines. Coral fungi is similar, but its teeth point upward. You should be careful of your identification when harvesting any wild mushrooms. Always consult a mushroom expert when you are unsure.

Edible Use: Lion's mane mushrooms are edible and tasty. The flavor and texture is like crab or lobster. The mushrooms can be eaten cooked, or dried and steeped into a tea.

Medicinal Use: I use Lion's mane daily as a double-extracted tincture. It can also be taken as a tea or in powdered form. It seems to work best with regular use.

Enhances Brain Function and Memory, Dementia, Alzheimer's, MS: Lion's mane mushrooms are known for their ability to enhance memory, stimulate cognitive function, prevent and treat neurodegenerative diseases, and encourage regrowth and recovery of nerve function. It slows down and is said to even reverse cell degeneration in the brain, which is important in diseases like Alzheimer's, Dementia, Parkinson's, Multiple Sclerosis and Diabetes, where nerve damage is a primary or secondary symptom of the disease. It also increases acetylcholine and choline acetyltransferase, which are severely depleted in Alzheimer's patients and necessary for nerve cell communication.

Heals the Nervous System, Stimulates Nerve Growth Factor: The nervous system is important to every bodily function and causes major problems when damaged. Lion's mane mushrooms can speed recovery to damaged nervous system tissue in the brain and spinal cord, and stimulate the repair of damaged nerve cells. Lion's mane has been shown to stimulate Nerve Growth Factor (NGF), which is important in the repair of the myelin sheath. Studies show great potential for myelination and regeneration of nerves. I feel so strongly about the regenerative properties of lion's mane on the nervous systems that I use it every day for Multiple Sclerosis.

Protects Against Cancer: Lion's mane has had good results in treating lung cancer, stomach cancer, esophageal cancer, liver cancer, leukemia, cervical cancer, stomach cancer, skin cancer, colon cancer, and breast cancer. I imagine it will be proven to be effective in treating other cancers as well. It stimulates the immune system and helps kill off cancer cells, controls tumor growth, and prevents cancer from spreading to other parts of the body.

Supports a Healthy Heart and Improved Circulation: Lion's mane mushrooms support the heart and circulatory system in many ways. It has been shown to lower LDL (bad) cholesterol and blood triglycerides, improve fat metabolism, and prevent blood clots, reducing the of risk heart attack or stroke. It also increases blood oxygenation and circulation.

Improves Digestive Health, Ulcers, and Leaky Gut: Lion's mane mushrooms are beneficial to the function of the digestive tract and aid leaky gut repair. It is used it to treat gastric ulcers, gastritis, inflammatory bowel disease, Crohn's disease, and colitis. Its anti-inflammatory effects provide most of the benefits, but the mushroom also soothes the gut and encourages a healthy gut environment. It also reduces intestinal bleeding and protects against H. pylori.

Reduces Inflammation and Oxidation, Autoimmune Diseases: Lion's mane is a powerful anti-inflammatory, which is useful in the prevention of most chronic disease, including heart disease, diabetes, autoimmune diseases, and cancer. It is also an antioxidant, reducing or preventing oxidative stress on the body. Chronic inflammation and oxidation are the cause of most symptoms of aging and the root cause of many diseases.

Anxiety, Stress, Depression, and Mental Health Issues: Lion's mane mushrooms are useful in improving a number of mental health issues, including insomnia, anxiety, depression, and slowing the progression of dementia. The mushrooms help regenerate brain cells and improve brain function. It is excellent for stress and anxiety, and helps with their symptoms, such as heart palpitations, irritation, and concentration.

Enhances the Intestinal Immune System: Lion's mane mushrooms enhance the function of the intestinal immune system, helping the body fight infection from bacteria, viruses, yeast, and fungi. It is especially beneficial in helping prevent infections.

Diabetes and Neuropathy: Lion's mane mushrooms have a variety of effects that are beneficial to diabetics. With consistent use, it lowers blood glucose levels and improves insulin sensitivity in type 2 diabetics. In lowering blood sugar levels, it helps prevent complications from kidney disease, eye damage, and nerve damage in the hands and feet. It also helps relieve the pain of diabetic neuropathy.

Strokes, Concussions, and Brain Injuries: Lion's mane is used to prevent strokes and after a stroke-related injury. Due to its neuroprotective effects it can help the nervous system deal with lack of oxygen, blood clots, memory issues, and more. Using it post-concussion makes sense since it is such an excellent healer for the brain and is a powerful anti-inflammatory.

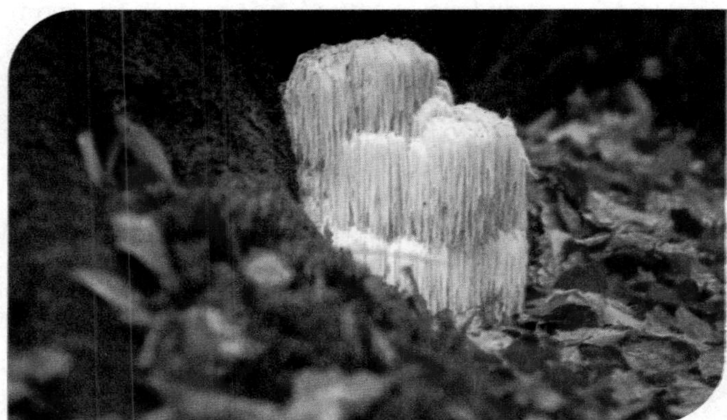

Increases Energy, Relieves Fatigue, and Enhances Athletic Performance: Lion's mane mushrooms are a rich source of antioxidants. They reduce lactic acid buildup in the blood, increase blood oxygen levels and reduce muscle fatigue. They also increase glycogen in tissues, providing a source of ready and sustainable energy for the body.

Harvesting: Harvest in late summer and autumn. Look for large mushrooms with multiple white spines hanging downward. If they have begun to turn pink, they are too mature and will not have good flavor if you are eating them. Cut the mushroom from the tree with a sharp knife, avoiding cutting into the wood of the tree. Leave some behind to establish a new crop for next year. Handle them gently.

Warning: Some people are allergic to mushrooms and thus should avoid lion's mane mushrooms as well. Symptoms of allergies can include skin rashes and difficulty breathing or even anaphylactic shock. If you have any burning, itching, swollen lips, or breathing difficulties, consult a doctor immediately.

Recipes. Lion's Mane Tea: Ingredients: ½ to 1 teaspoon Lion's mane powder, 1 cup water. Bring the water to a boil and turn off the heat. Put the lion's mane powder into an infuser or directly into the mug. Pour the hot water over the mushroom and allow the tea to steep for 10 minutes.

Lungwort Lichen, *Lobaria pulmonaria*

Lungwort lichen is a lobed lichen with leaf-like structures that resemble the human lung. It is known for its use in lung diseases but has many other uses. Lungwort lichen grows in old growth humid forests on conifers and hardwood trees. In its habitat, it is quite common to find the lichen hanging from trees and rocks. All lichens are organisms that were formed via symbiosis. Lungwort is actually a mutualistic relationship between three different organisms. It consists of an ascomycete fungus, a green alga, and a cyanobacterium. (Note this is different that the Common Lungwort plant, also in this book).

Identification: Lungwort lichen is large lichen with leaf-like lobed structures that measure 2 to 6 inches (5 cm to 7.5 cm) in length. The top of the lichen is bright green, while the underside is pale with dark pockets. It is leathery in texture with a pattern of ridges and creases on the surface. Its thallus is loosely attached to the growing surface. Lungwort turns brown when dried.

Medicinal Use: The leaf-like thallus is harvested and dried for medicine. I use it in its double-extracted, tinctured form (page 39 or page 268).

Respiratory Conditions, Asthma, Bronchitis, Whooping Cough, Tuberculosis, and Laryngitis: Lungwort lichen is mostly used to treat respiratory issues such as asthma, bronchitis, whooping cough, and tuberculosis. It is a natural antibiotic, and is ideal for treating bronchial and chest infections. It is excellent at clearing mucous from the bronchial passages. It reduces inflammation in the airways.

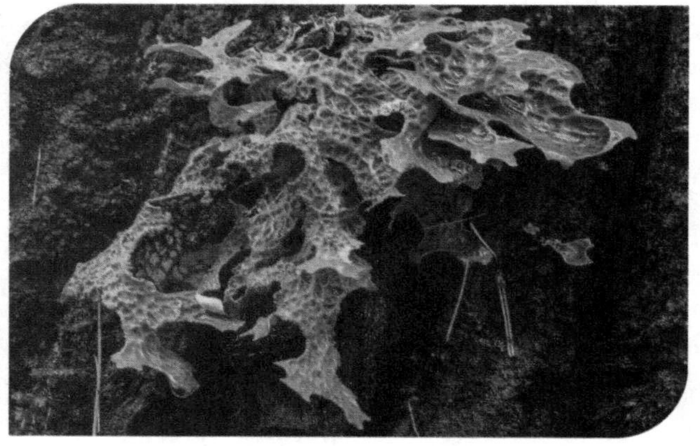

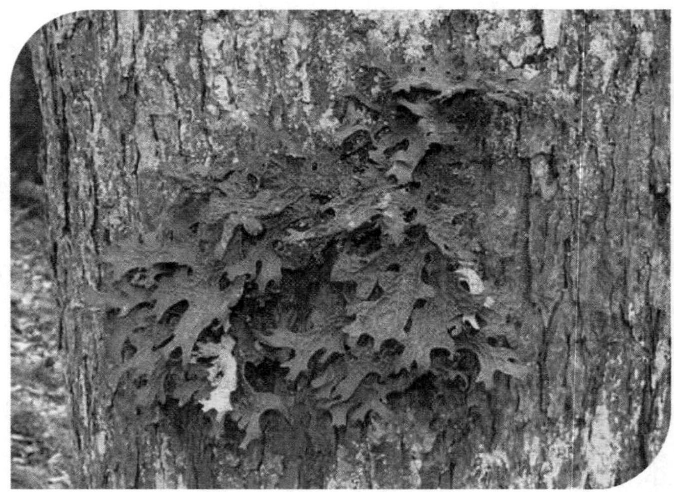

Lungwort Lichen,Bernd Haynold [CC BY-SA 3.0]

Lungwort lichen has high mucilage content and it is soothing on a sore throat or for laryngitis.

Antioxidant, Anti-Inflammatory, and Anti-Ulcer: Lungwort lichen contains high levels of antioxidants and anti-inflammatory compounds that work together to protect and heal the body. Antioxidants protect the body from free radicals that cause serious diseases like heart disease and cancer. Free radicals are also responsible for most of the symptoms of aging. Research on lungwort lichens as an anti-inflammatory show that, unlike many pharmaceutical anti-inflammatories (NSAIDs) it does not cause gastric distress. It even showed an anti-ulcer effect and may be useful for ulcerative colitis.

Degradation of Prions – Creutzfeldt-Jakob Disease: Creutzfeldt-Jakob Disease (CJD) is caused by prions. Prions also cause Mad Cow Disease in cattle and chronic wasting disease (CWD) in deer and elk (note that these are different diseases that CJD). The fungal part of the lungwort lichen has been shown to degrade prion proteins using a serine protease enzyme. This is a great find as prions are very hard to kill.

Anti-Bacterial: *Staphylococcus*, Pneumonia, TB, and *Salmonella*. Lungwort lichen contains powerful antibacterial agents. It is useful for treating staph infections and the bacteria that cause bacterial pneumonia and tuberculosis. It is also effective against *Salmonella* bacteria.

Digestive Health: Lungwort lichen is an effective remedy for digestive problems like constipation, stomach pain, indigestion, diarrhea, and bloating. It has mild diuretic properties that help remove excess fluid from the body. Best used as a tea for digestion.

Harvesting: Note: lungwort lichen is protected in some areas. Check your local laws before harvesting. Lungwort lichen grows very slowly and will not grow in heavily polluted areas, so it is becoming threatened in many environments. Harvest it carefully and do not take the whole plant. Only harvest in environmentally clean areas. The upper tissue edge must remain on the tree to regrow the lichen. Use a knife to slice off the outer lobes of the lichen, leaving the upper tissue attached to the tree. You do not need a large amount. Dry the lichen and store it in a sealed glass jar with a tight lid. Place the jar in a cool, dry place. Gathering after a windstorm is a great way to get fresh lungwort lichen that has blown down.

Warning: Do not use lungwort lichen if you are pregnant or breastfeeding, as safety is unknown.

Recipes. Lungwort Lichen Tea. Ingredients: 1 tablespoon dried lungwort lichen, 1 cup boiling water, 1 teaspoon raw honey, optional for sweetness.

Pour the boiling water over the herb and let it steep for 15 minutes. Strain and add raw honey, if desired.

Lungwort Tincture: Please follow our guide for a double-extraction like the one on page 39 or page 268. For most of the ailments above I use a dual-extracted tincture of Lungwort Lichen.

Reishi Mushroom, *Ganoderma lucidum*

The reishi mushroom is found on dead or dying trees, old stumps, and logs. They are quite easy to distinguish if you know your mushrooms well. They are also called *ling zhi,* the mushroom of immortality, and varnish conk, as they look like they have been painted with a clear coat of varnish or clear nail polish. Many places cultivate reishi for commercial use.

Identification: Always consult with an expert before using any mushrooms you find growing wild, though reishi mushrooms don't have any poisonous look-alikes. The cap of this polypore mushroom is fan or kidney-shaped, red to reddish-brown, and has a wet, varnished look when young. This shiny, reddish, bright yellow or white cap is the first identifying feature of reishi mushrooms. As they age, they become tougher, turn more of a reddish-brown, and the spores drop. These spores can end up on the top surface of the mushroom, making the cap lose its shiny luster. The pore surface on the underside of the mushroom bruises brown. The cap can grow to be a foot across and up to 2-inches (5 cm) thick. It may be attached to a stem, but not always. New growth appears along a whitish edge. The underside of the cap does not have gills. Instead, tiny brown spores come out of tiny pores on the underside. When stems are present, they are 1 to 6 inches (2.5 cm to 7.5 cm) long and almost 2 inches (5 cm) thick. They can be twisted or irregular, angling to one side of the cap. Like the cap, they are varnished and colored.

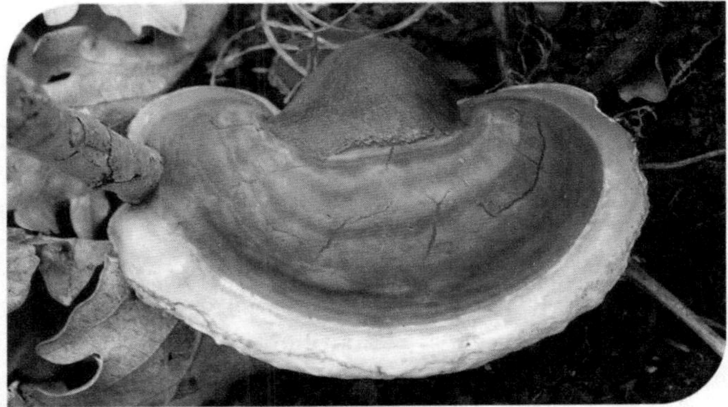

Reishi Mushrooms, photo by Eric Steinert [CC BY-SA 3.0]

Edible Use: While reishi mushrooms are technically edible when cooked, they have a bitter taste and are very tough, so they are rarely eaten. They can be used to season soups and are then strained out.

Medicinal Use and Adaptogenic Herb: I primarily use reishi mushrooms in their double-extracted tinctured form (page 39/268) to make available both the water-soluble and alcohol-soluble components. If you are only consuming reishi as a tea or a tea/coffee/hot chocolate-mixture you are missing out on a lot of the medicinal compounds. I take my reishi tincture every day.

It is an excellent adaptogenic herb. Adaptogens help our bodies deal with the negative aspects of stress, such as inflammation, hormonal imbalances, increased cortisol levels, fatigue, and low energy levels. They help with quality of sleep, adrenal fatigue, and with immune function.

Anti-Inflammatory Properties, Autoimmune Diseases, and Leaky Gut: Reishi mushrooms are a powerful anti-inflammatory both internally and externally. When applied topically, it relieves inflammation better than over the counter and many prescription steroid treatments. Because many autoimmune diseases are inflammatory in nature, reishi mushrooms are being used to slow or reverse the disease process. It also has immune modulating effects. I take it daily, along with Turkey Tail and Lion's Mane Mushroom Tinctures, for Multiple Sclerosis and believe that it greatly helps my condition. It is also indicated for Lupus, Myasthenia Gravis, Hashimoto's Thyroiditis, Crohn's, Inflammatory Bowel, Ulcerative Colitis, Guillain-Barre, Rheumatoid Arthritis, Psoriasis, Vasculitis, and Celiac Disease. It has been shown to have neuroprotective effects and is also good for treating Leaky Gut, a common cause of inflammation and immune response. Note that the anti-inflammatory properties in reishi (triterpenoids) are not water-soluble.

Anti-Aging and Anti-Oxidants: Reishi mushrooms are rich in antioxidants, which relieve oxidative stress in tissues and prevent age-related stress in the liver and body. It also has neuroprotective effects and is recommended for people with Alzheimer's and other nervous system diseases.

Cancer: Reishi mushrooms are used traditionally to prolong life in cancer patients and are currently used with modern cancer treatments to improve strength and stamina in patients. Reishi enhances immune system function and allows the body to better fight cancer. It has demonstrated significant anti-tumor and anti-cancer activity. They are also effective at alleviating nausea and kidney damage caused by cancer drugs and in reversing chemotherapy resistance. It can be used in tandem with traditional chemotherapy and radiation treatments in the same manner as Turkey Tail mushrooms are used.

Fatigue, Depression, Insomnia, Anxiety, and Adrenal Fatigue: People who regularly take reishi mushrooms report improvement in depression, fatigue, insomnia, anxiety, sense of wellbeing, and quality of life. Reishi is an adaptogenic herb and helps with adrenal fatigue.

Anti-Microbial, Anti-Fungal, Anti-Bacterial, and Anti-Viral: Reishi has anti-microbial, anti-fungal, anti-bacterial, and anti-viral effects. It regulates immune system activity and helps the body heal. These properties work together to help the body heal from wounds, infections, and diseases. It has been shown to be antiviral for HIV, HPV, herpes simplex 1 and 2, and influenza. It demonstrates antibacterial activity against *Streptococcus*, *Staphylococcus*, *Salmonella*, *Bacillus* (one of which causes anthrax), *E. coli*, and *Micrococcus*. It also works well for Urinary Tract Infections.

Liver Function, Hepatitis, Hormone Balance, Acne, PCOS, and Prostate: Reishi mushrooms have healing effects on the liver and help it release toxins that reduce its function. The mushrooms also speed up regeneration of healthy liver cells and promote overall liver health and whole-body vitality. It has shown great efficacy in the treatment of hepatitis. Through its help with liver function, hormones are better broken down and metabolized and hormonal balance is restored. It may be helpful for acne treatment, prostate health for men, and for women with PCOS due to its anti-androgenic effect.

Seizures, Convulsions, and Restless Legs Syndrome: Reishi mushrooms have been successfully used to relieve stress on the nervous system and reduce seizures and convulsions. Anticonvulsive and anti-inflammatory properties work together to calm the nervous system and help with recovery. It also helps people suffering from Restless Legs Syndrome (RLS).

Bronchitis, Allergies, and Asthma: Reishi is used to treat chronic bronchitis, allergies, and asthma. It helps prevent the release of histamines and reduces inflammation.

Blood Sugar Regulation: Reishi mushroom is known to improve symptoms of type II diabetes and to lower elevated blood sugar levels.

Heart Benefits, Blood Pressure, Blood Flow, and Cholesterol: Reishi mushrooms benefit the heart in several ways. They increase oxygenation of the blood, increase blood flow, lower cholesterol and fatty acids in the blood, and help lower blood pressure. People report improvement in symptoms of cardiovascular disease and improvement in heart function when taking reishi mushrooms regularly. It also seems to regulate irregular heartbeats. People also notice a drop in "Bad" LDL cholesterol and an increase in "Good" HDL cholesterol.

Altitude Sickness: Reishi mushroom's ability to increase blood flow and oxygenation of the blood is useful in treating altitude sickness. Breathing improves and dizziness is reduced. It is best to start taking reishi mushrooms before the trip and to continue use throughout.

Warning: Reishi mushrooms are safe, however it is possible to ingest too much. Use reishi mushrooms from a reputable source or consult an expert. Think about avoiding reishi mushrooms if you are pregnant or breastfeeding, since there is no information on their safety. Consult a doctor before using reishi mushrooms if you have a bleeding disorder. Do not use before surgery, as reishi is a vasodilator.

Recipes. Reishi Mushroom Tincture Double-Extraction: Use the double-extraction method found on page 39 or page 268 to make your tincture so that you extract all of the medicinal compounds from your mushrooms. If you have a cloudy solution in your finished product that is a good thing – it is the water-soluble polysaccharides coming out of solution as they are mixed back with the alcoholic part of the tincture. Just shake before using. The alcoholic portion has the triterpenoids, which lend the reishi its bitter taste, as well as other compounds. Note that you can also do the alcoholic extraction first and follow up with the water extraction.

Turkey Tail Mushroom, *Trametes versicolor* or *Coriolus versicolor*

Turkey Tail Mushrooms have been in use for many years in Japanese and Chinese Medicine; they are called *Yun Zhi* in China. They are commonly used as an adjunct cancer therapy as they complement both radiation and chemotherapy. This polypore mushroom is found around the globe.

Identification: Turkey tail mushrooms grow in colonies on tree stumps or fallen logs. The caps are multicolored with concentric circles of alternating colors. Bands may be black, brown, tan, gray, blue, red, orange, or white. The edges of the cap form wavy ripples like the outside edge of a turkey's tail and they can grow up to 4 inches (10 cm) wide, though I usually find them around 1.5 to 2 inches (3.75 cm to 5 cm) wide. They are stemless. The cap of the turkey tail mushroom is velvety or fuzzy, thin, and flexible. It has pores on the underside that are evenly spread out (3 to 5 pores per mm). They do not have gills. The wavy growing edges are white or nearly white.

Gathering wild mushrooms without expert knowledge can make you violently ill, or worse. Always consult with an expert before eating any wild mushroom. Look for these identifying characteristics and have an expert verify the mushroom's identity before using it.

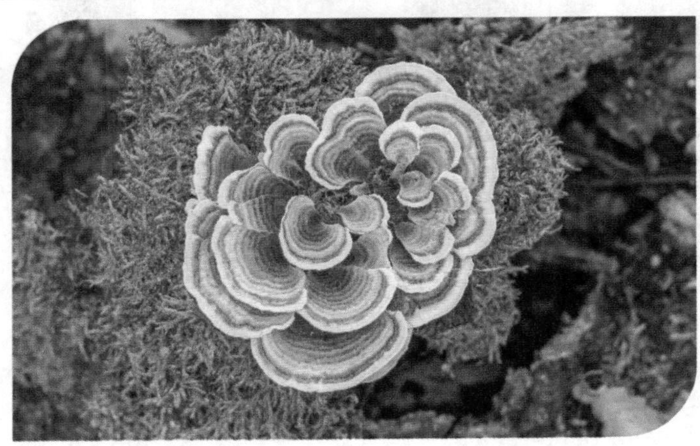

Turkey Tail Mushrooms, photo by Jerzy Opioła [CC BY-SA 3.0]

Edible Use: Turkey tail mushrooms are very nutritious and full of vitamins and minerals. However, they do not digest well, so they are rarely eaten.

Medicinal Use: I use turkey tail in tincture form and take this daily as part of my daily health routine. They are also taken in dry, powdered form or as Turkey Tail Tea. I use a double-extraction method to access all of its medicinal properties (see page 38 or page 268).

Regulates the Immune System, Prevents and Treats the Cold and Flu: The nutrients, antioxidants, and anti-inflammatory components in turkey tail mushrooms regulate the immune system and help fight off diseases. It is a very good anti-viral.

Fights Cancer and Supports Cancer Patients: Turkey tail mushrooms are often used for cancer patients to kill cancer cells and tumors and to support the immune system while undergoing chemotherapy. It strengthens the immune system, helping your body fight the disease and also protects the body from additional infections. Its anti-cancer properties help prevent the spread of the cancer and have been shown to augment the effects of Western cancer therapies. The two primary compounds in it for cancer are Polysaccharide -K (PSK) or Krestin and Polysaccharopeptide (PSP). PSK has been in common clinical use in Japan since the 1970s. The research on turkey tail mushrooms and cancer is too extensive to outline here

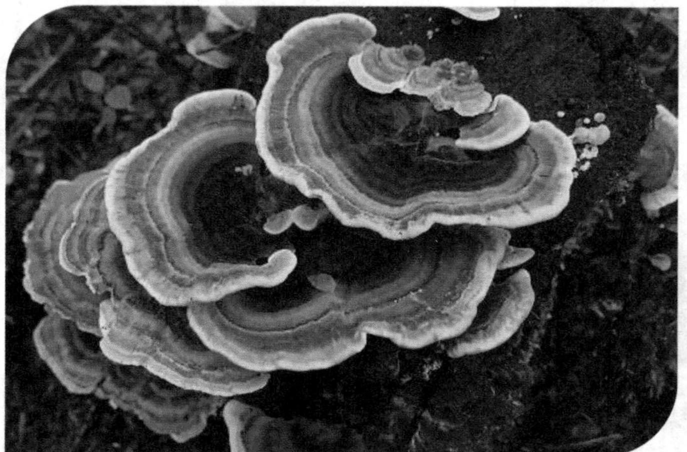

but it is very effective for treating many types of cancers, and in greatly reducing relapse rates.

Treats HPV, Cervical Dysplasia, Herpes, and Shingles: Turkey tail mushrooms fight infections of bacteria and viruses. It is effective in treating the human papillomavirus (HPV) and fighting the cancers that HPV sometimes triggers. Use turkey tail along with reishi mushrooms to treat viral infections like HPV, herpes, and shingles.

Improves Digestion and Leaky Gut: Digestive disorders respond well to treatment with turkey tail mushrooms. Turkey tail increases the levels of vitamins and minerals in the diet and supports healthy gut flora. Turkey tail helps Leaky Gut due to its prebiotic effects on the gut's microbiome (they feed the beneficial gut bacteria).

Helps Prevent and Treat HIV/AIDS and Kaposi's Sarcoma: There has been much research done on HIV and AIDS and turkey tail mushrooms have shown a remarkable ability to strengthen the immune system of these patients and help them fight the disease. It has been successfully used to treat Kaposi's Sarcoma, a skin cancer that affects AIDS patients. It stimulates interferon production and the probable mechanism of turkey tail for HIV is via the inhibition of the binding of HIV to lymphocytes. Lymphocyte depletion is the cause of the "acquired immunodeficiency" in AIDS.

Diabetes: Turkey tail mushrooms help lower the levels of glucose in the bloodstream and can be helpful in managing blood sugar levels in diabetics.

Reducing Inflammation, Autoimmune Diseases, and Chronic Inflammatory Diseases: Many modern diseases are caused by out of control inflammation in the body. These diseases are usually chronic and can become severe. Turkey tail mushrooms are high in anti-inflammatory properties and help reduce internal inflammation. It is also effective when applied to the skin to reduce rashes, swellings, and other external inflammations. Immune modulation coupled with its anti-inflammatory effects is most likely responsible.

***Candida* Overgrowth:** Turkey Tail helps with overgrowth of *Candida* as well as other bacterial flora in the small intestine.

Malaria: Turkey tail has been shown to be effective against malaria, including the chloroquine-resistant strain of Plasmodium.

Chronic Fatigue: Turkey tail has shown great efficacy in treating chronic fatigue syndrome.

Heart Health, Lowers Cholesterol and Blood Pressure: Turkey tail mushrooms are helpful in lowering LDL cholesterol levels in the body. It also reduces blood pressure in patients with hypertension. The mushrooms should be taken daily for full effects. By lowering cholesterol and reducing hypertension, it also reduces the risks of heart disease.

Harvesting: Choose mushrooms with clean white pore surfaces. Snip off the rough tissue where the mushroom was attached with a pair of clean scissors. Gather in environmentally clean areas.

Warning: Turkey Tail mushrooms are considered to be very safe. There are no known negative side effects but it is always a good idea to consult with a medical professional.

Usnea Lichen

Also known as Old Man's Beard, Usnea lichen grows in a similar fashion as Spanish Moss. Once you get to know this lichen, you will not mistake it for anything else. Usnea has a distinguishing characteristic of a white, rubber-band-like core, so always look for this. Usnea is an indicator of a healthy ecosystem with clean air. The lichen will not grow in heavily polluted areas and is now considered endangered in many areas. If I had to pick only one medicine to have available to me this would be the one. All Usnea species are medicinal.

Identification: Usnea can be found hanging from the bark of trees like long strands of an old man's beard. It can be distinguished from other lichens by its stretchy inner fibers and its exclusive white core. It is gray-green in color and can take many different forms. It prefers to grow in areas with a lot of rainfall.

Edible Use: Usnea is considered edible when leached a few times, but it is not very palatable. It can cause great stomach upset and I don't eat it. It is, however, one of my favorites go to medicinal plants.

Medicinal Use: Usnea lichen is a powerful antibiotic, antifungal, antimicrobial, and antiviral. I always carry Usnea and Blue Elderberry tinctures when I travel on airplanes and when I am around people who may be ill, as they both prevent and cure illness. I often put Usnea in a spray bottle for this use. I find that a spray of Usnea Tincture in the back of the throat helps prevent illnesses from taking hold. It is also a handy delivery mechanism to spray on to a wound or skin condition. Usnea extracts well in oil and as a double extracted tincture in alcohol and water.

Antibiotic Use: Strep, Staph, MRSA, Tuberculosis: The outer portion of the Usnea lichen contains antibiotic compounds that rival penicillin. For gram-positive bacteria like *Streptococcus*, *Pneumococcus*, MRSA, and tuberculosis, it works extremely well. I use it topically as well as internally. It doesn't seem to work as well for gram-negative bacteria like *E. coli*.

A Powerful Antiviral: Epstein-Barr, Herpes, HPV: Usnea lichen is effective in treating viral infections such as herpes simplex and the Epstein Barr virus that is implicated in so many modern diseases. Douching with Usnea can help with cervical dysplasia.

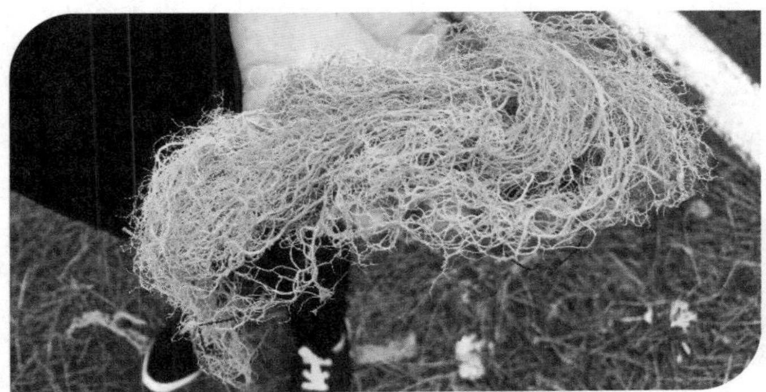

Respiratory System, Urinary Tract, Bladder, and Kidney Infections: Usnea helps heal respiratory problems such as bronchitis, pneumonia, sinus infections, strep throat, colds, flus, and other respiratory complaints. It is very effective in healing urinary tract, bladder, and kidney infections. Its antibiotic and antiviral properties help eliminate the infections while the immune system helps the body heal. I primarily use it in the form of a double-extracted Usnea tincture.

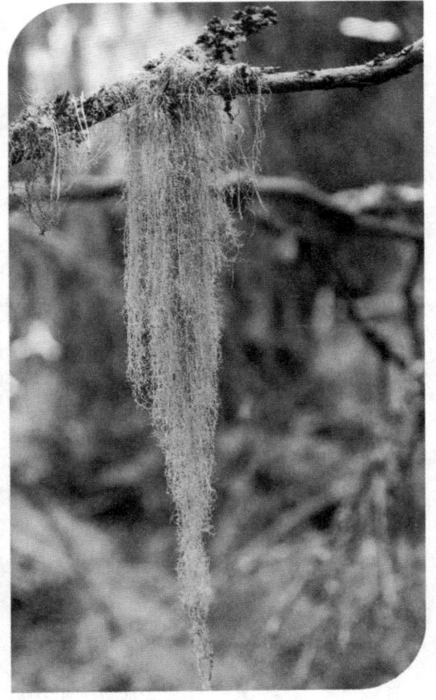

Skin Problems, Wounds, and Infections: Usnea's antibiotic and healing properties work on wounds and skin problems when it is applied as a poultice, salve, or tincture directly on the affected skin. This lichen also has analgesic and anti-inflammatory properties that help relieve pain.

Yeast Infections, Thrush, Athlete's Foot, Jock Itch, Ringworm, Dandruff, and Other Fungal Infections: Usnea is a powerful antifungal and treats yeast infections in women. It is also effective against the fungi causing athlete's foot, jock itch, ringworm, dandruff, and other common fungal infections. For vaginal use, dilute the tincture in boiled water and use as a douche. For thrush, put your tincture in a spray bottle and spray on the affected area. This is such a relief to cancer patients experiencing thrush.

Conjunctivitis: Usnea can be used in a cooled down tea as an eyewash along with other herbs (Yarrow, Chamomile, Plantain, raw honey) for conjunctivitis.

Stops Bleeding: When applied to wounds, this lichen quickly facilitates clotting and controls bleeding. Apply the lichen directly to the wound and bind in place with a gauze bandage for best results.

Harvesting: I like to harvest Usnea just after a storm has just passed. At this time, tree branches have broken and are lying on the ground, just waiting for me to collect Usnea. In this way, I do not have to struggle to reach high branches or harvest from live trees. Usnea, like other lichens, grows slowly, so only collect from downed branches. Lichens are used as pollution indicators so make sure you collect from very environmentally clean areas.

Pull on the lichen strands to find its white core. In this way, you'll have confirmation that you have the right lichen and good medicine. Use fresh or dry and store in a cool, dark place for future use.

Warning: Usnea lichen is a highly concentrated medicine and should not be taken continuously in large doses. Take it as needed for specific problems. I personally use a spray in my throat often as a preventative for illness but that is a very low dose (versus taking a large amount of internal tincture daily) and I have had no ill effects or abnormal liver enzyme readings. Do not use Usnea internally during pregnancy or breastfeeding, as safety is unknown. Usnea lichen absorbs pollutants and toxins from the environment. Do not harvest the lichen in areas exposed to heavy metals, roadway exhaust, industrial areas, or waste areas.

Recipes: Tea is ineffective as a delivery method to access all of the medicinally active compounds of Usnea. Personally, I use a tincture double-extracted in water and alcohol to access all of the medicinal compounds (p. 38). I do this for most lichen and mushroom extractions and also add a little heat. You can either extract it with water first as in the recipe below or else extract it in alcohol and then extract the Usnea in water afterwards, pouring the alcoholic tincture back in to your medicinal water in a ratio of 3 parts alcohol: 1-part water. If you have a cloudy solution in your finished product that is OK – it is the water-soluble polysaccharides coming out of solution as they are mixed back with the alcoholic part of the tincture. Simply shake before use. Usnea is also very soluble in oil for internal and external use – follow our recipe for oil infusions (page 38 or page 268) and grind the Usnea well before infusing in oil.

Usnea Lichen Tincture (Recipe can be scaled up or down as desired). *Note: I like to use a small crockpot for this recipe. You may also place the herbs and water into a jar, which is then covered and placed into the crockpot of water or a pot of water on low on the stove.

Double-extraction: You'll need: 8 ounces (230g) or more of dried Usnea Lichen, 24 ounces (710ml) of 80 to 100 proof alcohol, 8 ounces (250ml) distilled water.

Cut up the Usnea into very small pieces so that the core is also exposed to your solvent. Place the distilled water and the dried herbs into the crockpot and stir well. Cover and cook on the lowest possible setting for 3 days. Allow the herb and water mixture to cool and pour it into a glass jar. Add the alcohol while the mixture is still quite warm, but not hot. Cap the jar tightly, label and date the jar and allow it to macerate for 8 weeks, shaking the jar daily. Strain out the herb (cheesecloth works well for this). Store it in a tightly capped glass jar. Label and date. Note: If you are using this tincture internally, your alcohol must be drinking quality. See page 38 or page 268 for another way to double extract Usnea.

Water - Loving Plants

Cattails, *Typha* spp.

Traveling through wetlands, I am always happy to see cattail spikes growing near the water's edge. Practically the whole plant is edible, depending on the time of year. It is in the Typhaceae (Bulrush) Family.

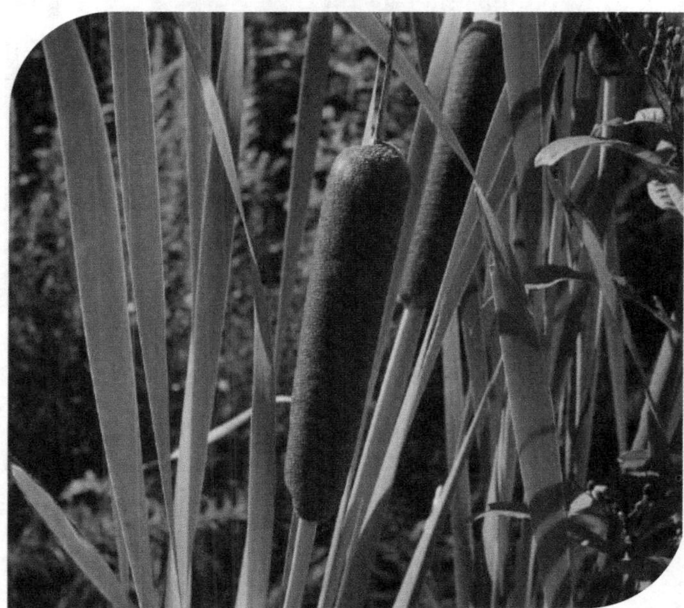

Identification: Cattails are common in and near marshes, ponds, and other wetland areas throughout the world. The sword-like leaves are similar to many grasses, but the plant is readily identifiable by its brown corndog-like flowerheads.

Cattails are perennials and grow 5 to 8 feet (1.5m to 2.4 meters) tall. The alternate leaves are spear-shaped and grow from a simple stem that terminates in a large number of male flowers forming a spike at the end of the stem. The flowers wither once the pollen is shed.

Cattails flower from May through July. Tiny female flowers form a dense, sausage-shaped structure just below the male spike. This structure can be up to a foot long and is 1 to 2 inches (2.5 cm to 5 cm) in diameter. Tiny seeds grow on fine hairs. When ripe, the cottony fluff blows away to disperse the seeds.

Edible and Other Use: Cattail rhizomes are edible and nutritious. They are made into a flour by scraping the starch from the fibers, drying, and pounding. They can also be boiled, steamed, or mashed and eaten like a potato. The small shoots on the rhizomes in early spring are good peeled and sliced. The flavor is mildly sweet.

In the spring, the outer part of the young plant can be peeled and eaten raw or cooked. In the summer, harvest the green flower spike and remove the outer sheath like you would shuck corn. Boil the flower spike and eat it like corn on the cob. The flavor is delicious.

In late summer, an abundance of pollen forms and can be harvested for edible and medicinal use. It is easy to collect quickly in a thick patch. Simply bend the pollen-laden stalk over and shake it into a bag or other container. This pollen makes an excellent thickener or flour extender for baking and for making cattail pancakes. The leaves are used for weaving mats and baskets.

Medicinal Use. Treating Skin Conditions: Every part of the cattail is useful for this purpose. The starchy root makes a healing poultice for burns, boils, sores, cuts, insect bites, and bruises. Pound the roots and use the pulp or split the root and bruise the fibers inside, then apply the exposed pulp to the wound. The fuzz from the flowers treats small burns and skin irritations. Apply it directly to the wound and cover with a clean cloth.

Treating Small Wounds, Insect Bites, Toothaches, and Relieving Pain: The jelly-like sap that seeps from the lower stems has antiseptic and analgesic properties. I can usually find it between young leaves and scrape it up with the back of a knife.

Use it for treating small wounds, especially when worried about infection. It also acts as a powerful pain killer when applied topically and can be ingested without harm. It is an ideal pain reliever for toothaches, teething pain, and sore gums, and it can also be used on insect bites and other skin irritations. Just rub a little on the sore spot for fast pain relief and to reduce inflammation.

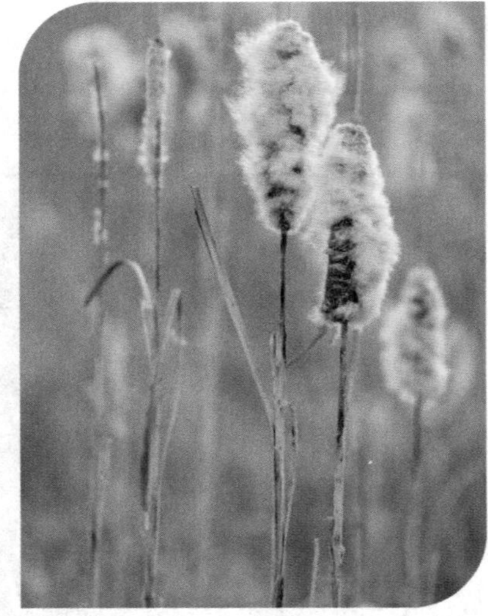

Abscesses and Infections: Clean abscesses with an antiseptic skin wash made by boiling the leaves. When the abscess is clean, combine cattail pollen with a small amount of raw honey and spread over the wound. Cover with a clean cloth and leave in place. Wash and replace the honey-pollen two to three times a day as needed.

Well Baby Care: Apply the fuzz from the flowers into skin folds to prevent chafing and diaper rash in babies. The jelly-like sap found between the lower stems numbs the gums and relieves teething pain when rubbed sparingly onto a baby's gums.

Cancer Prevention: Cattails are currently being researched as a cancer preventative. Cattail's anti-inflammatory and antioxidant properties may slow the growth and spread of cancer.

Antiseptic and Styptic Properties: Burned cattail leaf ash is an excellent styptic and antiseptic for wounds. To make the ash, build a small fire using cattail leaves. Allow the fire to burn completely, then scoop up the ash. Use when cool or store it in a dry place for future use. Cattail pollen, dusted on externally, is also good for bleeding. It speeds clotting and helps prevent infection. Once bleeding is no longer an issue, mix the pollen with raw honey and use it to prevent infection and speed healing.

Menstrual and Postpartum Bleeding: Cattail pollen, taken orally, lessens the severity of heavy menstrual bleeding and postpartum bleeding and pain. 5 to 10 grams is the usual dose.

Internal Bleeding: Both the pollen and the flower are useful for internal bleeding. It helps with bruising, vomiting blood, bloody stools, bloody urine, and uterine bleeding. It doesn't treat the cause of the bleeding but helps stop the bleeding.

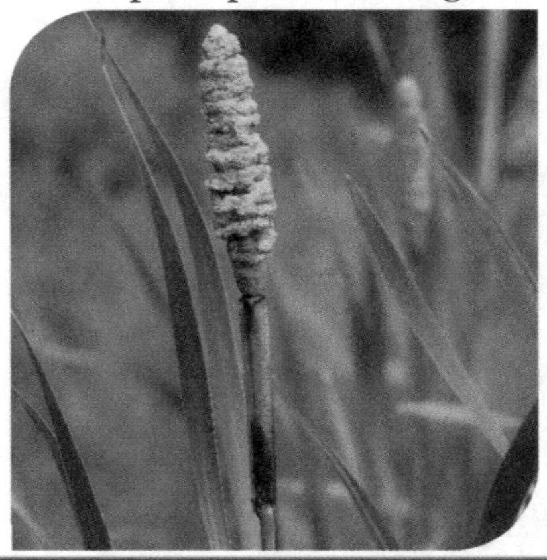

Warning: Its coagulant properties could be problematic for people with poor circulation, as it may slow down the blood even more and stimulate clotting in the skin. Pregnant women should not use cattail.

Cocoplum, *Chrysobalanus icaco*

The cocoplum is also called paradise plum and Icaco. It grows along beaches in tropical and subtropical areas. In North America it is found in Southern Florida, Mexico, and the Caribbean. It is in the Chrysobalanaceae Family.

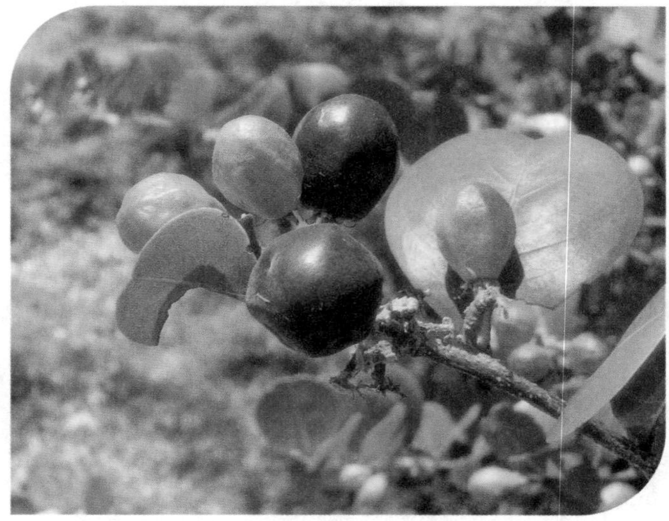

Cocoplum fruits, Ripe and immature. Daniel Di Palma, CC by SA 4.0

Identification: Along the shoreline and in cultivated situations, the cocoplum forms a shrub that is 4 to 8 feet (1.2m to 1.8m) tall, but inland the plant forms a bushy tree that grows to 20 to 30(6m to 9.1m) feet tall. There are three main types of Cocoplum. "Red Tip" and "Green Tip" varieties that grow inland, and a

"Horizontal" type that grows along the coast and is salt tolerant.

While all three varieties have a similar medicinal use, I am most familiar with the coastal-horizontal type. It sends down roots from branches that creep along the soil or sand. The leaves are alternate and egg-shaped with a small indentation at the tip. Each is about 1 1/2 inch to 3 inches (3.75 to 7.5 cm) long and has a tough, leathery texture and glossy appearance. New leaves can be yellow-green to reddish; mature leaves are light green in color. Small white flowers appear in clusters at the end of the stems. The thick-skinned fruit can be white, yellow, red, or purple. They usually bear crops in the spring and another in later fall. The fruits are oval shaped and about 1-inch (2.5 cm) long. The bark is grey to reddish brown with white flecks.

Edible and Other Use: The cocoplum fruit is often eaten raw or made into jams and syrups. The seed is also edible raw or cooked after the hard shell is removed. The seeds can be pressed and used like almond oil. The leaves are used to make a black dye that is decay resistant, and are used to treat cloth and fishing nets. The seeds within the fruit are very oily and can be used as a light or heat source.

Medicinal Use. Eye Health: Cocoplums fruits are an excellent source of beta-carotene and vitamin A, useful for treating night blindness and macular degeneration. It also helps protect the eyes from harmful UV rays. Eat the fruits either raw or cooked.

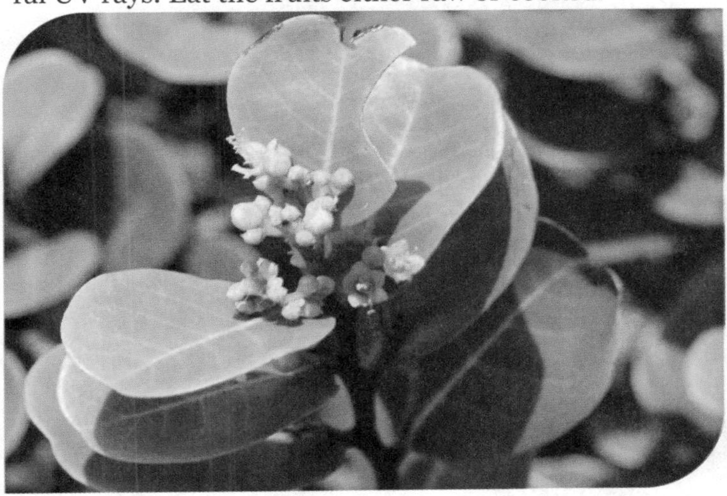

By © Hans Hillewaert /, CC BY-SA 3.0

Heart Health and Weight Loss: Cocoplums help treat atherosclerosis and reduce the risk of heart attack and strokes. It prevents fat accumulation and may help prevent weight gain.

Healthy Immune System: In addition to its vitamin A content, cocoplums also contain high levels of vitamin C, K, and the building blocks that your body uses to make vitamin D. They are also rich in minerals and antioxidants. Eating cocoplum fruits strengthens the immune system and helps prevent degenerative diseases.

Duckweed, *Lemna minor*

Duckweed, also called water lens and bayroot, is a fast-growing perennial aquatic plant that floats on or just below the surface of still or slow-moving water. It is in the Lemnaceae (Duckweed) Family. It is found throughout the world.

Identification: Duckweed is a small floating plant. Each plant is actually only one small flat floating modified stem, which looks like a leaf, and is 1/16 to 1/2 inch (1.25 cm) across, A single root hair protrudes down from each floating frond. They usually grow in large fresh water colonies.

The entire plant is less than 1/2 inch (1.25 cm) from the root tip to the top of the floating frond. While the plant does produce flowers, reproduction is mostly by asexual budding, which occurs at the base of the frond. Miniscule flowers occasionally appear, in groups of three, in summer.

Edible Use: It is eaten in some parts of the world as a vegetable. It is an excellent protein source, and contains more protein than soybeans. It is a good food

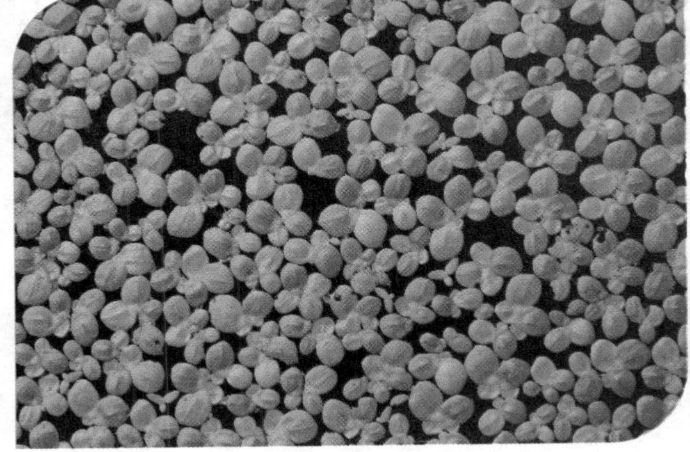

source as it grows very quickly. Be careful to harvest from clean water.

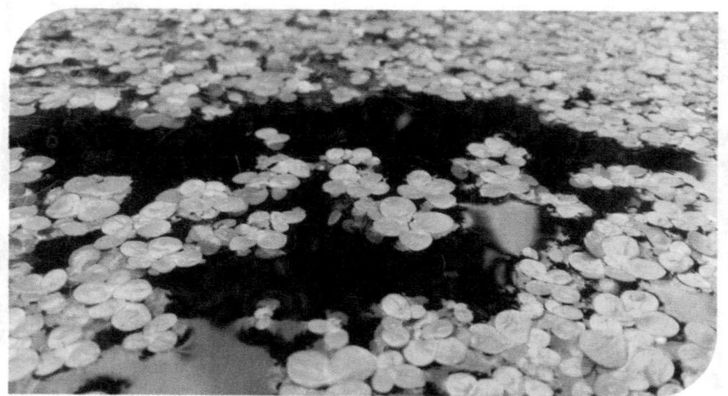

Medicinal Use: The entire plant is used and can be dried or used fresh. Both water and alcohol extractions work well, as does fresh consumption or juicing.

Anti-Bacterial and Anti-Fungal: Duckweed helps cure bacterial and yeast infections. It works for many different bacterial infections including *Staphylococcus, Streptococcus, Bacillus, Citrobacter*, and *Neisseria*, and also against *Candida* with great success.

Jaundice and Detox: Duckweed juice is said to absorb toxins and help detox the blood and liver.

Headaches, Swelling, and Body Aches: Duckweed juice treats aches and pains including headaches and body aches. Its anti-inflammatory properties help relieve swelling and inflammation in the muscles and joints, and help with arthritis and gout. For muscle and joint pain, make a poultice of crushed plants and apply it to the painful area.

Harvesting: Avoid harvesting duckweed from roadsides and polluted waters. It is known to accumulate heavy metals and other toxins. It is fairly easy to grow your own supply in clean water.

To grow duckweed, take a few plants from a clean water supply and move them into a pool or other container with a non-chlorinated clean water supply. They reproduce and grow quickly. To harvest, scoop the plant from the water and use it fresh or dry for later use.

Warning: Duckweed contains high levels of calcium oxalate, which can contribute to the formation of kidney stones.

Watercress, *Nasturtium officinale*

Watercress is an aquatic plant in the Brassicaceae (Mustard) Family. It is related to mustard and horseradish. Even though it bears the name Nasturtium, do not confuse it with the garden plant with the common name of nasturtium, which is in the genus *Tropaeolum*. It is a fast growing, aquatic or semi-aquatic, perennial plant that grows in clumps. Watercress was introduced to North America from Europe and is now found in almost every state and province. It is especially prevalent in the Pacific Northwest.

Identification: Watercress leaves are compound with 3 to 7 wavy-edged, oval leaflets that grow from a central stalk. The spicy leaves have a strong taste of pepper. Leaves are 2 to 5 inches (5 cm to 12.5 cm) long. Its flowers are at the top of these stems and are less than 1/5-inch-(0.5 cm) long with four white petals. Watercress fruits are thin, slightly curved, and measure less than 1 inch (2.5 cm) long and about 1/10 of an inch (0.25 cm) wide. They are borne on short stalks and contain 4 rows of small, round seeds.

Edible Use: The peppery leaves and seeds are edible and are used mainly as a condiment or a garnish in salads.

Medicinal Use: The leaves are used for arthritis, as a diuretic, a purgative, an expectorant, and have stimulant properties. It is very rich in vitamins and minerals. It is an effective cleansing herb, and is high in Vitamin C. It can be eaten fresh or taken as an infusion. It is best used fresh, but can also be dried for future use.

Immune Booster: The high nutrition and medicinal properties of watercress make it an excellent treatment for restoring immune function and health to the body. Eat watercress raw, drink the juice or the infusion, or cook. All provide the necessary nutrients and healing benefits.

Treating Tuberculosis: The freshly pressed juice of watercress is used to treat tuberculosis. Healers who use it report that they have patients drink one cup of watercress juice daily, in divided doses. Large doses taken all at once can cause stomach upset.

Swellings of the Lymphatic Systems: Make a poultice by crushing fresh watercress leaves to help drain swollen glands.

Headaches and Anxiety: Use Watercress Tincture made with vinegar to treat headaches and anxiety.

Saturate a handkerchief or a piece of cotton cloth in the tincture and wring it out. Place the cloth on your forehead and relax.

Mouth Sores, Swollen Gums, Bad Breath, and Hot Flashes: Watercress Soup is used for many mouth and gum issues as well as to cure hot flashes caused by menopause. Soup recipe below.

Dermatitis, Eczema, and Chronic Skin Diseases: For chronic skin conditions, watercress juice or Watercress Infusion is very effective. It is not an immediate fix. You will get a boost to the immune system, added nutrition, and gradual healing. Drink one cup of the infusion daily and use it to wash the affected areas twice a day.

Gout, Kidney Stones, Water Retention, and Expelling Mucous: Watercress is a diuretic. An infusion treats swelling in the body and helps expel mucous. Watercress Infusion also encourages the dissolution of kidney stones so that they can be flushed from the body.

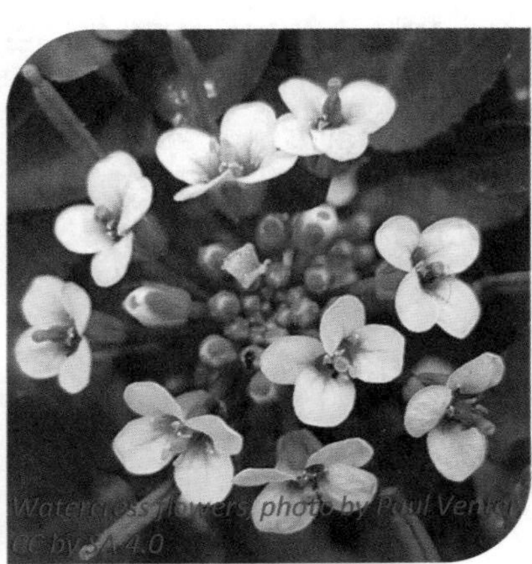
Watercress flowers, photo by Paul Venter CC by SA 4.0

Harvesting: The leaves of watercress can be harvested most of the year and are used fresh. Snip the tops of stems when they are about 6 inches (15 cm) long. Never take more than a third of the plant at any one time to protect the future supply. Do not pull on the stems of the plant directly as you may uproot the entire plant. This plant wilts quickly, so it is best harvested for immediate use. It can stay in the fridge for up to 3 days in a plastic bag or submerged in water. Harvest watercress only from known clean water supplies.

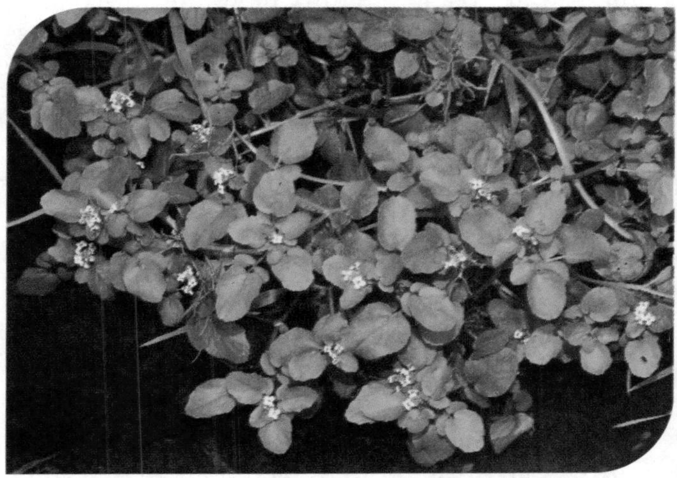

Warning: Collect your watercress from clean water sources. Fouled water can contaminate the herb. Excessive use of this plant can lead to stomach upset.

Recipes. Watercress Tincture: Rinse freshly picked watercress thoroughly and pack it into a clean and sterile glass jar with a tight lid. Bring some apple cider vinegar to a low boil and pour it over the watercress to fill the jar. Let the watercress steep for 6 to 8 hours, then strain it through a coffee filter. Pour it back into the glass jar and cap it tightly for long-term storage.

Watercress Soup: 1/2 cup loosely packed watercress, washed thoroughly, 1/2 cup sliced carrots, 1-quart (1 Liter) of water, salt and pepper to taste. Simmer the watercress and carrots in the water slowly over low heat for about 45 minutes or until the water is reduced by half. You may put it in a blender or eat as is (I prefer it blended). Consume it all. Makes one serving (it is easy to scale up this recipe).

Watercress Infusion: Gather a saucepan full of watercress and clean. Place the watercress in a ceramic or stainless-steel pot. Add enough cold water to barely cover the watercress. Bring the herbs to a boil and lower the heat. Simmer the herbs until they are soft. Filter the herbs out and store the infusion in the refrigerator for up to 3 days. The flavor can be enhanced if needed by mixing it with tomato juice or other vegetable juices.

Water Plantain, *Alisma subcordatum*

Southern water plantain grows in swamps, wetlands, lakes, marshes, and coastal areas. It is also known as *Alisma lantago-aquatica var. parviflorum*. It is in the Alismataceae (Water Plantain) Family. It grows in eastern North America.

Identification: Water plantain grows from 1 to 3 feet (0.3m to 0.9m). The broad leaves may float on the water surface but are often submerged. The leaves are widest at or near the middle and taper at the ends. Underwater leaves are often long, and ribbon-like.

The flowers are highly branched with whorls of white or pink to pink-purple flowers. Flowers have three petals and six stamens, and many carpels. Each carpel has one ovule and style. Flowers bloom all summer and seeds ripen from July to September.

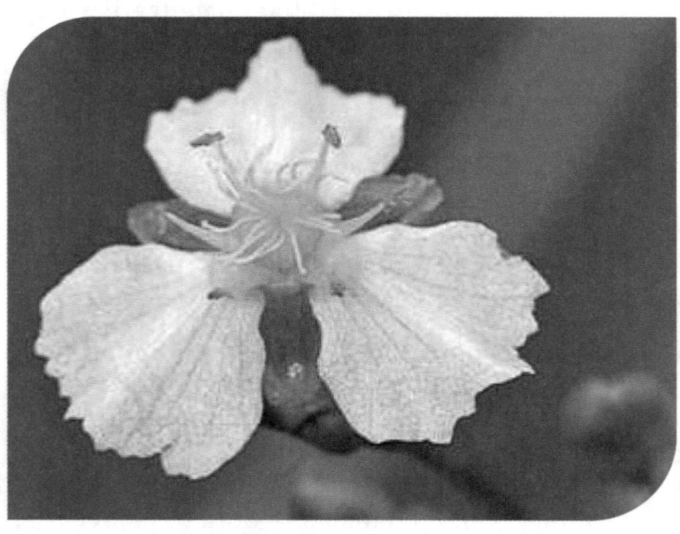

Christian Fischer, CC by SA 3.0 Unported

Edible Use: Boil the leaves and petioles of water plantain to eat. The leaves and root are toxic raw, but the poisons are destroyed by heat and drying. Cook them for a long time to make sure all toxins are destroyed.

The cooked roots are salty and rich in starch. They are a good starch source in the winter when wild food supplies are low.

Medicinal Use: Most of water plantain is used medicinally, including the fresh and dried roots, leaves, and seeds.

The easiest way to use it is to eat it as part of a daily diet. Make sure it is thoroughly cooked before use.

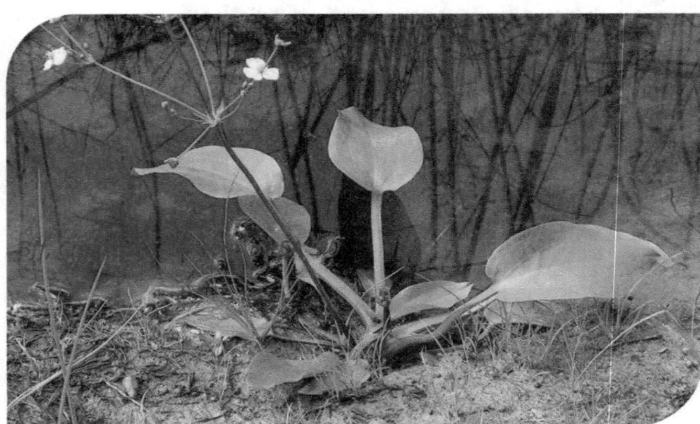

Diuretic, Kidney Stones, and Cystitis: Dried water plantain root is a diuretic and helps the body get rid of excess water (edema). The leaves treat cystitis (bladder infection) and kidney stones.

Powdered Water Plantain Seed for Bleeding: Dried and powdered water plantain seed is a good astringent and helps control bleeding. Apply it directly to the wound to disinfect the area and stop bleeding.

Digestive Ailments: Water plantain is a good source of dietary fiber (cook it well!). It also treats digestive issues such as cramps, stomach flu, bloating, and heartburn.

Lowers Cholesterol and Blood Pressure: Water plantain lowers blood pressure and cholesterol levels. It is heart healthy.

Poultice for Bruising and Swelling: Water plantain contains anti-inflammatories that work to reduce swelling and bruising. It is also a rubefacient. Crush the fresh leaves and use them as a poultice. Cover it with a clean cloth and replace as needed.

Harvesting: Harvest the roots in winter and boil for immediate use, or dry them for the future. Harvest leaves in spring and summer.

Warning: Water plantain can cause skin irritation in some people. While water plantain is considered safe, it can irritate the digestive tract with long-term use.

Western Skunk Cabbage, *Lysichiton americanus*

This plant is aptly named skunk cabbage because of its odor when crushed. It is very easy to identify by its physical characteristics, like its bright yellow spathe (leaf-like bract) surrounding a dense flower spike. This member of the Araceae (Arum) Family is also known as Swamp Lantern and Meadow Cabbage.

Identification: One of the first plants to bloom in the spring, it grows low to the ground in wet and swampy areas. The bright yellow spathe appears around the flower spike from February to May. Shiny large waxy green leaves appear after the flowers and can have a putrid smell. Skunk cabbage attracts flies, which facilitates pollination. The leaves are large, and can grow up to a few feet in length.

Edible Use: Do not consume raw due to calcium oxalate crystals. When boiled for long periods, traditionally 3 days or longer, the roots are edible. Boiling with multiple changes of water is necessary to remove the toxic substances, so routine use is not recommended. They are mostly known as a starvation food. The young leaves, thoroughly cooked with at least one change of water, are edible and have a pleasant peppery flavor. I use the large leaves as a wax paper for pit roasts or to wrap my fish in prior to cooking over a fire.

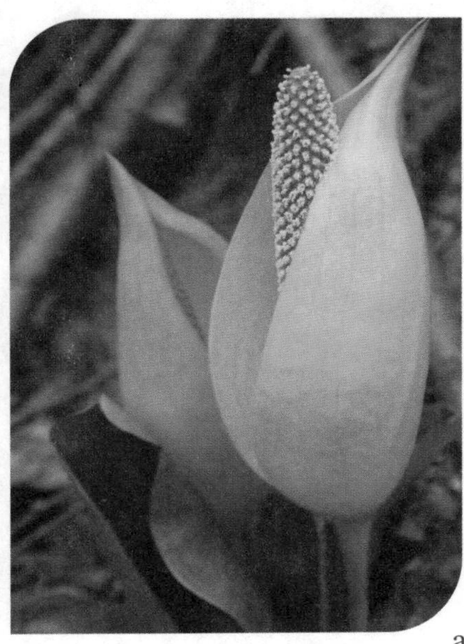

It does not impart a skunky smell or flavor and it holds in moisture nicely.

Medicinal Use: The root is toxic raw and must be thoroughly cooked or dried and aged to remove the toxin.

I dry my roots in a dehydrator and store them in a cool, dry, and dark place for at least 6 to 8 weeks before use.

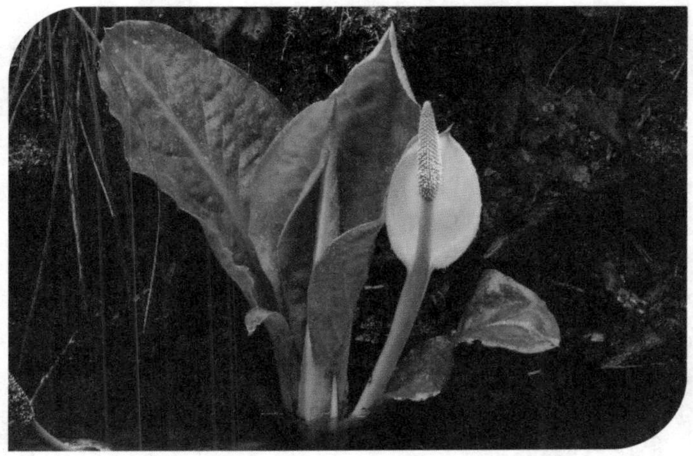

Use aged skunk cabbage root dried and powdered or apply the leaves directly to the skin as a poultice, compress, or wash.

Skin Infections, Wounds, Rashes, Burns, Bruises, and Insect Bites: Skunk cabbage is an anti-inflammatory and anti-infective.

Use it in a poultice to draw out infection or treat an insect bite, and as a wash to treat burns, bruises, rashes, poison ivy, and psoriasis.

Carpal Tunnel, Arthritis, Sore Muscles and Joints: A skunk cabbage poultice or compress made with Skunk Cabbage Tea placed on the joint or aching muscle helps reduce inflammation and pain.

Bronchitis, Asthma, Tuberculosis, and Anti-Spasmodic: Skunk cabbage root is an expectorant and antispasmodic, making it useful in treating bronchitis and asthma as it calms inflammation and bronchial spasms, while also helping to expel mucus. It also treats the underlying infection.

Nervous System: Aged skunk cabbage root is slightly narcotic. It calms the nervous system and treats headaches, vertigo, and some nervous conditions. It has been used to treat epilepsy and convulsions with mixed success.

Pregnancy and Labor: Skunk cabbage is beneficial during pregnancy and labor, promoting normal function of the nervous system and reproductive system. It soothes irritation and promotes efficient muscle contractions.

Consult a medical professional before using during pregnancy or breastfeeding.

Harvesting: Skunk cabbage contains crystals of calcium oxalate, which can be irritating on the skin. Wear gloves to handle the plant. Harvest the leaves and dig up the roots. Bring a good shovel as the roots are hard to dig up. Boil for several days, changing the water often, or dry the herb and age for at least 6 to 8 weeks before using. Boiling or drying destroys the calcium oxalate crystals.

Warning: Skunk cabbage contains large amounts of calcium oxalate, a toxin that is very irritating if ingested. Calcium oxalate is destroyed by cooking or by drying and aging the plant. Excess doses of skunk cabbage can cause side effects such as nausea, vomiting, dizziness, impaired vision, headaches, and vertigo. Some people may have allergic reactions to skunk cabbage. The fresh plant is extremely irritating and can cause itching, blistering of the skin, and redness when touched. If not treated properly the plant can irritate the mouth and throat. Never eat it raw, cook it as directed above.

Recipes. Skunk Cabbage Tincture: You'll need: dried and aged skunk cabbage root, 80 proof or higher vodka and a clean, sterile glass jar

Chop or grind the dried and aged root into small pieces and place it into a sterile jar, filling 1/3rd of it. Cover the root with vodka and fill to within ½ inch (1.25 cm) of the top of the jar. Cap the jar tightly, label and date it. Shake the jar to mix well and store the jar in a cool, dark place. Shake every few days for 6 to 8 weeks. Strain the herb out and store the tincture in a clean, labeled jar for up to 5 years.

Household Remedies

Activated Charcoal

Activated charcoal is very fine and porous. It is an effective way to remove toxins and poisons from the body. It reduces bloating, traps toxins and gases so they don't get absorbed by the body, and acts as an antidote to some poisons.

Medicinal Use. Detoxify the Body: Activated charcoal has tiny pores throughout that attract and traps toxins in the body. The toxins bind to the activated charcoal and pass through the body. To use activated charcoal to detoxify the body, take 10 grams of activated charcoal approximately 1 to 2 hours before each meal. Do this for two to three days. Drink 12 to 15 glasses of water per day during your cleanse. If you become constipated, drink a glass of warm water with lemon and raw honey every half hour until the constipation is gone.

Poisoning: Activated charcoal is useful for removing chemical poisons that have been ingested. Organic poisons such as pesticides, fertilizer, bleach, and mercury bind to the surface of the charcoal, preventing absorption in the body. It is also used it to prevent the absorption of an accidental or intentional overdose of drugs. It is effective against the ingestion of overdoses of aspirin, acetaminophen, opium, cocaine, and morphine. Charcoal must be administered quickly, within an hour of ingestion, and in quantity. The sooner the better and get medical help immediately. For adults, a large dose of 50 to 100 grams is required and 10 to 25 grams for children. Charcoal must be taken with a large quantity of water.

Food Poisoning: Many people do not realize that activated charcoal is useful for the treatment of nausea and diarrhea in cases of food poisoning. Adults take 25 grams of activated charcoal and children need 10 grams. Take the charcoal with large quantities of water immediately upon suspicion of food poisoning. Larger doses may be needed.

Snake Bites, Poisonous Spider Bites, and Insect Stings: For snake and poisonous spider bites, including bites from the black widow spider and the brown recluse, use a mixture of equal parts activated charcoal and coconut oil. Mix them together and cover the bite and a wide surrounding area with the mixture. Cover with a bandage to prevent staining clothes. The poison from the bites moves into the tissue surrounding the bites, so a wide area around the bite needs to be covered with the activated charcoal. After two to three hours, rinse the area well and reapply. Repeat the application until the inflammation is gone and the wound is healing. For insect bites, apply a small dab of the mixture, repeating every hour until the sting is gone. If it's a serious poisonous bite be sure to seek medical attention.

Acne: Treat acne with activated charcoal mixed with aloe vera gel. Smooth the mixture over the affected areas and let dry. Then rinse off completely. I prefer to treat the entire area, but it can also be used for spot treatments. Activated charcoal can also be mixed into soap and body wash for use in affected areas.

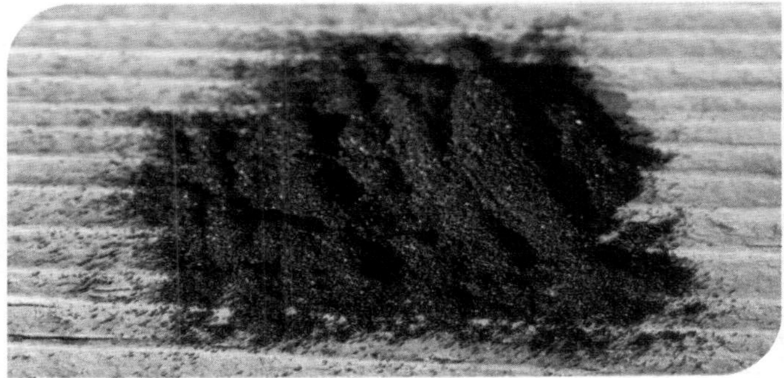

When to Avoid Activated Charcoal: Do not use activated charcoal in cases of poisoning by petroleum, alcohol, lye, acids and other corrosive chemicals. Do not take activated charcoal if you are taking prescription medications. It can interfere with some medications. Consult your doctor for more information on your medication.

Warning: Activated charcoal is not the same as barbecue charcoal. Barbecue charcoal should never be consumed. Drink 12 to 15 glasses of water daily when taking activated charcoal. The water prevents dehydration and constipation caused by the activated charcoal.

Bleach

Bleach is a good disinfectant for most household surfaces. It kills most bacteria, viruses, and fungi. Use it to sanitize surfaces in treatment areas, disinfect laundry, decontaminate blood spills, and disinfect equipment. In addition, it has medicinal uses for treating skin.

Medicinal Use. Bed Sores, Diabetic Ulcers, Eczema, and Inflammatory Skin Conditions: Soaking skin in a very dilute bleach solution is effective to treat bed sores, diabetic ulcers, eczema, and other inflammatory skin conditions. Use one tablespoon of regular strength bleach per gallon (per 4 liters) of water. The bleach solution is dilute enough not to harm the skin while calming inflammation and killing bacteria on the skin. Do not use undiluted bleach or bleach in higher concentrations. I prefer herbal medicine to bleach but it is a good remedy to know. You can also follow up a bleach treatment with soothing herbal oils specific to your condition and needs.

For a full 40-gallon (151 Liters) tub, use ½ cup of household bleach in warm water. Soak in the water for five to ten minutes, then rinse the skin completely with fresh water. Pat dry. Apply lotions, emollients, or medications after a bath. Repeat two to three times weekly, or as needed.

Sanitizing Water for Drinking: Unscented bleach is suitable for sanitizing water for drinking purposes. Add two drops of bleach per quart (liter) of water or 8 drops of bleach per gallon (4 liters) of water. Stir thoroughly and allow it to sit for at least one hour before drinking. If the water is cloudy, filter it before adding the chlorine. This treatment kills most bacteria and viruses found in water, but may not kill all. It does not remove chemicals or other toxins from water.

Using Bleach for Disinfecting: For disinfecting surfaces, use a higher concentration of bleach: 1/4 to 3/4 cup of bleach added to 1 gallon (4 liters) of water (1 to 3 tablespoons per quart (liter) of water). Let the bleach water stand on the surface for at least 2 minutes, then wipe dry or allow to air dry. This solution needs to be made fresh daily.

Warning: Do not use undiluted bleach or high concentrations of bleach directly on the skin. Bleach can cause dryness of skin irritations. Do not use with patients who have an allergy to chlorine.

Boric Acid

Boric acid is useful for a number of different purposes. It is especially effective for treating fungal infections of all kinds. Boric acid is not the same as borax. For medicinal use, always use therapeutic grade or pharmaceutical grade boric acid. Boric acid is a white crystalline acid (H3BO3) containing boron. It is sometimes called hydrogen borate or orthoboric acid. It is usually used as a dry powder, although it can be mixed with water to make a dilute acid for sanitizing purposes. Boric acid should never be taken orally.

Medicinal Use. Treating Yeast Infections: Boric acid suppositories are an excellent treatment for vaginal yeast infections. They are particularly useful for treating people who have had multiple yeast infections that keep returning because the boric acid can be used regularly as a preventative once the infection is cured.

Usual dose is 600mg of boric acid per suppository. Stuff the boric acid into a size "00" gelatin capsule and place the cap on it securely. Insert one suppository into the vagina every night just before bed. Patients should be warned that they may experience irritation or a burning sensation, but it will quickly pass. There will also be a discharge. Use one suppository each night for one week if this is an isolated yeast infection. If a person has been having problems with recurring infections, use the suppository every night for two weeks and then continue using one suppository twice a week for a year. This long-term use kills off the roots of the infection before it can reinfect the person.

As an Eyewash: Boric acid makes an easy eyewash for treating even serious and contagious eye infections. It can also be used for minor eye irritations and common childhood infections such as pink eye and conjunctivitis. It kills the bacterial infection and reduces inflammation. Before using the eyewash, make sure all of your materials are sterile including they eyedropper or eyecup. Sterilize before every use. Follow the recipe below to make the eyewash. Use an eyedropper or eye cup to wash the eye with the sterile eyewash. Blink several times and roll the eyes to be sure the eyewash gets into all the corners of the eye. Repeat three times a day until the infection is cleared.

Athlete's Foot, Nail Fungus: Boric acid is an excellent remedy for athlete's foot and toenail fungus. Dust the boric acid powder onto the foot or nail and put a few sprinkles into your socks each morning. At night, use the Boric Acid Foot Cure (recipe below.) The boric acid kills the infection, neutralizes the odor, and eases the associated itching. Continue to use daily until the infection is completely gone.

Jock Itch: Jock itch also responds well to a dusting of boric acid over the affected area. Apply boric acid in a light dusting, but make sure the entire area is covered. Repeat the application morning and night until the infection is completely cured.

Swimmer's Ear, Ear Infections: To treat swimmer's ear, mix two tablespoons of rubbing alcohol with ¼ teaspoon of boric acid. Mix thoroughly until all the boric acid is dissolved, then drop into the ear. Fill the ear canal, then drain it completely. Treat both ears, even if only one is infected. Do not use for a punctured eardrum.

Recipes. Boric Acid Foot Cure: 1 cup rubbing alcohol, 2 teaspoons of boric acid. Mix the ingredients in a sterile jar with a tight-fitting lid. Apply to the feet with a cotton ball or swab every night. No double dipping. Allow the alcohol to dry on the feet and leave on until morning.

Boric Acid Eye Wash: 1/8 teaspoon pharmaceutical grade boric acid powder. One cup distilled water, boiling. Sterilized jar, lid, and spoon sterilize in a pressure cooker (best), or by boiling for 10 minutes. Place the boiling water into the sterile jar and allow it to cool. Mix the boric acid into the sterilized water and stir it with the sterilized spoon until it is completely dissolved. Use the eyewash up to three times a day, as needed. Always use sterile tools with each use.

Cayenne Pepper

Cayenne is used sparingly as a seasoning agent because of its spicy heat. It is a spice found in most home spice cabinets and has significant medical benefits

Medicinal Use: Cayenne is a warming herb, heart tonic, and digestive aid. It also releases hormones that improve the mood. It is rich in vitamins and minerals that support the immune system. Use cayenne as a powder, in capsules, added to water for soaking, in rubs, and in salves.

Cayenne is a powerful stimulant and consuming too much can cause stomach problems. A small amount goes a long way with this herb.

Stops Bleeding: Cayenne is a powerful styptic. It helps blood to clot both internally and externally. For small cuts put a thick layer of cayenne directly onto the cut. Large wounds benefit from both external administration and internal use. As soon as the wound is covered in cayenne, drink a glass of water containing one teaspoon of cayenne pepper. It helps the blood clot quickly.

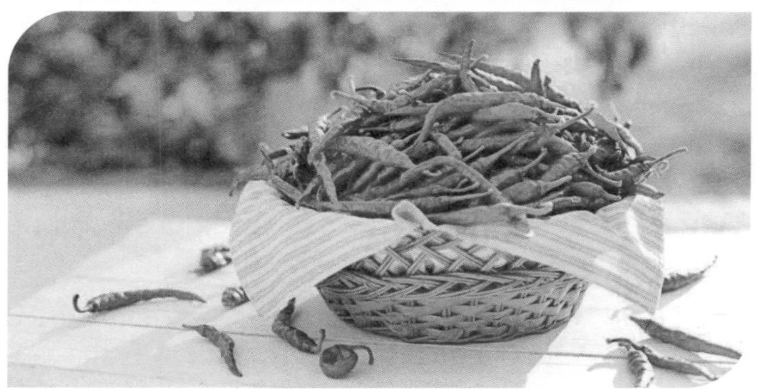

Sore Throats: At the first sign of throat irritation, gargle several times a day with 10 to 20 drops of Cayenne Infusion mixed into a glass of water. It works if you can stand the heat.

Colds and Flu: Cayenne is an excellent supportive preventative and remedy for colds and the flu. I help bring down fevers and expel mucus. It works best in combination with other herbs such as Echinacea, goldenseal, and marshmallow.

Poor Circulation, Warming the Hands and Feet: Cayenne is an effective herb for increasing circulation and for warming cold hands and feet.

Sprinkle a powder made from equal parts cayenne and dried ginger powder into your shoes or socks. Cayenne can be used alone, but it is often too irritating. Use only a pinch, approximately 1/8 teaspoon at most.

Another remedy is to add five drops of Cayenne Infusion to a foot bath of warm water. You can also rub Cayenne Oil or Salve on the hands and feet, taking care not to touch your eyes.

Achy Joints, Arthritis, and Muscle Strains: Cayenne salve works well for achy muscles and joints. The pepper increases blood circulation to the area and warms it naturally. It soothes and relaxes the muscles and helps relieve pain. Rub a small amount of Cayenne Salve over ache muscles and painful joints regularly for relief.

General Tonic and Immune Booster: Take Cayenne Infusion added to a cup of vegetable juice or water as a general tonic. It improves whole body blood circulation and gives the immune system a boost. Take the infusion once or twice a day, as needed.

Diabetes and Blood Sugar Control: Cayenne has a significant effect on blood sugar levels and can help bring them down in diabetic patients. Take one capsule of cayenne powder with each meal. The cayenne must be taken regularly to give the best effects, which increase over time. Hypoglycemic patients should avoid the use of cayenne in foods and supplements.

Warning: Use gloves when preparing this herb. Do not touch your eyes after using it.

Recipes. Cayenne Infusion: 1 teaspoon dried cayenne powder, 1-pint (0.5 Liters) water. Mix the cayenne powder and water together in a small pot and bring to a boil. Turn off the heat and let the infusion cool. This infusion should always be used diluted. For most uses, a few drops of Cayenne Infusion added to a cup of water is enough. It can also be used topically.

Cold and Flu Prevention Capsules: Mix together thoroughly. Not to be used by people with Autoimmune Issues due to the Echinacea and Goldenseal. 1/4 cup Echinacea root powder, 1/4 cup goldenseal root powder, 2 tablespoons marshmallow root powder, 1 to 2 tablespoons cayenne powder. Pack the powder into large gelatin or vegetable capsules. I use the "00" size. If you use smaller capsules, increase the dosage. Store the capsules in a glass jar with a tight lid. To Use: Take 2 capsules every 2 to 3 hours at the first sign of symptoms. Continue this dosage for the first two days, then reduce the dosage to 2 capsules, 3 times daily until all symptoms are gone.

Cayenne Salve: Use this salve with care. Wash your hands very well after applying it and do not touch your eyes! ½ cup olive oil, 1 tablespoon dried cayenne pepper flakes, 2 tablespoons beeswax, 3 to 4 drops wintergreen essential oil. Place the olive oil and cayenne flakes into the top of a double boiler. Bring the water in the bottom of the double boiler to a simmer.

Simmer the pepper and oil mixture for 60 minutes, keeping an eye on the water levels in the bottom of the double boiler. Remove the oil from the heat and allow it to cool slightly, strain the pepper flakes out and discard. Return the oil to the heat and add the beeswax. Stir until the beeswax is completely melted, then remove from the heat. Add the wintergreen essential oil and stir well. Pour the salve into a suitable container with a tight-fitting lid.

Warming Ginger Cayenne Salve and Massage Oil: This salve is a great choice for muscle pains, arthritis and achy joints, bruises, and other deep tissue pains.

Warming Ginger Cayenne Massage Oil: 1 cup of olive oil, coconut oil, or other carrier oil, 1 tablespoon cayenne pepper powder, 1 tablespoon ginger root, dried and powdered, 1 tablespoon arnica flowers. Add the cayenne, ginger root, and arnica to the oil in a jar with a tight-fitting lid. Shake well. Place the jar in a warm place like a sunny window for 4 to 6 weeks, shaking daily. Strain the oil through a coffee filter to remove the herbs.

Warming Ginger Cayenne Salve: 1 cup Warming Ginger Cayenne Massage Oil, ¼ cup beeswax, shaved, chopped, or shredded. Combine the beeswax and massage oil in the top of a double boiled. Warm gently until the beeswax is melted. Stir the salve to completely combine the wax and oil. Pour into widemouth jars or tins to cool. When hardened, cover and store in a cool, dark place.

Massage a small amount of salve into sore muscles and joints 2-3x/day. It can take a few weeks to get maximum results. Do not use on face or mucous membranes or open cuts or wounds. Do not use with pregnant or nursing patients. Wash your hands thoroughly with soap after use.

Cinnamon

Cinnamon is a spice taken from the inner bark of various species of the Cinnamon tree (genus *Cinnamomum*). There are two different kinds of cinnamon: Cassia and Ceylon. Both are beneficial, but the type you should use is controversial. Cassia cinnamon contains coumarin in higher amounts, which can be harmful in high doses. For this reason, Ceylon is often preferred as a supplement.

In my research and experience, Ceylon cinnamon may have more antioxidants and is often touted as the best for medicinal use; however, Cassia has more benefits for treating diabetes and controlling blood sugar. For general use, I prefer Ceylon, but for diabetes control, I prefer Cassia.

Medicinal Use: For medicinal use and preventative care, the common suggested dose for "true cinnamon" (Ceylon) is 1-2 grams of cinnamon with each meal. You can add it to a smoothie or food, use it in tea, or put it in capsules for easy consumption. Each capsule will hold about 500 mg, tightly packed, so take 2-4 capsules with each meal if needed.

Diabetes and Blood Sugar Control: Cassia cinnamon dramatically lowers fasting blood sugar levels and improves insulin sensitivity with consistent use. Taking 1 to 6 grams of cinnamon daily is enough to show beneficial effects immediately and full effects over time (6 grams is approximately 2 teaspoons). See warning section below.

Cinnamon improves sensitivity to insulin, a key hormone in regulating metabolism and blood sugar. In some metabolic conditions, the body may become insulin resistant. By increasing insulin sensitivity, cinnamon lowers blood sugar levels and helps prevent or treat diabetes. Additionally, cinnamon decreases the amount of glucose that enters your bloodstream after a meal. It slows the breakdown of carbohydrates and prevents blood sugar spikes. Another compound in cinnamon acts like insulin to improve glucose uptake in the cells. Care is needed as cinnamon may cause blood sugar levels to drop too low.

Reduces Triglycerides and Cholesterol: 1 to 6 grams of cinnamon lowers triglycerides and "bad" LDL-cholesterol. The full effects are seen over time, but one to two months of use should bring triglyceride and cholesterol levels down significantly.

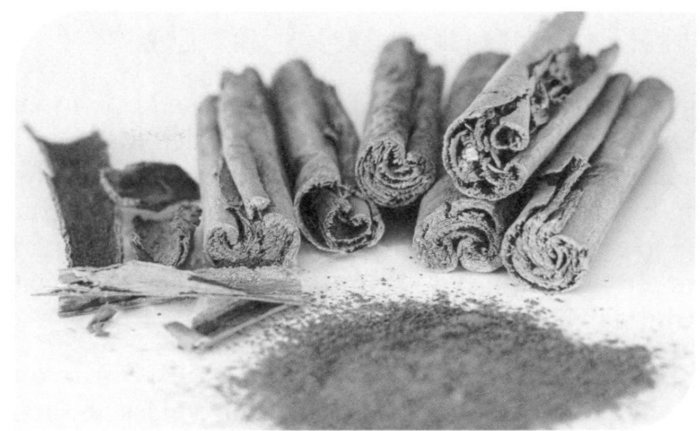

Neurodegenerative Diseases: Parkinson's and Alzheimer's: Cinnamon has been shown to protect the neurons in the brain. Animal studies have found that it helps normalize neurotransmitter levels, which could help improve motor function in Parkinson's patients. It also has two compounds (cinnamaldehyde and epicatechin) that inhibit the buildup of brain proteins (called "tau") that are found in Alzheimer's patients. We do not have human research on these processes yet; however, it is easy to add cinnamon, along with turmeric and other brain protecting herbs, to the daily diet.

Anti-Inflammatory: Cinnamon is loaded with antioxidants and anti-inflammatory compounds that fight free radicals and help lower your risk of disease.

Heart Disease: Because of its antioxidants and anti-inflammatory compounds, cinnamon can help reduce the risk of heart disease. It reduces blood pressure, triglycerides, and cholesterol, which contribute to heart disease.

HIV: Cassia cinnamon helps the body's fight against HIV-1, the most common HIV form in humans.

Anti-Bacterial and Anti-Fungal: Evidence shows that cinnamon inhibits the growth of some bacteria, including Salmonella and Listeria on surfaces, especially when cinnamon oil is used. We have no data on whether cinnamon will treat internal infections.

Warning: Coumarin may increase cancer risk in animals. More research in needed for humans. Coumarin may also cause liver damage in large amounts. Some people have an allergy to cinnamaldehyde, a compound found in cinnamon. The reaction usually presents as mouth sores. As always, please check with your doctor for possible medication interactions.

Diatomaceous Earth

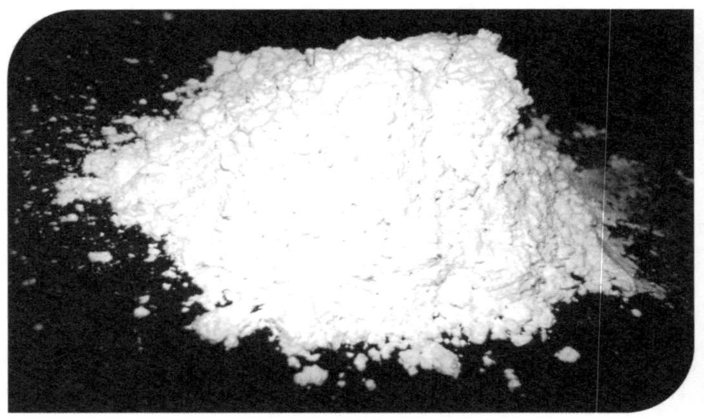

Diatomaceous earth (DE) is composed of fossils formed by tiny algae-like organisms called diatoms. It is a slightly abrasive powder that is safe for consumption by humans and animals. It has health and medicinal benefits to the body. Be sure that your DE is marked as food-grade. Non-food grade DE is not safe for human consumption.

How to Take Diatomaceous Earth: Mix one teaspoon full of diatomaceous earth in a glass of water. Drink it one hour before eating or two hours after eating. Repeat this dose for 10 days, then wait another 10 days before repeating the cycle. Do this for 5 full cycles of 10 days on and 10 days off. Diatomaceous earth can also remove medications from the body, so check with your doctor before use if you are taking medications.

Medicinal Use. Diatomaceous Earth Detoxifies the Body: Diatomaceous earth holds a negative ionic charge. This causes it to attract positively charged toxins and heavy metals, helping to flush them out of the bloodstream and the body.

Kills Parasites: Diatomaceous earth naturally kills parasites and viruses in the digestive tract. By using the 10 days on and 10 days off schedule, it kills parasites in all stages of the reproductive cycle, ending the infestation.

Improves Joint and Bone Health: DE is a natural source of silica and other trace minerals required by the body. Silica is essential for healthy joints, ligaments, and bones.

Encourages Heart Health: Diatomaceous Earth helps lower cholesterol and blood pressure, which encourages a healthy heart and circulatory system.

Clean Teeth: DE is an abrasive that is safe to use as a toothpaste.

Other Uses: Diatomaceous earth has many uses around the home. One of its most valuable household and garden uses is in killing fleas, bedbugs, cockroaches, spiders and other insects. You only need to dust it in the areas where infestations exist. It is completely safe with kids and pets. It is also valuable as an abrasive cleanser, an absorbent, deodorizer, and in water filtration.

Warning: Diatomaceous earth is a fine abrasive powder. It can be harmful if inhaled or if it gets in the eyes. Wear proper protective clothing when using.

Recipes. DE Toothpaste: ½ cup of diatomaceous earth, ½ cup coconut oil, 1 to 2 drops peppermint essential oil, vegetable glycerin, as desired for texture. Mix together and use as toothpaste.

Epsom Salts

Epsom salts is a crystalline mineral salt with the chemical formula $MgSO_4$. When mixed with water, the salt breaks down into magnesium, sulfur, and oxygen.

All of these are beneficial for the body and can be absorbed through the skin, one of the reasons that Epsom salt baths and foot soaks are so popular. It is also a powerful anti-inflammatory used to treat muscle soreness and skin inflammations.

Medicinal Use. Epsom Salts Treat Magnesium Deficiency, Stress, and Benefits the Body Systems and Chronic Diseases: An Epsom salt bath is a good way to de-stress and treat a number of health issues at the same time. Magnesium is a mineral that is vital to health, yet many people are deficient. An Epsom salt bath allows the magnesium to be absorbed by the body and is beneficial for the heart, bones, muscles, and other organs.

Epsom salt baths are beneficial for treating any disease that might cause or result from a magnesium deficiency, especially chronic diseases like heart disease and arrhythmias, osteoporosis, chronic fatigue syndrome, arthritis, and some mental illness.

Detoxifying the Body: The dissolved sulfur in an Epsom salt bath helps the body flush out toxins. It pulls toxins and heavy metals out of the body.

Reduces Inflammation: A soak in Epsom salt also reduces inflammation and pain in sore muscles, swellings, and skin inflammations. A long soak has the ability to reduce swelling and pain almost immediately.

To Benefit from an Epsom Salt Soak: To receive all of these benefits, soak in an Epsom salt bath for at least 40 minutes to 1 hour. Use two cups or more of Epsom salt in a full bath tub of warm water. For a foot soak, add 2 tablespoons of Epsom salt per gallon (4 Liters) of warm water. To aid the detoxifying process, drink plenty of water before, during, and after the soak.

Listerine

Listerine is a combination of alcohol and essential oils that are good for killing bacteria and fungus on the body. In addition to sanitizing the mouth and sweetening the breath, it is useful for killing bacteria and fungus in wounds and on the skin.

Medicinal Use. Get Rid of Lice: Listerine can be used to kill lice in the hair. Apply Listerine to the scalp and hair, soaking it well. Cover it with a disposable shower cap and leave it on for 2 hours. Wash and rinse like usual. Use a lice comb to remove the nits.

Get Rid of Ticks: To get a tick to turn loose soak a cotton ball or pad with Listerine and use it to cover the tick for 10 to 15 seconds. The tick will usually let go quickly and can be removed with tweezers.

Treat Itchy Skin: Listerine treats pain and itchy skin caused by bug bites, bee stings, poison ivy, allergies, psoriasis, and acne. It sanitizes the area, reduces pain, and relieves the itch temporarily.

Clean Blisters and Wounds: Clean wounds and blisters with Listerine to keep them from getting infected. The Listerine kills bacteria on the skin surface. Repeat several times daily to keep the wound clean.

Toe and Nail Fungus: Add a cup of Listerine to your foot soak to treat nail fungus. Soak daily until the fungus clears up completely.

Other Uses. Kills Mold and Mildew: Listerine also kills molds and mildew. Use it in a spray bottle to kill small spots of mold and mildew. Spray the area thoroughly and let it soak in.

Potassium Permanganate

Potassium permanganate is a chemical compound with medicinal use for the cleaning of wounds, treating skin conditions, and disinfecting water. It is a strong oxidizer, capable of starting fires when in contact with oxidizable materials.

Medicinal Use. Skin Infections: Potassium permanganate can irritate or even burn the skin when used in strong solutions. It must be carefully prepared into very dilute solutions before use. Only a small amount is needed to provide relief from skin infections including canker sores, ulcers, abscesses, acne, dermatitis, eczema, vaginal thrush, and vulvovaginitis.

Apply a small amount on small wounds and soak larger areas in a very dilute solution. If necessary, a dilute potassium permanganate water bath can be used. Compresses can also be used.

Wound Cleansing: Cleaning wounds with dilute concentrations of potassium permanganate kills bacteria, funguses, and viruses. This prevents wound infections.

Fungal Infections: Fungal infections such as athlete's foot is easily treated by soaking the foot in a dilute solution of potassium permanganate for about 15 minutes, twice a day, for two or three weeks. These soaks kill or inhibit the growth of the fungus. The patient should be aware that the treatment will temporarily stain the foot brown, but normal color will return when the soaks are finished.

Cholera Prevention: Potassium permanganate is an effective way to sanitize water for drinking.

Clean food and drinking water is necessary to prevent infective diseases such as cholera and dysentery. To prepare water for drinking with potassium permanganate, add permanganate granules to 1 gallon (4 Liters) of water, one or two at a time, until the water turns pink. Allow the water to sit for 30 minutes before drinking or using. The water is safe to drink while the pink color remains. If the color is purple, you have added too much permanganate and the water is unsafe for drinking. Add more water to dilute it until the color is pink.

How to Prepare: Potassium permanganate must be dissolved and diluted by clean water before using.

Dissolve one 400 mg tablet or granules in 1 gallon (4 liters) of water. Use the water to soak weeping skin wounds and infections for 1 hour, but no more.

Use potassium permanganate as a short-term solution while treating the underlying conditions. Do not use potassium permanganate internally or in the eyes.

Other Uses: Water purification, as described above under preventing cholera. Potassium permanganate is also useful for starting fires.

Warning: Potassium permanganate is an aggressive oxidizer and will readily start fires when in contact with suitable materials. It must be stored in a non-reactive plastic bottle. Strong solutions can cause burns. Dilute the solutions as recommended. Potassium permanganate will stain almost everything it comes into contact with a nice shade of pink or purple.

Raw Honey

Honey is made by bees. It is made up of concentrated flower nectar that bees break down into simple sugars using an enzyme in their salivary glands (invertase). It is then deposited into honeycomb for long-term storage. Honey contains many medicinal qualities taken from the flower. Once the honey has been cooked or diluted, these properties may no longer exist in beneficial quantities. I prefer to use undiluted raw honey, as it contains pollen and parts of the waxen honeycomb in addition to the honey itself.

Honey has a rich medicinal history. It has been used since ancient times for the dressing of wounds and as a cough suppressant.

Medicinal Use. Burn and Wound Healing: The antibacterial and anti-inflammatory properties of raw honey make it a natural for wound care. It kills germs and helps the wound heal. Use it applied directly to burns, infected wounds, diabetic foot ulcers and other skin conditions such as psoriasis and herpes. You can apply it in a layer directly on the skin or apply it to the bandage before use.

For especially difficult infections and ulcers, the use of Manuka honey is recommended, if available.

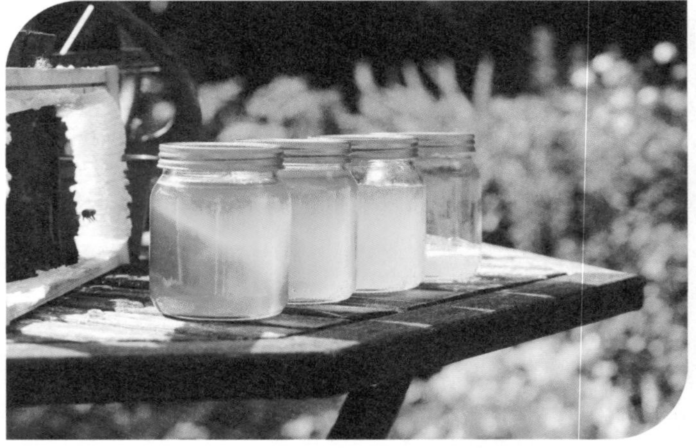

Antibacterial, Antimicrobial, and Anti-Inflammatory: Some kinds of honey have more intense antibacterial and anti-inflammatory properties than others. In particular, Manuka Honey from New Zealand is known to be very high in these active compounds. However, any natural raw honey has these properties in varying amounts.

Cough Suppressant: Honey is a natural cough suppressant. Take a spoonful of honey straight or use it to make a cough syrup infused with beneficial herbs.

Allergies: Local raw honey may help with seasonal allergies. I use it in conjunction with stinging nettle tincture.

Lowers Blood Pressure: When used moderately, in place of sugar, honey may help lower blood pressure. Because of its antioxidant compounds, modest blood pressure reductions can occur when reducing sugar use and replacing it with a small amount of honey. Instead of sucrose, honey is made up of glucose and fructose, and has a lower glycemic index than sugar.

Lowers Cholesterol and Triglycerides: High LDL-cholesterol is a strong risk factor for heart disease and plays a major role in atherosclerosis. Honey can improve cholesterol levels, lowering the dangerous LDL-cholesterol and increasing the beneficial HDL-cholesterol ratio. Additionally, replacing sugar with honey lowers triglyceride levels, which are associated with insulin resistance and type 2 diabetes.

Warning: Never give raw honey to an infant or child under 1 year old. Their immature immune systems cannot handle the botulism spores, where older children and adults have a natural immunity.

While honey is considered a "healthy" sugar, it is still a sugar and should be used in moderation. It will affect blood sugar and contains the same calories as sugar.

Choose high quality, raw honey. Lower quality brands may be mixed with syrup and may contain very little honey. Unless your honey is marked as "raw", assume that it has been pasteurized.

Turmeric/Curcumin

Turmeric is a spice used to give flavor and color to curry and other foods. It has many known medicinal uses, most derived from the curcuminoid compounds it contains. The main active ingredient in turmeric is curcumin and some brands list the curcumin content on the label, usually around 3% by weight. You can also buy curcumin extracts.

Turmeric, because of its curcumin and other curcuminoid compounds, is a powerful anti-inflammatory and a strong antioxidant. Unfortunately, the curcumin is not well absorbed into the bloodstream. Absorption is helped by the presence of piperine, a compound found in black pepper. Using turmeric with black pepper increases the absorption of curcumin by 2,000 percent.

Medicinal Use: Using turmeric in food is beneficial, but food consumption alone is not enough to get the amounts of curcumin needed. For this reason, I mix turmeric with finely ground black pepper when taking it as a supplement. I pack the mixture into capsules and take 1 to 4 grams (2 to 8 capsules) daily.

Anti-Inflammatory: Acute, short-term inflammation is beneficial and helps signal your body of an invading virus or bacterium. However, when inflammation becomes chronic, it is the root of many modern chronic illnesses. Calming chronic inflammation is vitally important.

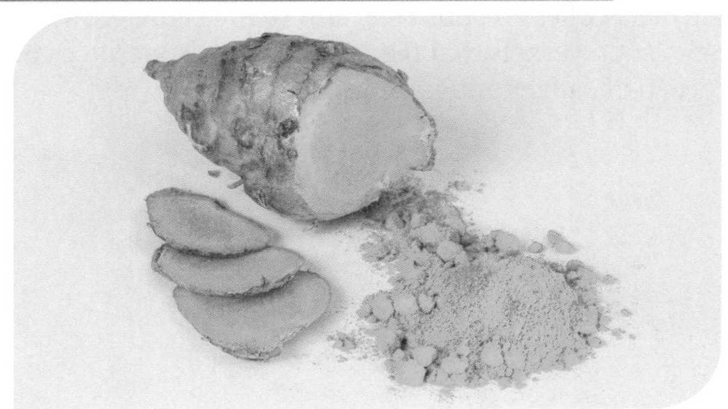

Turmeric is strongly anti-inflammatory and is as effective as many anti-inflammatory drugs, without their side effects. It is my # 1 go to for internal inflammation.

Antioxidant: Oxidative damage is one of the mechanisms that promotes aging and many diseases. Curcumin fights free radicals that cause oxidative damage and protects the body. It also boosts the body's own antioxidant enzymes.

Improves Brain Function and Lowers Risk of Brain Diseases, Including Alzheimer's Disease & Depression. Curcumin can increase the levels of brain-derived neurotrophic factor (BDNF), which is a growth hormone for the brain. Many brain diseases, including Alzheimer's Disease and depression, are linked to decreasing levels of the BDNF hormone. Increasing BDNF levels with curcumin can effectively delay or possibly reverse many age-related brain function diseases.

By increasing BDNF, curcumin may also improve memory and cognitive performance by increasing the growth of new neurons and fighting degenerative processes in the brain.

Alzheimer's disease is characterized by a buildup of amyloid plaques in the brain. Curcumin crosses the blood-brain barrier and helps clear these plaques. Long-term use is required.

Arthritis and Pain: Curcumin supplements are beneficial in reducing the inflammation in arthritis and slowing or stopping the progress of the disease. Patients report the improvement of symptoms and a reduction in joint inflammation, as well as a reduction in pain.

Cancer. Prevention and Treatment: Studies show that curcumin affects cancer growth, development, and spread at the molecular level. It promotes the death of cancerous cells and reduces the growth of new blood vessels that feed tumors. It also reduces the spread of cancer and inhibits its growth.

Lowers the Risk of Heart Disease: Because of its powerful anti-inflammatory properties, turmeric can lower your risk of heart disease. It improves the function of blood vessels, the regulation of blood pressure, and blood clotting. Studies show that taking 4 grams of curcumin per day decreases the risk of a heart attack.

Reduces Cholesterol Levels: Using turmeric, especially when eating fatty foods, helps reduce blood cholesterol levels, including the dangerous LDL cholesterol levels.

Promotes Wound Healing: Turmeric is effective as a disinfectant and reduces healing time in wounds. Apply turmeric as a powder, directly to the wounded area.

Warning: Turmeric may slow the clotting of the blood. People taking blood-thinners and pregnant women should be especially careful.

Appendix

A

B

C

D

E

F

G

H

I

N

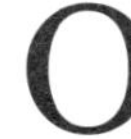

P

U

V

W

X

Y

Z